Vaccine Design and Technology: Advances in Veterinary Medicine

Vaccine Design and Technology: Advances in Veterinary Medicine

Edited by Isabel Myers

MURPHY & MOORE
www.murphy-moorepublishing.com

Published by Murphy & Moore Publishing,
1 Rockefeller Plaza,
New York City, NY 10020, USA
www.murphy-moorepublishing.com

Vaccine Design and Technology: Advances in Veterinary Medicine
Edited by Isabel Myers

International Standard Book Number: 978-1-63987-564-1 (Hardback)

Cataloging-in-Publication Data

Vaccine design and technology : advances in veterinary medicine / edited by Isabel Myers.
p. cm.
Includes bibliographical references and index.
ISBN 978-1-63987-564-1
1. Veterinary vaccines. 2. Vaccination of animals. 3. Vaccines--Design.
4. Veterinary vaccines--Biotechnology. 5. Veterinary medicine. I. Myers, Isabel.
SF918.V32 V33 2022
636.089 537 2--dc23

TABLE OF CONTENTS

Preface IX

Chapter 1 **Impact of maternally derived immunity on piglets' immune response and protection against porcine circovirus type 2 (PCV2) after vaccination against PCV2 at different age** 1
Paolo Martelli, Roberta Saleri, Giulia Ferrarini, Elena De Angelis, Valeria Cavalli, Michele Benetti, Luca Ferrari, Elena Canelli, Paolo Bonilauri, Elena Arioli, Antonio Caleffi, Heiko Nathues and Paolo Borghetti

Chapter 2 **Efficacy of one dose vaccination against experimental infection with two *Mycoplasma hyopneumoniae* strains** 13
Annelies Michiels, Ioannis Arsenakis, Filip Boyen, Roman Krejci, Freddy Haesebrouck and Dominiek Maes

Chapter 3 **A proteomic approach to the development of DIVA ELISA distinguishing pigs infected with *Salmonella* Typhimurium and pigs vaccinated with a *Salmonella* Typhimurium-based inactivated vaccine** 23
Jan Gebauer, Hana Kudlackova, Marcel Kosina, Kamil Kovarcik, Radek Tesarik, Alena Osvaldova, Martin Faldyna and Jan Matiasovic

Chapter 4 **Sero-prevalence of virus neutralizing antibodies for rabies in different groups of dogs following vaccination** 34
R. M. S. Pimburage, M. Gunatilake, O. Wimalaratne, A. Balasuriya and K. A. D. N. Perera

Chapter 5 **Field evaluation of the efficacy of *Mycobacterium bovis* BCG vaccine against tuberculosis in goats** 44
Enric Vidal, Claudia Arrieta-Villegas, Miriam Grasa, Irene Mercader, Mariano Domingo and Bernat Pérez de Val

Chapter 6 **Evaluation of serological response to foot-and-mouth disease vaccination in BLV infected cows** 50
Rodrigo Puentes, Laureana De Brun, Agustina Algorta, Valeria Da Silva, Florencia Mansilla, Gustavo Sacco, Silvia Llambí and Alejandra V. Capozzo

Chapter 7 **Methodology for the assessment of brucellosis management practices and its vaccination campaign** 57
M. N. Aznar, M. Arregui, M. F. Humblet, L. E. Samartino and C. Saegerman

Chapter 8 **Preparation and evaluation of goose reovirus inactivated vaccine** 68
Xiaoyu Niu, Bingqian Zhang, Xianglong Yu, Xin Zhang, Yanguo Dou, Yi Tang and Youxiang Diao

Chapter 9 **Comparative efficacy of the Leucofeligen™ FeLV/RCP and Purevax™ RCP FeLV vaccines against infection with circulating feline Calicivirus** 76
T. Almeras, P. Schreiber, S. Fournel, V. Martin, C. S. Nicolas, C. Fontaine, C. Lesbros and S. Gueguen

Chapter 10 **Nitric oxide-generating compound GSNO suppresses porcine circovirus type 2 infection in vitro and in vivo** ... 86
Chuanmin Liu, Libin Wen, Qi Xiao and Kongwang He

Chapter 11 **Evaluation of ELISA for the detection of rabies virus antibodies from the thoracic liquid and muscle extract samples in the monitoring of fox oral vaccination campaigns** ... 95
Tomislav Bedeković, Ivana Šimić, Nina Krešić, Ivana Lojkićs, Željko Mihaljević, Ivica Sučec, Ivana Lohman Janković and Peter Hostnik

Chapter 12 **Evaluation of spray and oral delivery of Newcastle disease I2 vaccine in chicken reared by smallholder farmers** ... 102
Kibrom Mebrahtu, S. Teshale, Wendimeneh Esatu, Tadios Habte and Esayas Gelaye

Chapter 13 **A randomized controlled study on the efficacy of a novel combination vaccine against enzootic pneumonia (*Mycoplasma hyopneumoniae*) and porcine Circovirus type 2 (PCV2) in the presence of strong maternally derived PCV2 immunity in pigs** ... 109
Panagiotis D. Tassis, Ioannis Tsakmakidis, Vassileios G. Papatsiros, Dimitrios Koulialis, Tom Nell, Georgia Brellou and Eleni D. Tzika

Chapter 14 **Comparative innocuity and efficacy of live and inactivated sheeppox vaccines** ... 118
Zineb Boumart, Samira Daouam, Imane Belkourati, Lamya Rafi, Eeva Tuppurainens, Khalid Omari Tadlaoui and Mehdi El Harrak

Chapter 15 **The immune mechanism of *Mycoplasma hyopneumoniae* 168 vaccine strain through dendritic cells** ... 124
Yumeng Shen, Weiwei Hu, Yanna Wei, Zhixin Feng and Qian Yang

Chapter 16 **Safety and immunogenecity of a live attenuated Rift Valley fever vaccine (CL13T) in camels** ... 131
S. Daouam, F. Ghzal, Y. Naouli, K. O. Tadlaoui, M. M. Ennaji, C. Oura and M. EL Harrak

Chapter 17 **Safety studies with the oral rabies virus vaccine strain SPBN GASGAS in the small Indian mongoose (*Herpestes auropunctatus*)** ... 136
Steffen Ortmann, Ad Vos, Antje Kretzschmar, Nomusa Walther, Christiane Kaiser, Conrad Freuling, Ivana Lojkic and Thomas Müller

Chapter 18 **Nutrient digestibility, organ morphometry and performance in vaccinated or non-vaccinated *Lawsonia intracellularis* infected piglets** ... 143
Christian Visscher, Jasmin Mischok, Saara Sander, Marion Schmicke, Eva-Ursula Peitzmeier, Isabel von dem Busche, Karl Rohn and Josef Kamphues

Chapter 19 **Exploratory field study on the effect of Porcine circovirus 2 (PCV2) sow vaccination on serological, virological and reproductive parameters in a PCV2 subclinically infected sow herd** ... 153
Salvador Oliver-Ferrando, Joaquim Segalés, Sergio López-Soria, Antonio Callén, Olivier Merdy, François Joisel and Marina Sibila

Chapter 20 **Responses to dietary levels of methionine in broilers medicated or vaccinated against coccidia under *Eimeria tenella*-challenged condition** 163
Anqiang Lai, Guozhong Dong, Daijun Song, Tan Yang and Xiaolong Zhang

Chapter 21 **Efficacy of an adenovirus-vectored foot-and-mouth disease virus serotype: a subunit vaccine in cattle using a direct contact transmission model** 174
John G. Neilan, Christopher Schutta, José Barrera, Melia Pisano, Laszlo Zsak, Ethan Hartwig, Max V. Rasmussen, Barbara J. Kamicker, Damodar Ettyreddy, Douglas E. Brough, Bryan T. Butman and David A. Brake

Chapter 22 **On-farm storage of livestock vaccines may be a risk to vaccine efficacy: a study of the performance of on-farm refrigerators to maintain the correct storage temperature** 183
Paul D. Williams and Gustavo Paixão

Chapter 23 **Evaluation of the humoral immune response induced by vaccination for canine distemper and parvovirus** 190
Beatriz Vila Nova, Eva Cunha, Nuno Sepúlveda, Manuela Oliveira, Berta São Braz, Luis Tavares, Virgílio Almeida and Solange Gil

Chapter 24 **Safety and immunogenicity of an attenuated Chinese pseudorabies variant by dual deletion of TK&gE genes** 198
Jichun Wang, Zengcai Song, Aimin Ge, Rongli Guo, Yongfeng Qiao, Mengwei Xu, Zhisheng Wang, Yamei Liu, Yating Zheng, Hongjie Fan and Jibo Hou

Chapter 25 **Evaluation and optimization of a conventional SPCE for FMD post-vaccination monitoring** 209
Yeong-Lim Kang, Ji-Yun Jeong, Hwi-Yeon Choi, Yanhong Zhang, Yumei Liu, Ho-Jong Lee, Jong-Chul Choi, So-Hyun Lee, Beom-Joo Lee, Sang-Won Lee, Joong-Bok Lee, Ki-hyun Cho and Seung-Yong Park

Chapter 26 **Supplementation of dietary germanium biotite enhances induction of the immune responses by foot-and-mouth disease vaccine in cattle** 217
Myunghwan Jung, Min-Kyoung Shin, Seung-Bin Cha, Seung Won Shin, Anna Yoo, Won-Jung Lee, Hong-Tae Park, Jong-Hyeon Park, Byounghan Kim, Yeon-Kwon Jung and Han Sang Yoo

Chapter 27 **Efficacy of multivalent, modified-live virus (MLV) vaccines administered to early weaned beef calves subsequently challenged with virulent *Bovine viral diarrhea virus* type 2** 227
Manuel F Chamorro, Paul H Walz, Thomas Passler, Edzard van Santen, Julie Gard, Soren P Rodning, Kay P Riddell, Patricia K Galik and Yijing Zhang

Permissions

List of Contributors

Index

PREFACE

Over the recent decade, advancements and applications have progressed exponentially. This has led to the increased interest in this field and projects are being conducted to enhance knowledge. The main objective of this book is to present some of the critical challenges and provide insights into possible solutions. This book will answer the varied questions that arise in the field and also provide an increased scope for furthering studies.

The immunization of animals has long been an effective and sustainable method of controlling and preventing infectious diseases and increasing livestock production. Vaccine has served as an important component in the field of veterinary medicine to improve the animal health. Appropriate administration of specific antigens which are present in vaccines can provide persistent and effective immunity against infections in animals. Feline vaccination, canine vaccination, farm animal vaccination and equine vaccination are some types of vaccinations which are used within this discipline. This book is meant for students who are looking for an elaborate reference text on vaccine design and technological advances in veterinary medicine. It aims to equip students and experts with the advanced topics and upcoming concepts in this area. Through this book, we attempt to further enlighten the readers about the new concepts in this field.

I hope that this book, with its visionary approach, will be a valuable addition and will promote interest among readers. Each of the authors has provided their extraordinary competence in their specific fields by providing different perspectives as they come from diverse nations and regions. I thank them for their contributions.

Editor

1

Impact of maternally derived immunity on piglets' immune response and protection against porcine circovirus type 2 (PCV2) after vaccination against PCV2 at different age

Paolo Martelli[1*], Roberta Saleri[1], Giulia Ferrarini[1], Elena De Angelis[1], Valeria Cavalli[1], Michele Benetti[1], Luca Ferrari[1], Elena Canelli[1], Paolo Bonilauri[2], Elena Arioli[3], Antonio Caleffi[3], Heiko Nathues[4] and Paolo Borghetti[1]

Abstract

Background: This study was aimed at evaluating the clinical protection, the level of *Porcine circovirus* type 2 (PCV2) viremia and the immune response (antibodies and IFN-γ secreting cells (SC)) in piglets derived from PCV2 vaccinated sows and themselves vaccinated against PCV2 at different age, namely at 4, 6 and 8 weeks. The cohort study has been carried out over three subsequent production cycles (replicates). At the start/enrolment, 46 gilts were considered at first mating, bled and vaccinated. At the first, second and third farrowing, dams were bled and re-vaccinated at the subsequent mating after weaning piglets. Overall 400 piglets at each farrowing (first, second and third) were randomly allocated in three different groups (100 piglets/group) based on the timing of vaccination (4, 6 or 8 weeks of age). A fourth group was kept non-vaccinated (controls). Piglets were vaccinated intramuscularly with one dose (2 mL) of a commercial PCV2a-based subunit vaccine (Porcilis® PCV). Twenty animals per group were bled at weaning and from vaccination to slaughter every 4 weeks for the detection of PCV2 viremia, humoral and cell-mediated immune responses. Clinical signs and individual treatments (morbidity), mortality, and body weight of all piglets were recorded.

Results: All vaccination schemes (4, 6 and 8 weeks of age) were able to induce an antibody response and IFN-γ SC. The highest clinical and virological protection sustained by immune reactivity was observed in pigs vaccinated at 6 weeks of age. Overall, repeated PCV2 vaccination in sows at mating and the subsequent higher levels of maternally derived antibodies did not significantly interfere with the induction of both humoral and cell-mediated immunity in their piglets after vaccination.

Conclusions: The combination of vaccination in sows at mating and in piglets at 6 weeks of age was more effective for controlling PCV2 natural infection, than other vaccination schemas, thus sustaining that some interference of MDA with the induction of an efficient immune response could be considered. In conclusion, optimal vaccination strategy needs to balance the levels of passive immunity, the management practices and timing of infection.

Keywords: *Porcine circovirus* type 2 (PCV2), Vaccine efficacy, Protection, Immune response

* Correspondence: paolo.martelli@unipr.it
[1]Department of Veterinary Science, University of Parma, Via del Taglio, 10 - 43126 Parma, Italy
Full list of author information is available at the end of the article

Background

The control of *Porcine circovirus* type 2 (PCV2) associated diseases (PCVD) is based on management strategies, control of coinfections, and vaccination. At present, different commercial PCV2 vaccines are available, licenced for use in piglets most often from three weeks of age and all of them have been described to be effective in controlling the disease [4, 6, 9, 15, 29]. In fact, the PCV2 vaccines are able to reduce the viral burden and viral-induced specific lesions in the lymphoid tissue, but the potential interference of vaccines with maternally derived immunity and the optimization of the vaccination timing are still worth investigating. Deeper understanding is required with regard to the age-related maturity and responsiveness of piglets' immune system towards PCV2 vaccines and the extent of passive immunity either from sows' PCV2 infection or vaccination. Several studies showed that vaccination against PCV2 in piglets with high levels of maternally derived antibodies (MDA) can result in clinical protection [4, 9, 14, 15, 22]. However, in some of these studies, maternal immunity apparently interfered with the humoral immune response after vaccination [9, 22]. Most of the authors characterised the humoral immunity towards PCV2 by determination of total PCV2-specific antibodies and/or by demonstration of an increase of the concentration showing seroconversion that occurs either in subclinically infected or clinically affected pigs, e.g. PMWS-affected pigs [10, 26, 30]. Apart from the humoral immunity, previous reports based on laboratory trials demonstrated that cell-mediated immunity measured as levels of PCV2-specific interferon-γ (IFN-γ) secreting cells (SC) may play a role in mediating viral clearance in combination with neutralising antibodies and that the intensity of the cell-mediated immune response may be influenced by the load and the extent of viral replication [7, 18, 19]. These features were investigated under field conditions both in diseased pigs naturally infected with PCV2 in combination with coinfections and in vaccinated animals showing no or only a few clinical signs [5, 16, 23, 31].

Previous studies showed that high levels of MDA in piglets do not allow eliciting seroconversion after vaccination. Conversely, when the level of passively acquired antibodies is lower than a certain titre (exact value is depending on the serological method), the vaccine administration induces a marked seroconversion [8, 9, 15, 16]. Usually, in piglets vaccinated in the face of a high level of passive immunity, a decline of antibody is observed similarly to the decline in unvaccinated animals. Moreover, Haake and others [11] suggested that vaccination at one week of age clearly affects the induction of an active humoral immunity in piglets. In contrast, the cell-mediated immune response is not affected by MDA levels and contributes to the long-lasting protection [5, 7, 8, 15].

This study was aimed at investigating the clinical protection (vaccine efficacy) and the immune responses (both humoral and cell-mediated) of a one-dose PCV2 subunit vaccine administered in piglets. In particular, identifying the ideal time of vaccination (4, 6 or 8 weeks of age), also in respect to their levels of passively acquired immunity being derived from gilts and sows repeatedly vaccinated at mating against the same antigen, was of interest. The outcome parameters were comprised by clinical (morbidity and mortality), productive (average daily weight gain - ADWG), and virological (PCV2 viremia and viral load) parameters. The immune response in piglets was assessed in terms of development of humoral (total antibodies) and cell-mediated (PCV2-specific IFN-γ secreting cells) immunity.

Methods

Clinical history of the herd

The study was carried out in the Northern part of Italy at a farm selected with regard to its history of PCVD. The farm was constituted of a 1200-sow farrow-to-finish herd that, in the previous years, had experienced mortality in the nursery and fattening periods due to PCVD. This diagnosis was based on clinical signs, gross lesions, histopathological findings, and presence of PCV2 in lesions of the lymphoid tissue, all together typical for PCVD in accordance to Sorden [32]. Seropositivity to PCV2 in all categories of animals (replacement gilts, sows, nursery, growing and finishing pigs) was demonstrated by enzyme-linked immune sorbent assay (ELISA). Since the occurrence of the disease, the piglets have been vaccinated at three weeks of age, whereas gilts and sows were vaccinated at each mating. At the time of start of the study no clinical signs of PCV2-SD (PCV2-systemic disease; [28]) were noted. Diagnostic investigations performed on dead pigs older than 15 weeks of age demonstrated no PCV2-specific lesions in the lymphoid tissue. Instead very low titres of the virus determined by PCR were suggestive for PCV2 subclinical infection in several pigs (PCV2-SI).

The involvement of *Porcine reproductive and respiratory syndrome virus* (PRRSV) in the clinical problems of the herd was demonstrated by repeated detection of the virus by PCR in nursery and growing pigs that were suffering from respiratory disease. However, based on diagnostics the herd had been classified as "positive - stable" for PRRS according to Holtkamp and others [13]. The presence of the most common secondary bacteria (*Streptococcus* spp., *Pasteurella multocida*) was confirmed in animals also tested infected by PRRSV. The farm was seronegative for *Aujeszky's disease virus* (ADV) and *Actinobacillus pleuropneumoniae* and seropositive for *Mycoplasma hyopneumoniae*. Sows were vaccinated against ADV (three times per year), *Porcine parvovirus*, *Erysipelothrix rhusiopathiae* (both at mid-lactation) and *Swine influenza virus* (SIV). Piglets were vaccinated against *M. hyopneumoniae* once at one week of age and ADV according to the National Control Program of Italy.

Experimental design

This study was a double-blind, randomised, controlled field trial performed in accordance to the principles of "Good Clinical Practice" with the consent of animals' owner and the protocol had been previously evaluated and approved by the Ethical Committee for Animal Experimentation of the University of Parma (23/12). The work has been carried out over three subsequent production cycles (replicates). At the beginning, 46 commercial hybrid gilts at 230 to 260 days of age, were included at their first mating. Replacement gilts were produced into the farm. They were individually identified by numbered ear tagging and a blood sample of approx. 10 mL was obtained by puncture of the *Vena jugularis externa* from each animal. Subsequently the gilts were vaccinated with one dose (2 mL) of a commercial PCV2a-based subunit vaccine (Porcilis® PCV, MSD Animal Health, Boxmeer, The Netherlands) via intramuscular injection in the neck (off-label use). At day 113 of the first, second and third gestation period, these animals were bled; i.e. two days prior to expected farrowing date. The sows were re-vaccinated against PCV2 at the same day of subsequent mating after their piglets had been weaned. The day of inclusion of suckling pigs was at their weaning (D -1). On this day, suckling pigs of each farrowing (first, second and third parity) were identified, double ear-tagged (both ears) and randomly assigned to one of the treatment groups. The treatment groups with 100 animals each differed in the time when vaccination was applied to the piglets. Namely, animals in the first group were vaccinated at four weeks of age (weaning age) (group A), six weeks of age (group B) or eight weeks of age (group C). One group of piglets was kept non-vaccinated (group D) as placebo/control. The animals were assigned to the different groups as they came to hand sequentially using a randomized block design ($n = 4$) across litters. The identification of the sow and the date of birth of the piglets were recorded.

The piglets were vaccinated with 2 mL of a commercial PCV2 vaccine (Porcilis PCV®) administered intramuscularly according to the manufacturer's recommendations. The non-vaccinated control pigs received the same amount of adjuvant (2 mL) by injection in the neck at four weeks of age. The recording of the clinical signs was performed by a veterinarian, who was blinded regarding the treatments. At weaning, all piglets under investigation were moved to the nursery unit and kept commingled in pens of 25 pigs per pen each, all constructed in a unique barn. Upon each accommodation change, pigs were commingled according to usual farm procedures. Treatments, housing, husbandry and feeding were in accordance to the European Union Guidelines on Animal Husbandry and were identical for all experimental groups.

During the first week post-vaccination, pigs were monitored daily for side reactions. At weaning (four weeks of age) and at vaccination (four, six or eight weeks of age), blood samples were collected from 20 piglets per treatment group. These piglets were identified by their number and a differently coloured ear tag. Further sets of blood samples were then taken every four weeks until slaughter (eight [group A only]), 12, 16, 20, 24, 28 and 32 weeks of age in groups A and C, and 10, 14, 18, 22, 26, 30 and 34 in group B). The 20 pigs of the control group were blood sampled four weeks after they had received only the adjuvant (at the time of weaning) and then on a two week interval until slaughter (10, 12, 14, 16, 18, 20, 22, 24, 26, 28, 30, 32 and 34 weeks of age). The same procedures were applied in all three replicates (litters).

Clinical signs (morbidity) and mortality recording

The individual treatment of every pig was recorded on a daily basis and considered as a parameter for the measurement of morbidity. Dead pigs or those that had to be euthanized for reasons of animal welfare were recorded and immediately submitted to pathological investigations.

Body weight and average daily weight gain (ADWG)

Individual body weights of the pigs enrolled in the study were measured at inclusion, at 12 and at 24 weeks of age. The ADWG was calculated based on the daily weight gain of all the animals being alive at the end of each weighing period.

Gross pathology and histopathology

All pigs that died spontaneously and those needing euthanasia underwent gross pathological examination and histopathology within 24 h after death. Samples from inguinal, mesenteric and mediastinic lymph nodes were removed and fixed in 10 % buffered formalin. For routine histopathology, 5-µm thick sections of the lymph nodes were stained with haematoxylin-eosin and examined for lesions compatible with PCV2-SD. The diagnosis of PCV2-SD was concluded, when all the three criteria for the disease were present [28] including moderate-to-high amounts of PCV2 in the lesions determined by quantitative real-time PCR (qPCR) as described by Olvera and others [21].

DNA extraction and qPCR to detect PCV2 nucleic acid in tissues and serum samples

In order to detect and to quantify the viral DNA by qPCR, DNA was firstly extracted from 200 μL of serum and 200 μL of 1:10 PBS homogenate of lymph node tissue, by using TRIzol LS (Invitrogen–San Diego, CA-USA) following the manufacturer's instructions. The DNA obtained was suspended in 50 μL of DEPC-treated water. A qPCR was carried out using primers and probes according to Olvera and others [21] on a LightCycler 1.5 thermocycler (Roche Diagnostics–Basel, CH). The results were expressed as number of PCV2 genome copies per millilitre of serum or gram of tissue.

Serology

Detection of PCV2 antibodies

For the detection of PCV2-specific antibodies, a commercially available indirect enzymatic immunoassay (INGENZIM CIRCO–INGENASA, Madrid, Spain) was used according to the manufacturer's instructions. The titre of each sample was calculated as follows: titre = 53 ($e^{3.2x}$) where **e** is the natural logarithm base and **x** is the S/P of the sample (S/P = sample O.D./positive control O.D.; O.D.: optical density).

Retrospective analysis of the courses of PCV2 antibodies after grouping the animals according to maternally derived antibodies at vaccination

The animals of the three replicates taken together were retrospectively grouped based on the value of the S/P ratio at PCV2 vaccination considering a high S/P value (≥ the median S/P ratio of all piglets at 4 weeks of age) and a low S/P value (< the median).

Detection of antibodies against other infections

Antibodies against *M. hyopneumoniae* were evaluated by a commercially available ELISA kit (Herd Check® *M. hyopneumoniae,* IDEXX Laboratories). The presence of antibodies against the gE glycoprotein of ADV was measured using a commercially available ELISA kit (HerdChek® PRV g1 (gE) test kit, IDEXX Laboratories) according to the manufacturer's instructions. Another commercial ELISA kit (CHEKIT-APP-ApxIV ELISA test kit, IDEXX Laboratories) was used for the detection of antibodies against *A. pleuropneumoniae.* Antibodies to different SIV sub-types (H1N1, H1N2 and H3N2) were determined by a haemoagglutination inhibition (HI) assay, using a standard method [2]. The presence of antibodies to PRRSV were determined using a commercially available ELISA kit (HerdChek® Porcine Reproductive and Respiratory Syndrome Antibody Test Kit, IDEXX Laboratories, Westbrook, ME, USA) according to the manufacturer's instructions.

Quantification of PCV2-specific IFN-γ secreting cells

The frequencies of PCV2-specific IFN-γ secreting cells (SC) in the peripheral blood of pigs were determined according to Martelli and others [15] with minor modifications. Peripheral blood mononuclear cells (PBMCs) were isolated by Histopaque-1.077® gradient and plated at 4 × 10^5 cells/well in complete RPMI-1640 (cRPMI-1640) supplemented with 10 % foetal bovine serum (FBS) into 96-well plates (MultiScreen®$_{HTS}$-IP, Millipore) coated overnight at 4 °C with 5 μg/mL anti-pig IFN-γ mAb (P2G10, BD, Biosciences, Franklin lakes, NJ - USA) and blocked with cRPMI-1640 + 10 % FBS for 2 h at 37 °C. For the PCV2 antigen recall, an elaborate on the whole strain (I12/11) at 0.1 multiplicity of infection (MOI) was used as stimulus, in cRPMI-1640 + 10 % FBS, for 20 h at 37 °C, 5 % CO_2. In all samples, >98 % of PBMCs were viable as confirmed by Trypan blue. Afterwards, plates were incubated for 1 h at 37 °C with 0.5 μg/mL anti-pig IFN-γ biotin-labelled mAb (P2C11, BD) and then with 1:750 AP-conjugated anti-biotin mAb in PBS + 0.5 % BSA. Plates were finally incubated for 7 min with a BCIP/NBT solution (BioRad, Hercules, CA - USA) and the reaction was stopped with distilled water. The frequencies of PCV2-specific IFN-γ SC were determined using an AID® ELISpot Reader (AID® ELISpot Software v.3.5 - AID). As a positive control, 4 × 10^5 PBMCs/well were incubated with PHA (5 μg/mL); as a negative control, 4 × 10^5 PBMCs were incubated without antigen (PCV2 mock stimulus: supernatant of non-PCV2-infected PK-15 cells). The background values (number of spots in negative control wells) were subtracted from the respective counts of the stimulated cells and the immune responses were expressed as number of IFN-γ SC per million PBMCs (IFN-γ SC/10^6 PBMCs).

Statistical analysis

All statistical analyses were carried out using the STATA/IC 12.1 for Windows (64-bit ×86-64; StataCorp LP, College Station, TX, USA). For all analyses, the individual pig was considered as the experimental unit.

Descriptive analysis was performed for all individual parameters from pigs stratified according to replicate and group. Outcome of continuous variables (ADWG, PCV2 ELISA S/P, IFN-γ SC and PCV2 viral loads) were tested for normality (Shapiro-Wild test) and further analyzed by either one way ANOVA (normally distributed data) or Kruskall–Wallis test (non-normally distributed data). Differences between groups were further evaluated by pairwise comparisons of marginal linear predictions. Moreover, piglets were re-grouped according to their level of MDAs into two groups: 'Low level of MDA' (S/P ratio < median S/P ratio of all piglets at 4 weeks of age) or 'High level of MDA' (S/P ratio ≥ median). A chi-square test was used to evaluate differences between groups in mortality, the number of animals with a PCV2 viral load higher than 10^6 PCV2 copies/mL, and the number of animals needing an individual treatment. The correlation between ELISA S/P at the time of vaccination and four weeks later was tested employing linear regression analysis. The significance level (α) for all analyses was set at 0.05.

Results

The results of this field trial are described for each of the three replicates, namely for pigs from nursery to the finishing phase and derived from the three consecutive litters (1st, 2nd and 3rd parity) of vaccinated sows.

Morbidity and mortality

Morbidity in pigs of the three replicates is shown in Table 1. Among pigs of the first replicate, morbidity was significantly higher in those of groups C and D ($p < 0.05$). None of the recorded clinical signs that needed treatment was associated with or typical for PCVD. In the second replicate, a high proportion of treatments was needed in all groups and no statistical difference was observed. All the individual treatments were applied in the post-weaning period concomitantly with the occurrence of a severe outbreak of PRRSV infection and associated clinical signs. In the third replicate, morbidity in group B was significantly lower as compared to the other groups ($p < 0.05$). In particular, it is worth mentioning that the majority of the individual treatments in groups A, C and D were needed from 12 weeks of age until slaughter. Pigs belonging to group D had a very high percentage of diseased pigs (18 %) concomitantly with the high proportion of PCV2 viremic animals and high titres of viral burden (see the paragraph about PCV viremia) even if overt clinical signs compatible with PCV2-SD were not observed.

Dead pigs, animals needing euthanasia, and runt non-marketable pigs (lost pigs) underwent pathological and virological investigations to be categorised as PCVD and non-PCVD affected. None of the investigated pigs fulfilled the diagnostic criteria for PCV2-SD. The mortality rate in the first replicate was significantly lower in group B (vaccinated at 6 weeks of age) ($p < 0.05$) in both of the considered periods of observation, namely from weaning to 12 weeks of age and from then to slaughter. In the second replicate, production cycle mortality was significantly lower in group C in the period from weaning to 12 weeks. In contrast, in the fattening period (from 12 weeks to slaughter), groups A and B had less mortality than other groups. None of the fatality cases fulfilled the diagnostic criteria of PCVD. In the last replicate, the mortality was significantly lower in groups B and C until 12 weeks and in group B only from 12 weeks of age to slaughter. The higher mortality in group D was associated with PCV2 viremia. Details are reported in the paragraph regarding PCV2 viremia.

Average Daily Weight Gain (ADWG)

The ADWG is considered a useful parameter for measuring the effect of PCVD both in clinical and in subclinical cases. Table 2 shows the ADWG in vaccinated and placebo/control animals for the two intervals among the three different weighing time points. The ADWG of the four groups was not significantly different in any period of the three considered replicates.

PCV2 viremia

The course of PCV2 viremia was different in the three replicates. In the first replicate (litters from gilts, i.e. 1st parity sows), PCV2 viremia was detected in some pigs of all groups (from 5 % to 25 %). The viral burden was always $<10^6$ PCV2 genome copies/mL of serum. In the second replicate (litters from 2nd parity sows), groups A, C and D had different proportions of viremic pigs, and the viral burden in vaccinated animals (groups A and C, but not B) and controls was

Table 1 Morbidity (parenteral injections) and mortality in the four groups under study for each replicate

	REPLICATE		GROUP			
			A	B	C	D
MORBIDITY*	1st		6.2^a	5.4^a	14.7^b	18.9^b
	2nd		22.7^a	20.7^a	21.3^a	22.4^a
	3rd		10.3^a	0^b	8.3^a	18.2^a
MORTALITY*	1st	from weaning to 12 weeks of age	3.1^a	1.6^b	3.1^a	3.6^a
		from 12 weeks to slaughter	3.9^a	1.6^b	4.7^a	3.1^a
	2nd	from weaning to 12 weeks of age	5.3^a	4.0^a	2.7^b	4.3^a
		from 12 weeks to slaughter	2.7^a	2.7^a	4.0^b	5.4^b
	3rd	from weaning to 12 weeks of age	5.7^a	1.9^b	2.0^b	3.8^a
		from 12 weeks to slaughter	14.0^a	7.7^b	18.0^a	20.0^a

Legend: * proportion of pigs; Different superscript letters indicate statistically significant differences ($p < 0.05$)
Group A: pigs vaccinated at 4 weeks; group B: pigs vaccinated at 6 weeks; group C: pigs vaccinated at 8 weeks; group D: non-vaccinated placebo/controls

Table 2 Average daily weight gain (ADWG) ± STD in the four groups under study for each replicate

	REPLICATE		GROUP			
			A (100)[b]	B (100)[b]	C (100)[b]	D (100)[b]
ADWG[a]	1st	from weaning to 12 weeks of age	317 ± 78	303 ± 92	310 ± 69	325 ± 71
		from 12 weeks to 24 weeks of age	681 ± 129	649 ± 131	633 ± 98	683 ± 132
	2nd	from weaning to 12 weeks of age	244 ± 92	308 ± 72	255 ± 83	304 ± 75
		from 12 weeks to 24 weeks of age	613 ± 97	683 ± 115	623 ± 125	696 ± 104
	3rd	from weaning to 12 weeks of age	391 ± 72	410 ± 89	420 ± 91	363 ± 88
		from 12 weeks to 24 weeks of age	741 ± 110	740 ± 107	704 ± 124	730 ± 121

[a]average daily weight gain: grams/day; [b]number of pigs at enrolment (first weighing)
Group A: pigs vaccinated at 4 weeks; group B: pigs vaccinated at 6 weeks; group C: pigs vaccinated at 8 weeks; group D: non-vaccinated placebo/controls

confirmed to be always <10^6 PCV2 genome copies/mL of serum. In the last replicate (litters from 3rd parity sows), PCV2 viremia was detected in group D (placebo/control) from 16 weeks of age to the end of the experiment, and the proportion of viremic animals ranged from 47 % to 100 %. The high proportion of PCV2 viremia was associated with a viral burden >10^6 PCV2 genome copies/mL of serum in at least one sampling per pig during the whole period of positivity.

Serology

Serologic response to PCV2 vaccination and infection

The course of serology for PCV2 in the three replicates is shown in Fig. 1 (a-c). In the first replicate, pigs of groups B and C had an increase of the S/P ratio after vaccination, whereas pigs in group A and non-vaccinated pigs showed a decline during the four weeks post-vaccination. In the second replicate, no increases of S/P values were recorded in any group after vaccination. From 12 weeks of age onwards in both replicates (1 and 2), all vaccinated groups showed significantly higher values of S/P compared to the controls (group D). The same course of ELISA antibodies in vaccinated pigs was observed in the third replicate. In fact, the values of the S/P ratio in vaccinated animals (all groups) did not increase after vaccination and kept a stable course over the threshold of positivity. At 16 to 18 weeks of age the non-vaccinated control pigs (group D) seroconverted shown by an increase of the average S/P ratio.

Retrospective analysis of the courses of PCV2 antibodies after grouping animals according to the levels of maternally derived antibodies at vaccination

The values of the S/P ratio are also presented (Fig. 2). Animals with high S/P ratios due to MDA demonstrated an identical decline of PCV2 antibodies. In vaccinated animals, 4 weeks after vaccination, the decline stopped and remained in a stable state for the whole duration of the study. Conversely, in non-vaccinated animals having high S/P values, the decline was longer reaching values below the threshold of seropositivity (<0.4) at 12 weeks. The animals with low S/P values at vaccination showed no decline of antibodies and a stable course that was not significantly different compared to the levels in vaccinated pigs with high S/P values. In the low S/P value non-vaccinated group, the levels of antibodies declined promptly, reaching a negative value in 4 weeks. Similarly to the non-vaccinated group with high S/P value, the viremic pigs of this group seroconverted later in their life.

The antibody course in non-vaccinated groups declined and maintained values below the threshold of seropositivity for the whole duration of the study. In contrast, vaccination in animals with high S/P values did not induce seroconversion but only a decline followed by a stable state. In animals with low S/P values, the course of antibodies was characterized by a marked seroconversion and the S/P values shown for the whole duration of the trial were not different as compared to those of animals with high S/P values at vaccination.

A correlation between S/P values at the time of vaccination and four weeks later could be confirmed for pigs in group A and group D (Table 3). In contrast to this, no correlation were observed when pigs were vaccinated with 6 or 8 weeks of age.

Serologic response to other infections

Serologic investigations performed to monitor the most frequently occurring infections in the herds (PRRSV and *M. hyopneumoniae*) found that the prevalence of PRRSV infection was 100 % at 12-15 weeks of age in all groups and replicates. Concomitantly, *M. hyopneumoniae* seroconversion was also observed. For the latter antigen, seroprevalence continued to increase in the subsequent period in all replicates (data not shown).

Low titres of antibodies (at HI) to SIV were detected in some samples and were inconclusive. Antibodies to ADV were not detected in any sample at any time point.

a)

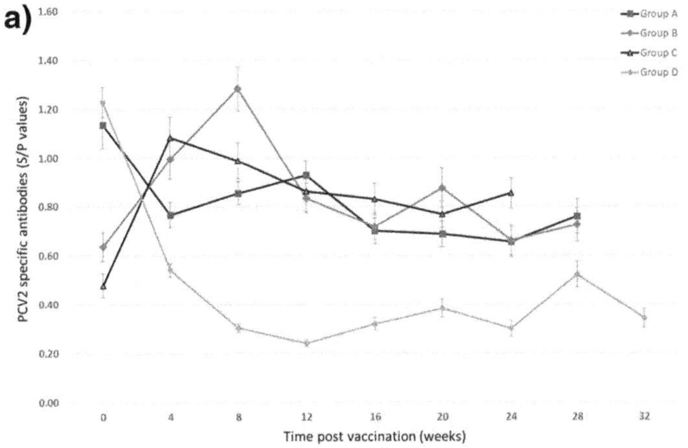

	0	4	8	12	16	20	24	28	32
Group A	a	a	a	a	a	a	a	a	
Group B	b	b	b	a	a	b	a	a	
Group C	b	b	a	a	a	ab	b		
Group D	a	c	c	b	b	c	c	b	

b)

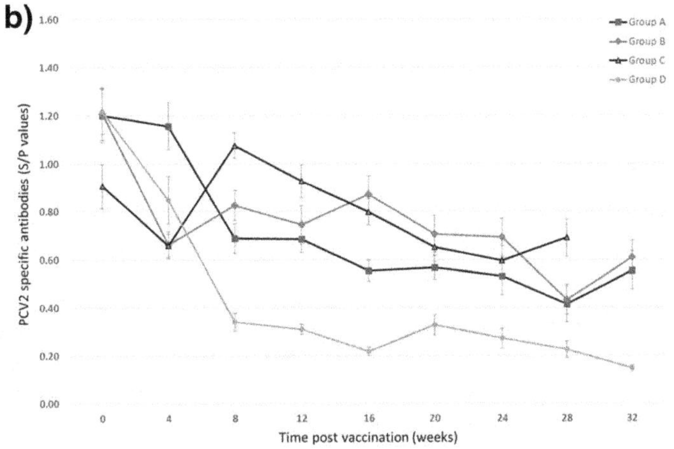

	0	4	8	12	16	20	24	28	32
Group A	a	a	a	a	a	a	a	a	a
Group B	a	b	a	a	b	a	a	a	a
Group C	b	b	b	b	b	a	a	b	
Group D	a	b	c	c	c	b	b	c	b

c)

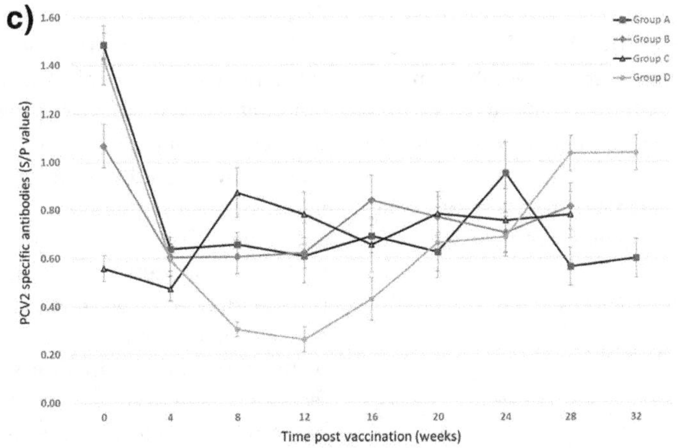

	0	4	8	12	16	20	24	28	32
Group A	a	a	a	a	a	a	a	a	a
Group B	b	ab	a	a	a	a	a	bc	
Group C	c	ab	b	a	ab	a	a	ab	
Group D	a	b	c	b	b	a	a	c	b

Fig. 1 Course of the serologic response to PCV2 (Mean ± STD anti-PCV2 ELISA antibodies) in the four groups under study (PCV2-vaccinated and unvaccinated) for each consecutive replicate (**a**, **b**, **c**). Group A: pigs vaccinated at 4 weeks; group B: pigs vaccinated at 6 weeks; group C: pigs vaccinated at 8 weeks; group D: non-vaccinated placebo/controls

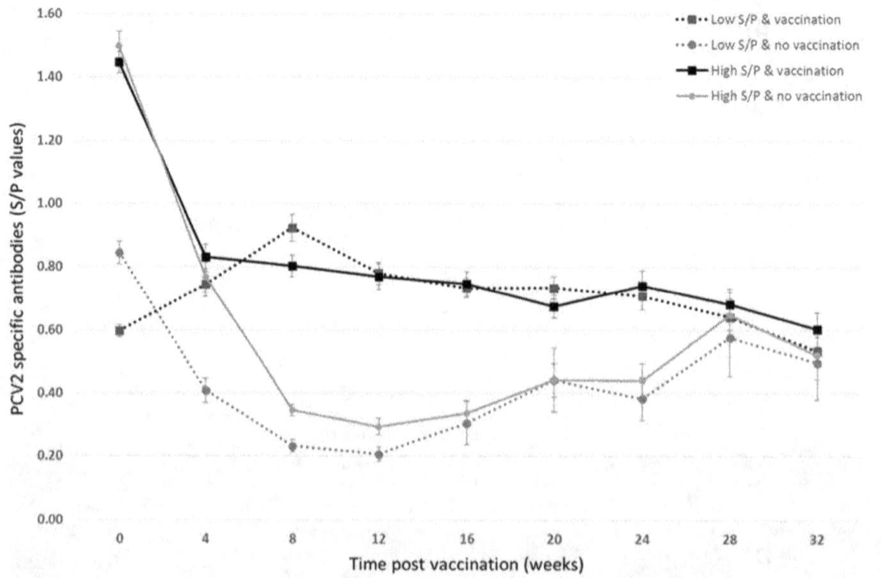

Low S/P & vaccination	a	a	a	a	a	a	a	a
Low S/P & no vaccination	b	b	b	b	b	b	a	a
High S/P & vaccination	a	c	a	a	a	a	a	a
High S/P & no vaccination	a	b	b	b	b	b	a	a

Fig. 2 Course of the serologic response to PCV2 (Mean ± STD anti-PCV2 ELISA antibodies) according to the levels of maternal derived antibodies (MDA) at vaccination and PCV2 infection (viremia) occurred at 20 weeks of age. Overall, the animals of the 3 replicates were divided based on a low (≤0.9) or high (≥1.2) S/P value at 4 weeks of age when vaccinated animals were inoculated with the vaccine ("HIGH S/P vac" and "LOW S/P vac" groups) while unvaccinated animals were inoculated with the adjuvant alone ("HIGH S/P NV" and "LOW S/P NV" groups)

Cell-mediated immune response to PCV2 vaccination and infection

In the first and second replicates, in all vaccinated groups, an increase of the PCV2-specific IFN-γ SC levels was observed after vaccination regardless of the vaccination timing (4, 6 or 8 weeks of age). For the whole duration of the study, the frequencies of IFN-γ SC remained stable with some non-significant variations. Control animals (group D) concomitantly showed an increase with PCV2 infection in some animals. Notably, in the second replicate, the values of IFN-γ SC after vaccination were lower as compared to those recorded in the first replicate (Fig. 3a-c).

In the third replicate, the increase of IFN-γ SC post-vaccination was numerically higher in comparison with the previous replicates. Moreover, the IFN-γ SC maintained high levels during the whole period of infection concomitantly with the onset and increase of the response in the control group (group D) between 20-22 and 34 weeks of age.

Table 3 Correlation of PCV2-specific antibodies in piglets at the time of vaccination and 4 weeks later in the four groups under study for each replicate

	Regression coefficient	Lower CI	Upper CI	p-value
Group A	0.521	0.218	0.825	<0.001
Group B	−0.088	−0.474	0.299	0.651
Group C	0.038	−0.215	0.290	0.766
Group D	0.777	0.500	1.055	<0.001

Group A: pigs vaccinated at 4 weeks; group B: pigs vaccinated at 6 weeks; group C: pigs vaccinated at 8 weeks; group D: non-vaccinated placebo/controls

Discussion and conclusions

The present study is aimed at assessing the efficacy of and the immunological response to a commercial PCV2a sub-type based subunit vaccine when administered at different ages (4, 6 and 8 weeks of age) in pigs with theoretically higher and more homogeneous levels of maternally derived immunity obtained by repeated vaccinations in the population of the matching mothers (gilts and sows). Thus, this purpose could allow defining and evaluating a delayed vaccination scheme of piglets (vaccination at 6 or 8 weeks of age) in respect to the conventional timing (3 weeks of age or earlier) in order to optimize the vaccination scheme. To evaluate the effects of vaccination, clinical, pathological and virological outcomes as well as some aspects of the humoral and cell-mediated immune response towards PCV2 were studied. Under the conditions of this study, the onset of the clinical signs related to PCV2-SD did not occur in the first two replicates as demonstrated by the relatively low PCV2 natural challenge in the blood of vaccinated and particularly of non-vaccinated and more susceptible

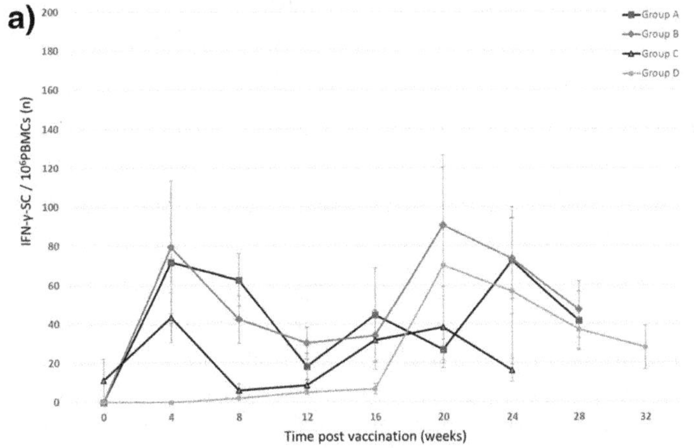

	0	4	8	12	16	20	24	28	32
Group A	a	a	a	ab	a	a	a	a	
Group B	a	a	a	b	a	a	a	a	
Group C	a	ab	b	a	a	a	a		
Group D	a	b	b	a	a	a	a	a	

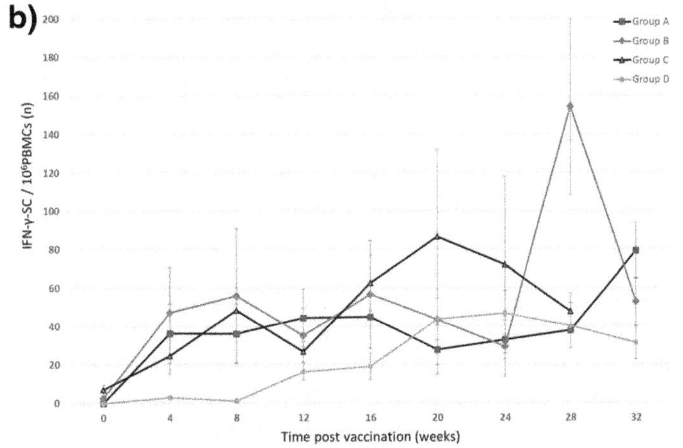

	0	4	8	12	16	20	24	28	32
Group A	a	ab	a	a	a	a	a	a	a
Group B	a	a	a	a	a	a	a	b	ab
Group C	b	ab	a	a	a	a	a	a	
Group D	a	b	a	a	a	a	a	a	b

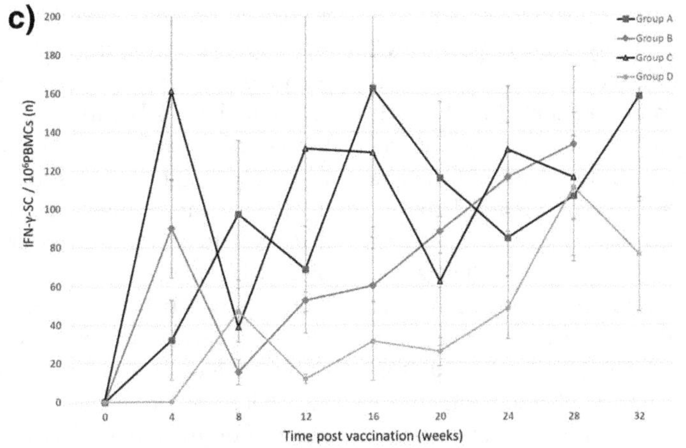

	0	4	8	12	16	20	24	28	32
Group A	a	ab	a	ab	a	a	a	a	a
Group B	a	bc	b	ab	a	a	a	a	
Group C	b	c	ab	a	a	a	a	a	
Group D	a	a	ab	b	a	a	a	a	a

Fig. 3 Course of PCV2-specific IFN-γ SC number (Mean ± STD) in the four groups under study (PCV2-vaccinated and unvaccinated) for each consecutive replicate (**a**, **b**, **c**). Group A: pigs vaccinated at 4 weeks; group B: pigs vaccinated at 6 weeks; group C: pigs vaccinated at 8 weeks; group D: non-vaccinated placebo/controls

pigs. In the third replicate, PCV2 infection and morbidity were detected from 16 weeks of age to the end of the observation period in controls in conjunction with a more intense PCV2 natural challenge.

The present data clearly indicates that vaccination against PCV2 at different ages induces a statistically significant reduction of the proportion of viremic animals and also of the viral load in the blood compared to placebo/controls ($p < 0.05$).

Vaccination with a single dose of the test vaccine administered intramuscularly at 3 weeks of age consistently reduced the clinical signs attributed to PCVD as well as mortality and PCV2 viral load and viremia [7, 15, 16]. More recently, the effect of sow and piglet vaccination under the same field conditions was proven [9].

Overall in the three replicates, it was confirmed that mortality was numerically reduced in vaccinated animals when PCV2 infection occurred and, under the conditions of this study, statistically significant differences were observed in animals vaccinated at 6 weeks of age. To measure morbidity, the number of individual treatments in unvaccinated and vaccinated animals was recorded throughout the study. After intense PCV2 natural challenge, morbidity was significantly higher in the placebo/control group compared to all vaccinated animals.

Average daily weight gain was also evaluated as an efficacy parameter for the vaccination schedule under investigation. Both before the onset of PCV2 viremia and associated disease (from 4 to 12 weeks of age), and from 12 to 24 weeks (the period when PCV2 viremia occurred in the third replicate), the ADWG was not positively affected in vaccinated animals. This result is not in accordance with previous studies [4, 12, 14, 15, 27] supporting a positive effect of vaccination on this parameter. The inability to detect any influence of PCV2 viremia on the productive performance of vaccinated animals compared to controls can be attributed to the early measurement of body weight (24 weeks of age) in respect to the occurrence of viremia detected until the end of the study. Thus control animals experienced the effects of PCV2 viremia after the last weighing. These results highlight the fact that PCV2 natural challenge can occur late in the fattening period and, particularly, that viremia can last very long until the slaughter time.

The improved clinical parameters (morbidity and mortality) are associated with a significant reduction in the proportion of infected pigs and in the viral load in the blood. Particularly, in the third replicate, when PCV2 natural challenge overtly occurred (from 16 weeks of age onward), a high number of placebo/control pigs had high viral loads in serum ($>10^6$ DNA copies/mL), whereas in vaccinated pigs the duration of viremia and the viral load were markedly lower (A and C) or neglectable (group B). It is remarkable that pigs vaccinated at 6 weeks of age (group B) never became PCR-positive for PCV2 in all replicates. It is also notable that, in an almost one year and half time period of observation in the field conditions of this study, PCV2 infection was undetectable for a certain time period (two replicates) and suddenly re-appeared without any evident and expected reason.

All tested animals were PCV2 negative by PCR at the time of vaccination so that the antibody titres detected were most likely of maternal origin also in pigs vaccinated at 8 weeks of age. Overall, the S/P ratio in piglets at 4 weeks of age increased in the three subsequent replicates as a consequence of the effect of repeated vaccination of the corresponding dams at mating. Thus, in the 1st replicate, even if the S/P ratios were the lowest within the three considered replicate, no seroconversion was measured overall in piglets vaccinated at 4 weeks of age as a consequence of some interference of the MDA passively transferred by colostrum on seroconvertion by vaccination. This result is in accordance with a previous study [15]. Conversely, seroconversion could be measured in animals vaccinated at 6 and 8 weeks of age (group B and C, respectively) as a direct consequence of the decline of MDA occurring within 2-4 weeks. In the 2nd and 3rd replicates this reduction of MDA was delayed because of the higher level of the S/P ratio at 4 weeks of age. However, upon vaccination, even when seroconversion did not occur, the S/P ratios remained above the threshold of positivity (S/P >0.4) throughout the study. On the other hand, the placebo/controls had a continuous decline of MDA reaching negative values (S/P <0.4) at 10 weeks of age. The retrospective analysis of the course of PCV2 antibodies after grouping animals according to maternally derived antibody levels measured as S/P ratios at vaccination supports that animals with high values of S/P ratio do not seroconvert whereas vaccinated animals with low S/P values do. Interestingly, the course of the S/P ratios for the whole duration of the study maintained at stable levels with no differences in the absolute values comparing the two groups (high S/P vs. low S/P). Moreover, non-vaccinated animals, both with high and low MDA, experience a decline reaching negative values during the second month of life. Non-vaccinated animals grouped according to the occurrence of PCV2 natural challenge seroconvert soon after viremia. Vaccinated animals either seroconverting because of low levels of MDA or not due to high MDA, maintain stable and efficient, protective values of antibodies for the whole production cycle even when PCV2 natural exposure occurs relatively late in their life (from 16 weeks onward). Thus, these results make clear that the degree of protection is not higher in animals with low S/P values at vaccination compared to those with high values. It has been shown that in Group A and D antibody concentration at the time of vaccination significantly correlates with the antibody concentration four weeks later, which was always lower than the value before. This underlines the hypothesis that high concentration of MDA prevent seroconversion in vaccinated pigs (Group A), whereas low to medium concentration (Group B and C, being two and four weeks, respectively, older at the time of vaccination) does not interfere with the humoral immune response. The latter assumption of no correlation between these levels of MDA and the individual response to vaccination is confirmed by the absence of any significant correlation of S/P values in Group B and C during four weeks following vaccination.

Some studies investigated the influence of age on the efficacy of one-dose PCV2 vaccination in piglets with high levels of maternally derived antibodies. A recent paper studied the efficacy of vaccination at one and three weeks of age under field conditions [11]. Similarly to this study, we detected mean values of MDA in piglets that increased in parallel with the parity of the sows [17].

A previous study [15] demonstrated that PCV2 vaccine efficacy is also sustained by the development of the cellular immune response and this is confirmed by the increased levels of IFN-γ SC in pigs soon after vaccination, supporting the capacity of the PCV2 subunit vaccine to induce cellular immunity which response is not negatively influenced by the presence of high MDA. The age-dependent induction of the cellular response and the influence of the MDA in vaccinated animals are important features to evaluate since different outcomes (extent and duration of the recalled immunity) can be observed in different species and in relation to the challenge conditions [1, 3, 24, 25]. The data of the present paper confirm that the cell-mediated immunity to PCV2 measured as IFN-γ SC was induced within 4 weeks post-vaccination in all replicates and all vaccinated groups. The levels of IFN-γ SC are maintained stable throughout the study (34 weeks of age) and are at the highest levels during the period of late infection that occurred in the third replicate.

In conclusion, the present study demonstrates the beneficial effect of vaccination with a single dose of a PCV2 Cap-based vaccine against PCVD under field conditions even in the presence of high levels of MDA at the time of vaccination, particularly when the experimental animals (all groups) were exposed to a "robust" PCV2 natural infection.

The effects of vaccination at different ages are strictly associated with virological and clinical protection as a result of the immunogenicity of the tested vaccine measured as activation of both the humoral and cellular immune response. This trial demonstrates that even in a condition of high levels of MDA, piglets vaccination at 4, 6 or 8 weeks of age confer a protective immune response characterized by cellular immunity and a stable and long-lasting (until 34 weeks of age) antibody response. However, in the conditions of this study, the combination of vaccination in sows at mating and in piglets at 6 weeks of age was more effective for controlling PCV2 natural infection, than other treatment schemas, thus sustaining that some interference of MDA with the induction of an efficient immune response could be considered. These evidences are in agreement with the conclusion of a research based on experimentally PCV2 infected pigs with or without MDA' [20]. In conclusion, optimal vaccination strategy needs to balance the levels of passive immunity, the management practices and timing of infection.

Competing interests
The authors state they have no conflict of interest.

Authors' contributions
EC: carried out virological investigations and serology; EDA: carried out data analysis and coordinated laboratory investigations; GF: carried out flow data analysis and laboratory investigations; HN: participated in the design of the study, performed the statistical investigations and finalized the manuscript; LF: carried out laboratory investigation and data analysis; MB, AC and EA supported the clinical investigations; PB: conceived the study, participated in its design and coordination, and finalized the manuscript; PBo: performed the virological investigations; PM: conceived the study, participated in its design and coordination, and finalized the manuscript. RS: carried out serology; VC: carried out serology; All authors read and approved the final version of the manuscript.

Acknowledgements
The PhD studies of Dr. Giulia Ferrarini and Dr. Michele Benetti are funded by a pre-doctoral grant of the University of Parma, Italy (PhD Course in Veterinary Science). Dr. Luca Ferrari and Dr. Elena Canelli are funded by grants of the Department of Veterinary Science, University of Parma and partially with funds from MSD Animal Health.

Funding
MSD Animal Health, manufacturer of the vaccine, funded the study.

Author details
[1]Department of Veterinary Science, University of Parma, Via del Taglio, 10 - 43126 Parma, Italy. [2]Istituto Zooprofilattico Sperimentale della Lombardia e dell'Emilia Romagna (IZSLER), Via Pitagora, 2-42100 Reggio, Emilia, Italy. [3]Veterinary Practitioner, 46100 Mantua, Italy. [4]Swine Clinic, Department of Clinical Veterinary Medicine, Vetsuisse Faculty, University of Bern, Bremgartenstrasse 109a, CH-3012 Bern, Switzerland.

References
1. Bandrick M, Theis K, Molitor TW. Maternal immunity enhances Mycoplasma hyopneumoniae vaccination induced cell-mediated immune responses in piglets. BMC Vet Res. 2014;10:124.
2. De Jong JC, De Ronde-Verloop FM, Dorpema JW. Testing of the strain identity of influenza vaccines by haemagglutination inhibition. J Biol Stand. 1982;10:175–83.

3. Endsley JJ, Roth JA, Ridpath J, Neill J. Maternal antibody blocks humoral but not T cell responses to BVDV. Biologicals. 2003;31:123–5.
4. Fachinger V, Bischoff R, Jedidia SB, Saalmuller A, Elbers K. The effect of vaccination against porcine circovirus type 2 in pigs suffering from porcine respiratory disease complex. Vaccine. 2008;26:1488–99.
5. Ferrari L, Borghetti P, De Angelis E, Martelli P. Memory T cell proliferative responses and IFN-γ productivity sustain long-lasting efficacy of a Cap-based PCV2 vaccine upon PCV2 natural infection and associated disease. Vet Res. 2014;45:44.
6. Fort M, Sibila M, Allepuz A, Mateu E, Roerink F, Segales J. Porcine circovirus type 2 (PCV2) vaccination of conventional pigs prevents viremia against PCV2 isolates of different genotypes and geographic origins. Vaccine. 2008;26:1063–71.
7. Fort M, Sibila M, Pérez-Martín E, Nofrarías M, Mateu E, Segalés J. One dose of a porcine circovirus 2 (PCV2) sub-unit vaccine administered to 3-week-old conventional piglets elicits cell-mediated immunity and significantly reduces PCV2 viremia in an experimental model. Vaccine. 2009;27:4031–7.
8. Fort M, Fernandes LT, Nofrarias M, Diaz I, Sibila M, Pujols J, Mateu E, Segalés J. Development of cell-mediated immunity to porcine circovirus type 2 (PCV2) in caesarean-derived, colostrum-deprived piglets. Vet Immunol Immunopathol. 2009;129:101–7.
9. Fraile L, Sibila M, Nofrarías M, López-Jimenez R, Huerta E, Llorens A, López-Soria S, Pérez D, Segalés J. Effect of sow and piglet porcine circovirus type 2 (PCV2) vaccination on piglet mortality, viraemia, antibody titre and production parameters. Vet Microbiol. 2012;161:229–34.
10. Grau-Roma L, Hjulsager CK, Sibila M, Kristensen CS, López-Soria S, Enøe C, Casal J, Bøtner A, Nofrarías M, Bille-Hansen V, Fraile L, Baekbo P, Segalés J, Larsen LE. Infection, excretion and seroconversion dynamics of porcine circovirus type 2 (PCV2) in pigs from post-weaning multisystemic wasting syndrome (PMWS) affected farms in Spain and Denmark. Vet Microbiol. 2009;135:272–82.
11. Haake M, Palzer A, Rist B, Weissenbacher-Lang C, Fachinger V, Eggen A, Ritzmann M, Eddicks M. Influence of age on the effectiveness of PCV2 vaccination in piglets with high levels of maternally derived antibodies. Vet Microbiol. 2014;168:272–80.
12. Horlen KP, Dritz SS, Nietfeld JC, Henry SC, Hesse RA, Oberst R, Hays M, Anderson J, Rowland RR. A field evaluation of mortality rate and growth performance in pigs vaccinated against porcine circovirus type 2. J Am Vet Med Assoc. 2008;232:906–12.
13. Holtkamp DJ, Polson DD, Torremorell M, Morrison B, Classen DM, Becton L, Henry S, Rodibaugh MT, Rowland RR, Snelson H, Straw B, Yeske P, Zimmerman J; American Association of Swine Veterinarians; United States Department of Agriculture PRRS-Coordinated Agricultural Project. Terminology for classifying swine herds by porcine reproductive and respiratory syndrome virus status. J Swine Health Prod. 2011;19(1):44–56.
14. Kixmoller M, Ritzmann M, Eddicks M, Saalmuller A, Elbers K, Fachinger V. Reduction of PMWS-associated clinical signs and co-infections by vaccination against PCV2. Vaccine. 2008;26:3443–51.
15. Martelli P, Ferrari L, Morganti M, De Angelis E, Bonilauri P, Guazzetti S, Caleffi A, Borghetti P. One dose of a porcine circovirus 2 subunit vaccine induces humoral and cell-mediated immunity and protects against porcine circovirus-associated disease under field conditions. Vet Microbiol. 2011;149:339–51.
16. Martelli P, Ardigò P, Ferrari L, Morganti M, De Angelis E, Bonilauri P, Luppi A, Guazzetti S, Caleffi A, Borghetti P. Concurrent vaccinations against PCV2 and PRRSV: study on the specific immunity and clinical protection in naturally infected pigs. Vet Microbiol. 2013;162:558–71.
17. Martelli P, Ferrari L, Ferrarini G, De Angelis E, Catella A, Benetti M, Nathues H, Canelli E, Borghetti P. Influence of repeated porcine circovirus type 2 vaccination on sows' immune response. Veterinary Record. 2015. doi:10.1136/vr.103322.
18. Meerts P, Misinzo G, Lefebvre D, Nielsen J, Bøtner A, Kristensen CS, Nauwynck HJ. Correlation between the presence of neutralizing antibodies against porcine circovirus 2 (PCV2) and protection against replication of the virus and development of PCV2-associated disease. BMC Vet Res. 2006;2:6.
19. Oh Y, Seo HW, Han K, Park C, Chae C. Protective effect of the maternally derived porcine circovirus type 2 (PCV2)-specific cellular immune response in piglets by dam vaccination against PCV2 challenge. J Gen Virol. 2012;93:1556–62.
20. Oh Y, Seo HW, Park C, Chae C, Chae C. Comparison of sow and/or piglet vaccination of 3 commercial porcine circovirus type 2 (PCV2) single-dose vaccines on pigs under experimental PCV2 challenge. Vet Microbiol. 2014; 172:371–80.
21. Olvera A, Sibila M, Calsamiglia M, Segalés J, Domingo M. Comparison of porcine circovirus type 2 load in serum quantified by a real time PCR in postweaning multisystemic wasting syndrome and porcine dermatitis and nephropathy syndrome naturally affected pigs. J Virol Methods. 2004;117:75–80.
22. Opriessnig T, Patterson AR, Elsener J, Meng XJ, Halbur PG. Influence of maternal antibodies on efficacy of porcine circovirus type 2 (PCV2) vaccination to protect pigs from experimental infection with PCV2. Clin Vaccine Immunol. 2008;15:397–401.
23. Opriessnig T, Shen HG, Pal N, Ramamoorthy S, Huang YW, Lager KM, Beach NM, Halbur PG, Meng XJ. A live-attenuated chimeric porcine circovirus type 2 (PCV2) vaccine is transmitted to contact pigs but is not upregulated by concurrent infection with porcine parvovirus (PPV) and porcine reproductive and respiratory syndrome virus (PRRSV) and is efficacious in a PCV2b-PRRSV-PPV challenge model. Clin Vaccine Immunol. 2011;18:1261–8.
24. Pomorska-Mól M, Markowska-Daniel I. Interferon-gamma secretion and proliferative responses of peripheral blood mononuclear cells after vaccination of pigs against Aujeszky's disease in the presence of maternal immunity. FEMS Immunol Med Microbiol. 2010;58:405–11.
25. Pomorska-Mól M, Markowska-Daniel I, Pejsak Z. Effect of age and maternally-derived antibody status on humoral and cellular immune responses to vaccination of pigs against Erysipelothrix rhusiopathiae. Veterinary Journal. 2012;194:128–30.
26. Rodríguez-Arrioja GM, Segalés J, Balasch M, Rosell C, Quintant J, Folch JM, Plana-Durán J, Mankertz A, Domingo M. Serum antibodies to porcine circovirus type 1 (PCV-1) and type 2 (PCV-2) in pigs with and without postweaning multisystemic wasting syndrome (PMWS). Vet Rec. 2000;146: 762–4.
27. Segalés J, Urniza A, Alegre A, Bru T, Crisci E, Nofrarías M, López-Soria S, Balasch M, Sibila M, Xu Z, Chu HJ, Fraile L. A genetically engineered chimeric vaccine against porcine circovirus type 2 (PCV2) improves clinical, pathological and virological outcomes in postweaning multisystemic wasting syndrome affected farms. Vaccine. 2009;27:7313--7321.
28. Segalés J. Porcine circovirus type 2 (PCV2) infections: clinical signs, pathology and laboratory diagnosis. Virus Res. 2012;164:10–9.
29. Seo HW, Han K, Oh Y, Park C. Efficacy of a reformulated inactivated chimeric PCV1-2 vaccine based on clinical, virological, pathological and immunological examination under field conditions. Vaccine. 2012;30:6671–7.
30. Sibila M, Calsamiglia M, Segalés J, Blanchard P, Badiella L, Le Dimna M, Jestin A, Domingo M. Use of a polymerase chain reaction assay and an ELISA to monitor porcine circovirus type 2 infection in pigs from farms with and without postweaning multisystemic wasting syndrome. Am J Vet Res. 2004;65:88–92.
31. Steiner E, Balmelli C, Gerber H, Summerfield A, McCullough K. Cellular adaptive immune response against porcine circovirus type 2 in subclinically infected pigs. BMC Vet Res. 2009;5:45.
32. Sorden SD. Update on porcine circovirus and postweaning multisystemic wasting syndrome (PMWS). Swine Health Production. 2000;8:133–6.

2

Efficacy of one dose vaccination against experimental infection with two *Mycoplasma hyopneumoniae* strains

Annelies Michiels[1*], Ioannis Arsenakis[1], Filip Boyen[2], Roman Krejci[3], Freddy Haesebrouck[2] and Dominiek Maes[1]

Abstract

Background: *Mycoplasma hyopneumoniae* (*M. hyopneumoniae*) is the primary agent of enzootic pneumonia in pigs. Pigs are often infected with different *M. hyopneumoniae* strains. This study assessed the efficacy of vaccination against experimental infection with two genetically different *M. hyopneumoniae* strains in weaned piglets. At 33 days of age (D0), 45 *M. hyopneumoniae*-free piglets were randomly assigned to three different groups: 1) negative control group (NCG; $n = 5$): not vaccinated, not infected, 2) positive control group (PCG; $n = 20$): not vaccinated, infected, and 3) vaccination group (VG; $n = 20$): single vaccination with an inactivated whole-cell *M. hyopneumoniae* vaccine (Hyogen®, Ceva) (D1), infected. The PCG and VG were endotracheally inoculated with 7×10^7 CCU in 7 ml of the highly virulent *M. hyopneumoniae* strain F7.2C (D24) and 7×10^7 CCU in 7 ml low virulent strain F1.12A (D25). A respiratory disease score (RDS) was assessed from D24 until D53. At D53 (euthanasia), macroscopic lung lesions (MLL) were scored, log copies of *M. hyopneumoniae* DNA (qPCR) and IL-1 and IL-6-concentrations (ELISA) on bronchoalveolar lavage fluid were determined.

Results: The RDS and MLL at euthanasia were respectively 0, 1.20 and 0.55 ($P < 0.001$) and 0, 7.56 and 0.68 ($P < 0.001$) for NCG, PCG and VG, respectively. The qPCR results for PCG and VG were 3.99 and 1.78 log copies ($P < 0.001$), respectively, with a significant difference between PCG and VG. The IL-1 and IL-6 results at euthanasia for NCG, PCG and VG were 17.61, 1283.39 and 53.04 pg/ml ($P < 0.001$) and 148.10, 493.35 and 259.80 pg/ml ($P = 0.004$), respectively with a significant difference between PCG and VG.

Conclusions: Vaccination with Hyogen® in pigs was efficacious against an experimental challenge with both a low and highly virulent *M. hyopneumoniae* strain as the vaccinated pigs coughed significantly less, and showed significantly less lung lesions compared to the non-vaccinated challenged pigs: the vaccinated animals showed a 52.9% lower RDS and 91.0% lower MLL compared to the PCG. In the bronchoalveolar lavage fluid collected at the necropsy of the vaccinated pigs, a significantly lower amount of *M. hyopneumoniae*-DNA and a significantly lower IL-1 and IL-6 concentration was found compared to the pigs of the PCG.

Keywords: *Mycoplasma hyopneumoniae*, Double challenge, Vaccination

Background

Mycoplasma hyopneumoniae (*M. hyopneumoniae*) is the causative agent of enzootic pneumonia [1]. The disease has a worldwide impact on intensive swine production and causes substantial losses due to reduced growth of the pigs, poor feed conversion ratio, higher antimicrobial use and increased susceptibility to secondary respiratory agents [1–3]. Previous research has shown that most pigs are infected with more than one *M. hyopneumoniae* strain [4, 5], and recently, Michiels et al., [6] showed that a higher severity and prevalence of *Mycoplasma*-like lung lesions was found in batches of slaughter pigs with detection of more than one *M. hyopneumoniae* strain [6]. It is generally accepted that control of *M. hyopneumoniae* is critical for reducing economical losses in infected swine operations [7]. This is achieved by optimizing housing conditions, management practices, antimicrobial therapy and vaccination against *M. hyopneumoniae* [8]. It is

* Correspondence: Annelies.Michiels@UGent.be
[1]Department of Reproduction, Obstetrics and Herd Health, Faculty of Veterinary Medicine, Ghent University, Merelbeke, Belgium
Full list of author information is available at the end of the article

estimated that 70% of swine herds are practising vaccination against *M. hyopneumoniae* worldwide [9]. Vaccination reduces clinical signs, lung lesions and improves performance, although colonization is not prevented and there is no significant reduction in transmission [3, 8, 10–12]. The benefits obtained through vaccination can vary from herd to herd [13]. Most commercially available bacterin vaccines are based on an adjuvanted whole-cell preparation of an inactivated *M. hyopneumoniae* strain [8]. This strain is mostly the J-strain of *M. hyopneumoniae*, which was isolated in 1958 [14, 15]. Recently a commercial bacterin became available, using *M. hyopneumoniae* strain 2940, isolated in the 1999's from a farm in the United States facing a severe outbreak of enzootic pneumonia. Also, most vaccination studies so far used one single strain for experimental infection. As most pigs are infected with more than one *M. hyopneumoniae* strain [4–6], it may be more appropriate to challenge the pigs with different *M. hyopneumoniae* strains.

The aim of the present study was to determine the efficacy of a commercial vaccine (Hyogen®) against an experimental challenge with two genetically different (low and highly virulent) *M. hyopneumoniae* strains.

Methods

Study animals and experimental design

The study was performed after approval by the Ethical Committee for Animal Experiments of the Faculty of Veterinary Medicine, Ghent University (approval number EC2014/165). Forty-five *M. hyopneumoniae*-free Rattrelow-Seghers (RA-SE Genetics NV, Ooigem, Belgium) piglets were enrolled in the study. The herd of origin has been free of *M. hyopneumoniae* for many years based on repeated serological testing, absence of clinical signs and pneumonia lesions, and nPCR testing on tracheobronchial swabs. The piglets were free of following pathogens as well: porcine reproductive and respiratory syndrome virus, *Pasteurella multocida* and *Actinobacillus pleuropneumoniae*. The piglets were weaned at 28 days of age and moved to the experimental facilities of the Faculty of Veterinary Medicine, Ghent University, Belgium. They were housed in experimental chambers with absolute filters (HEPA U15) and were fed ad libitum using a non- antimicrobial supplemented diet. At 33 days of age (D0), the piglets were randomly allocated to three different groups (D0): 1) negative control group (NCG; $n = 5$): not vaccinated, not infected, 2) positive control group (PCG; $n = 20$): not vaccinated, infected, and 3) vaccination group (VG; $n = 20$): single vaccination with a one- dose commercial vaccine (Hyogen®, CEVA Santé Animale, Libourne Cedex, France) (D1), infected.

Hyogen® is a whole-cell bacterin based on strain BA 2940–99, oil adjuvanted with paraffin and *Escherichia coli* J5 LPS with thiomersal as excipient. The animals of the VG were intramuscularly vaccinated with two ml of the commercial vaccine. The animals of the PCG and NCG were injected intramuscularly with two mL of phosphate-buffered saline (PBS).

Mycoplasma hyopneumoniae strains and challenge infection

The highly virulent F7.2C and the low virulent *M. hyopneumoniae* strain F1.12A were used for challenge infection [16]. The pigs were anesthesized with 0.22 ml/kg of a mixture of Zoletil 100® (Virbac, Louvain la Neuve, Belgium) and Xyl-M® 2% (VMD, Arendonk, Belgium). The pigs of the PCG and VG were endotracheally inoculated with 7×10^7 CCU in 7 ml inoculum of strain F7.2C at D24 and with 7×10^7 CCU in 7 ml inoculum of strain F1.12A at D25. Pigs of the NCG were endotracheally inoculated with 7 ml sterile culture medium (Friis medium) at D24 and D25. At four weeks post-inoculation (PI) (D53), all piglets were euthanized. Therefore, deep anaesthesia was applied by intramuscularly administrating 0.3 ml/kg of a mixture of Zoletil 100® (Virbac, Louvain la Neuve, Belgium) and Xyl-M® 2% (VMD, Arendonk, Belgium), followed by exsanguination.

Clinical and performance parameters

The piglets were observed for at least half an hour daily from D0 until D53. Body condition, appetite, manure consistence, and presence of dyspnea or tachypnea were evaluated. A respiratory disease score (RDS) was recorded daily by the same person at eight a.m. from D1 until D53 and could range from 0 to 6 with 0 (no coughing), 1 (mild coughing after encouraged move), 2 (mild coughing in rest), 3 (moderate coughing after encouraged move), 4 (moderate coughing in rest), 5 (severe coughing after encouraged move), 6 (severe coughing in rest) [17]. The daily RDS values were averaged for the following periods: D1- D23, D24– D53, D1-D53. All pigs were weighed at D0, the day of the first inoculation (D24) and the day of euthanasia (D53), to calculate the anesthesia dose discussed above. The pigs were weighed at D0, D24 and D53 (g). The average daily gain (ADG) (g/pig/d) from day 0–24, 24–53 and from day 0–53 was calculated according to Del Pozo Sacristán et al. (2014), [18] by subtracting the starting weights from the final weights divided by the number of days during the respective periods.

Macroscopic and histopathologic lung lesions

The lungs were collected and scored for macroscopic lung lesions (MLL) (0–35) according to Hannan et al. (1982) [19]. Samples from the right apical, cardiac and diaphragmatic lung lobe were collected. If lesions were present, the samples were collected from the border of a lesion. Samples were fixated in 10%

neutral formalin and processed and embedded in paraffin for histopathological examination. The samples were stained with hematoxylin and eosin and scored using light microscopy according to the degree of peribronchiolar and perivascular lymphohistiocytic infiltration and nodule formation (cuffing) [20]. The scoring system ranged from 1 to 5 with 1) limited infiltration of macrophages and lymphocytes around bronchioles, with airways and alveolar spaces free of cellular exudates; score 2) light to moderate infiltrates with mild diffuse cellular exudates into airways; score 3, score 4 and score 5 (respectively mild (score 3), moderate (score 4) and severe (score 5) lesions characteristic of broncho-interstitial pneumonia, centered around bronchioles but extending to the interstitium, with lymphofollicular infiltration and mixed inflammatory cell exudates. Scores 1 and 2 are considered not to be related with *M. hyopneumoniae* infection, while scores 3 to 5 are presumptive of a *M. hyopneumoniae* infection. The percentage of lung area occupied by air (percentage air) was examined by means of an automated image analysis system (Leica application suite AF Lite (Diegem, Belgium) and image J (Bethesda, Maryland, USA)) [21]. This parameter is inversely proportional to the lymphohistiocytic infiltration in the lung tissue and the intrabronchiolar- and bronchial exudate.

Quantitative PCR for f *M. hyopneumoniae*

Bronchoalveolar lavage fluid was collected from all animals two weeks PI (D39) by inserting a catheter (Portex® Dog Catheter with Female Luer Mount, Smiths Medical International Ltd. Kent, United Kingdom) in the trachea by means of a mouth gag and whilst snaring the pigs. Next, the lungs were flushed with 20 mL sterile PBS to collect the bronchoalveolar lavage fluid. Additionally, during necropsy (D53), bronchoalveolar fluid was collected from the left part of the lung before collection of the histopathological samples by flushing the head bronchus of the left part of the lung with 20 mL sterile PBS. The bronchoalveolar lavage fluid was divided into seven aliquots and stored at −70 °C awaiting analysis. From one aliquot of the bronchoalveolar lavage samples, DNA was extracted with the QIAGEN protocol (QIAGEN, DNeasy Blood & Tissue kit, Belgium) and quantitative PCR (qPCR) was performed as previously described to detect the numbers of *M. hyopneumoniae* organisms [22]. A tenfold dilution series of *M. hyopneumoniae* DNA of strain F7.2C was used to convert the threshold values to the number of *M. hyopneumoniae* organisms. Values below the dilution of 1.50×10^1 (1.18 log copies) were considered as negative.

Immunological parameters on bronchoalveolar lavage fluid

M. hyopneumoniae-specific antibodies in bronchoalveolar lavage fluid

The isotype of *M. hyopneumoniae*-specific antibodies in bronchoalveolar lavage fluid collected at D39 and D53 was determined via an indirect ELISA (expressed in optical density "OD"-values) according to the protocol of Bereiter et al. [23, 24]. Briefly, a Nunc Maxisorp® flat-bottom 96 well plate (eBioscience, Vienna, Austria) was coated with Tween® 20 extracted *M. hyopneumoniae* antigens on which the bronchoalveolar lavage fluid (D39, D53) was added, undiluted. Peroxidase labeled goat anti-porcine Ig A or Ig G polyclonal antibodies (Bethyl Laboratories, Texas, TX, USA) were added and the OD at 450 nm was measured.

Cytokines in bronchoalveolar lavage fluid

The bronchoalveolar lavage fluid collected at D39 and D53 was tested undiluted for presence of porcine TNF-α (TNF-α Swine Antibody Pair, Invitrogen), IL-1 (Porcine IL-1 beta/IL-1F2 DuoSet, R&D Systems) and IL-6 (Porcine IL-6 DuoSet, R&D Systems). A sandwich ELISA was performed according to the manufacturers' recommendations. The sample reactions were measured using OD at 450 nm and quantified by the use of a standard curve as described in the manual.

Serology

At D1, D24 and at euthanasia (D53), blood was collected from all pigs and tested for the presence of antibodies against *M. hyopneumoniae* with a blocking ELISA (IDEIA™ *Mycoplasma hyopneumoniae* EIA kit, Oxoid Limited, Hampshire, UK), according to the protocol manual. Sera with optical density < 50% of the average value of the OD-buffercontrol were considered to be positive. All values above or equal to 50% of the average value of the OD-buffercontrol were classified as negative.

Routine bacteriological culture on bronchoalveolar lavage fluid

For the bacteriological examination, ten µL of bronchoalveolar lavage fluid collected on D53 of each pig was inoculated on Columbia agar supplemented with 5% sheep blood (Oxoid, Hampshire, UK) with a *Staphylococcus pseudintermedius* streak [25]. Plates were incubated overnight in a 5% CO_2-enriched environment at 35 °C for 48 h for identification of respiratory bacteria in the lungs.

Statistical analysis

Descriptive statistics were performed in order to check the normality of the data. One-way analysis of variance (ANOVA) was used to analyse weight and ADG. Repeated measurements ANOVA was performed to analyze the RDS data. Scheffé's post hoc test was used to make pairwise group comparisons. The parameters MLL, histopathological lesions, percentage air analysis, ELISA *M. hyopneumoniae*, TNF-α, IL-1, IL-6, Ig A, Ig G and qPCR results were analyzed using a non-parametric Kruskal-Wallis, as the data did not fulfil the assumptions of normality. Theses analyses were performed with SPSS 22 for Windows (SPSS inc. Illinois, USA). Percentage of seropositive pigs and percentage of pigs testing positive with qPCR in each group were analyzed using binomial logistic regression (R version 3.3.1) [26]. Results were considered to be statistically significant when $P < 0.05$.

Results

No animals died during or shortly after the inoculations. One out of 45 piglets in the NCG was euthanized (D22) (Release®300 mg/ml, WDT, Garbsen, Germany) due to nervous symptoms and lateral decubitus. Necropsy was performed and *Haemophilus parasuis* was isolated in pure culture from the meninges and pericardium. All animals in the PCG coughed, showed macroscopic lung lesions and seroconverted. *Mycoplasma hyopneumoniae*-DNA was detected in 19 out of 20 animals from this group.

Clinical and performance parameters

The results of the clinical parameters are summarized in Table 1. There was no coughing in the NCG throughout the study. The RDS_{24-53} was 1.20 ± 0.83 and 0.55 ± 0.42 for the PCG and VG ($P < 0.001$), respectively. This corresponds with a reduction of 52.9% in RDS when vaccinating the piglets compared to the PCG. All groups significantly differed from each other. These results and the RDS_{1-53} and RDS_{1-23} results are shown in Table 1 and Fig. 1.

The average group weight at D0, D24 and D53 and the ADG calculated during these three periods (0–24, 24–53 and 0–53 days of age) for each group are shown in Table 1.

Macroscopic and histopathologic lung lesions

There were no macroscopic lung lesions in the NCG. The MLL of the PCG and VG was 7.56 ± 4.73 and 0.68 ± 0.73, respectively ($P < 0.001$) (Table 1). A reduction of 91.0% in MLL of the VG was observed compared to the PCG. The histopathological lung lesion scoring in the NCG, PCG and VG was 1.31 ± 0.18, 3.32 ± 0.85 and 1.92 ± 0.47 ($P < 0.001$), respectively. The percentage of lung area occupied by air (percentage air) was 47.72 ± 7.29, 34.49 ± 8.22 and 45.23 ± 5.99% for the NCG, PCG and VG ($P < 0.001$), respectively. For the MLL and percentage of air analysis, the PCG was significantly different from the VG and NCG. For the histopathology score, all groups significantly differed from each other (Table 1).

Quantitative PCR for detection of *M. hyopneumoniae* DNA

The samples of the NCG remained negative throughout the study. The number of log copies of *M. hyopneumoniae* detected in the bronchoalveolar lavage fluid with qPCR in the PCG and VG were: 3.99 ± 1.20 (PCG) and 1.78 ± 1.36 (VG) ($P < 0.001$) at D53 (Table 1). The results of D39 and the percentage of animals that tested positive by qPCR are also shown in Table 1.

Immunological parameters on bronchoalveolar lavage fluid

All results of the immunological parameters on D39 and D53 are summarized in Table 2.

Detection of M. hyopneumoniae-specific antibodies in bronchoalveolar lavage fluid

There were no significant differences in the Ig G and Ig A results between the three groups at D39 (Table 2).

At D53, the Ig G values were 0.38 ± 0.17, 2.25 ± 0.91 and 2.41 ± 0.88 for the NCG, PCG and VG, respectively ($P = 0.005$). At D53, the results for Ig A were 0.18 ± 0.14, 2.10 ± 0.75, 2.08 ± 0.58 for the NCG, PCG and VG, respectively ($P = 0.005$). Both the Ig G and Ig A concentrations at D53 of the PCG and VG differed significantly from the NCG.

Detection of cytokines in bronchoalveolar lavage fluid

The TNF-α, IL-1 and IL-6 results at D39 and D53 are shown in Table 2. There were no significant differences obtained in the TNF-α- results (pg/ml) at D39, nor at D53.

At D53, the IL-1 concentration in the bronchoalveolar lavage fluid was 17.61 ± 1.98, 1283.39 ± 1075.65 and 53.04 ± 54.23 pg/ml in the NCG, PCG and VG, respectively ($P < 0.001$).

At D39, the IL-6 concentration was significantly different between the PCG and VG (Table 2). At D53, the IL-6 concentration was 148.10 ± 8.89, 493.35 ± 494.70 and 259.80 ± 333.38 for the NCG, PCG and VG, respectively ($P = 0.004$) with significantly higher concentrations in the PCG compared to the NCG and VG.

Serology

The serological results are presented in Table 1. All pigs of the NCG remained serologically negative throughout the study at D53 all pigs of the PCG and VG were serologically positive for *M. hyopneumoniae*. The OD values at D53 were 0.90 ± 0.10, 0.23 ± 0.11 and 0.087 ± 0.041 in the NCG, PCG and VG, respectively ($P < 0.001$). In the VG significantly lower OD-values were detected, thus higher *M. hyopneumoniae* specific antibodies compared to the PCG and NCG (Table 1).

Table 1 Results of different parameters in the different experimental groups

Parameter	Experimental Groups			
	NCG (# = 5)	PCG (# = 20)	VG (# = 20)	*P*-value
RDS				
D1–53	0 ± 0 [a]	0.68 ± 0.41 [b]	0.32 ± 0.86 [c]	*<0.001*
D1–23	0 ± 0 [a]	0 ± 0 [a]	0.017 ± 0.060 [a]	0.983
D24–53	0 ± 0 [a]	1.20 ± 0.83 [b]	0.55 ± 0.42 [c]	*<0.001*
Weight ± SD				
D0	7.04 ± 1.22 [a]	6.97 ± 0.84 [a]	7.04 ± 1.02 [a]	0.966
D24	15.25 ± 3.96 [a]	16.39 ± 2.16 [a]	15.61 ± 2.96 [a]	0.581
D53	36.51 ± 8.63 [a]	34.63 ± 6.63 [a]	34.27 ± 5.35 [a]	0.808
ADG (g/pig/d)				
D0–24	357 ± 123 [a]	393 ± 62.8 [a]	357 ± 92.0 [a]	0.372
D24–53	733 ± 194 [a]	629 ± 199 [a]	643 ± 102 [a]	0.504
D0–53	563 ± 144 [a]	522 ± 121 [a]	514 ± 87.0 [a]	0.714
MLL, histopathology and air analysis D53				
MLL	0 ± 0 [a]	7.56 ± 4.73 [b]	0.68 ± 0.73 [a]	*<0.001*
Histopathology	1.31 ± 0.18 [a]	3.32 ± 0.85 [b]	1.92 ± 0.47 [c]	*<0.001*
Percentage of air (%)	47.72 ± 7.29 [a]	34.49 ± 8.22 [b]	45.23 ± 5.99 [a]	*<0.001*
log copies of *M. hyopneumoniae* DNA/ml BALF (qPCR) ± SD				
D39	0.36 ± 0.64 [a]	1.81 ± 1.32 [a]	1.23 ± 1.61 [a]	0.062
D53	0.40 ± 0.43 [a]	3.99 ± 1.20 [b]	1.78 ± 1.36 [a]	*<0.001*
Percentage of *M. hyopneumoniae* qPCR positive samples in BALF (#positive samples/total number of samples)				
D39	(0/4) 0 [a]	(14/20) 70 [b]	(7/20) 35 [c]	*<0.01*
D53	(0/4) 0 [a]	(19/20) 95 [b]	(12/20) 60 [c]	*<0.001*
M. hyopneumoniae specific AB expressed in OD-values ± SD in serum				
D1	1.51 ± 0.037 [a]	1.48 ± 0.058 [a]	1.48 ± 0.16 [a]	0.578
D24	0.91 ± 0.044 [a]	0.95 ± 0.069 [a]	0.50 ± 0.17 [b]	*<0.001*
D53	0.90 ± 0.10 [a]	0.23 ± 0.11 [a]	0.087 ± 0.041 [b]	*<0.001*
Percentage of ELISA *M. hyopneumoniae* positive samples in serum				
D1	(0/5) 0 [a]	(0/20) 0 [a]	(0/20) 0 [a]	1.000
D24	(0/4) 0 [a]	(0/20) 0 [a]	(15/20) 75 [b]	*<0.001*
D53	(0/4) 0 [a]	(20/20) 100 [b]	(20/20)100 [b]	*<0.001*

The respiratory disease score (RDS), body weight, average daily gain (ADG), *M. hyopneumoniae* specific antibodies, macroscopical lung lesions (MLL), histopathology and air analysis, log copies of *M. hyopneumoniae* DNA (qPCR), percentage of of *M. hyopneumoniae* qPCR positive samples, *M. hyopneumoniae* specific AB expressed in OD-values and Percentage of ELISA *M. hyopneumoniae* positive samples

[a,b,c]Different superscripts in one row are statistically different ($P < 0.05$)

NCG negative control group, *PCG* positive control group, *VG* vaccination group, *SD* standard deviation, *D* Day of the study, *ADG* average daily gain, *kg* kilogram, *RDS* respiratory disease score, *M. hyopneumoniae Mycoplasma hyopneumoniae*, *AB* antibodies, *OD* optical densities, *#* number, *MLL* macroscopic lung lesions, *qPCR* quantitative polymerase chain reaction, *DNA* DeoxyriboNucleic Acid, *BALF* bronchoalveolar lavage fluid

Bacteriological culture

Streptococcus suis was isolated in only one pig of the PCG. No relevant bacterial growth was observed in all other lung samples.

Discussion

This study showed that the vaccine was efficacious for the most part against an experimental challenge with both a low and highly virulent *M. hyopneumoniae* strain. The vaccinated pigs coughed significantly less, showed significantly less lung lesions, a significantly lower number of log copies in the bronchoalveolar fluid at euthanasia was shown and the IL-1 and IL-6 concentrations at euthanasia were lower compared to the non-vaccinated inoculated pigs.

The challenge infection was performed with two genetically different [27] *M. hyopneumoniae* isolates. The virulence of these strains was evaluated by Vicca et al.

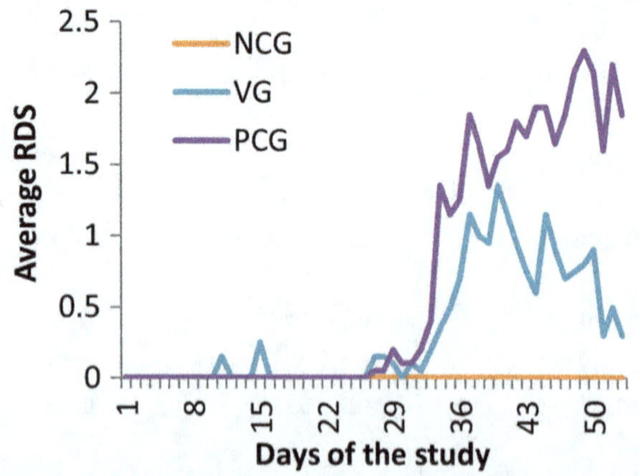

Fig. 1 Average respiratory disease score (RDS) during the trial for the negative control group (NCG), positive control group (PCG) and vaccination group (VG). The average RDS was assessed daily from day 1 until day 53. The piglets were vaccinated at D1 and the inoculations were performed at D24 and D25

[16] and both strains were characterised at proteomic and genomic level by Calus et al. [28], Vranckx et al. [4] and Stakenborg et al. [29], respectively. The double challenge infection model was successful as all animals in the PCG showed lung lesions, coughed and seroconverted. In 19 out of 20 animals of the PCG at euthanasia, DNA of *M. hyopneumoniae* was detected in the bronchoalveolar lavage fluid. It is well known that there can be quite some variation between pigs in terms of responses to an experimental infection. Why this particular pig tested negative is not known. Possibly, the conditions for multiplication of the *M. hyopneumoniae* strains were not optimal in that pig. Although bronchoalveolar fluid is an appropriate sampling technique to detect *M. hyopneumoniae* during the early stages of infection, it fails to recover some positive animals in case of chronic infection [30]. Taken these factors into consideration, this might be the reason why, although the pig was challenged, it did not test positive. Although comparing to other experimental settings should be done with caution, clinical symptoms and lung lesions were comparable or more severe than the single F7.2C challenge model performed in our research group [12, 16, 24, 25, 31–38] and the standard deviation was lower [16, 31–35]. It was shown that most pigs in the field are simultaneously infected with two or sometimes three genetically different *M. hyopneumoniae* strains and that when batches of slaughter pigs are infected with more than one *M. hyopneumoniae* strain, this can result in more (severe) pneumonia lesions and fissures [6]. The current experimental setting might therefore better resemble the field situation than infection with a single strain. Finally, it was shown that anesthetizing and inoculating the piglets with seven ml of inoculum on two consecutive days is feasible, as none of the piglets showed adverse reactions or died during or shortly after the inoculations.

Table 2 Immunological parameters measured in the BALF at D39 and D53

Parameter	Experimental groups			
	NCG (# = 5)	PCG (# = 20)	VG (# = 20)	*P*-value
Ig G ± SD (OD-values)				
D39	0 ± 0 ^{a}	0.069 ± 0.14 ^{a}	0.31 ± 0.65 ^{a}	0.366
D53	0.38 ± 0.17 ^{a}	2.25 ± 0.91 ^{b}	2.41 ± 0.88 ^{b}	*0.005*
Ig A ± SD (OD-values)				
D39	0 ± 0 ^{a}	0.067 ± 0.18 ^{a}	0.55 ± 0.99 ^{a}	0.359
D53	0.18 ± 0.14 ^{a}	2.10 ± 0.75 ^{b}	2.08 ± 0.58 ^{b}	*0.005*
TNF-α ± SD (pg/ml)				
D39	23.61 ± 1.74 ^{a}	18.56 ± 4.40 ^{a}	21.12 ± 4.56^{a}	*0.029*
D53	16.03 ± 1.10 ^{a}	14.53 ± 5.95 ^{a}	15.15 ± 2.40^{a}	0.065
IL-1 ± SD (pg/ml)				
D39	32.47 ± 1.77 ^{a}	239.63 ± 511.35 ^{a}	247.13 ± 606.71^{a}	0.367
D53	17.61 ± 1.98 ^{a}	1283.39 ± 1075.65 ^{b}	53.04 ± 54.23 ^{a}	*<0.001*
IL-6 ± SD (pg/ml)				
D39	130.33 ± 18.65 ^{ab}	242.24 ± 122.23 ^{a}	164.64 ± 84.48 ^{b}	0.03
D53	148.10 ± 8.89 ^{a}	493.35 ± 494.70 ^{b}	259.80 ± 333.38 ^{a}	*0.004*

D39: two weeks after challenge
D53: necropsy
^{a,b}Different superscripts in one row are statistically different ($P < 0.05$)
NCG negative control group, *PCG* positive control group, *VG* vaccination group, *SD* standard deviation, *D* Day of the study, *OD* optical densities, # number

The pigs in the vaccinated group coughed significantly less (−53%) from inoculation until euthanasia compared to the positive control group, demonstrating the efficacy of the vaccine. The degree of coughing is an important efficacy parameter [39, 40] not only under experimental but also under field conditions. A coughing index can be used to estimate if a higher prevalence of enzootic pneumonia in a herd might be present [41] and to determine the most optimal timing of serological sampling of the pigs or collecting bronchoalveolar fluid to be tested with PCR [41, 42]. In this study, no statistical significant differences were observed in the parameters weight and ADG, although the pigs in the VG grew slightly faster compared to the PCG from day of inoculation until day of euthanasia onwards. Although the parameter weight and ADG are of great use to evaluate in field circumstances, in experimental trials they are merely of descriptive value as the low number of animals used, the duration of the trial and the sometimes high standard deviations are the reason why only numerical differences are found [10, 16, 31].

The MLL score in the vaccinated pigs was very low (0.68) and statistically different from the PCG (7.56), implying a reduction with 91%, and demonstrating the efficacy of the vaccine. A recent field study showed that when pigs are infected with more strains, more lung lesions are detected [6]. When comparing the MLL scores from the double inoculated challenge in PCG with those from challenged unvaccinated pigs in the single inoculation model from previous studies (highest MLL was 6.69 for F7.2C challenge in Villarreal et al., [25]), higher MLL in this study are obtained. However, comparing different experimental settings, should be done with caution. To make a true comparison, the resulting MLL from the double infection model should be compared with the single inoculation model from both strains F7.2C and F1.12A in one experimental setting.

In the vaccinated animals significantly less lymphohistiocytic infiltration (1.92) was observed compared to the PCG (3.32). These results are in accordance with the results of previous studies [25, 31, 32]. Although many aspects of the effect of vaccination on the immunological response remain unclear [43], the present results confirm that vaccination has a regulating function on the immune system, causing less infiltration of macrophages in the lung tissue [34]. A significantly lower area occupied by air or air percentage was measured in the non-vaccinated animals of PCG (34.49%) compared to VG (45.23%). Infection with *M. hyopneumoniae* results in intrabronchiolar- and bronchial exudate and infiltration of lymphohistiocytic cells in the lung tissue. These responses may result in compressing the airways and alveoli, leading to less air volume in the lungs [15]. Vaccination also significantly reduced the log copies of *M. hyopneumoniae* DNA in the bronchoalveolar lavage fluid compared to the non-vaccinated animals (1.78 versus 3.99), which may lead to less shedding of *M. hyopneumoniae* in vaccinated pigs. Similar reductions were found in previous studies [34, 44]. These results, although very promising, confirm once more that vaccination is not able to prevent pigs from being colonized as commonly known [8].

Mycoplasma hyopneumoniae-specific antibody (Ig G and Ig A) levels in tracheo-bronchial washings were not significantly different between vaccinated and non-vaccinated pigs. Our findings are in accordance with Djordevic et al. (1997) [24, 45], but Thacker et al. (2000) suggested that secretion of *M. hyopneumoniae-* antibodies induced by vaccination into the bronchoalveolar washings might be implied in resolving mycoplasmal pneumonia [43, 46, 47]. Further research is needed to clarify a possible protective role of *M. hyopneumoniae*-specific antibodies in trachea-bronchial washings.

There were no significant differences between the vaccinated and non-vaccinated animals for the TNF-α concentration in the bronchoalveolar fluids. In the study of Marchioro et al. [24], vaccination significantly decreased TNF-α concentrations, but the difference was small and only borderline significant. This highlights the need to further elucidate the pathogenesis of *M. hyopneumoniae* and the exact mechanisms in which way *M. hyopneumoniae*-bacterins provide protection to the animal.

The cytokines IL-1 and IL-6, next to TNF-α are pro-inflammatory cytokines [48]. Previous research stated that they mediate lymphocyte infiltration and activation in the pneumonic lung [49, 50], and thus are associated with the induction of pneumonia lesions [24, 51, 52]. The pro-inflammatory cytokines TNF-α, IL-1 and IL-6 were correlated with MLL at D39 and D53. The parameter TNF-α was weakly and not significantly correlated with MLL on both sampling days (D39 and D53). Interleukin 1 was strongly and significantly correlated with MLL at euthanasia, and IL-6 was moderately and significantly correlated with MLL on D39 and D53. This suggests that the vaccine shows a protective effect mainly by modulation of the pro-inflammatory cytokines IL-1 and IL-6, but not TNF-α (data not shown). The IL-1 concentration and the standard deviation in the non-vaccinated pigs was very high. This result is in accordance with the result of Meyns et al. [38] at 28 days post inoculation with the F7.2C isolate. One can conclude that a part of the piglets in the non- vaccinated group showed very high IL-1 levels. The reason why this occurred is not clear, however the individual susceptibility of the pig to an *M. hyopneumoniae* infection must be kept into account causing the challenge infection to be more successful. The IL-1 and IL-6 concentrations at necropsy in the vaccinated pigs were significantly lower than in the non-vaccinated pigs and not significantly different from the levels in negative control group. These results substantiate the statement that was made in Marchioro et al. [24] based on the IL-1 result of the vaccinated pigs at D36 that IL-1 and IL-6 may have a regulatory role upon *M. hyopneumoniae* vaccination [24].

In this study, the pigs were vaccinated approximately 4 weeks before challenge, as vaccination is most likely to be effective if active immunity is established before the piglets are exposed to the pathogen. Under field conditions, however, the time between vaccination and infection is not known, and very likely highly variable between pigs. Hence, it is possible that the vaccine used in the field is less efficacious when the timing of vaccination is not optimal. As this is an experimental study, the results cannot be extrapolated as such to field conditions. Under field circumstances, more factors challenging the efficacy of a vaccine are present, compared to the controlled environment of an experimental facility. First, multi-factorial and multi-pathogen enzootic pneumonia outbreaks are typically found in the field, rather than isolated *M. hyopneumoniae* outbreaks [2]. The piglets originated from a herd free of important diseases which can influence the outcome of an *M. hyopneumoniae* infection, such as PRRSv *Pasteurella multocida*, and *Actinobacillus pleuropneumoniae*. [1, 53, 54] and according to some authors infection with certain pathogens can determine the effectiveness of *M. hyopneumoniae* vaccination as well [54–56]. Second, the impact of weaning stress should be taken into account when vaccinating piglets at weaning age in the field. Although the impact of weaning stress on vaccine efficacy might not be clear [31], it could not have influenced the efficacy of the vaccine, as the pigs were transported and vaccinated some days after weaning. Thirdly, passively acquired maternal derived immunity could not have influenced the efficacy of the vaccine as these piglets were originating from a herd free of *M. hyopneumoniae* and no vaccinations against *M. hyopneumoniae* in the sows, nor the piglets were performed. This is a double sided given. On the one hand, Hodgins et al. [57] stated that maternal antibodies in the piglets were associated with reduced antibody responses to vaccination. On the other hand, the piglets in the study could not benefit from the passively transferred cell-mediated immunity. Bandrick et al. [30] showed that vaccination of piglets against *M. hyopneumoniae* in the face of antigen-specific maternal-derived immunity results in cell-mediated immunity priming and anamnestic cell-mediated immunity responses following the exposure *to M. hyopneumoniae* antigen. On the other hand, some factors in the experimental study were comparable to field circumstances or challenged the vaccine more. First, although the piglets were free from certain pathogens, other than that, the piglets were originating from a conventional farm. Second: the piglets were transported from the herd of origin to the experimental facilities and the piglets needed to establish a new hierarchy after comingling. These events are associated with stress, which might influence the efficacy of the vaccine. This can resemble the stress that piglets experience in the field, when sorted and moved from one facility to another in a multi-site production system. Thirdly: the vaccine was highly challenged in this experimental study, because as stated by Villarreal et al., [35] and Meyns et al. [37], it can be assumed that the *M. hyopneumoniae* challenge dose used to infect the pigs was higher than might be reached under natural conditions resulting in a faster and higher colonization level and presumably challenging the vaccine more than under field circumstances [35, 37]. Although extrapolation of the efficacy testing of the vaccine results obtained in experimentally *M. hyopneumoniae* infected pigs should be done with caution, this infection model enabled to study the effect of the vaccine in *M. hyopneumoniae* infected pigs in a reproducible and standardized way.

Conclusion

Using a double challenge infection model with a low and highly virulent *M. hyopneumoniae* strain, one-dose vaccination of piglets was efficacious for the most part, as coughing was reduced by more than 50% and macroscopical lung lesions by 91%. In addition, the lymphohistiocytic infiltration in lung tissue was lower, the number of log copies of *M. hyopneumoniae* DNA detected in bronchoalveolar lavage fluid and the IL-1 and IL-6 concentrations at euthanasia were lower in the vaccinated animals compared to non-vaccinated animals.

Abbreviations

#: Number; ADG: Average daily gain; ANOVA: Analysis of variance; BALF: Bronchoalveolar lavage fluid; D: Day of the study; DNA: DeoxyriboNucleic Acid; *M. hyopneumoniae*: *Mycoplasma hyopneumoniae*; MLL: Macroscopic lung lesions; NCG: Negative control group; OD: Optical density; PBS: Phosphate-buffered saline; PCG: Positive control group; PI: Post-inoculation; qPCR: Quantitative polymerase chain reaction; RA-SE genetics: Rattrelow-Seghers genetics; RDS: Respiratory disease score; SD: Standard deviation; VG: Vaccination group

Acknowledgements

The authors are grateful to Marleen Foubert for the assistance with the laboratory analyses and to Pieter-Jan De Temmerman for the assistance with the binary data analysis.

Funding

The study was funded by CEVA Santé Animale, Libourne Cedex, France. CEVA Santé Animale participated in the study design, and in the review of the final manuscript.

Authors' contributions

AM designed the study protocol, wrote the ethical application, performed the trial, performed the laboratory analyses, performed the statistical analyses, interpreted the data and wrote the manuscript. IA reviewed the study protocol, assisted with performing the trial, assisted with interpretation of the data and reviewed the manuscript. FB reviewed the study protocol, the ethical application dossier, assisted with interpretation of the data and reviewed the manuscript and helped with the laboratory analysis. RC, FH and DM designed the study protocol, reviewed the ethical application dossier and the manuscript and assisted with interpretation of the data. All authors gave their final approval for publication of the study.

Consent for publication

Not applicable

Competing interests

The study was funded by CEVA Santé Animale, Libourne Cedex, France.

Author details

[1]Department of Reproduction, Obstetrics and Herd Health, Faculty of Veterinary Medicine, Ghent University, Merelbeke, Belgium. [2]Department of Pathology, Bacteriology and Avian Diseases, Faculty of Veterinary Medicine, Ghent University, Merelbeke, Belgium. [3]CEVA Santé Animale, Cedex, Libourne, France.

References

1. Maes D, Segales J, Meyns T, Sibila M, Pieters M, Haesebrouck F. Control of *Mycoplasma hyopneumoniae* infections in pigs. Vet Microbiol. 2008;126:297–309.
2. Maes D, Deluyker H, Verdonck M, Castryck F, Miry C, Vrijens B, et al. Effect of vaccination against *Mycoplasma hyopneumoniae* in pig herds with an all-in/all-out production system. Vaccine. 1999;17:1024–34.
3. Villarreal I, Meyns T, Dewulf J, Vranckx K, Calus D, Pasmans F, et al. The effect of vaccination on the transmission of Mycoplasma hyopneumoniae in pigs under field conditions. Vet J. 2011;188:48–52.
4. Vranckx K, Maes D, Calus D, Villarreal I, Pasmans F, Haesebrouck F. Multiple locus variable number of tandem repeats analysis is a suitable tool for the differentiation of *Mycoplasma hyopneumoniae* strains without cultivation. J Clin Microbiol. 2011;49:2020–3.
5. Vranckx K, Maes D, Del Pozo SR, Pasmans F, Haesebrouck F. A longitudinal study of the diversity and dynamics of *Mycoplasma hyopneumoniae* infections in pig herds. Vet Microbiol. 2011;156:315–21.
6. Michiels A, Vranckx K, Piepers S, Del Pozo SR, Arsenakis I, Boyen F, et al. Impact of diversity of *Mycoplasma hyopneumoniae* strains on lung lesions in slaughter pigs. Vet Res. 2017;48:1–14.
7. Pointon AMD, Byrt D, Heap P. Effect of enzootic pneumonia of pigs on growth performance. Aust Vet J. 1985;62:13–8.
8. Haesebrouck F, Pasmans F, Chiers K, Maes D, Ducatelle R, Decostere A. Efficacy of vaccines against bacterial diseases in swine: what can we expect? Vet Microbiol. 2004;100:255–68.
9. Martelli P, Saleri R, Cavalli V, De Angelis E, Ferrari L, Benetti M, et al. Systemic and local immune response in pigs intradermally and intramuscularly injected with inactivated *Mycoplasma hyopneumoniae* vaccines. Vet Microbiol. 2014;168:357–64.
10. Jensen CS, Ersbøll AK, Nielsen JP. A meta-analysis comparing the effect of vaccines against *Mycoplasma hyopneumoniae* on daily weight gain in pigs. Prev Vet Med. 2002;54:265–78.
11. Kyriakis SC, Alexopoulos C, Vlemmas J, Sarris K, Lekkas S, Koutsoviti-Papadopoulou M, et al. Field study on the efficacy of two different vaccination schedules with HYORESP® in a *Mycoplasma hyopneumoniae*-infected commercial pig unit. J Vet Med. 2001;48:675–84.
12. Meyns T, Dewulf J, de Kruif A, Calus D, Haesebrouck F, Maes D. Comparison of transmission of *Mycoplasma hyopneumoniae* in vaccinated and non-vaccinated populations. Vaccine. 2006;24:7081–6.
13. Martelli P, Terreni M, Guazzetti S, Cavirani S. Antibody response to *Mycoplasma hyopneumoniae* infection in vaccinated pigs with or without maternal antibodies induced by sow vaccination. J Vet Med. 2006;53:229–33.
14. Goodwin RFW, Whittlestone P. Production of enzootic pneumonia in pigs with an agent grown in tissue culture from the natural disease. Br J Exp Pathol. 1963;44:291–9.
15. Marchioro SB, Maes D, Haesebrouck F, Dellagostin OA. Immune responses following vaccination of pigs and mice against *Mycoplasma hyopneumoniae*. Ghent: Ghent Univeristy; 2013.
16. Vicca J, Stakenborg T, Maes D, Butaye P, Peeters J, de Kruif A, et al. Evaluation of virulence of *Mycoplasma hyopneumoniae* field isolates. Vet Microbiol. 2003;97:177–90.
17. Halbur PG, Paul PS, Meng XJ, Lum MA, Andrews JJ, Rathje JA. Comparative pathogenicity of nine US porcine reproductive and respiratory syndrome virus (PRRSV) isolates in a five-week-old cesarean-derived, colostrum-deprived pig model. J Vet Diagn Investig. 1996;8:11–20.
18. Del Pozo SR, Sierens A, Marchioro SB, Vangroenweghe F, Jourquin J, Labarque G, et al. Efficacy of early *Mycoplasma hyopneumoniae* vaccination against mixed respiratory disease in older fattening pigs. Vet Rec. 2014;174
19. Hannan PC, Bhogal BS, Fish JP. Tylosin tartrate and tiamutilin effects on experimental piglet pneumonia induced with pneumonic pig lung homogenate containing mycoplasmas, bacteria and viruses. Res Vet Sci. 1982;33:76–88.
20. Morris C, Gardner I, Hietala S, Carpenter T, Anderson R, Parker K. Seroepidemiologic study of natural transmission of *Mycoplasma hyopneumoniae* in a swine herd. Prev Vet Med. 1995;21:323–37.
21. Rasband WS. ImageJ U. S. National Institutes of Health, Bethesda. 1997–2016. https://imagej.nih.gov/ij/. Accessed 17 Aug 2017.
22. Marois C, Dory D, Fablet C, Madec F, Kobisch M. Development of a quantitative real-time TaqMan PCR assay for determination of the minimal dose of *Mycoplasma hyopneumoniae* strain 116 required to induce pneumonia in SPF pigs. J Appl Microbiol. 2010;108:1523–33.
23. Bereiter M, Young TF, Joo HS, Ross RF. Evaluation of the ELISA and comparison to the complement-fixation test and radial immunodiffusion enzyme assay for detection of antibodies against *Mycoplasma hyopneumoniae* in swine serum. Vet Microbiol. 1990;25:177–92.
24. Marchioro SB, Maes D, Flahou B, Pasmans F, Del Pozo SR, Vranckx K, et al. Local and systemic immune responses in pigs intramuscularly injected with an inactivated *Mycoplasma hyopneumoniae* vaccine. Vaccine. 2013;31:1305–11.
25. Villarreal I, Maes D, Vranckx K, Calus D, Pasmans F, Haesebrouck F. Effect of vaccination of pigs against experimental infection with high and low virulence *Mycoplasma hyopneumoniae* strains. Vaccine. 2011;29:1731–5.
26. Team RC. R: A language and environment for statistical computing. Vienna, Austria. 2016. URL https://www.R-project.org/. Accessed 17 Aug 2017.
27. Stakenborg T, Vicca J, Butaye P, Maes D, Peeters J, de Kruif A, et al. The diversity of *Mycoplasma hyopneumoniae* within and between herds using pulsed-field gel electrophoresis. Vet Microbiol. 2005;109:29–35.
28. Calus D, Baele M, Meyns T, de Kruif A, Butaye P, Decostere A, et al. Protein variability among *Mycoplasma hyopneumoniae* isolates. Vet Microbiol. 2007;120:284–91.
29. Stakenborg T, Vicca J, Maes D, Peeters J, de Kruif A, Haesebrouck F, et al. Comparison of molecular techniques for the typing of *Mycoplasma hyopneumoniae* isolates. J Microbiol Methods. 2006;66:263–75.
30. Moorkamp L, Nathues H, Spergser J, Tegeler R, Grosse Beilage E. Detection of respiratory pathogens in porcine lung tissue and lavage fluid. Vet J. 2008;175:273–5.
31. Arsenakis I, Panzavolta L, Michiels A, Del Pozo SR, Boyen F, Haesebrouck F, et al. Efficacy of *Mycoplasma hyopneumoniae* vaccination before and at weaning against experimental challenge infection in pigs. BMC Vet Res. 2016;12:1–7.
32. Marchioro SB, Del Pozo SR, Michiels A, Haesebrouck F, Conceição FR, Dellagostin OA, et al. Immune responses of a chimaeric protein vaccine containing *Mycoplasma hyopneumoniae* antigens and LTB against experimental *M. hyopneumoniae* infection in pigs. Vaccine. 2014;6:4689–94.
33. Del Pozo SR, Thiry J, Vranckx K, López Rodríguez A, Chiers K, Haesebrouck F, et al. Efficacy of florfenicol injection in the treatment of Mycoplasma hyopneumoniae induced respiratory disease in pigs. Vet J. 2012;194:420–2.
34. Vranckx K, Maes D, Marchioro SB, Villarreal I, Chiers K, Pasmans F, et al. Vaccination reduces macrophage infiltration in bronchus-associated lymphoid tissue in pigs infected with a highly virulent *Mycoplasma hyopneumoniae* strain. BMC Vet Res. 2012;8:1–7.
35. Villarreal I, Maes D, Meyns T, Gebruers F, Calus D, Pasmans F, et al. Infection with a low virulent *Mycoplasma hyopneumoniae* isolate does not protect piglets against subsequent infection with a highly virulent *M. hyopneumoniae* isolate. Vaccine. 2009;27:1875–9.
36. Vicca J, Maes D, Jonker L, De Kruif A, Haesebrouck F. Efficacy of in-feed medication with tylosin for the treatment and control of *Mycoplasma hyopneumoniae* infections. Vet Rec. 2005;156:606–10.
37. Meyns T, Maes D, Dewulf J, Vicca J, Haesebrouck F, de Kruif A. Quantification of the spread of *Mycoplasma hyopneumoniae* in nursery pigs using transmission experiments. Prev Vet Med. 2004;66:265–75.

38. Meyns T, Maes D, Calus D, Ribbens S, Dewulf J, Chiers K, et al. Interactions of highly and low virulent *Mycoplasma hyopneumoniae* isolates with the respiratory tract of pigs. Vet Microbiol. 2007;120:87–95.
39. Baskerville A. Development of the early lesions in experimental enzootic pneumonia of pigs: an ultrastructural and histological study. Res Vet Sci. 1972;13:570–8.
40. Sarradell J, Andrada M, Ramirez AS, Fernández A, Gómez-Villamandos JC, Jover A, et al. A morphologic and Immunohistochemical study of the bronchus-associated lymphoid tissue of pigs naturally infected with *Mycoplasma hyopneumoniae*. Vet Pathol. 2003;40:395–404.
41. Nathues H, Spergser J, Rosengarten R, Kreienbrock L, Grosse Beilage E. Value of the clinical examination in diagnosing enzootic pneumonia in fattening pigs. Vet J. 2012;193:443–7.
42. Leon EA, Madec F, Taylor NM, Kobisch M. Seroepidemiology of *Mycoplasma hyopneumoniae* in pigs from farrow-to-finisch farm. Vet Microbiol. 2001;78: 331–41.
43. Thacker EL, Thacker BJ, Kuhn M, Hawkins PA, Waters WR. Evaluation of local and systemic immune responses induced by intramuscular injection of a *Mycoplasma hyopneumoniae* bacterin to pigs. Am J Vet Res. 2000;61:1384–9.
44. Woolley LK, Fell SA, Gonsalves JR JR, BBA R, Collins D, Kuit TA, et al. Evaluation of recombinant Mycoplasma hyopneumoniae P97/P102 paralogs formulated with selected adjuvants as vaccines against mycoplasmal pneumonia in pigs. Vaccine. 2014;32:4333–41.
45. Djordjevic SP, Eamens GJ, Romalis LF, Nicholls PJ, Taylor DJ, Chin J. Serum and mucosal antibody responses and protection in pigs vaccinated against *Mycoplasma hyopneumoniae* with vaccines containing a denatured membrane antigen pool and adjuvant. Aust Vet J. 1997;75:504–11.
46. Thacker EL, Thacker BJ, Young TF, Halbur PG. Effect of vaccination on the potentiation of porcine reproductive and respiratory syndrome virus (PRRSV)-induced pneumonia by *Mycoplasma hyopneumoniae*. Vaccine. 2000;18:1244–52.
47. Thacker E, Strait EL, Ruebling K, Nilubol D, Erickson B, White R. Evaluation of organism number and the immune response to one dose *Mycoplasma hyopneumoniae* vaccines. In: Blaha T, Pahlitzsch C, editors. 18th IPVS Congress. Hamburg, Germany; 2000.
48. Yang J, Hooper WC, Phillips DJ, Talkington DF. Cytokines in Mycoplasma pneumoniae infection. Cytokine Growth Factor Rev. 2004;15:157–68.
49. Van Reeth K, Van Gucht S, Pensaert M. In vivo studies on cytokine involvement during acute viral respiratory disease of swine: troublesome but rewarding. Vet Immunol Immunopathol. 2002;87:161–8.
50. Ahn KK, Kwon D, Jung K, Ha Y, Seo MJ, Kim S-H, et al. Identification of interleukin-1, tumor necrosis factor-α, and interleukin-6 expression in lungs from pigs naturally infected with *Mycoplasma hyopneumoniae* by in situ hybridization. J Vet Med Sci. 2009;71:441–5.
51. Asai T, Okadaa M, Onoa M, Irisawaa T, Morib Y, Yokomizob Y, et al. Increased levels of tumor necrosis factor and interleukin 1 in bronchoalveolar lavage fluids from pigs infected with *Mycoplasma hyopneumoniae*. Vet Immunol Immunopathol. 1993;38:253–60.
52. Rodriguez F, Ramireza GA, Sarradell J, Andradaa M, Lorenzo H. Immunohistochemical Labelling of cytokines in lung lesions of pigs naturally infected with *Mycoplasma hyopneumoniae*. J Comp Pathol. 2004;130:306–12.
53. Sibila M, Pieters M, Molitor T, Maes D, Haesebrouck F, Segalés J. Current perspectives on the diagnosis and epidemiology of *Mycoplasma hyopneumoniae* infection. Vet J. 2009;181:221–31.
54. Steenhard NR, Jungersen G, Kokotovic B, Beshah E, Dawson HD, Urban JFJ, et al. *Ascaris suum* infection negatively affects the response to a *Mycoplasma hyopneumoniae* vaccination and subsequent challenge infection in pigs. Vaccine. 2009;27:5161–9.
55. Stevenson GW. Bacterial pneumonia in swine. In: Done S, Thomson J, Varley M, editors. 15th IPVS congress. Birmingham: Nottingham University Press; 1998.
56. Martinod S. Protection against *Mycoplasma hyopneumoniae* and *Actinobacillus pleuropneumoniae* infections using a mycoplasma inactivated vaccine Respisure under field conditions. In: Moneti G, Vignola G, editors. 14th IPVS congress. Bologna: Press point-Abbiategrasso, Bologna; 1996.
57. Hodgins DC, Shewen PE, Dewey CE. Influence of age and maternal antibodies on antibody responses of neonatal piglets vaccinated against *Mycoplasma hyopneumoniae*. J Swine Health Prod. 2004;12:10–6.

3

A proteomic approach to the development of DIVA ELISA distinguishing pigs infected with *Salmonella* Typhimurium and pigs vaccinated with a *Salmonella* Typhimurium-based inactivated vaccine

Jan Gebauer[1,2*], Hana Kudlackova[1], Marcel Kosina[3], Kamil Kovarcik[4], Radek Tesarik[1], Alena Osvaldova[1,5], Martin Faldyna[1] and Jan Matiasovic[1]

Abstract

Background: *Salmonella enterica* serovar Typhimurium is one of the most common enteropathogenic bacteria found in pigs in Europe. In our previous work, we demonstrated the protective effects in suckling piglets when their dams had been vaccinated with an *S.* Typhimurium-based inactivated vaccine. This study is focused on a procedure leading to serological discrimination between vaccinated and infected pigs. As we supposed, distinct environment during natural infection and in bacterial cultures used for vaccine preparation led to a slightly different spectrum of expressed *S.* Typhimurium proteins. The examination of porcine antibodies produced after the experimental infection with *S.* Typhimurium or after vaccination with *S.* Typhimurium-based inactivated vaccine by affinity chromatography and mass spectrometry revealed differences in antibody response applicable for serological differentiation of infected from vaccinated animals.

Results: Antibodies against *Salmonella* SipB, SipD and SseB proteins were detected at much higher levels in post-infection sera in comparison with control and post-vaccination sera. On the other hand, proteins BamB, OppA and a fragment of FliC interacted with antibodies from post-vaccination sera with a much higher intensity than from control and post-infection sera. In addition, we constructed ELISA assays using post-infection antigen - SipB protein and post-vaccination antigen - FliC-fragment and evaluated them on a panel of individual porcine sera.

Conclusions: The analysis of antibody response of infected and vaccinated pigs by proteomic tools enabled to identify *S.* Typhimurium antigens useful for distinguishing infected from vaccinated animals. This approach can be utilized in other challenges where DIVA vaccine and a subsequent serological assay are required, especially when genetic modification of a vaccine strain is not desirable.

Keywords: Porcine, *Salmonella* Typhimurium, DIVA vaccine, Recombinant protein, Mass spectrometry

* Correspondence: gebauer@vri.cz
[1]Department of Immunology, Veterinary Research Institute, Hudcova296/70, 62100 Brno, Czech Republic
[2]Department of Experimental Biology, Faculty of Science, Masaryk University, Kotlarska267/2, 611 37 Brno, Czech Republic
Full list of author information is available at the end of the article

Background

Infections caused by non-typhoid *Salmonella enterica* serovar Typhimurium (*Salmonella* Typhimurium) constitute a persistent problem in human and veterinary medicine. *Salmonella* Typhimurium is the most frequent serotype found in pigs. Contaminated pork and porcine products are thus a source of infection for human consumers [1]. A possible way to moderate the *Salmonella* burden in pigs is vaccination. A successful and widely used vaccine should allow distinguishing vaccinated animals from those that were naturally infected, so-called DIVA approach (Differentiating Infected from Vaccinated individuals) [2]. Available diagnostic serological tests for the evaluation of *Salmonella* infections in pigs are based on measurements of the level of antibodies induced by O-antigens, the outer segment of bacterial lipopolysaccharide (LPS) [3]. These assays do not allow us to distinguish infected and vaccinated animals when *Salmonella* strain without any deletion in genes responsible for lipopolysaccharide formation is used for vaccination [4]. On the other hand, LPS plays a role as an inducer of the immune response, which might be beneficial for the vaccination itself [5, 6]. Selke et al. [7] introduced a live negative-marker vaccine based on *Salmonella* Typhimurium strain with deleted gene for the outer membrane protein *ompD*. Bearson et al. [8] prepared a similar attenuated live negative-marker vaccine with a deletion of multiple small regulatory RNAs combined with *rfaH* mutation. However, using a genetically modified live bacterial strain as a vaccine may be questionable because of current regulation and public non-acceptance of genetically modified organisms in Europe.

With an unmodified inactivated *Salmonella* Typhimurium-based vaccine for pigs developed in our previous work we achieved a similar level of protectivity for suckling piglets [9] as Selke et al. [7]. In this study, we extend the development of this vaccine to include DIVA testing. We took advantage of the fact that *Salmonella* express virulence factors (proteins from SPIs - *Salmonella* pathogenicity islands) in an environment-dependent manner. We thus expected differences in bacterial protein expression under in vitro and in vivo conditions. We analysed the antibody response to the vaccine based on inactivated *Salmonella* Typhimurium cultivated in vitro and the antibody response of animals infected with live bacteria.

Based on this, we introduced a method for discovering *Salmonella* proteins able to induce condition-specific antibody production, which allows us to serologically distinguish animals that were vaccinated from those infected with *Salmonella* Typhimurium.

Methods

Bacterial strain

Salmonella enterica serovar Typhimurium phage type DT104 strain (strain number 1A5, from bacterial collection at Veterinary Research Institute, originally isolated from healthy sow), hereinafter referred to as *Salmonella* Typhimurium, was used in this experiment. Bacteria were cultivated overnight at 37 °C in Miller's LB Broth Base (Invitrogen, USA) or brain heart infusion (BHI) broth (Oxoid, UK) for certain analyses as described below.

Vaccination and infection of pigs

Three groups of animals consisting of twelve white mixed-breed piglets (bought from a commercial stud) weaned 21 days after birth were used in the experiment. Pigs in the first group remained serologically negative for anti-*Salmonella* antibodies (determined by Pig Screen ELISA, Qiagen, Germany). Another twelve animals were orally infected one week after housing with 1×10^8 CFU of *Salmonella* Typhimurium grown in BHI medium and blood was collected 28 days after the infection. The last group of animals was vaccinated intramuscularly into the neck with 1 ml of a vaccine prepared from 1×10^9 CFU of *Salmonella* Typhimurium grown in BHI medium, inactivated with formaldehyde and adjuvanted with Montanide ISA50V2 (Seppic, France). The first dose was administered one week after housing and the second dose two weeks later. Blood was collected 14 days after the second dose of a vaccine.

Antibody fraction preparation

Serum samples from three random animals from each group were pooled together and IgG fractions were isolated using Protein G columns (HiTrap Protein G HP, GE Healthcare, UK) according to the manufacturer's protocol. Affinity chromatography was performed on an FPLC instrument (Pharmacia, Sweden).

Antigen preparation

The same procedure of preparing bacterial protein lysate was used for the comparison of *Salmonella* Typhimurium protein expression when cultivated in LB or BHI medium using MS and for immunoaffinity chromatography.

Salmonella Typhimurium was grown overnight at 37 °C in LB and BHI medium, as noted above. The culture was then centrifuged (3,500 × g, 10 min), and a cell pellet was washed 3 times in PBS (Dulbecco's, Lonza, Switzerland). The cell pellet was resuspended in PBS and sonicated (Sonopuls HD 3100, Bandelin, Germany) with zirconia/silica beads (BioSpec Products, USA). The sonicate was centrifuged at 20,000 × g and the supernatant with proteins was taken. The pellet was then resuspended in 8 M urea (Serva, Germany), 0.1 % SDS (Carl Roth, Germany), 2 % Triton X-100 (Serva, Germany) and 25 mM triethylammonium bicarbonate (Sigma-Aldrich, USA) and centrifuged at 20,000 × g again. The supernatant was mixed with the supernatant from the previous step and together used as an antigen for subsequent analysis.

Immunoaffinity chromatography

IgGs from all three sample groups were covalently bound to CNBr-activated Sepharose (GE Healthcare, UK) according to the manufacturer's protocol. Sepharose with bound immunoglobulins was loaded into 3 plastic cartridges (BioRad, USA) creating liquid chromatography columns. The same antigen (protein lysate from *Salmonella* Typhimurium grown in LB) was used for all three IgG columns - column with antibodies from negative control animals, from vaccinated animals and from infected animals. 20 mM sodium phosphate buffer, pH 7.0 (Serva, Germany) served as a binding buffer. 0.1 M glycine-HCl (Serva, Germany), pH 2.7 was used for elution of bound proteins and 1 M Tris–HCl (Carl Roth, Germany), pH 9.0, was added to collection tubes for pH adjustment. Protein eluates were then used for analysis by mass spectrometry.

LC-MS/MS analysis

100 µg of proteins (measured with Pierce™ BCA Protein Assay Kit, Thermo Scientific, USA) was used for each sample preparation with the FASP (filter-aided sample preparation) method [10]. Each sample was washed five times with 8 M urea (Serva, Germany) in Vivacon 500 centrifugal tubes (Sartorius Stedim, Germany) with 10,000 MWCO membrane filter. Dithiothreitol (10 mM, Sigma-Aldrich, USA) and iodoacetamide (50 mM, Serva, Germany) in triethylammonium bicarbonate buffer (25 mM, Sigma-Aldrich, USA) were used for reduction and alkylation, respectively. Proteins were then digested with trypsin (Promega, USA) in 1:50 ratio, for one hour, at 37 °C and then overnight at 25 °C. After centrifugation, the eluate with digested peptides was evaporated (DNA120 SpeedVac, Thermo Savant, USA), peptide pellet was resuspended in 0.1 % aqueous formic acid (Sigma-Aldrich, USA) which serves as a mobile phase for liquid chromatography (UltiMate 3000 RSLCnano, Dionex -Thermo Scientific, USA). For separation and elution of peptides, 2-h gradient with increasing (0 min - 4 %, 4 min - 4 %, 98 min - 45 %, 98.5 min - 90 %, 112 min - 90 %, 112.5 min - 4 %, 120 min - 4 %) concentrations of acetonitrile (0.1 % formic acid in acetonitrile, Sigma-Aldrich, USA) at a flow rate of 300 nl/min was used. Peptides were separated on a 25 cm column (Acclaim PepMap RSLC C18, 2 µm, 100 Å, 75 µm I.D., Thermo Scientific, USA). uHPLC was connected to EASY-Spray ion source and Orbitrap Velos Pro mass spectrometer (Thermo Scientific, USA). A survey scan over the m/z range 390–1700 was used to identify protonated peptides with charge states of at least 2, which were automatically selected for data-dependent MS/MS analysis and fragmented by collision with helium gas. Ten fragment mass spectra after each full scan were recorded. Measured spectra were then searched using Proteome Discoverer (version 1.4, Thermo Scientific, USA) software with Mascot (Matrix Science, USA) or Sequest HT (Thermo Scientific, USA) as a searching algorithm. Oxidation of methionine as a dynamic, and carbamidomethylation of cysteine as a static modification was used. Precursor and fragment mass tolerances were set up as 10 ppm and 0.5 Da, respectively. Swiss-Prot database for *Salmonella* strain was used (based on 2014/06 release) in Mascot and Uniprot database for *Salmonella* strain (from 2013/04) was used in Sequest HT. Only peptides with a false discovery rate less than 0.05 were considered as well identified. Proteins that were uniquely found in each sample - proteins bound to the IgG fraction from sera from either vaccinated or infected animals, but not from control pigs were then pinpointed as candidate antigens for serological discrimination.

Recombinant protein preparation and its purification

Appropriate primers (Tab. 1) for each selected protein were designed using NCBI/Primer-BLAST. PCR reaction with *Salmonella* DNA (supernatant from washed cell culture heated in distilled water for 10 min at 95 °C) as a template and Taq polymerase (Plain PP Master Mix, Top Bio, Czech Republic) was carried out. PCR products were purified (MinElute PCR Purification Kit, Qiagen, Germany), then cloned into the pTrcHis-TOPO vector (Invitrogen, USA) and recombinant proteins were expressed in TOP10 One Shot chemically competent *E. coli* cells (Invitrogen, USA). IPTG was used as an inducer of the expression. Recombinant proteins with N-terminal His-Tag were isolated on HiTrap Chelating HP columns (GE Healthcare, UK) with attached nickel ions. Briefly, an overnight *E. coli* culture in LB broth (Invitrogen, USA) was centrifuged and washed in PBS (Dulbecco's, Lonza, Switzerland) and cells were disrupted by sonication (Sonopuls HD 3100, Bandelin, Germany). After centrifugation, supernatant with proteins was transferred to a binding buffer (0.02 M sodium phosphate, 0.5 M NaCl, 5 mM imidazole, pH 7.4) using desalting columns (PD-10, Sephadex G-25 M, GE Healthcare, UK). Metal-chelate affinity chromatography was performed on an FPLC system (Pharmacia, Sweden). After washing with a buffer containing an increased concentration of imidazole (40 mM), His-Tagged proteins were finally eluted with the elution buffer (0.02 M sodium phosphate, 0.5 M NaCl and 250 mM imidazole, pH 7.4).

If further purification was needed, we performed a preparative electrophoresis in a polyacrylamide gel (Model 491 Prep Cell, BioRad, USA) according to the manufacturer's protocol. For protein expression and purity verification, SDS-PAGE and western blot with a mouse anti-

Table 1 Primer pairs of DNA sequences for used proteins (or polypeptide fragments) and their expected molecular weight including HisTag

Protein	Forward primer 5'-3'	Reverse primer 5'-3'	Expected protein molecular weight
BamB	ATGCAATTGCGTAAATTACTTCTGCC	TTAACGCGTAATCGCGTAGACC	45.8 kDa
FliC-frag	ACGCTGAATGTGCAACAAAAATATAAGGTC	ACCTTCGGCTTTACTTGCAGCG	25.8 kDa
MetQ	ATGGCGTTCAAATTCAAAACCTTTGCGG	TTACCAGCCTTTCACCGCGCC	33.3 kDa
PrgI	ATGGCAACACCTTGGTCAGGCTATC	TTAACGGAAGTTCTGAATAATGGCAGCATC	12.7 kDa
SipC	ATGTTAATTAGTAATGTGGGAATAAATCCCGCC	TTAAGCGCGAATATTGCCTGCGAT	46.8 kDa
SipD	ATGCTTAATATTCAAAATTATTCCGCT	TTATCCTTGCAGGAAGCTTTT	41.0 kDa
SseB	ATGTCTTCAGGAAACATCTTATGGGGAA	TCATGAGTACGTTTTCTGCGCTATC	25.4 kDa
SurA	ATGAAGAACTGGAAAACGCTGCTTC	TTAGTTACTCAAAATCTTAACGTAAGCGCTG	51.1 kDa
SipB	ATGGTAAATGACGCAAGTAGCATTAGCCG	TTATGCGCGACTCTGGCGCAGAATAAAAC	66.3 kDa
OppA	ATGTCTAACATCACGAAAAAAAGTTTG	TTAATGTTTGATAATATATAAGTTTTTCACATAAAT	65.1 kDa

HisTag antibody (Pierce, Thermo Scientific, USA) was used.

Western blot

Purified recombinant proteins were resolved on a 10 % SDS-PAGE gel and transferred to PVDF membranes (Amersham, GE Healthcare, UK), which were subsequently blocked in 1 % casein hydrolysate (Imuna, Czech Republic) overnight at 4 °C. The membranes were incubated with 100× diluted porcine sera for one hour at room temperature (RT), washed in PBS with 0.05 % Tween-20 (PBS/T, Serva, Germany) and then incubated (one hour, RT) with goat anti-pig IgG conjugated with HRP (Bethyl Laboratories, USA). After a washing step, the protein bands were visualized with diaminobenzidine (Sigma-Aldrich, USA). Western blots were performed with group-specific pooled sera samples.

ELISA assay

Purified recombinant proteins in 0.05 M sodium carbonate-bicarbonate buffer (pH 9.6) were coated (4 °C overnight) on microtiter plates (MaxiSorp, Nunc, Denmark) that were blocked afterwards with 1 % casein hydrolysate in PBS/T (30 min). The plates were subsequently incubated (one hour, RT) with 100× diluted porcine sera, washed with PBS/T and then incubated (one hour, RT) with goat anti-pig IgG conjugated with HRP (Bethyl Laboratories, USA). After a washing step, the colour was developed by adding the chromogenic substrate TMB Complete (Test-line, Czech Republic) and the reaction was stopped with 2 M sulfuric acid (Penta, Czech Republic). The absorbance was measured at 450 nm on Synergy H1 (Biotek, USA). IgG antibody response to LPS was determined by commercially available Pig Screen ELISA (Qiagen, Germany). The individual serum samples were tested in duplicate by ELISA. Positive thresholds in time course graphs were counted as an average plus three standard deviations of all control samples and time zero samples of respective groups [11]. Positive thresholds for LPS commercial kit were provided by a manufacturer.

Statistical evaluation

Densities of western blot bands were calculated using ImageJ software (ver. 1.48). Differences between groups in ELISA assays were evaluated by ANOVA with Dunn's post test using GraphPad Prism (ver. 5). All graphs were also made using GraphPad Prism software (GraphPad Software, USA).

Results

Protein expression profiles in different media

At first, we examined protein expression profiles of *Salmonella* growing in different cultivation media. LB broth was used as a standard growth medium for cultivation of bacteria. For comparison, brain heart infusion (BHI), a highly nutritious medium was used as a vaccine preparation medium when the vaccine was proved to be protective [9]. From the whole-proteome mass spectrometry analysis, we observed the differences in LB and BHI cultures in relative quantities of several proteins that belong to the SPI-1 and SPI-2 loci which are important for the virulence of *Salmonella.* Relative quantification was attained using spectral counting and, in Tab. 2, it is shown as PSMs (peptide spectrum matches) for all peptides which identify the protein. Since PSMs depend on the length of a protein, the comparison of PSM value for the same protein between each medium is more informative rather than the absolute number. Note that the shown proteins are only representatives of the SPI-1 and SPI-2 loci and not the complete list.

All selected SPI-1 proteins were expressed in much higher amounts in LB medium than in BHI medium while proteins belonging to the SPI-2 locus were not highly expressed in either of the media. Flagellar proteins that also play an important role in the first stages

Table 2 Several selected proteins belonging to SPI-1 and/or SPI-2 locus and their relative amounts produced by *S.* Typhimurium grown in LB and BHI medium, respectively

Locus	Protein	Accession number	PSMs	
			LB	BHI
SPI-1	SipA	P0CL52	37	2
SPI-1	SipB	Q56019	31	4
SPI-1	SipC	P0CL47	50	3
SPI-1	SipD	Q56026	10	0
SPI-1	PrgI	P41784	5	2
SPI-1	SptP	P74873	20	0
SPI-1	SopA	Q8ZNR3	16	5
SPI-1	SopB	O30916	38	0
SPI-1	SopE2	Q7CQD4	5	0
SPI-1 and-2	SteA	Q8ZPD7	0	0
SPI-1 and-2	SopD	P40722	5	0
SPI-2	SopD2	Q8ZQC8	3	0
SPI-2	SseB	Q7BVH7	0	3
SPI-2	PipB	Q8ZQ59	0	1
SPI-2	PipB2	Q8ZMM8	4	0
flagellar proteins	FliC	P06179	132	77
	FljB	P52616	107	61
reference proteins	PepN	Q8ZQ76	48	39
	GapA	P0A1P0	185	279

of an invasion were expressed in both media in high amounts. Proteins PepN (Aminopeptidase N) and GapA (Glyceraldehyde-3-phosphate dehydrogenase A) are mentioned only as reference proteins.

Mass spectrometry analysis of immunoaffinity chromatography samples

Salmonella protein lysates preparations and consecutive immunoaffinity chromatography analyses resulted in three sets of samples for MS identification (*Salmonella* proteins bound to antibodies from control, infected or vaccinated animals). While most of the proteins were identified in all three samples in similar proportion, we found several proteins that were identified in relatively higher amounts in "post-infection" or "post-vaccination" fraction (Tab. 3). Relative amounts are shown as peptide spectrum matches (PSMs). Proteins SipB and SipC from SPI-1 were found in eluates from the column with post-infection sera while several proteins (OppA, BamB and SurA) were predominantly bound to antibodies in post-vaccination sera. We also included the identification of proteins that were chosen for their involvement in the infection process (SipD, SseB, PrgI and FliC) rather than from immunoaffinity chromatography/MS analysis only.

Recombinant protein preparation

All proteins listed in Table 3 were prepared as recombinant proteins in an *E. coli* expression system. The sequences of all proteins containing signal peptides at their N-termini were designed without this peptide. Otherwise, they possessed an identical sequence as naturally occurring in *S.* Typhimurium except FliC protein. Due to an inability of full-length protein expression, flagellar protein FliC was expressed only as a 22 kDa fragment. The expression of proteins was endorsed by SDS-PAGE and confirmed by western blot with an anti-HisTag antibody (Fig. 1 and Additional file 1: Figure S1). Four out of ten selected proteins (MetQ, SurA, PrgI, SipC) were not expressed in sufficient amount or purity and were not included in subsequent serological testing.

Serological testing

Western blot

Purified recombinant proteins were then used as antigens for serological analysis. After western blot, PVDF membranes were incubated with pooled serum samples from three animals of each group (control, infected and vaccinated animals). As shown in Fig. 2, proteins SipB, SipD and SseB presumed to be "post-infection" antigens were detected by sera of infected animals with a higher intensity than by sera of control or vaccinated animals. On the other hand, proteins BamB, FliC-frag and OppA, supposed to be "post-vaccination" antigens, were detected by sera of vaccinated pigs with a higher intensity than by sera of control or infected animals. Anti-HisTag antibody was used as a positive control for recombinant protein presence (in Fig. 2D).

ELISA assay

Based on western blot results, proteins SipB and FliC-frag were selected for testing specific antibody response of individual animals by ELISA method. Serum samples from 12 animals in each group were used for measuring antibody levels against recombinant SipB and FliC-frag proteins.

Antibody levels against SipB protein in sera of control animals had the values of absorbance between 0.062 and 0.126; sera of vaccinated animals had the values of absorbance between 0.075 and 0.147. The difference in absorbance between these two groups was not statistically significant. Sera of infected pigs had the values of absorbance between 0.248 and 1.056. These values were significantly different ($P < 0.01$) from the two previous groups of animals.

Antibody levels against FliC-frag proteins in sera of control animals had the values of absorbance between 0.018 and 0.271; sera of infected animals had the values of absorbance between 0.060 and 0.891. The difference in absorbance between these two groups was not statistically

Table 3 Identification and relative quantification of chosen proteins in terms of Peptide Spectrum Matches for all three runs

Protein name	Accession number	PSMs (peptide spectrum matches)		
		Control	Post-infection	Post-vaccination
Cell invasion protein SipB	Q56019	3, 0, 22	29, 20, 27	13, 7, 25
Cell invasion protein SipC	P0CL47	5, 1, 22	30, 33, 31	7, 18, 26
D-methionine-binding lipoprotein MetQ	Q8ZRN1	3, 1, 0	12, 5, 11	0, 0, 9
Periplasmic oligopeptide-binding protein OppA	P06202	7, 0, 0	31, 0, 0	25, 16, 14
Outer membrane protein assembly factor BamB	H9L451	0, 2, 0	0, 0, 7	7, 10, 0
Chaperone SurA	Q7CR87	1, 5, 1	2, 0, 21	21, 15, 15
Cell invasion protein SipD	Q56026	7, 3, 0	4, 15, 0	4, 14, 1
Secreted effector protein SseB	Q7BVH7	0, 0, 0	2, 0, 0	1, 0, 1
Protein PrgI	P41784	0, 2, 0	1, 2, 0	2, 0, 1
Flagellin FliC	P06179	3, 22, 17	23, 29, 26	19, 17, 63

significant. Sera of vaccinated pigs had the values of absorbance between 1.727 and 2.159. These values were significantly different (P <0.01) from two previous groups of animals (Fig. 3). Hence, proteins SipB and FliC-frag may serve as marker proteins applicable for serological discrimination between vaccinated pigs, pigs after natural infection and pigs without any contact with *S.* Typhimurium.

When compared to a non-infected group, from graphs showing the time course of antibody response (Fig. 4) we

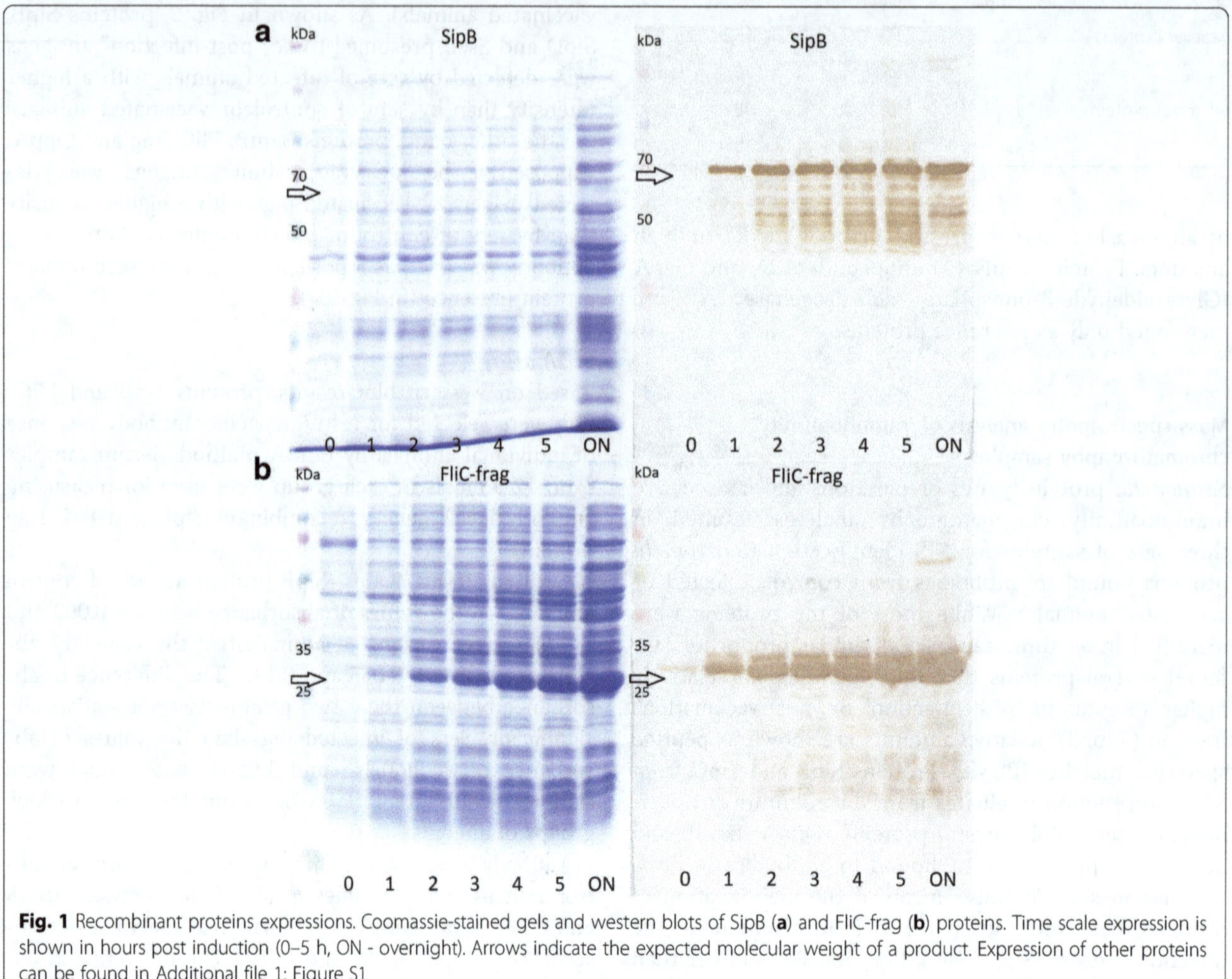

Fig. 1 Recombinant proteins expressions. Coomassie-stained gels and western blots of SipB (**a**) and FliC-frag (**b**) proteins. Time scale expression is shown in hours post induction (0–5 h, ON - overnight). Arrows indicate the expected molecular weight of a product. Expression of other proteins can be found in Additional file 1: Figure S1

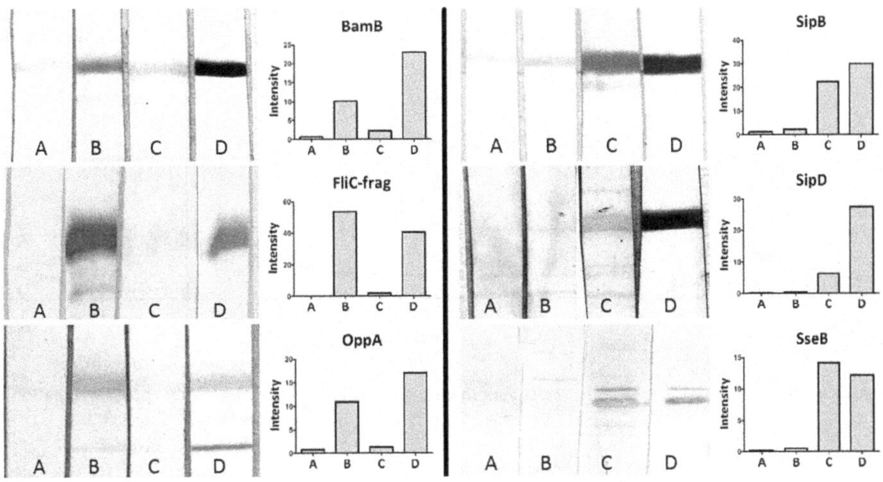

Fig. 2 Western blots of recombinant proteins with sera. Western blots with respective density graphs of purified recombinant proteins with **A** – control sera, **B** – post-vaccination sera, **C** – post-infection sera, and **D** – with anti-HisTag Ab

can see the increase of anti-SipB IgG level from the third week of infection but not significant differences for anti-FliC antibodies throughout the infection experiment (Fig. 4a, b). In contrary, the vaccination does not induce anti-SipB antibody production but anti-FliC IgGs are detectable after 14 days that is the time of revaccination (Fig. 4d, e). For comparison, we measured the level of post-infection and post-vaccination antibodies against O-antigens - the outer segments of surface lipopolysaccharides using commercially available ELISA kit (Fig. 4c, f). As expected, we found a similar pattern of immunoglobulin G production in both, infected and vaccinated groups. Additionally, a concentration of IgM antibodies against SipB protein did not exceed positive threshold after the infection. Anti-LPS IgMs were detectable on day 7 and 14 in two and four pigs respectively (see Additional file 1: Figure S2).

Discussion

Although the vaccination of animals against bacterial pathogens helps to moderate the severity of infection and is widely used in veterinary medicine, there are several issues that have to be solved during the development process and before introducing such vaccines to the market. Besides the induction of humoral and cellular immunity - the protectivity itself, in many cases, we must ensure a proper distinction between animals after the natural infection and vaccinated animals – i.e. DIVA vaccines [12]. We believe that using a vaccine with differentiability of infected and vaccinated animals enable establishment of *Salmonella* control programs in pig herds. This goal is currently not possible using the only licensed live attenuated vaccine [7]. In a case of *Salmonella* DIVA vaccines, several groups followed the path of a negative marker vaccine [7, 8], which uses a vaccine strain with a deleted gene for an antigenic protein. Host antibodies against this protein are thus found only in naturally infected animals and are absent in vaccinated animals. However, using live attenuated genetically modified *Salmonella* vaccine strains in pig herds is not straightforward. We proved inactivated *Salmonella* vaccine efficiently protects suckling piglets against infection [9] and further developed a DIVA method whereby there is no need for using a live genetically modified organism as an antigen for a vaccine. To develop DIVA assay, we decided to use a novel approach

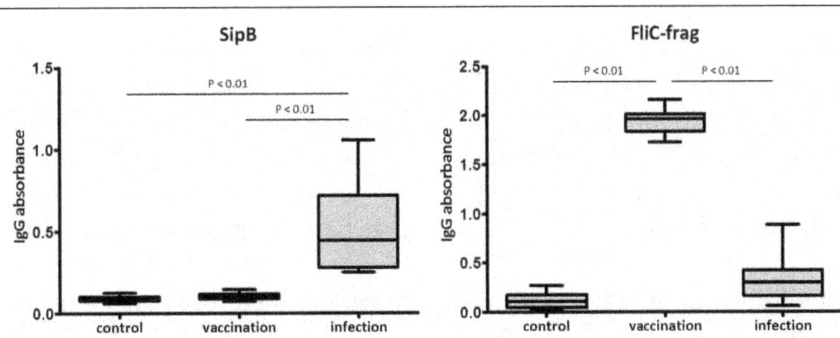

Fig. 3 ELISA assay of recombinant proteins. Graphs of IgG absorbance from ELISA assays of two recombinant proteins incubated with individual sera of control animals ($N = 12$), STM infected animals ($N = 12$) and animals after vaccination with STM-based vaccine ($N = 12$)

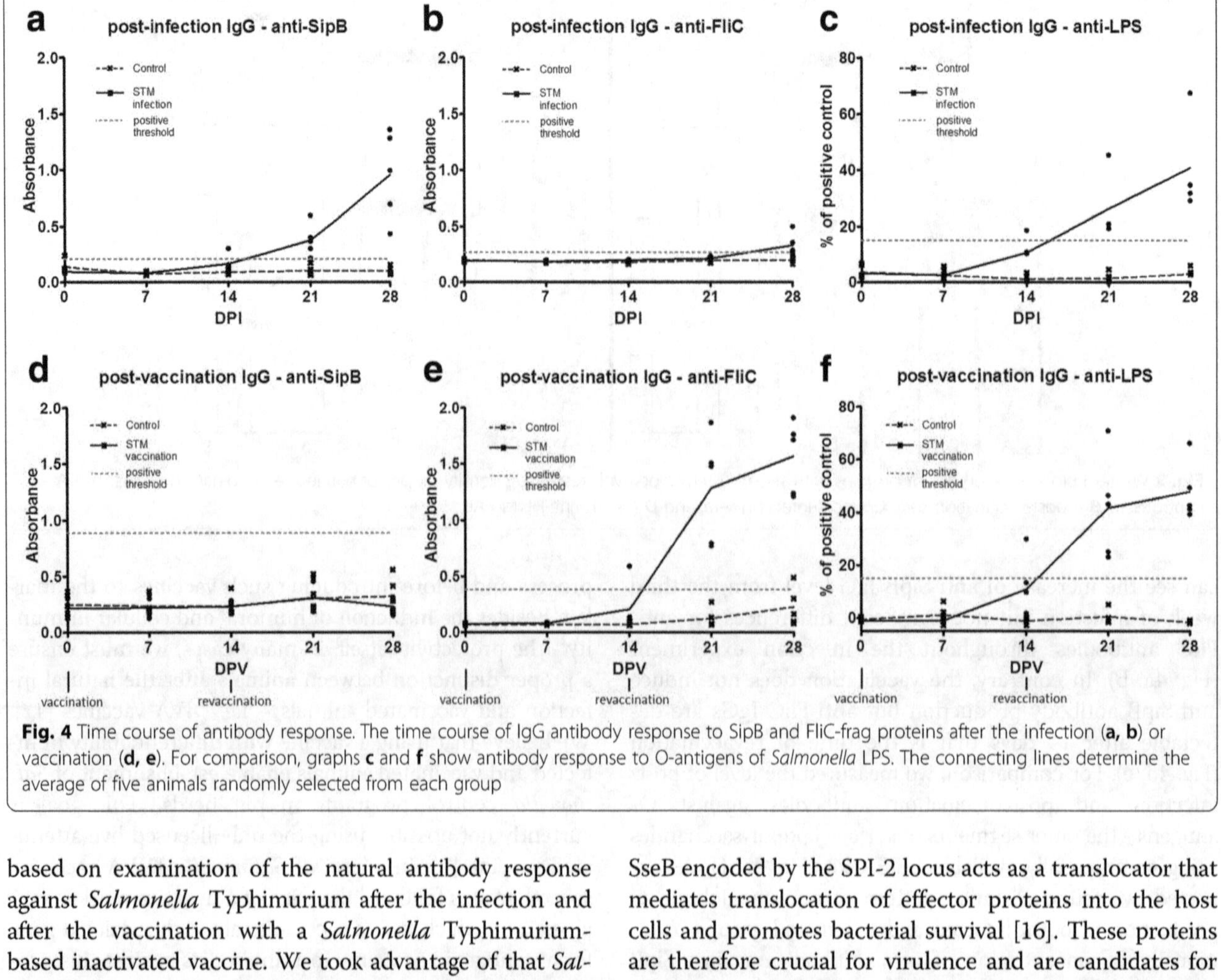

Fig. 4 Time course of antibody response. The time course of IgG antibody response to SipB and FliC-frag proteins after the infection (**a, b**) or vaccination (**d, e**). For comparison, graphs **c** and **f** show antibody response to O-antigens of *Salmonella* LPS. The connecting lines determine the average of five animals randomly selected from each group

based on examination of the natural antibody response against *Salmonella* Typhimurium after the infection and after the vaccination with a *Salmonella* Typhimurium-based inactivated vaccine. We took advantage of that *Salmonella* Typhimurium undergoes several different stages during the infection according to its localization and to the host immune response. Following these conditions, bacteria change the expression of virulence and protecting proteins [13, 14] that are subsequently exposed to the immune system.

Besides proven protectivity of the used vaccine in suckling piglets [9], we found that antibodies produced after the infection, are indeed different from those after the vaccination. From the immunoaffinity chromatography and mass spectrometry, we selected the following candidate proteins – SipB, SipC, MetQ, OppA, Bam and SurA. Then, we added some proteins that were not determined by the aforementioned method, but are known to be involved in the infection process as they belong to the SPI-1 or SPI-2 locus – SipD, SseB and PrgI and a highly immunogenic flagellar protein FliC.

Proteins SipB, SipC and SipD are representatives of the SPI-1 system which is responsible for invading the host cells. It is well established that these proteins form a tip of a needle structure of the type III secretion system complex that interacts with the eukaryotic cells [13, 15]. Protein SseB encoded by the SPI-2 locus acts as a translocator that mediates translocation of effector proteins into the host cells and promotes bacterial survival [16]. These proteins are therefore crucial for virulence and are candidates for inducing the antibody response that was also confirmed in this work. On the other hand, when *Salmonella* Typhimurium was cultivated *in vitro* in BHI culture medium as a vaccine batch, these proteins were not expressed in amounts able to induce antibody production. SPI-1 proteins were nevertheless found in high amounts when *Salmonella* had grown in LB medium. This medium is therefore not applicable for a vaccine batch preparation because it could induce production of the same antibodies as after a natural infection. Nutrient-limiting conditions provided by LB broth partially resemble *in vivo* environment and trigger SPI-1 proteins expression, while rich BHI medium does not induce production of *Salmonella* virulence factors. Jaradat and Bhunia [17] suggested a similar explanation as gained from their results in different growth conditions of *Listeria monocytogenes,* stating that bacteria produce more virulence factors in a nutritionally poor milieu in order to adapt to the new environment. On the other hand, bacterial virulence factors seem to be good candidates for antibody response induction and therefore for the vaccine protectivity in general. However, we showed that the efficacy of our vaccine prepared from a culture grown in a medium not inducing the expression of SPI proteins is high [9].

In spite of the fact that flagellin has powerful immunostimulatory properties and may play a role as a potent adjuvant in a variety of anti-bacterial vaccines [18–20], it was also shown that expression of flagellar proteins is selectively repressed when *Salmonella* is located intracellularly during the infection [21, 22]. The flagellum as an extracellular structure on the surface of a bacterium could be a good candidate as a post-vaccination antigen if an appropriate growth medium capable of promoting the expression of flagellar proteins is used. This was proved for FliC protein fragment by western-blot and ELISA but interestingly not by PSM spectra of immunoaffinity eluates. We speculate this was caused by overall high amount of anti-FliC antibodies in all samples and the capacity of immunoaffinity columns was probably saturated. Only western-blot and ELISA were able to show much higher anti-FliC antibody level in post-vaccination sera than in post-infection and control sera. PSM for FliC in control sample was probably caused by cross-reactivity of anti-flagellar antibodies induced by other bacteria in control animals. The other possible explanation is very high expression of FliC protein in cultures and possible unspecific binding in the chromatography column. Proteins BamB (Outer membrane protein assembly factor) and OppA (Periplasmic oligopeptide-binding protein) are located on the outer membrane and the periplasm, respectively, which makes them easy targets for the immune system. Although both proteins are involved in transmembrane transport (OppA as a permease [23] and BamB as a part of the outer membrane protein assembly complex involved in insertion of beta-barrel proteins [24]), their role in the infection is not known. Interestingly, both proteins are much less immunogenic during infection than after vaccination. This finding makes them together with FliC good candidates for serological differentiation between infected and vaccinated animals.

After successful isolation of recombinant proteins, we tested them using western blot and ELISA with post-infection, post-vaccination and control serum samples to prove their ability to distinguish between infected and vaccinated animals. Proteins SseB, SipB and SipD were confirmed to be highly immunogenic during the infection. This is in agreement with previous findings [25, 26]. The level of antibodies against these proteins, measured as a density of bands on western blots, was, at least, ten times higher in a group of infected animals than in a group of control or vaccinated animals. On the other hand, proteins BamB, OppA and FliC-frag were confirmed to be highly immunogenic during the vaccination of pigs. The level of antibodies against these proteins was, at least, ten times higher in a group of vaccinated animals than in a group of control or infected animals. As in the case of FliC, there is a partial discrepancy with immunoaffinity chromatography results in the case of SseB protein when it showed a similar level of binding to post-infection and post-vaccination antibodies. However, it can be explained by low expression of SseB in cultivation media and thus possible incomplete saturation of all specific antibodies present in the chromatography column.

Finally, proteins SipB and FliC-frag were selected for ELISA assays to examine the interaction with 36 porcine serum samples. All 12 post-infection sera exhibited higher absorbance with the SipB protein than 12 control and 12 post-vaccination sera. In contrast, all 12 post-vaccination sera exhibited higher absorbance with the FliC-frag protein than 12 control and 12 post-infection sera. All differences were statistically significant ($P < 0.01$). The time-dependent onset of IgG antibody levels against SipB after the infection, and against FliC after the vaccination imitates the increase of IgG against surface lipopolysaccharide. These two proteins are thus considered as useful antigens for serological differentiation of infected and vaccinated animals.

In general, induction of different protein expression profiles, their potential exposure to the immune recognition machinery and subsequent specific antibody production can be conveniently applied for the differentiation between infected and vaccinated animals without any intervention into the genome of an organism used as a vaccine strain.

Conclusions

Using antibodies from previously vaccinated and infected animals and using immunoaffinity chromatography and mass spectrometry tools, we identified *Salmonella* proteins that induce post-infection and post-vaccination specific antibody production. Gene cloning and recombinant protein expression techniques were used for antigen preparation that allows serological distinction between infected animals and animals vaccinated with a *Salmonella*-based inactivated vaccine.

This approach can be utilized in many other challenges where DIVA vaccine and a subsequent serological assay are required, especially when genetic modification of a vaccine strain is not desirable.

Additional files

Additional file 1: Figure S1. Recombinant proteins expressions. Coomassie-stained gels and western blots of recombinant proteins. Time scale expression is shown in hours post induction (0–5 h, ON - overnight). Arrows indicate the expected molecular weight of a product. **Figure S2.** IgM antibody response. The time course of IgM antibody response to SipB protein and to *Salmonella* LPS after the infection. The connecting lines determine the average of five animals randomly selected from each group. (PDF 434 kb)

Additional file 2: Identified *Salmonella* proteins from different media. Mass spectrometry identification of *Salmonella* proteins and a comparison of expression between two cultivation media (LB vs BHI). (XLSX 433 kb)

Additional file 3: Identified proteins from immunoaffinity chromatography. Mass spectrometry identification of *Salmonella* proteins bound to control, post-infection or post-vaccination serum. Immunoaffinity chromatography was made in triplicates. (XLSX 913 kb)

Abbreviations
BHI: Brain-heart infusion; CFU: Colony-forming unit; DIVA: Differentiation of infected and vaccinated animals; FASP: Filter-aided sample preparation; FPLC: Fast protein liquid chromatography; HRP: Horseradish peroxidase; LB: Lysogeny broth; LPS: Lipopolysaccharide; MS: Mass spectrometry; PSM: Peptide spectrum match; PVDF: Polyvinylidene difluoride; SPI: *Salmonella* pathogenicity island; TMB: 3,3′,5,5′-tetramethylbenzidine; uHPLC: Ultra-high pressure liquid chromatography

Acknowledgments
The authors wish to thank Dr. Ludmila Faldikova for correcting and proofreading of the manuscript.

Funding
This study was supported by the Ministry of Agriculture of the Czech Republic (QJ1210115, RO0516) and the Ministry of Education, Youth and Sports of the Czech Republic (LO1218 from the MEYS of the CR under the NPU I program).

Authors' contributions
JG carried out immunoaffinity chromatography, mass spectrometry, and the cloning and wrote the first and the final draft of the manuscript. HK performed all ELISA assays including their validation. MK contributed to culture media testing and in vaccination design. KK designed the serological assays. RT did the isolation and the purification of recombinant proteins. AO participated in the experimental infection and vaccination and sample collection. MF helped to design the animal experiments, obtained financial support and took part in the revising of the manuscript. JM was responsible for the whole project, generated the working hypothesis, designed the experiments, obtained financial support, revised the draft and wrote the final version of the manuscript. All authors read and approved the final manuscript.

Competing interests
Using SseB, Gene ID: 1252916; SipB, Gene ID: 1254408; SipD, Gene ID: 1254406; FliC, Gene ID: 1253480 and BamB, Gene ID: 1254042 proteins in serological methods differentiating infected and vaccinated pigs is covered by Czech patent number 305077. Except of Martin Faldyna, all authors are holders of 305077 patent rights. Marcel Kosina is an employee of Bioveta company which potentially may have a commercial benefit from results of this work. The authors declare that they have no competing interests.

Consent for publication
Not applicable

Author details
[1]Department of Immunology, Veterinary Research Institute, Hudcova296/70, 62100 Brno, Czech Republic. [2]Department of Experimental Biology, Faculty of Science, Masaryk University, Kotlarska267/2, 611 37 Brno, Czech Republic. [3]Bioveta a. s., Komenskeho212/12, 683 23 Ivanovice na Hane, Czech Republic. [4]Department of Virology, Veterinary Research Institute, Hudcova296/70, 62100 Brno, Czech Republic. [5]Faculty of Veterinary Medicine, University of Veterinary and Pharmaceutical Sciences, Palackeho 1/3, 612 42 Brno, Czech Republic.

References

1. Anonymous. Analysis of the baseline survey on the prevalence of Salmonella in holdings with breeding pigs in the EU, 2008 – Part A: Salmonella prevalence estimates. EFSA J. 2009;7:1377.
2. van Oirschot JT. Diva vaccines that reduce virus transmission. J Biotechnol. 1999;73(I2–3):195–205.
3. Vico JP, Engel B, Buist WG, Mainar-Jaime RC. Evaluation of three commercial enzyme-linked immunosorbent assays for the detection of antibodies against Salmonella spp. in meat juice from finishing pigs in Spain. Zoonoses Public Health. 2010;57 Suppl 1:107–14.
4. Leyman B, Boyen F, Van Parys A, Verbrugghe E, Haesebrouck F, Pasmans F. Salmonella Typhimurium LPS mutations for use in vaccines allowing differentiation of infected and vaccinated pigs. Vaccine. 2011;29(20):3679–85.
5. Zariri A, van der Ley P. Biosynthetically engineered lipopolysaccharide as vaccine adjuvant. Expert Rev Vaccines. 2015;14(6):861–76.
6. Arenas J. The Role of Bacterial Lipopolysaccharides as Immune Modulator in Vaccine and Drug Development. Endocr Metab Immune Disord Drug Targets. 2012;12(3):221–35.
7. Selke M, Meens J, Springer S, Frank R, Gerlach GF. Immunization of pigs to prevent disease in humans: construction and protective efficacy of a Salmonella enterica serovar Typhimurium live negative-marker vaccine. Infect Immun. 2007;75(5):2476–83.
8. Bearson BL, Bearson SMD, Kich JD. A DIVA vaccine for cross-protection against Salmonella. Vaccine. 2016;34(10):1241–6.
9. Matiasovic J, Kudlackova H, Babickova K, Stepanova H, Volf J, Rychlik I, Babak V, Faldyna M. Impact of maternally-derived antibodies against Salmonella enterica serovar Typhimurium on the bacterial load in suckling piglets. Vet J. 2013;196(1):114–5.
10. Wiśniewski JR, Zougman A, Nagaraj N, Mann M. Universal sample preparation method for proteome analysis. Nat Methods. 2009;6(5):359–62.
11. Jacobson RH. Factors in selecting serum samples for use in determining the positive/negative threshold (cut-off) in ELISA. Diagnosis and Epidemiology of Animal Disease in Latin America 1998. IAEA-TECDOC-1055, pp. 25–28. http://www-pub.iaea.org/books/IAEABooks/5352/Diagnosis-and-Epidemiology-of-Animal-Diseases-in-Latin-America.
12. Pasick J. Application of DIVA vaccines and their companion diagnostic tests to foreign animal disease eradication. Anim Health Res Rev. 2004;5(2):257–62.
13. Mirold S, Ehrbar K, Weissmüller A, Prager R, Tschäpe H, Rüssmann H, Hardt WD. Salmonella host cell invasion emerged by acquisition of a mosaic of separate genetic elements, including Salmonella pathogenicity island 1 (SPI1), SPI5, and sopE2. J Bacteriol. 2001;183(7):2348–58.
14. McGhie EJ, Brawn LC, Hume PJ, Humphreys D, Koronakis V. Salmonella takes control: effector-driven manipulation of the host. Curr Opin Microbiol. 2009;12(1):117–24.
15. Marlovits TC, Stebbins CE. Type III secretion systems shape up as they ship out. Curr Opin Microbiol. 2010;13:47–52.
16. Waterman SR, Holden DW. Functions and effectors of the Salmonella pathogenicity island 2 type III secretion system. Cell Microbiol. 2003;5(8):501–11.
17. Jaradat ZW, Bhunia AK. Glucose and nutrient concentrations affect the expression of a 104-kilodalton Listeria adhesion protein in Listeria monocytogenes. Appl Environ Microbiol. 2002;68(10):4876–83.
18. Smith KD, Andersen-Nissen E, Hayashi F, Strobe K, Bergman MA, Rassoulian Barrett SL, Cookson BT, Aderem A. Toll-like receptor 5 recognizes a conserved site on flagellin required for protofilament formation and bacterial motility. Nat Immunol. 2003;4:1247–53.
19. das Gracas Luna M, Sardella FF, Ferreira LC. Salmonella flagellin fused with a linear epitope of colonization factor antigen I (CFA/I) can prime antibody responses against homologous and heterologous fimbriae of enterotoxigenic Escherichia coli. Res Micribiol. 2000;151:575–82.
20. Honko AN, Sriranganathan N, Lees CJ, Mizel SB. Flagellin is an effective adjuvant for immunization against lethal respiratory challenge with Yersinia pestits. Infect Immun. 2006;74:1113–20.

21. Cummings LA, Rassoulian Barrett SL, Wilkerson WD, Fellnerova I, Cookson BT. FliC-specific $CD4^+$ T cell responses are restricted by bacterial regulation of antigen expression. J Immunol. 2005;174(12):7929–38.
22. Lai MA, Quarles EK, López-Yglesias AH, Zhao X, Hajjar AM, Smith KD. Innate immune detection of flagellin positively and negatively regulates Salmonella infection. PLoS One. 2013;8(8):e72047.
23. Hiles ID, Gallagher MP, Jamieson DJ, Higgins CF. Molecular characterization of the oligopeptide permease of Salmonella typhimurium. J Mol Biol. 1987; 195(I1):125–42.
24. Hagan CL, Silhavy TJ, Kahne D. β-Barrel Membrane Protein Assembly by the Bam Complex. Annu Rev Biochem. 2011;80:189–210.
25. Lee S-J, Liang L, Juarez S, Nanton MR, Gondwe EN, Msefula CL, Kayala MA, Necchi F, Heath JN, Hart P, Tsolis RM, Heyderman RS, Mac Lennan CA, Felgner PL, Davies DH, McSorley SJ. Identification of a common immune signature in murine and human systemic Salmonellosis. Proc Natl Acad Sci. 2012;109(13):4998–5003.
26. Desin TS, Mickael CS, Lam PK, Potter AA, Köster W. Protection of epithelial cells from Salmonella enterica serovar Enteritidis invasion by antibodies against the SPI-1 type III secretion system. Can J Microbiol. 2010;56(6):522–6.

4

Sero-prevalence of virus neutralizing antibodies for rabies in different groups of dogs following vaccination

R.M.S. Pimburage[1*], M. Gunatilake[2], O. Wimalaratne[3], A. Balasuriya[4] and K.A.D.N. Perera[3]

Abstract

Background: Mass vaccination of dogs is considered fundamental for national rabies control programmes in Sri Lanka, as dog is the main reservoir and transmitter of the disease.

Methods: Dogs were followed to determine the sero-prevalence of antibodies to the rabies virus. Altogether 510 previously vaccinated and unvaccinated dogs with owners (domestic dogs) and dogs without owners (stray dogs) of the local guard dog breed in different age groups recruited from Kalutara District, Sri Lanka. The dogs were vaccinated with a monovalent inactivated vaccine intramuscularly and serum antibody titres on days 0, 30, 180 and 360 were determined by the Rapid Fluorescent Focus Inhibition Test (RFFIT).

Results: The results indicated, a single dose of anti-rabies vaccination fails to generate a protective level of immunity (0.5 IU/ml) which lasts until 1 year in 40.42% of dogs without owners and 57.14% of previously unvaccinated juvenile (age: 3 months to 1 year) dogs with owners. More than one vaccination would help to maintain antibody titres above the protective level in the majority of dogs. The pattern of antibody titre development in annually vaccinated and irregularly vaccinated (not annual) adult dogs with owners is closely similar irrespective of regularity in vaccination. Previously vaccinated animals have higher (2 IU/ml) antibody titres to begin with and have a higher antibody titre on day 360 too. They show a very good antibody titre by day 180. Unvaccinated animals start with low antibody titre and return to low titres by day 360, but have a satisfactory antibody titre by day 180.

Conclusions: A single dose of anti-rabies vaccination is not sufficient for the maintenance of antibody titres for a period of 1 year in puppies, juvenile dogs with owners and in dogs without owners. Maternal antibodies do not provide adequate protection to puppies of previously vaccinated dams and puppies of previously unvaccinated dams. Immunity development after vaccination seems to be closely similar in both the groups of puppies.

Keywords: Antibody, Anti-rabies vaccine, Dogs, RFFIT, Sero-prevalence, Titre

Background

Rabies is a vaccine preventable, zoonotic disease [1]. Still it remains as a serious public health problem all over the world [2]. It is commonly transmitted to other animals and humans through close contact with saliva from infected animals [3]. It is estimated that 60,000 human rabies-related deaths occur worldwide each year [1, 4, 5].

Sri Lanka has invested a large amount of money to control dog rabies. Human deaths due to rabies were further decreased from 56 (2.8 per 1,000,000) in 2007 to 19 (0.05 per 1,000,000) in 2014. This was the lowest incidence reported in Sri Lanka. This reduction was mainly because of mass vaccination of dogs against rabies, mass Animal Birth Control (ABC) programmes, Post Exposure Prophylaxis (PEP) for rabid and rabies suspected animal bites and mass awareness programmes [6, 7]. Being an island once rabies is completely eradicated from Sri Lanka it should be easier to prevent re-introduction of rabies from other countries [7, 8].

The mass vaccination of dogs is considered fundamental in rabies control programmes in many countries including Sri Lanka [7, 9]. The total number of animal rabies cases

* Correspondence: ruwinipimburage@gmail.com
[1]Ministry of Health, No.555/5, Elvitigala Mawatha, Colombo 05, Sri Lanka
Full list of author information is available at the end of the article

reported during the 2014 was 746. The majority 81.7% (610) of the animal rabies were dogs. Nearly 50% of the total dog population in the country are vaccinated annually [10]. A strong body of theoretical and empirical evidence indicates that vaccinating 70% of the dog population during annual campaigns should be sufficient to control rabies [11, 12].

According to the vaccine schedule practice in Sri Lanka dogs are vaccinated against rabies at the age of 3 months if the dam is previously vaccinated. If dam is unvaccinated, the 1st vaccine is given to the pup at the age of 6 weeks with a booster at the age of 3 months and subsequently with annual boosters. The study carried out by Gunatilake et al. [13] showed that antibodies transferred from the dam is well below the protective level in the puppies of vaccinated dams at the age of 3 months.

As the government has been investing large amount of money on the treatment of dog bite victims, it is important to determine the ideal time period for the 1st Anti-rabies Vaccination (ARV) for puppies and the level of antibody titres in dogs until the time of revaccination. Measurement of humoral immune response (virus neutralizing antibody titres) in vaccinated dogs is helpful in judging the protectiveness of vaccinated dogs [14]. In a sero-survey carried out in Garborone, Bostwana, it was shown that dogs that had more than one successive vaccination against rabies had better antibody titres than that had received only one vaccination [15]. Another study carried out in Thailand suggested that one dose of tissue culture vaccine in dogs is not adequate to maintain rabies neutralizing antibody titre in serum for 1 year [16].

It is important to know whether dogs in a representative population (specially Sri Lankan local breed) have antibody titres above the protective level (higher than 0.5 IU/ml on WHO recommendation) after the 1st vaccination and whether the antibody titres are maintained above the protective level until the time of annual revaccination [17].

This study was carried out to determine the pattern of immunogenicity and the suitable time for booster vaccination among different age groups of dogs without owner and owned dogs, in order to make recommendations regarding dog vaccination for rabies control in Sri Lanka.

Methods

Study design and sample recruitment

This study was carried out in Kalutara district, Sri Lanka. It has 11 MOH (Medical Officer of Health) areas and consists of multi cultural, rural and urban human population. Out of nearly 2000 temporary vaccination centers distributed in 11 MOH areas in the district 37 temporary vaccination centers were randomly selected for the study. In 2014 the average number of confirmed rabies cases in animals throughout the district was 7 per year. Out of 19 total human deaths reported in Srilanka in 2014, one death was in Kalutara district [7].

A total of 510 apparently healthy dogs with owners and without owners of the local breed were recruited based on pre-defined age groups and previous vaccination history (Fig. 1 and Table 1). Previously vaccinated groups contain dogs with at least one vaccination with ARV.

To recruit dogs with owners, a message was sent through dog handlers from house to house requesting them to bring their dogs for vaccination with the vaccination card as evidence for previous vaccination. Dogs were recruited after general clinical examination, that was carried out by a veterinarian. Pedigreed dogs, pregnant or sick animals (e.g. with anorexia, pallor, large wounds), dogs with a known allergy to rabies vaccine were excluded. Vaccination history of domestic animals was noted down from their previous vaccination records.

Some areas in Kalutara district, which were not covered by the government anti-rabies programme were selected for the recruitment of unvaccinated dogs without owners. Previously vaccinated dogs without owners were identified by the presence of tattooing mark and/or red dog collar with a confirmation from villagers from the areas covered by the anti-rabies programme. The dogs without owners were caught and restrained by specially trained skilled dog catchers. A special tattooing number and a photograph were used for easy identification of dogs without owners for the follow up.

Anti-rabies vaccine and vaccination

A monovalent chemically inactivated vaccine (Nobivac® Rabies) recommended by the WHO for rabies control programmes was used to vaccinate all groups of dogs [7, 18]. This imported vaccine contained >1.0 IU antigenic content per 1 ml dose and the virus was grown on the Baby Hamster Kidney-21 (BHK-21) connective tissue cell line. As recommended by the manufacturer a single dose (1 ml) of vaccine was injected intramuscularly on day 0 (D0). After vaccination, the dogs without owners were released to their territories.

Collection of blood samples

A venous blood sample (2–3 ml) was collected from the cephalic vein of each animal on day 0 (D0) before vaccination and on day 30 (D30), 180 (D180), 360 (D360) post vaccination. Samples were kept for 1 h at room temperature for separation of serum and transported in ice to the Medical Research Institute (MRI), Colombo. Serum was separated and stored at −70 °C until analyzed by Rapid Fluorescent Focus Inhibition Test (RFFIT) to determine the titres of virus neutralizing antibodies [19].

Analysis of antibody titres

The antibody titres were analyzed using the Rapid Fluorescent Focus Inhibition Test (RFFIT). Rapid Fluorescent Focus Inhibition Test (RFFIT) is a tissue

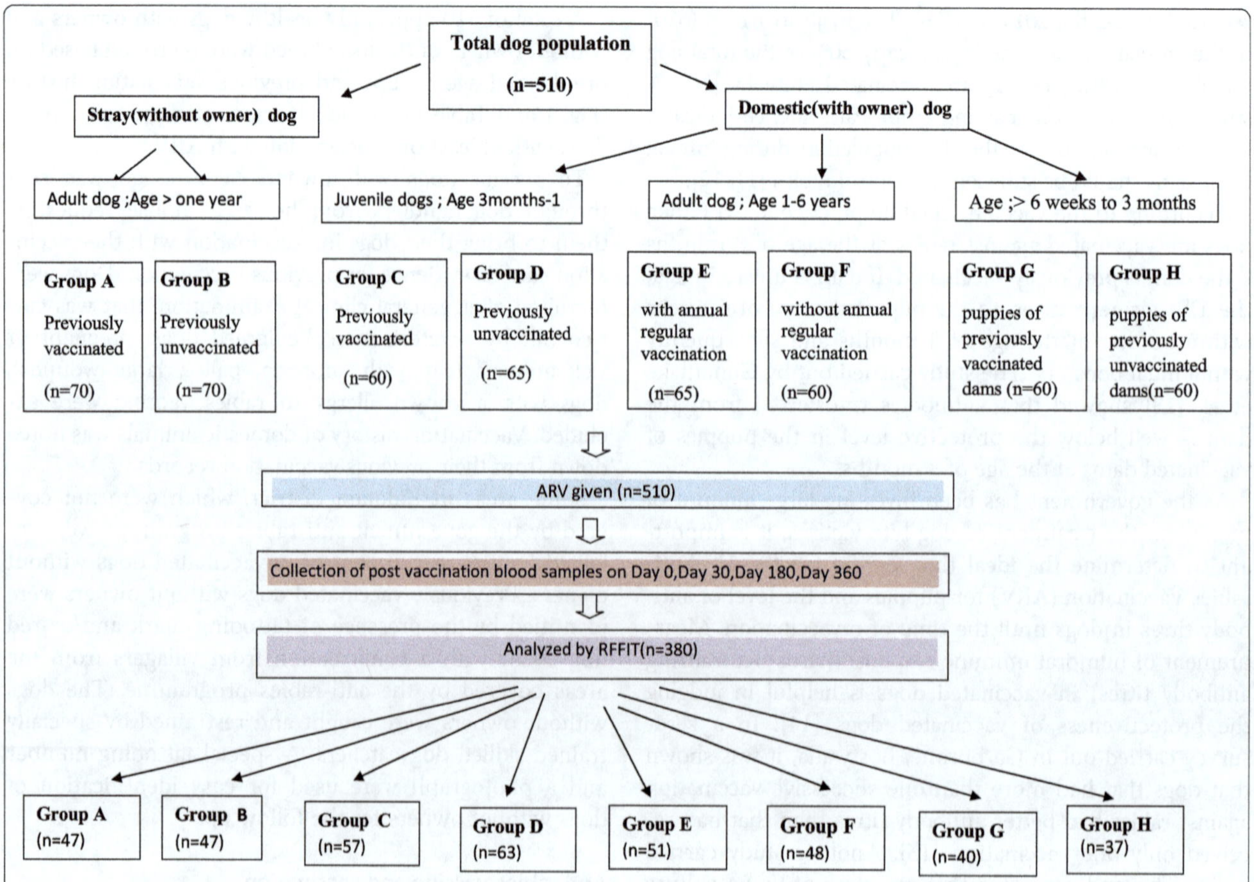

Fig. 1 Study Population

culture virus neutralization assay, which measures the level of protection against rabies in humans and animals and consider as the "Gold standard method". The assay measures the amount of antibodies present in serum that neutralizes and block rabies virus from infecting the cells [19]. Infected cells were then identified by fluorescent microscopy. The endpoint titer was calculated using Reed & Muench formula [20]. Serum of each animal was analyzed in the same run to minimize variation.

Statistical analysis

Antibody titres of dogs in different groups were presented as mean, median and inter quartile range (IQR). An antibody titer of 0.5 IU/ml was considered as the protective level [7, 8, 21] and the percentage of protected dogs in each category was calculated.

Difference between means in different groups according to age and vaccination status was calculated and compared. Multivariate analysis was applied to compare antibody titres and significance was considered at 0.05

Table 1 The groups included in the study under pre-defined criteria and the number of animals recruited for each group initially

Group		Age	Vaccination history against rabies	No. of Dogs recruited
A	Stray (dogs without owner)	> one year	With previous vaccination	70
B			Without previous vaccination	70
C	Domestic (dog with owners)	3 months –1 year	With previous vaccination	60
D			Without previous vaccination	65
E		>1to 6 years	With regular annual vaccination	65
F			Without regular annual vaccination	60
G		> 6 weeks to 3 months	Puppies of vaccinated dams	60
H			Puppies of unvaccinated dams	60
Total				510

level. Statistical analysis was done using a computer software package – SPSS version 10.

Results

Of the total recruited 510, 428 dogs were available in the follow up until D360 due to unavailability of recruited dogs. However 380 blood samples were available for analysis of antibody titres as some of the samples were haemolyzed.

The mean, 95% confidance intervals, median antibody titres, Inter Quartile Ranges (IQRs) are shown in Table 2. The comparision of protective levels (0.5 IU/ml) of rabies virus neutralization antibody titres of dogs in different age groups on D0, D30, D180 and D360 are shown in Tables 3, 4, 5 and 6. Comparison of median antibody titres of dogs in all groups is graphically presented in Fig. 2, with the removal of outliers. Median antibody titres of all groups with error bars is presented in Fig. 3.

Dogs in the previously vaccinated groups had higher (2 IU/ml) antibody levels to begin with and had a higher antibody level on day 360 than the unvaccinated groups. They showed a very good antibody level at day 180. Unvaccinated animals started with low antibody levels and returned to low levels by day 360, but had a satisfactory antibody level by day 180.

As per Table 2, the antibody titres in puppies of both vaccinated and unvaccinated dams were very low on day

Table 2 Comparison of mean, 95% confidence intervals, median, Inter Quartile Range in groups A to H

Group	Days	Mean	Median	Minimum	Maximum	IQR	% with protective titer
Group A (*n* = 47) Previously vaccinated Adult stray dogs	0	6.66 (4.05–9.92)	2 (1.32–8.74)	0.02	49.09	9.4	70.21
	30	51.85(35.90–71.27)	36.44 (13.74–49.05)	1.96	269.76	41.1	100
	180	22.89 (15.11–31.20)	10.53 (8.43–14.32)	0.4	100.4	31.17	100
	360	7.177 (4.25–10.88)	2 (1.62–4.01)	0.19	49.09	8.08	82.98
Group B (*n* = 47) Previously unvaccinated Adult stray dogs	0	0.13 (.08–.19)	0.65 (0.2–.08)	0.02	0.8	0.08	6.4
	30	12.61 (7.23–19.89)	4 (2.10–9.80)	0.02	102.6	11.68	87.24
	180	9.16 (4.74–15.29)	2.15 (1.78–5.48)	0.02	110.2	7.75	87.24
	360	3.89 (1.93)	0.67 (47–1.70)	0.02	50.24	1.85	59.82
Group C (*n* = 47) Previously vaccinated domestic juveniles	0	15.99 (8.06–26.10)	2.7 (1.63–6.78)	0.03	177.5	8.53	78.72
	30	34.77 (18.07–56.20)	10.74 (5.40–11.59)	0.03	269.79	25.11	95.74
	180	27.09 (13.40–45.05)	8.34 (2.90–13-84)	0.06	269.83	17.76	93.62
	360	21.59 (9.00–37.74)	2.90 (1.98–7.78)	0.08	229	8.31	78.72
Group D (*n* = 63) Previously unvaccinated domestic juveniles	0	0.11 (0.07–0.14)	0.06 (0.02–0.08)	0.02	0.8	0.07	1.59
	30	17.39 (11.34–24.13)	9.40 (4.07–10.74)	0.02	125	17.44	93.65
	180	11.21 (6.05–17.26)	2.50 (2.12–5.20)	0.02	124.02	6.34	93.65
	360	3.04 (1.53–4.71)	0.44 (0.28–0.52)	0.02	27.4	1.7	42.86
Group E (*n* = 51) Adult dogs with regular annual vaccination	0	13.62 (6.01–24-24)	29(.56–2.96)	0.03	214.63	7.28	76.47
	30	29.81 (14.55–46.80)	10.02 (2.50–11.04)	0.03	269.79	18.87	96
	180	39.47 (20.48–60.20)	10.50 (2.35–12.46)	0.06	269.83	18.03	88
	360	24.23 (11.11–40.90)	2.56 (2.19–8.93)	0.36	229	10.21	78
Group F (*n* = 48) Adult dogs without regular vaccination	0	6.84 (3.14–11.06)	0.93 (0.55–2.28)	0.03	51.41	5.6	77.08
	30	25.73 (15.20–40.34)	10.74 (4.30–19.54)	0.72	269.76	17.54	100
	180	16.95 (11.12–23.80)	9.41 (2.35–15.56)	0.06	96.5	17.85	95.84
	360	9.69 (5.91–13.97)	2.95 (2.07–8.93)	0.26	47.98	9.15	83.33
Group G (*n* = 40) Puppies of previously vaccinated dams	0	0.10 (0.07–0.14)	0.08 (0.08–0.08)	0.02	0.44	0.03	0
	30	10.66 (7.93–13.74)	9.80 (9.70–10.20)	0.4	49.09	6.3	97.5
	180	4.63 (3.16–6.46)	3.31 (2.00–5.35)	0.04	32.5	5.64	82.5
	360	0.23 (0.15–0.35)	0.09 (0.08–0.19)	0.04	1.8	0.32	7.5
Group H (*n* = 37) Puppies of previously unvaccinated dams	0	0.07 (0.06–0.09)	0.08 (0.04–0.08)	0.02	0.38	0.04	0
	30	12.56 (8.32–17.15)	8.50 (4.70–10.45)	0.08	51.45	9.75	94.59
	180	4.76 (3.00–6.80)	2.09 (0.59–5.40)	0.08	25.6	7.31	78.38
	360	0.32 (0.21–0.44)	0.19 (0.09–0.40)	0.04	1.5	0.36	10.81

Table 3 Comparison of protective levels and percentage of rabies virus neutralization antibody (different age groups A to B) titers in previously vaccinated and unvaccinated adult stray dogs

Day	Group A Stray (ownerless) dogs with previous vaccination history;Age > one year (n = 47)		Group B Stray (ownerless) dogs without previous vaccination history;Age > one year (n = 47)		*P* value
	No. with antibody titre ≥0.5 IU/ml	% with antibody titre ≥0.5 IU/ml	No. with antibody titre ≥0.5 IU/ml	% with antibody titre ≥0.5 IU/ml	
0	33	70.21	3	6.4	0.000*
30	47	100	41	87.23	0.026*
180	47	100	41	87.23	0.059
360	39	82.98	28	59.57	0.041*

*Indicates the significance level at 0.05 when groups A (Stray dogs with previous vaccination history) & B (Stray dogs without previous vaccination history) are compared

0. Irrespective of the presence of maternal antibodies, titres in puppies after the first vaccination, came only to very low levels by day 360. Data in group G (previously vaccinated dams) indicates that puppies in that group do not have protection by maternal antibodies until the time of primer vaccination.

Discussion

This is the first comparative study conducted to investigate virus neutralizing antibody titre development (humoral immunity) in stray and domestic dogs and in puppies of vaccinated and unvaccinated dams after an anti-rabies vaccination compared to the antibody titre on the day of vaccination. Previous studies indicate that peak titre of antibodies is generally reached between 4 to 6 weeks after vaccination if the antigenic response is stimulated for the first time [22]. If it is a subsequent stimulation, the time taken for the development of peak titres should be less than this [23]. As per the results of groups A to F, animals with previous vaccination history have antibody titres above the protective level (> 0.5 IU/ml) on D0 and have a higher antibody titre on D360 too (Table 2). Animals without previous vaccination history start with low antibody titres and return to low titres by D360, but have a satisfactory antibody titre at D180. Antibody titre development observed in domestic dogs and puppies in the preliminary study conducted in Kotte, Sri Lanka by Gunatilake et al. [13] was almost similar to the present study. A study done by Seghaier et al. [24] in Tunisia, showed a similar pattern when serum samples of vaccinated dogs against rabies were analyzed. Similarly, Adeyemi et al. [25] compared single vaccination and booster coverage and noted that booster vaccination developed significantly higher level of antibodies. Bunn [26] and Sage et al. [27] reported that single injection of rabies vaccine did not produce a long lasting protective level of antibody titre in a significant number of animals.

Antibody titres on D30 of 5 dogs in group A were between 269 IU/mL to 123 IU/mL which resulted an unusual peak in the median value and therefore to minimize this deviation, these outliers were removed during analysis. This deviation in the antibody titres in individual dogs specially in the stray population could have been resulted due to various reasons such as interval between vaccinations, health or nutrition status, sex and age of the animal (1 to 6 years) and sub-clinical infections. We conducted this study in their natural environment without any intervention which mimics the similar situation in mass vaccination programmes. Also, it was not an objective of our study to find out reasons for individual variation in antibody titres following vaccination.

Table 4 Comparision of protective levels and percentage of rabies virus neutralization antibody (different age groups C to D) titers in previously vaccinated and unvaccinated domestic juvenile dogs

Day	Group C Domestic juvenile dogs with a previous vaccination history: Age 3 months – 1 year, (n = 47)		Group D Domestic juvenile dogs without a previous vaccination history: Age 3 months – 1 year (n = 63)		*P* value
	No. with antibody titre ≥0.5 IU/ml	% with antibody titre ≥0.5 IU/ml	No. with antibody titre ≥0.5 IU/ml	% with antibody titre ≥0.5 IU/ml	
0	37	78.72	1	1.59	0.000*
30	45	95.74	59	93.65	0.487
180	44	93.62	59	93.65	0.643
360	37	78.72	27	42.86	0.000*

*Indicates the significance level at 0.05 when groups C (domestic juvenile dogs with a previous vaccination history) & D (domestic juvenile dogs without a previous vaccination history) are compared

Table 5 Comparision of protective levels and percentage of rabies virus neutralization antibody (different age groups E to F) titers in regular annual and without regular annual vaccinated adult domestic dogs

Day	Group E Adult domestic dogs with regular annual vaccination history: Age 1 to 6 years (*n* = 51)		Group F Adult domestic dogs without regular annual vaccination history: Age 1 to 6 years (*n* = 48)		*P* value
	No. with antibody titre ≥0.5 IU/ml	% with antibody titre ≥0.5 IU/ml	No. with antibody titre ≥0.5 IU/ml	% with antibody titre ≥0.5 IU/ml	
0	39	76.47	37	77.08	0.566
30	49	96	48	100	0.133
180	45	88.23	46	95.84	0.095
360	40	78.43	40	83.33	0.275

Antibody titres of dogs and puppies on D30 in all groups except dogs in group A show that 8.4% of animals have not achieved protective levels of titres. The lack of proper protective antibody level after the vaccination of dogs against rabies was reported by Tepsumathanon et al. [29] and Sage et al. [27]. In contrast, Chomel et al. [28] found that 97% of the animals had titres above 0.5 IU/ml D360 after vaccination.

When considering the number of animals in group D (previously vaccinated), only 42.7% of animals had protective antibody titres at D360. Authorities should pay more attention during vaccination programmes to animals in group D which included juvenile dogs without previous vaccination history; aged 3 months-1 year and who are more active and have closer contacts with humans. They carry the greatest risk similar to the puppies in groups G and H. Of the human rabies cases in Thailand, 57% were bitten by puppies under 3 months of age [29]. More than 50% of dogs in group D and more than 80% of puppies in groups G and H did not have antibody titres on D360. Kasempimolporn et al. [22] analyzed serum antibody titres to rabies virus in 32 puppies before primary vaccination and only five showed protective level of antibody [30]. Jakel et al. [31] reported that low levels of neutralizing antibodies (less than 0.5 IU/ml) did not protect the animals. Therefore, it is necessary to give two anti-rabies vaccines to animals in groups D, G and H at a suitable interval with annual boosters. The recommendation of Adeyemi et al. [23], is to give 2 vaccines 1–3 months apart with annual boosters after that to all newly acquired pet dogs and cats in canine endemic regions [25].

Although the dogs in groups B and D were without previous vaccination history, the development and maintenance of antibody titres above the recommended protective level could be acquired by a primary vaccination in majority of dogs until D180. This is an indirect evidence for the efficacy of the vaccine used in the study. However, 40.42% and 57.14% dogs in groups B and D out of 47 and 63 recruited for those groups did not have protective level of antibody titres by D360. According to Cliquet et al. [24] the number of dogs who had antibody titres below the protective level was 7.8% after two months, 19.1% between 2 and 4 months, 25% between 4 to 6 months, 22% more than 6 months after the primovaccination in 1351 dogs [32]. The very low humoral response observed in the present study on D0 in unvaccinated dogs could be a technical issue with the RFFIT as it compares antibody titre with a reference sera sample.

However, we observed a large individual variation in the humoral response in animals irrespective of previous vaccination (e.g. *minimum* and maximum titres were

Table 6 Comparision of protective levels and the percentage of rabies virus neutralization antibody (different age groups G to H) titers in puppies of previously vaccinated and unvaccinated dams

Day	Group G Puppies of vaccinated domestic dams: Age > 6 weeks to 3 months (*n* = 40)		Group H Puppies of unvaccinated domestic dams:Age > 6 weeks to 3 months (*n* = 37)		*P* value
	No. with antibody titre ≥0.5 IU/ml	% with antibody titre ≥0.5 IU/ml	No. with antibody titre ≥0.5 IU/ml	% with antibody titre ≥0.5 IU/ml	
0	0	0	0	0	
30	39	97.5	35	94.59	0.470
180	33	82.5	29	78.38	0.433
360	3	7.5	4	10.81	0.203

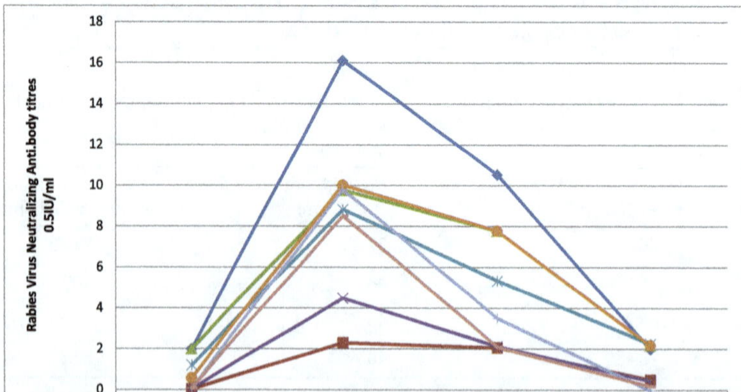

	Day 0	Day 30	Day 180	Day 360
Group A	2	16.11	10.53	2
Group B	0.04	2.29	2.06	0.51
Group C	2	9.76	7.78	2.19
Group D	0.06	4.47	2.12	0.45
Group E	1.2	8.82	5.34	2.25
Group F	0.58	10.02	7.78	2.19
Group G	0.08	9.8	3.5	0
Group H	0.08	8.5	2.09	0.19

Fig. 2 Comparison of median antibody titres of all groups (A-H) without outliers. (Group A- Stray dogs with previous vaccination history; Age > one year, Group B- Stray dogs without previous vaccination history; Age > one year, Group C- Domestic juvenile dogs with a previous vaccination history: Age 3 months – 1 year, Group D- Domestic juvenile dogs without a previous vaccination history: Age 3 months – 1 year, Group E- Adult domestic dogs with regular annual vaccination history :Age 1 to 6 years, Group F- Adult domestic (dogs with owner) dogs without regular annual vaccination history: Age 1 to 6 years, Group G- Puppies of vaccinated domestic dams: Age > 6 weeks to 3 months, Group H- Puppies of unvaccinated domestic dams: Age > 6 weeks to 3 months)

between 1.96 and 269.76 IU/ml compared to 0.02 and 102.6 IU/ml on D30 of dogs in groups A and B respectively). Similar results were observed by Cliquet et al. [24] in the study carried out using 25,000 sera samples of dogs and cats vaccinated against rabies [32]. We used a monovalent anti-rabies vaccine recommended by WHO and used by the Government Rabies Control Programme for many years. After purchasing from the local supplier vaccine was stored under recommended conditions of the manufacturer until it is used. Therefore, type and efficacy of vaccine could not be a major cause for the variation in the humoral response that we observed as there is a good response by the animals in certain groups for the vaccination. We made every effort to recruit healthy dogs after a general examination of the animal which is the accepted method in mass vaccinations. It is difficult to comment about the physical status of the animal by the general examination if it is not very obvious. Therefore, whether the discrepancy observed in the humoral response in dogs in different groups is due to the nutritional status of individual animals or not cannot be ruled out. When grouping animals we considered similar age categories; even with this categorization we observed discrepancies in the humoral response. However, Cliquet et al., [24] had observed a significant difference in the humoral response in dogs between primo-vaccinated and multi-vaccinated groups while it was not significant among similar groups of cats [32]. The method we used for the determination of humoral response is RFFIT which has a higher sensitivity recommended by the WHO and well established at the MRI. Therefore, sensitivity of RFFIT is not a factor for the differences observed in the humoral response among animals for the anti-rabies vaccination.

Humoral response induced by vaccination has been identified as an important method of control and prevention of rabies which is a deadly zoonotic disease. Considering the cut off value of 0.5 IU/ml for antibody titres as recommended by the WHO for human sera, our results show that a single vaccination to dogs without owner and owned dogs without a previous vaccination history and to puppies fails to produce an adequate immune response on D360 in many dogs. There were animals in other groups with past vaccination history who did not have adequate protection. Similar patterns of data had been observed by research groups in other countries as well [33–35]. However, Barth et al., indicates by analyzing many experimental results that dogs have a very high probability of survival after a later rabies infection, even if serum does not contain detectable anti-rabies antibodies irrespective of the period of time elapsed since the vaccination [18].

Without measuring immunogenecity (both humoral and cell mediated) in an animal following vaccination and without doing challenge studies it is difficult to consider whether an animal is well protected or not. Irrespective of this hypothesis, based on the results of our study, it is necessary to vaccinate puppies at an early

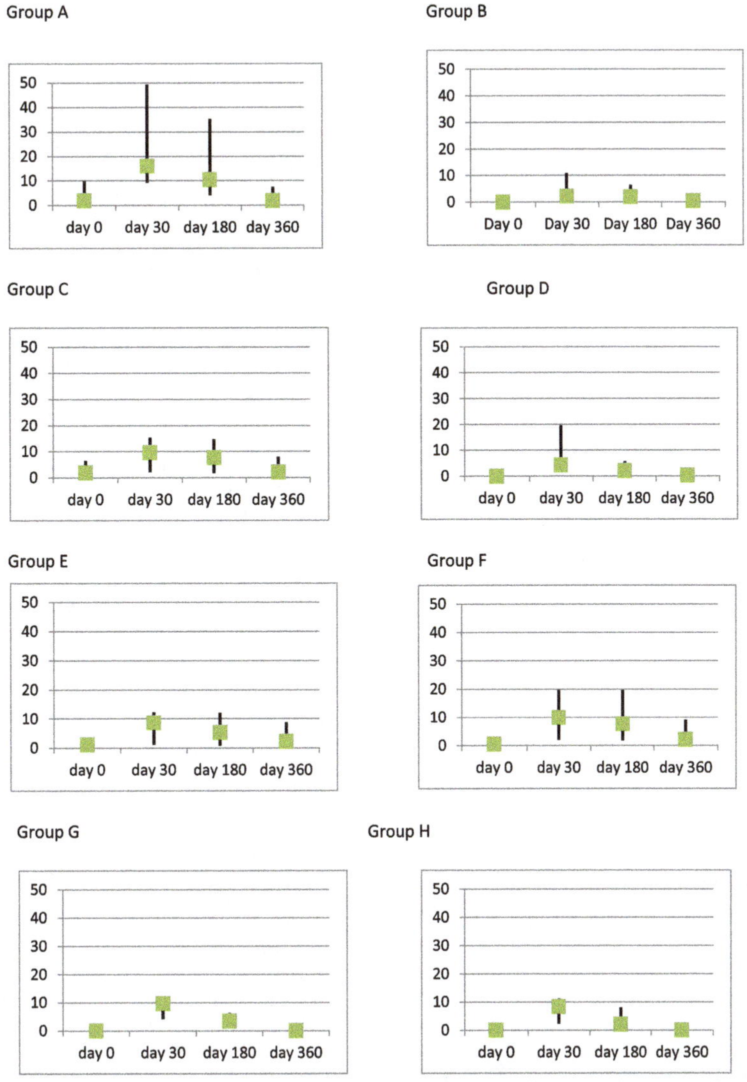

Fig. 3 Median antibody titers of all groups A-H with error bars. Green boxes represent medians, error bars range from 25th quartile to 75th quartile. (**Group A**- Stray dogs with previous vaccination history;Age > one year, **Group B**- Stray dogs without previous vaccination history; Age > one year, **Group C**- Domestic juveniles dogs with a previous vaccination history: Age 3 months – 1 year, **Group D**- Domestic juveniles dogs without a previous vaccination history: Age 3 months – 1 year, **Group E**- Adult domestic dogs with regular an nual vaccination history: Age 1 to 6 years, **Group F**- Adult domestic dogs without regular an nual vaccination history: Age 1 to 6 years, **Group G**- Puppies of vaccinated domestic dams: Age > 6 weeks to 3 months, **Group H**- Puppies of unvaccinated domestic dams: Age > 6 weeks to 3 months)

stage with a booster at a suitable interval with annual boosters thereafter, in order to improve herd immunity. This could interrupt rabies transmission by both urban and sylvatic cycles. By this way vaccination could take the lead role in eradicating rabies from Sri Lanka.

Conclusion

A single dose of anti-rabies vaccination is not sufficient for the maintenance of antibody titres for a period of 1 year in 40.42% of canines in group B. Median antibody titres of dogs in groups C and D indicate immune responsiveness in animals in group C with previous vaccination history is higher than the animals in group D without vaccination history. Irrespective of whether previously vaccinated dogs in groups E and F were regularly vaccinated or not, antibody titres were above the protective level in most of the dogs on day 60, 180 and 360. Maternal antibodies do not provide adequate protection to puppies in group G (puppies from previously vaccinated dams) until the first anti-rabies vaccination. Immunity development after vaccination seems to be closely similar in both the groups of puppies. There seem to be many factors which affect development of antibodies following vaccination against rabies. Based on these findings, we recommend that puppies should be given two anti-rabies vaccines in the first year of life at suitable time intervals with annual revaccinations. It is necessary to

conduct further studies to determine the exact time interval for the first booster vaccine for puppies.

Abbreviations

ABC: Animal birth control; ARV: Anti-rabies vaccination; IQR: Inter quartile ranges; MOH: Medical officer of health; MRI: Medical research institute; PET: Post exposure treatment; RFFIT: Rapid fluorescent focus inhibition test; WHO: World health organization

Acknowledgements

We gratefully acknowledge the financial support given by the National Science Foundation of Sri Lanka for this study.

Funding

Financial support given by the National Science Foundation of Sri Lanka this study.

Authors, contributions

RMSP, Designed the study, analyzed serum samples, complied results, carried out statistical analysis, wrote the paper. MG, Designed and supervised the study, helped in drafting the paper and corrections. OW and KADNP, Collaborated and guided RMSP for doing RFFIT. AB, helped in statistical analysis. All authors read and approved the final manuscript.

Competing interests

The authors declare that they have no competing interests.

Consent for publication

Not applicable.

Ethics approval and consent to participate

This research project was carried out according to International and local guidelines for animal research after obtaining ethical clearance from the Ethics Review Committees of the Faculty of Medicine, University of Colombo (EC/06/75) and the Medical Research Institute, Sri Lanka (17/2006). Animals were recruited with the owners' consent after obtaining permission from the Regional Director of Health Services, Kalutara to recruit dogs to the study. All personnel involved in the study during handling, collecting and processing of blood samples from animals were given pre-exposure vaccination against rabies. Handling of animals for blood collection was done with care to minimize pain and discomfort to animals [36].

Author details

[1]Ministry of Health, No.555/5, Elvitigala Mawatha, Colombo 05, Sri Lanka. [2]Department of Physiology, Faculty of Medicine, University of Colombo, No.25, Kynsey Road, Colombo 08, Sri Lanka. [3]Department of Rabies Research and Vaccine Quality Control, Medical Research Institute, Colombo 08, Sri Lanka. [4]Faculty of Medicine, General Sir John Kotelawala Defense University, Kandawala Road, Rathmalana, Sri Lanka.

References

1. Knobel D, Cleaveland S, Coleman PG, Fevre EM, Meltzer MI, Miranda MEG, Shaw A, Zinsstag J, Meslin FX. Re-evaluating the burden of rabies in Africa and Asia. Bulletin World Health Organization. 2005;83:360–8.
2. Rozario M. Rabies in India. CMAJ. 2008;178(5):64–566.
3. Wandeler AI, Budde A, Capt S, Kappeler A, Matter H. Dog ecology and dog rabies control. Rev Infect Dis. 1988;10:684–8.
4. Hampson K, Laurent C, Tiziana L, Maganga S, Alexia K, Michaël A, Jacques B, Jesse D. Blanton, Estimating the Global Burden of Endemic Canine Rabies. PLOS Negl Trop. 2015.
5. Sudarshan MK, Madhusudana SN, Mahendra BJ, Rao NS, Ashwath NDH, Abdul Rahman S. Assessing the burden of human rabies in India: results of a national multi-center epidemiological survey. Intl J Infect Dis. 2007;11(1):29–35.
6. Touihri L, Zaouia I, Elhili K, Dellagi K, Bahloul C. Evaluation of mass vaccination campaign coverage against rabies in dogs in Tunisia. Zoonoses Public Health. 2011;58(2):110–8.
7. Epidermiology unit, Ministry of Health. http://www.epid.gov.lk/web/index.php?option=com_content&view=article&id=163&Itemid=450&lang=en.
8. Prevention and Control of Rabies in the South-East Asia Region World Health Organization, Regional Office for South–East Asia. July 2004; New Delhi. http://apps.searo.who.int/PDS_DOCS/B0216.pdf.
9. Coleman PG, Dye C. Immunization coverage required to prevent outbreaks of dog rabies. Vaccine. 1996;14:185–6. [PubMed] https://www.ncbi.nlm.nih.gov/pubmed/8920697.
10. Public Health Veterinary Services, Ministry of Health. Prevention and Control of Rabies in the South-East Asia Region. https://www.google.lk/#q=www.rabies.gov.lk. Accessed 11 Jan 2015.
11. Vigilato MA, Clavijo A, Knobl T, Tamayo HM, Cosivi O, Schneider MC, et al. Progress towards eliminating canine rabies: policies and perspectives from Latin American and the Caribbean. Phil Trans R Soc B. 2013;368:20120143.
12. WHO. Rabies vaccines: WHO position paper-recommendations. Vaccine. 2010;28:7140–2.
13. Gunatilake M, Wimalaratne O, Perera KADN. Persistence of antibody titres in adult dogs and puppies following the anti-rabies immunization. Ceylon J Med. 2003;46(2):67–72.
14. Cleaveland S, Kaare M, Tiringa P, Mlengeya T, Barrat J. A dog rabies vaccination campaign in rural Africa: impact on the incidence of dog rabies and human dog-bite injuries. Vaccine. 21:2003, 1965–1973.
15. Tk S, Ndabambi N, Mpuchane S. A seroservey of Rabies antibodies in Dogs in Gaborone, Botswana. J Anim Vet Adv. 2007;6(4):549–52.
16. Kamoltham T, Singhsa J, Promsaranee U, Sonthon P, Mathean P, Thinyounyong W. Elimination of human rabies in a canine endemic province in Thailand: five-year programme. Bull WHO. 2003;81(5):375–81.
17. WHO. Expert consultation on rabies First report, WHO Technical Report Series No. 931. Geneva: World Health Organization; 2004.
18. Barth R, Gruschkau H, Jaeger O. Chick embryo cell inactivated rabies vaccine for veterinary use. Laboratory and field experience. In: Kuwert E, Merieux C, Koprowski H, Bogel K, editors. Rabies in the tropics. Berlin: Springer Verlag; 1985. p. 241–8.
19. Smith JS, Yager PA, Bear GM. A rapid reproducible test for determining rabies neutralizing antibody. Bull WHO. 1973;48:535–41.
20. Reed LJ, Muench H. A simple method of estimating fifty percent endpoints. Am J Hyg. 1938;27:493–7.
21. Feyssaguet M, Dacheux L, Audry L, Compoint A, Morize JL, Blanchard I, Bourhy H. Multicenter comparative study of a new ELISA for the detection and titration of anti-rabies glycoprotein antibodies and comparison with the rapid fluorescent focus inhibition test (RFFIT) on human samples from vaccinated and non- vaccinated people. Vaccine. 2006;25:2244–51.
22. Kasempimolporn S, Jitapunkul S, Sitprija V. Moving towards the elimination of rabies in Thailand. J Med Assoc Thail. 2008;91:433–7.
23. Aliye Ebru GAZI, Seyyal AK. Detection of neutralizing antibody titration in vaccinated owned and stray dogs against rabies virus. J Fac Vet Med Istanbul Univ. 2011;37(2):97–106.
24. Seghaier C, Cliquet F, Hammami S, Aouina T, Tlatli A, Aubert M. Rabies mass vaccination campaigns in Tunisia: are vaccinated dogs correctly immunized? AmJTrop Med Hyg. 1999;61(6):879–84.
25. Adeyemi IG, Adetunji VO, James VO, Alonge DO Ten Year. 1993–2002, Retrospective Evaluation of Vaccination of Dogs against Rabies at the University of Ibadan, Nigeria. Afr J Biomed Res. 2004;8(1):71–7.
26. Bunn TO. Canine and feline vaccines, past and present. In: Baer CM, editor. The Natural History of Rabies. 2nd ed; 1991. p. 415–25.
27. Sage G, Khawplod P, Wilde H, Lobaugh C, Hemachudha T, Tepsumethanon W, Lumlertdaecha B. Immune response to rabies vaccine in Alaskan dogs: failure to achieve a consistently protective antibody response. Trans Roy Soc Trop Med Hyg. 1993;87:593–5.
28. Chomel B, Chappi G, Bullon F, Cardenas E, De BT, Lombard M, Giambrun E. Mass vaccination campaign against rabies: are dogs correctly protected? The Peruvian experience. Revised. Infect Dis. 1988;10(4):697–02.
29. Wilde H, Khawplod P, Khamoltham T, Hemachudha T, Tepsumethanon V, Lumlerdacha B, Mitmoonpitak C, Sitprija V. Rabies control in South and Southeast Asia. Vaccine. 2005;23:2284–9.
30. Kasempimolporn S, Sichanasai B, Saengseesom W, Puempumpanich S, Chatraporn S, Sitprija V. Prevalence of rabies virus infection and rabies antibody in stray dogs: A survey in Bangkok, Thailand. Prev Vet Med. 2007;78(3–4):325–32.

31. Jakel V, Konig M, Cussler K, Hanschmann K, Thiel HJ. Factors influencing the antibody response to vaccination against rabies. Dev Biol. 2008;131:431–6.
32. Cliquet F, Aubert M, Sagne L. Development of a fluorescent antibody virus neutralization test (FAVN test) for the quantification of rabies-neutralizing antibody. J Immunol Meth. 1998;212:79–87.
33. Suzuki KET, Gonzalez G, Ascarrunz A, Loza A, Ascarrunz G, Loza M, et al. Antibody response to an anti-rabies vaccine in a dog population underfield conditions in Bolivia, Zoonosis. Public Health. 2008;55(8–10):414–20.
34. Ogawa T, Gamoh K, Kanda K, Suzuki T, Kawashima A, Narushima R, Shimazaki T. Rabies immune status of dogs brought into the Hyogo Prefecture Animal Well-being Center, Japan. J Vet Med Sci. 2009;71(6):825–6.
35. Rigo L, Honer MR. Rabies virus antibody titers in dogs in Campo Grande, Mato Grosso do Sul State, during the anti-rabies campaign, 2003. Rev Soc Bras Med Trop. 2006;39(6):553–5.
36. Rowan AN. Animals, science, and ethics – Section IV. Ethical review and the animal care and use committee. Hast Cent Rep. 1990;20(3):S19–24.

5

Field evaluation of the efficacy of *Mycobacterium bovis* BCG vaccine against tuberculosis in goats

Enric Vidal[1*], Claudia Arrieta-Villegas[2], Miriam Grasa[3], Irene Mercader[4], Mariano Domingo[1,2] and Bernat Pérez de Val[1]

Abstract

Background: Control of animal tuberculosis (TB) through vaccination has emerged as a long-term strategy to complement test and slaughter control strategy. A pilot trial under field conditions was conducted in a goat herd with high TB prevalence to assess the efficacy of the *Mycobacterium bovis* BCG vaccine.

Results: Twenty-three goat kids vaccinated with BCG and other 22 unvaccinated control kids were euthanized at 18 months post-vaccination. Gross pathological and histopathological examination of target tissues was performed for detection of tuberculous lesions and assessment of vaccine efficacy. Mycobacterial culture and DNA detection were used to confirm *Mycobacterium caprae* infection. Vaccination significantly reduced the number of animals with TB lesions compared to unvaccinated controls (35% and 77%, respectively; $P < 0.01$). This reduction was even higher if only extra-pulmonary infection was considered (17% and 68%, respectively; $P < 0.001$).

Conclusions: This trial demonstrates that BCG vaccination of goats can significantly reduce the TB lesion rates in high disease exposure conditions, indicating that vaccination could contribute to the control of TB in domestic goats.

Keywords: BCG, Efficacy, Field study, Goats, Tuberculosis, Vaccine

Background

Animal tuberculosis (TB) is a chronic infectious disease caused by mycobacteria of the *Mycobacterium tuberculosis* complex (MTBC), mainly *M. bovis* and *M. caprae*, which affects a wide range of domestic and wild animals. TB in goats causes economic losses in endemic areas due to trade limitations, and depopulation of positive herds, when test and slaughter strategy fails [1, 2]. Furthermore, infected goats have been identified as a source of bovine TB in mixed goats-cattle herds or nearby cattle farms in non-officially bovine TB-free EU countries [3, 4]. Unlike TB in cattle, no official EU policy exists for TB control in goats, thus hindering the success of bovine TB eradication programs.

Vaccination may be a control option to reduce disease prevalence in animals in high-prevalent herds where the test and slaughter strategy could be inefficient, expensive in terms of cost-benefit, logistically demanding or could threaten valuable genetic resources [5, 6]. Also, vaccination could be an affordable tool to control TB in underdeveloped countries unable to afford conventional test and slaughter protocols [7–9].

M. bovis bacillus Calmette-Guérin (BCG) is an appealing vaccine for use in livestock and wildlife as its use is licensed for humans, has an excellent safety record and is relatively inexpensive to manufacture [10]. The efficacy of BCG in the field has been assessed in cattle [7, 11] and in wildlife TB hosts, such as possums or badgers [12, 13]. Furthermore, our research group has also recently demonstrated that BCG vaccination of goats affords a degree of protection against experimental challenge with *M. caprae* [14, 15].

Even though vaccination of cattle with mycobacterial vaccines is at present prohibited in EU counties, the implementation of vaccination campaigns in goats is not expressly prohibited and would not require national and EU laws and directives. Here we report the first trial to assess the efficacy of BCG vaccination of goat kids under field conditions.

* Correspondence: enric.vidal@irta.cat
[1]IRTA, Centre de Recerca en Sanitat Animal (CReSA, IRTA-UAB), Campus de la Universitat Autònoma de Barcelona, Bellaterra, 08193 Barcelona, Catalonia, Spain
Full list of author information is available at the end of the article

Methods

Herd and experimental schedule

A TB positive herd of Murciana-Grandina goats, located in Catalonia, with confirmed *Mycobacterium caprae* (spoligotype profile SB0416) infection and a reactor rate of 79% to the single intradermal comparative cervical tuberculin (SICCT) test, was selected for this study. A lot of 45 new born, approximately 1 month old, goat kids (16 males and 29 females) from the herd reposition were included in the study. Animals were randomly divided in two groups of 23 (8 males and 15 females) and 22 (8 males and 14 females), respectively. This sample size was deemed appropriate to estimate differences of proportions between treatment groups, i.e. 25% and 66% estimated proportion of infection in vaccinated and unvaccinated groups respectively (95% confidence interval, 90% statistical power, one-tailed test; source: www.winepi.net, University of Zaragoza).

At day 0, all experimental animals were negative to the SICCT test and the IFN-γ release assay (Bovigam™, Thermo Fisher Scientific, Schlieren, Switzerland). Twenty three animals were vaccinated subcutaneously with approximately 10^5 colony forming units (CFU) *M. bovis* BCG Danish strain (ATCC, Ref. 35,733™), prepared as previously described [16], and the other 22 remained as unvaccinated controls. Two months after vaccination, the kids were mixed with the rest of the herd and remained exposed to natural infection for 16 months, after this period, all the animals included in the study were humanely sacrificed.

All animals were fed following the regular farm conditions throughout the study (i.e. colostrum/milk initially, followed by forage supplemented with feed). Animals were followed-up for clinical signs every two months approximately.

Necropsy, tissue sampling and histopathology

The 45 experimental animals were euthanized by intravenous sodium pentobarbital overdose and carefully post-mortem examined in order to detect tuberculous lesions. Euthanasia was performed at 18 months after BCG vaccination. A complete necropsy procedure was conducted as previously described [17]. Briefly, tracheobronchial and mediastinal lymph nodes (LN) were aseptically removed making sure that the pleural lung surface was not sectioned, were sliced and examined for the presence of TB-like gross lesions, and then were stored at −20 °C as a pulmonary LN pool. Whole lungs were fixed with 10%-buffered formalin by pouring the fixative into the trachea. One month later, lungs were sliced at 1 cm thick intervals for TB-like gross lesion examination. All remaining viscera were also examined and all TB-like gross lesions detected in other tissues were collected at necropsy and subsequently fixed with 10%-buffered formalin, embedded in paraffin and examined by histopathology (haematoxylin and eosin and Ziehl Neelsen staining). For each animal at least one section of any tissues with visible lesions was included in the paraffin block, samples of the mesenteric lymph node and ileum were always included regardless whether lesions were observed or not macroscopically. The whole slide was evaluated under the microscope using the different magnification available in the microscope (4×, 10×, 20 x and 40× and, in the case of the Ziehl Neelsen Staining, the 100× magnification with immersion oil was used). The slides were analysed blindly by a pathologist. TB indicative lesions were set when the following histopathological features were observed: Presence of granulomas, with or without central necrosis and mineralization, surrounded by macrophages, multinucleated giant cells, sometimes partially or completely encapsulated. Enumeration (when present) of acid fast bacilli (AFB) was also performed. Four different categories were defined: None detected (no AFB detected after evaluation of the whole lesion under 100× magnification); 1 (observation of one AFB in at least one 100× field); 2–5 (observation of 2 to 5 AFB in at least one 100× field), >5 (observation of more than 5 AFB in at least one 100×).

MTBC culture

For microbiological culture, the pulmonary LN pools were thawed and a quantitative mycobacterial culture was subsequently carried out following the procedure described in previous studies [17]. Briefly, LN pools were homogenized, decontaminated, suspended and 100 μl of this suspension were twice serial diluted 1:10. Afterwards, 100 μl of each suspension dilution (1:100, 1:1000 and 1:10,000) were inoculated onto 7H11 agar plates (BD Diagnostics, MD, USA). The inoculated media were incubated at 37 °C. Bacterial counts were performed after 28 days and total CFUs in each pool of pulmonary LN were calculated. Isolates were confirmed as MTBC by multiplex PCR [18]. Then, DNA samples from MTBC isolates were analysed by DVR-spoligotyping [19].

Direct DNA detection

Once TB lesions were confirmed in non-respiratory tissues by histopathology, DNA extraction was carried out as following: Excess paraffin was trimmed off the sample block using a scalpel, and then 10 μm thick sections were obtained and dewaxed with xylene and absolute ethanol. Once the ethanol supernatant was removed and the remaining ethanol had evaporated the tissue was weighed to obtain an amount of 25 mg. Afterwards, DNA from resulting tissue powder was extracted using a DNA purification kit (Promega Biotech Iberica, Madrid, Spain). A semi-nested PCR, targeted to the MTBC-specific IS*6110* sequence [17] was run under standard conditions and a *M. avium* subsp. *paratuberculosis*

(*MAP*)-specific Real Time PCR (Vacunek, Derio, Spain) was run following the manufacturer instructions.

Serology

Blood samples were collected from all experimental animals at the end point of the study. Sera from all animals were analysed by ELISA to detect antibodies against MTBC as previously described [17] and against *MAP* (ID Screen® Paratuberculosis indirect, ID.vet, Grabels, France).

Data analysis

Differences in presence of TB lesions and histopathological parameters between groups were assessed by chi-square test. Significance was set at P value <0.05. Statistical analysis was performed with R package v2.15.0 (R Foundation for Statistical Computing, Vienna, Austria).

Results

Besides occasional coughing, experimental animals did not show remarkable clinical signs throughout the experiment. No adverse reactions at BCG injection site were observed at necropsy.

A total of 25 out of 45 goats showed gross and histopathological TB lesions. The proportion of animals with TB lesions was significantly higher in unvaccinated (77%, 95% CI: 54–91) than in vaccinated goats (35%, 95% CI: 17–57; $P < 0.01$). There were no significant differences between sex categories (Table 1).

Ten goats, 6 vaccinated and 4 unvaccinated, showed pulmonary lesions (Fig. 1a-b, Table 1). MTBC were isolated from pulmonary LN (10^2 CFU/pooled LN) in 2 of them (both vaccinated). In both cases the strain isolated was identified as *M. caprae* with the spoligotype profile SB0415 (www.Mbovis.org). Nineteen goats showed extra-pulmonary TB lesions confirmed by histopathology (Fig. 1c-d, Table 1). The proportion of goats with extra-pulmonary lesions was significantly higher in unvaccinated than in vaccinated goats (68% and 17%, respectively; $P < 0.001$). All these animals ($N = 19$) showed TB lesions in mesenteric LN. The proportion of AFB positive results in mesenteric LN was significantly lower in BCG vaccinated compared to control animals (25% and 80%, respectively; $P < 0.05$). BCG vaccinated animals also showed a higher (yet not statistically significant) proportion of granulomas in mesenteric LN without necrosis, mineralization or fibrotic capsule compared to control animals (50% and 13%, respectively). A characterization of granulomas in mesenteric LN for each group is shown in Table 2. MTBC DNA was detected in one of them, whereas *MAP* DNA was not detected in any sample. In addition, 5 (2 vaccinated and 3 unvaccinated) and 3 (1 vaccinated and 2 unvaccinated) animals showed TB lesions in retropharyngeal LN and ileum wall, respectively (data not shown).

At the end of the study, 5 out of 22 unvaccinated goats were positive to the MTBC ELISA (four of them with TB visible lesions), whereas none of the unvaccinated goats were positive to the *MAP* ELISA. Within the BCG vaccinated group, 16 out of 23 goats were positive to the MTBC ELISA (only one with TB visible lesions), and one of them (which had no visible TB lesions) was also positive to the *MAP* ELISA.

Discussion

We report herein, for first time, a pilot vaccination trial under field conditions that has demonstrated a degree of protection of goats vaccinated with BCG against natural exposure to MTBC. Similar field studies conducted in cattle also showed protective efficacy of BCG seen as a reduction of pathological scores and the number of animals positive to bacteriological culture or immunological tests [7, 11].

Our results are also consistent with those obtained in previous laboratory BCG efficacy studies in goats experimentally infected with *M. caprae* [14, 15], that showed reduction of extra-pulmonary TB cases in vaccinated goats. Unfortunately the quantitative culture method carried out, which started by platting a 1/100 dilution of the pool of whole lymph node homogenates, irrespectively of the extension or localization of lesions, and also

Table 1 Distribution of TB cases by experimental groups, sex and lesion location

		No. of goats with TB lesions (%)[a]			
Group	Sex	Only pulmonary lesions[b]	Only extra-pulmonary lesions[c]	Both pulmonary and extra-pulmonary lesions	Total
BCG	Male ($N = 8$)	1 (13)	0 (0)	2 (25)	3 (38)
($N = 23$)	Female ($N = 15$)	3 (20)	2 (13)	0 (0)	5 (33)
	Total	4 (17)	2 (9)	2 (9)	8 (35)
Control	Male ($N = 8$)	0 (0)	5 (63)**	1 (13)	6 (75)
($N = 22$)	Female ($N = 14$)	2 (14)	8 (57)*	1 (7)	11 (79)
	Total	2 (9)	13 (59)***	2 (9)	17 (77)**

[a]TB lesions were determined by histopathology
[b]Lungs and mediastinal and tracheobronchial lymph nodes
[c]Ileum and mesenteric and retropharyngeal lymph nodes
*$P < 0.05$, **$P < 0.01$, ***$P < 0.001$; Chi-square test

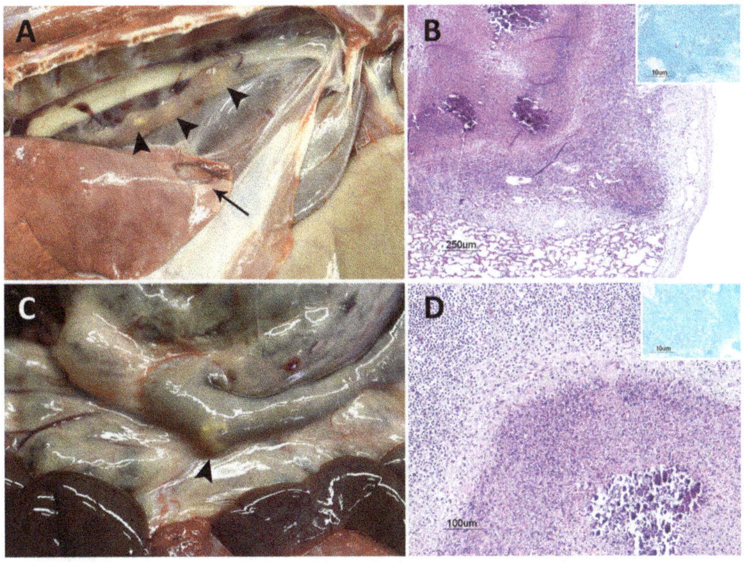

Fig. 1 Study of tuberculous lesions. **a** Goat showing a pulmonary tuberculous granuloma (*arrow*) and tuberculous lesions in the mediastinal lymph node (*arrowheads*). **b** Histopathological study of the lung lesion observed in **a**. The insert shows Ziehl-Neelsen stained mycobacteria. **c** Goat with tuberculous granulomatous lymphadenitis lesions in the mesenteric lymph node (*arrowhead*). **d** Histopathology of the lesions observed in C, showing paubacillary tuberculous granulomatous lymphadenitis. The insert shows a Ziehl-Neelsen positive bacillus

included a sample freezing and defrosting step, may have hampered the mycobacterial detection by culture. Thus, even though *M. caprae* infection was confirmed in the herd and in 2 experimental animals (with the same spoligotype profile previously identified in the herd), the vaccine efficacy assessment had to rely on histopathological results.

Interestingly, in the present study most unvaccinated animals showed only extra-pulmonary lesions, mainly in mesenteric LN. In all these cases the lesions showed consistent histopathological features that are strongly indicative of TB. MTBC DNA was detected in one of these lesions confirming the ethiology. Even though other diseases, such as paratuberculosis might occasionally induce similar lesions, the possibility that extra-pulmonary lesions were caused by *MAP* was ruled out: No diffuse granulomatous infiltrates (the most frequent lesions in paratuberculosis infection) were observed in any animal, *MAP* DNA was not detected from any extra-pulmonary lesion, and the 13 goats that only showed extra-pulmonary lesions were all negative to *MAP* ELISA, whereas 5 of them were positive to MTBC ELISA at the end point of the study. Thus the possibility that extra-pulmonary lesions were caused by *MAP* was ruled out. The location of TB lesions in unvaccinated animals suggests that the digestive route of infection could be particularly important in the studied farm, probably due to shared feed and water points with the rest of the farmed animals. These results suggest that BCG vaccination might reduce the number of animals infected through the oral route, and non-respiratory bacterial shedding from infected animals, thus leading to a lower risk of horizontal transmission within the herd.

In high caprine TB prevalent regions, where infected goats may act as domestic reservoirs of TB in cattle [3], the ultimate goal should be to eradicate the disease in goats, along with the eradication of TB in cattle. Hence, our results indicate that vaccination of the entire herd, or at least of the rearing kids, could be useful in reducing the intra-herd prevalence. This strategy could be combined with slaughtering of goats positive to ante-

Table 2 Histopathological analysis of granulomas in mesenteric lymph nodes

Parameter		Group	
		BCG ($N = 4$)	Control ($N = 15$)
		No. (%)	No. (%)
Capsule	Absent	2 (50)	2 (13)
	Partial	1 (25)	3 (20)
	Complete	1 (25)	10 (67)
Necrosis	Absence	2 (50)	2 (13)
	Presence	2 (50)	13 (87)
Mineralization	None	2 (50)	2 (13)
	Low	0 (0)	9 (60)
	High	2 (50)	4 (27)
No. of AFB	None detected	3 (75)	3 (20)
	1	1 (25)	3 (20)
	2–5	0 (0)	5 (33)
	>5	0 (0)	4 (27)

AFB Acid fast bacilli

mortem DIVA tests until all infected goats are removed from the flock. Accordingly, some authors have suggested that the effect of BCG vaccination in a targeted population of badgers would result in a gradual decrease in the number of infected individuals leading to a reduction in interspecies transmission, and, if the aim of the vaccination was to eradicate TB from badgers, it would need to be continued until the last infected badger was removed from the population [10, 20].

Conclusion

The results of this study demonstrate that BCG vaccinated goats in field conditions showed not only reduced MTBC infection rates, but also a significant reduction of extrapulmonary TB. These results indicate that vaccination may be a long-term prospect to reduce the prevalence in herds with a high number of infected animals. A vaccination program, in addition to other disease reduction practices, such as good herd management, biosafety practices and an efficient DIVA tests, may contribute to eradicate caprine TB in endemic areas.

Abbreviations

BCG: Bacillus Calmette-Guérin; DIVA: Differention of Infected and Vaccinated Animals; IFN-γ: Interferon gamma; LN: lymph nodes; MAP: *M. avium* subsp. *paratuberculosis*; MTBC: *Mycobacterium tuberculosis* complex.; SICCT: single intradermal comparative cervical tuberculin; TB: Tuberculosis

Acknowledgements

DVR-spoligotyping analyses were conducted at VISAVET Health Surveillance Centre, Universidad Complutense of Madrid, Spain. We are grateful to Mónica Pérez, Júlia Vergara-Alert, Núria Galofré, Maite Martín, Zoraida Cervera, Maria Jesus Navas, the CReSA-IRTA Field Studies Unit staff, and the goat farm staff, for their technical assistance.

Funding

This work was funded by the project AGL2012-36171 of the Spanish Ministry of Economy and Competitiveness (MINECO), by the Department of Agriculture, Livestock, Fisheries and Food (DARP) and the CERCA Programme of the Generalitat de Catalunya.

Authors' contributions

MD, IM and BP conceived the study. EV, CA, MG, BP and MD performed the experiments (vaccination, bleeding, necropsies, laboratory analysis) and analysed the data. All authors read and approved the final manuscript.

Consent for publication

Not applicable.

Competing interests

The authors declare that they have no competing interests.

Author details

[1]IRTA, Centre de Recerca en Sanitat Animal (CReSA, IRTA-UAB), Campus de la Universitat Autònoma de Barcelona, Bellaterra, 08193 Barcelona, Catalonia, Spain. [2]Departament de Sanitat i Anatomia Animals, Universitat Autònoma de Barcelona, Bellaterra, 08193 Barcelona, Catalonia, Spain. [3]Associació de Ramaders de Cabrum de Catalunya, 25400 Les Borges Blanques, Lleida, Catalonia, Spain. [4]Departament d'Agricultura, Ramaderia, Pesca i Alimentació de la Generalitat de Catalunya, 08007 Barcelona, Catalonia, Spain.

References

1. Daniel R, Evans H, Rolfe S, de la Rua-Domenech R, Crawshaw T, Higgins RJ, Schock A, Clifton-Hadley R. Outbreak of tuberculosis caused by Mycobacterium Bovis in golden Guernsey goats in great Britain. Vet Rec. 2009;165:335–42.
2. Seva J, Menchén V, Navarro JA, Pallarés FJ, Villar D, Vásquez F, Bernabé A. Caprine tuberculosis eradication program: an immunohistochemical study. Small Rumin Res. 2002;46:107–14.
3. Napp S, Allepuz A, Mercader I, Nofrarías M, López-Soria S, Domingo M, Romero B, Bezos J, Pérez de Val B. Evidence of goats acting as domestic reservoirs of bovine tuberculosis. Vet Rec. 2013;172:663.
4. Zanardi G, Boniotti MB, Gaffuri A, Casto B, Zanoni M, Pacciarini ML. Tuberculosis transmission by Mycobacterium Bovis in a mixed cattle and goat herd. Res Vet Sci. 2013;95:430–3.
5. Krebs JR, Group TISR. Bovine tuberculosis in cattle and badgers. London: Minist Agric Fish Food Publ London, UK; 1997.
6. Vordermeier HM, Pérez de Val B, Buddle BM, Villarreal-Ramos B, Jones GJ, Hewinson RG, Domingo M. Vaccination of domestic animals against tuberculosis: review of progress and contributions to the field of the TBSTEP project. Res Vet Sci. 2014;97(Supple):S53–60.
7. Ameni G, Vordermeier M, Aseffa A, Young DB, Hewinson RG. Field evaluation of the efficacy of Mycobacterium Bovis Bacillus Calmette-Guerin against bovine tuberculosis in neonatal calves in Ethiopia. Clin Vaccine Immunol. 2010;17:1533–8.
8. Conlan AJK, Brooks Pollock E, McKinley TJ, Mitchell AP, Jones GJ, Vordermeier M, Wood JLN. Potential benefits of cattle vaccination as a supplementary control for bovine tuberculosis. PLoS Comput Biol. 2015;11:e1004038.
9. Murphy D, Corner LAL, Gormley E. Adverse reactions to Mycobacterium Bovis bacille Calmette-Guérin (BCG) vaccination against tuberculosis in humans, veterinary animals and wildlife species. Tuberculosis (Edinb). 2008;88:344–57.
10. Buddle BM, de Lisle GW. The role of vaccination in the control of tuberculosis in badgers. Vet J. 2014;200:349–50.
11. Lopez-Valencia G, Renteria-Evangelista T, Williams J de J, Licea-Navarro A, la M-VAD, Medina-Basulto G. Field evaluation of the protective efficacy of Mycobacterium Bovis BCG vaccine against bovine tuberculosis. Res Vet Sci. 2010;88:44–9.
12. Chambers MA, Rogers F, Delahay RJ, Lesellier S, Ashford R, Dalley D, Gowtage S, Dave D, Palmer S, Brewer J, Crawshaw T, Clifton-Hadley R, Carter S, Cheeseman C, Hanks C, Murray A, Palphramand K, Pietravalle S, Smith GC, Tomlinson A, Walker NJ, Wilson GJ, Corner LA, Rushton SP, Shirley MD, Gettinby G, McDonald RA, Hewinson RG. Bacillus Calmette-Guerin vaccination reduces the severity and progression of tuberculosis in badgers. Proc Biol Sci / R Soc. 2011;278:1913–20.
13. Tompkins DM, Ramsey DS, Cross ML, Aldwell FE, de Lisle GW, Buddle BM. Oral vaccination reduces the incidence of tuberculosis in free-living brushtail possums. Proc Biol Sci / R Soc. 2009;276:2987–95.
14. Pérez de Val B, Villarreal-Ramos B, Nofrarías M, López-Soria S, Romera N, Singh M, Abad FX, Xing Z, Vordermeier HM, Domingo M. Goats primed with Mycobacterium Bovis BCG and boosted with a recombinant adenovirus expressing Ag85A show enhanced protection against tuberculosis. Clin Vaccine Immunol. 2012;19:1339–47.
15. Pérez de Val B, Vidal E, Villarreal-Ramos B, Gilbert SC, Andaluz A, Moll X, Martí-n M, Nofrarías M, McShane H, Vordermeier HM, Domingo M. A multi-antigenic adenoviral-vectored vaccine improves BCG-induced protection of goats against pulmonary tuberculosis infection and prevents disease progression. PLoS One. 2013;8:e81317.
16. Pérez de Val B, Vidal E, López-Soria S, Marco A, Cervera Z, Martín M, Mercader I, Singh M, Raeber A, Domingo M. Assessment of safety and interferon gamma responses of Mycobacterium Bovis BCG vaccine in goat kids and milking goats. Vaccine. 2016;34:881–6.
17. Pérez de Val B, López-Soria S, Nofrarías M, Martín M, Vordermeier HM, Villarreal-Ramos B, Romera N, Escobar M, Solanes D, Cardona PJ, Domingo

M. Experimental model of tuberculosis in the domestic goat after Endobronchial infection with Mycobacterium Caprae. Clin Vaccine Immunol. 2011;18:1872–81.
18. Wilton S, Cousins D. Detection and identification of multiple mycobacterial pathogens by DNA amplification in a single tube. Genome Res. 1992;1:269–73.
19. Kamerbeek J, Schouls L, Kolk A, van Agterveld M, van Soolingen D, Kuijper S, Bunschoten A, Molhuizen H, Shaw R, Goyal M, van Embden J. Simultaneous detection and strain differentiation of mycobacterium tuberculosis for diagnosis and epidemiology. J Clin Microbiol. 1997;35:907–14.
20. Gormley E, Corner LAL. Control of tuberculosis in badgers by vaccination: where next? Vet J. 2011;189:239–41.

6

Evaluation of serological response to foot-and-mouth disease vaccination in BLV infected cows

Rodrigo Puentes[1*†], Laureana De Brun[1†], Agustina Algorta[1], Valeria Da Silva[1], Florencia Mansilla[3], Gustavo Sacco[4], Silvia Llambí[2] and Alejandra V. Capozzo[3,5]

Abstract

Background: Bovine Leukemia Virus (BLV) produces disorders on the immune system in naturally infected animals, which may counteract the development of immunity after vaccination. The aim of this study was to investigate whether healthy and BLV infected cattle elicited similar humoral responses after foot and mouth disease (FMD) immunization. In a field study, 35 Holstein heifers were selected based on their BLV serological status and immunized with a single dose of a commercial bivalent oil-based FMD vaccine. Serum samples were collected at 0, 15, 60, 165 and 300 days post vaccination (dpv).

Results: Total anti-A24/Cruzeiro antibodies, IgM, IgG1, IgG2 titers and avidity index of specific antibodies were determined by ELISA. Although only marginally significant differences were found between groups in terms of total antibodies, anti-FMD IgM and IgG1 titers were significantly lower in heifers infected with BLV at the 15 dpv ($p < 0.01$). Animals that became infected during the study did not show differences to the BLV negative group.

Conclusions: Cattle infected with BLV at the time of immunization may elicit a low-magnitude serological response to a commercial Foot-and-mouth disease vaccine.

Keywords: Immune response, BLV, Serology, FMD, Immunization, Dairy cattle

Background

Enzootic bovine leucosis is a contagious disease of cattle induced by an exogenous retrovirus, bovine leukemia virus (BLV). It is worldwide distributed and only 20 countries had been able to eradicate the disease. Approximately 60 % of infected animals do not display clinical signs of disease, and these animals are referred to as asymptomatic or aleukemic. Approximately 30–40 % of BLV carriers will develop a persistent lymphocytosis, while fewer than 5 % develop malignant lymphosarcoma [1].

BLV positive animals at early stages of infection develop a cellular response mediated mainly by T helper 1 lymphocytes (Th1) producing IL-2, IL-12 and IFN-γ. Disease progression, together with persistent lymphocytosis produces changes on the T-cells profile towards a Th2 response [2]. In this phase, there is a dramatic increase in the B-lymphocyte populations and a decrease in the percentages of both CD4+ and CD8+ T lymphocytes [3]. The altered cytokine production was suggested to be responsible for the suppressed mitogen-induced T lymphocyte proliferation in BLV-infected animals [3, 4].

Current literature discuses if these BLV-induced immune mechanisms have a detrimental impact on the ability of cattle to resist the progression of infectious disease [5–7]. Considering that BLV is endemic in many countries and approximately 60 % of the animals are asymptomatic, it is important to know how BLV infection interacts with the immunogenicity of those vaccines usually used in bovines. An early study reported a possible impairment of immune responses against rotavirus in BLV-positive animals [8]. Recently, Erskine et al. [1] verified that dairy cows that were infected with BLV had decreased antibody responses to J5 *E. coli* bacterin as compared to non-infected cows.

* Correspondence: rpuentes@adinet.com.uy
†Equal contributors
[1]Immunology Area - Department of Microbiological Sciences, Faculty of Veterinary, University of the Republic (UdelaR), Montevideo, Uruguay
Full list of author information is available at the end of the article

Foot and mouth disease (FMD) is a highly contagious acute vesicular viral disease that affects cloven-hoofed animals and is mainly controlled by vaccination. The circulation of FMD virus (FMDV) in susceptible livestock imposes severe restrictions on the movement and trade of animals and derived products, causing serious economic loss to the affected countries [9]. FMD is endemic in many parts of Asia, Africa, and South America, where vaccination of susceptible populations is widely used as a major control measure. Commercial formulations usually contain more than one virus strain, as immune responses induced by vaccination are strain-specific [10]. Protection is mediated by specific antibodies. IgG1 has been related with protection in vaccinated cattle [11–14] while IgM mediates protection in naïve-infected cattle [15]. Maintaining high levels of total antibodies against FMDV is paramount to prevent outbreaks, keeping the OIE free-with-vaccination status and thus, the international markets.

There is no information on how the application of FMD vaccine in BLV infected animals may interfere with the immune response against FMDV. Considering the critical role that T- and B-cell populations play in humoral immunity and the immune-modulation caused by BLV in cattle, the purpose of this study was to investigate whether BLV natural infection may counteract the serological response to FMD primo- vaccination.

Methods

Animals

Thirty-five animals 6 to 10 months old Heifers were selected from a herd of 73 heifers according to their BLV antibodies status measured by ELISA twice (4 weeks and 1 week) before vaccination against FMD. The animals had not received anti-FMDV vaccine until the beginning of the experiment. They received one dose of FMD vaccine throughout the study, corresponding to FMD vaccination campaign of February 2014. Animals were housed in the same farm situated in the Department of Florida-Uruguay.

Vaccine

A commercial oil-adjuvanted (water-in-oil) vaccine against FMD was used in this study. This is an oil-adjuvanted vaccine that contains two inactivated FMDV strains: O1/Campos and A24/Cruzeiro, produced by a Paraguayan manufacturer. This vaccine was approved by the "Ministerio de Ganadería Agricultura y Pesca" (MGAP) according to the current national regulations of Uruguay.

Experimental design

The selected heifers were divided into 2 groups: BLV seropositive (BLV+, $n = 20$) and BLV seronegative (BLV–, $n = 10$). There were 5 seronegative animals at the day of vaccination (Day 0) seroconverted throughout the study, they were considered in a third group: Seroconverted (SC). Furthermore, all seropositive animals were tested by hemogram in peripheral blood mononuclear cell (PBMC) to detect leukocytosis or lymphocytosis at the beginning of the experiment using the protocol described by Marshak et al. [16]. All the selected animals were negative against anti FMDV antibodies at 0 dpv (liquid phase blocking ELISA titers ≤ 1.5).

All animals received one dose of 3 mL of FMD vaccine applied subcutaneously in the left side of the neck, according to current regulation in Uruguay [17]. Serum samples (2 aliquots of 2 mL each per animal) obtained at 0, 15, 60, 165 and 300 dpv were stored at −20 °C for further serological assessments.

BLV antibody detection by ELISA

A commercial kit was used for detection of BLV specific antibodies in bovine sera (IDEXX, REF P02110-10 LOT 4155 N, The Netherlands. Samples were processed according to manufacturer's instructions and the reading was performed at 450 nm in a visible range spectrophotometer (Thermo Fisher Scientific Inc., USA). Two weak positive controls were used per plate and interpretation was made according to manufacturer's protocol.

Liquid phase blocking ELISA (LPBE)

Total anti-FMDV A24/Cruzeiro antibody responses were assessed in serum samples by LPBE performed as stated by the OIE Manual using a rabbit antiserum to capture inactivated whole 140S viral particles, and a guinea-pig antiserum as detector antibody, both of them strain-specific as described before [18]. Antibody titers were expressed as the reciprocal Log10 of serum dilutions giving the 50 % of the absorbance recorded in the virus control wells without serum.

Single dilution avidity ELISA

Avidity assessment of specific antibodies was performed at 15 dpv as described before [12]. The Avidity Index (AI) was calculated as the percentage of residual activity of the serum sample after a 20 min urea washing step, relative to that of untreated sample: AI% = (OD sample with urea/OD sample without urea) × 100.

Isotype ELISAs

Isotype ELISAs were performed as reported before [12, 18] using HRP-conjugated antibodies anti IgG1 (1:750), IgG2 (1:750) and IgM (1:500) (AbD Serotec, Oxford, UK). Briefly, 96 well flat bottom well plates (MICROLON®, Greiner Bio-One, Monroe, NC) were coated with 50 µl per well of a dilution that contained 15 ng/well of sucrose-gradient purified FMDV 146S particles of A24 Cruzeiro strain, and blocked with dilution buffer. Individual serum samples were run in two-fold serial dilutions starting at 1:50. Titers were expressed as the inverse dilution reaching the cut off value (0.2) calculated as mean OD + 2SD achieved by the FMDV-negative Patagonian bovine serum samples ($n = 25$). Titers were expressed as the dilution factor reaching the cut-off value [12].

Data analysis

The "expected protection percentage" (EPP) was used as a reference to protective vaccine-induced responses. The EPP relates antibody titers measured by LPBE at 60 dpv, with the percentages of protection achieved for the same groups of animals after in vivo challenge experiments performed at 90 dpv following the "protection against generalized foot infection" (PGP) test. LPBE titers corresponding to EPP values = 75 % (EPP-75 %) are 1.90 for A24/Cruzeiro strain [19, 20].

Time-course titers obtained by LPBE, AI and IgG-subtype ELISAs were plotted and results between the three experimental groups were compared by ANOVA 2-factor repeated measures followed by Bonferroni multiple comparisons test. Mann-Whitney test was used when data from the groups were compared. The confidence interval was 95 %. Statistical analyses were carried out using GraphPad Prism v5.0 (GraphPad Software).

Results

Total antibodies against BLV and hemogram results

Groups BLV+ and BLV- remained seropositive and seronegative respectively, whereas the SC group seroconverted during the study between day 15 and 150 of the experiment (Fig. 1). Any animal showed leukocytosis or lymphocytosis at the beginning of the experiment, which was confirmed by hemogram in PBMC.

Total FMDV antibodies

LPBE kinetics curves were similar between the three groups up to day 300 of the assay. Total antibody titers increased after vaccination in all the animals and this difference was significant at 15 dpv for each group compared to titers measured at 0 dpv ($p <$ 0,01). After that, the titers decreased and remained at low levels up to the end of the experiment. Antibody levels fell below the EPP 75 %- protective levels for FMD after 60 dpv (Maradei, et al. [19]) (Fig. 2a). Total FMD LPBE titers 15 dpv were not significantly different between groups ($p > 0.05$), although titers were higher in the BLV-compared with BLV+ group (Fig. 3a).

Avidity indexes kinetic curves were comparable between the groups. Antibody avidity was boosted 15 dpv, and the tendency seemed to be higher for BLV-animals, however, though differences were not significant compared to BLV+ animals (Fig. 3e).

The SC group behaved as the BLV-animals, both for total antibodies and avidity.

Isotype responses

We then studied the isotype composition of the induced antibodies, to verify the primary (IgM) response and the switch towards IgG isotypes, indicative of T-cell collaboration. IgM, IgG1 and IgG2 titer against A24/Cruzeiro strain were measured in serum samples from the different groups along time.

An increase in IgM anti-FMDV serum titers was observed at 15 dpv in all groups, being significantly higher in BLV negative animals (Fig. 3c). IgG1 titers were also higher for BLV negative compared to BLV positive animals at 15 dpv ($p < 0{,}01$), with a mean titer of 287,1 y 127,8 respectively (Fig. 3b). At longer time-points, however, no significant differences were

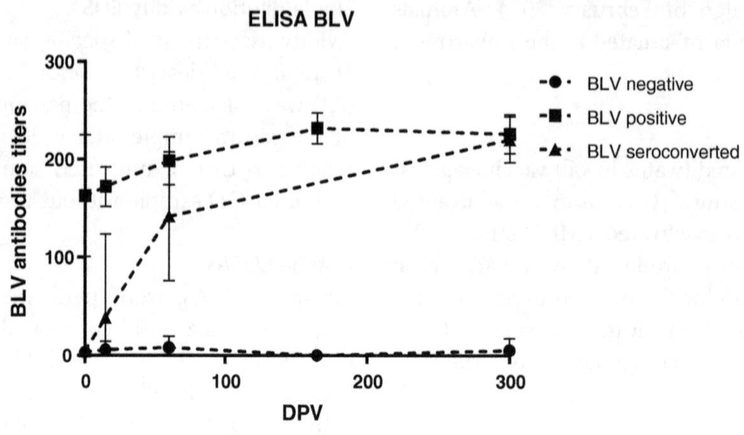

Fig. 1 Kinetics of BLV Ab titers of each group of animals throughout the study measured by indirect ELISA. Mean titers standard errors (SEM) are depicted. BLV – and BLV+ animals were negative and positive respectively throughout the experiment. The "BLV seroconverted" group corresponds to animals that were seronegative at the beginning of the experiment and became seropositive to BLV at 60 dpv

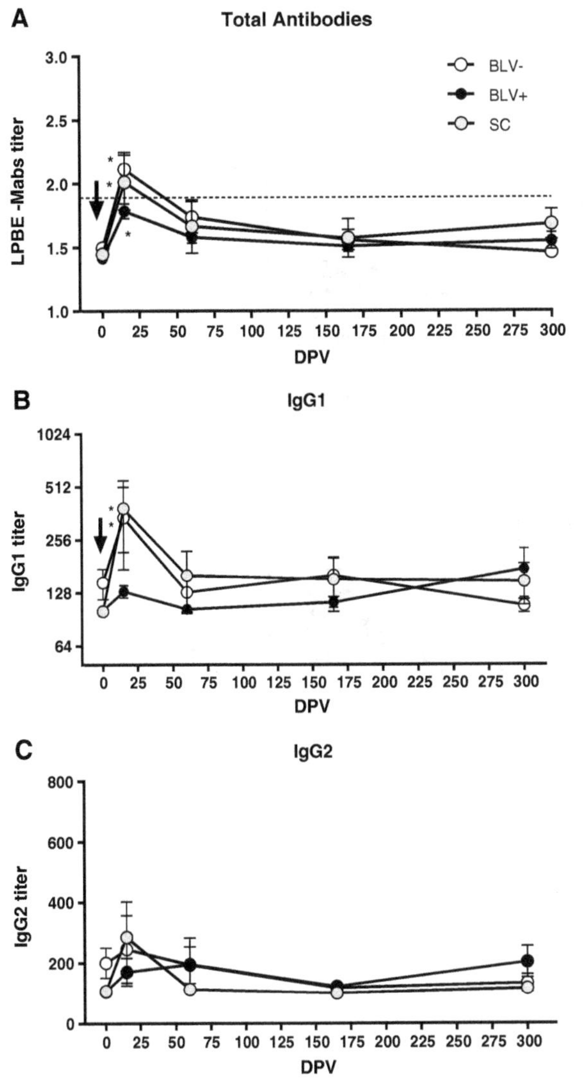

Fig. 2 Kinetics of antibody titers against A24/Cruzeiro strain in BLV seronegative (BLV-; $n = 10$; white circles), BLV seropositive (BLV+; $n = 20$; black circles) and seroconverted groups (SC; $n = 5$; gray circles). Mean titers standard errors (SEM) are depicted. A) Total antibody measured by LPBE. **a** titer of 1.90 (dotted line) is considered to be related to an EPP 75 % for A24/Cruzeiro strain. **b** IgG1 and **c** IgG2 measured by ELISA. All animals received one dose of a commercial bivalent FMD vaccine at 0 dpv. Titers against A24/Cruzeiro were significantly higher in all groups at 15 dpv compared to 0 dpv ($p < 0.01$)

detected (Fig. 2b). IgG2 titers and kinetics were similar in all groups (Fig. 2c). Higher antibody titers were observed at 15 dpv in BLV negative animals, with a mean titer of 229.3 compared with 174.6 of BLV positive animals (Fig. 3d), although this differences were not significant ($p > 0,05$). In all cases, the SC group behaved as the BLV-animals in terms of isotype responses.

Discussion

FMD has global consequences, costing an estimated USD \$6–\$21 billion each year in prevention expenditures and agricultural damage [9]. A significant portion of this cost is shouldered by the world's poorest countries, which experience major economic losses from trade restrictions [21]. Uruguay, a small country where the main economy comes from agriculture and depends heavily on the export of products of animal origin, was free from FMD without vaccination until 2000. Later, after clinical signs manifestations in cattle, government turned to compulsory vaccination in all the country. Uruguay is actually classified as free from FMD with vaccination and invests millions of dollars to assure the maintenance of the FMD-free status granted by the World Organization for Animal Health.

On the other hand, BLV is another main virosis of dairy cattle, produces chronic infections with high percentage of asymptomatic animals. BLV infection reduces expression of type 1 cytokines from CD4+ T lymphocytes, and cytokine profiles from all peripheral blood mononuclear cell populations, suggesting that both type I and II cytokines are altered with increases in IL10 and IL4, and decreases in IL2, IL12, and IFN-γ [5, 22]. The progression of BLV is also known to disrupt the homeostasis of lymphocyte proliferation and cell death, in both B-cells and T-cells [1, 3, 4, 6].

Here we evaluated if the application of a bivalent FMD vaccine in BLV infected animals modify the humoral responses against A24/Cruzeiro strain included in the FMD vaccine. The study was designed to assess the FMD responses to match the practical approach applied in the field, where the probability of heifers to be infected with BLV at the moment of vaccination is very high, mainly in Uruguay, where the seroprevalence may reach 77 % in dairy cattle [23].

FMD immune response to vaccination is currently assessed using Liquid phase blocking ELISA (LPBE), and there are published curves relating LPBE titers with protection. An EPP of 75 % has been estimated to correspond to LPBE titers equal to 1.90 for A24/Cruzeiro strain [19, 20]. The animals included in this study presented low levels of antibody titers between 1.4 and 1.5 for A24/Cruzeiro at Day 0 of assay. This basal response could be associated to maternal antibodies transferred by colostrum because animals used were from 6 months age [24]. Even though, this response would not be interfering with oil emulsified vaccine applied in this assay [25].

After vaccination, every animal seroconverted at 15 dpv, with an average titer of 1.76 and 2.12 in BLV+ and BLV−, respectively. Although a greater response in non-infected heifers with titers higher than 1.90 (EPP of 75 %) was observed, this difference was not significant

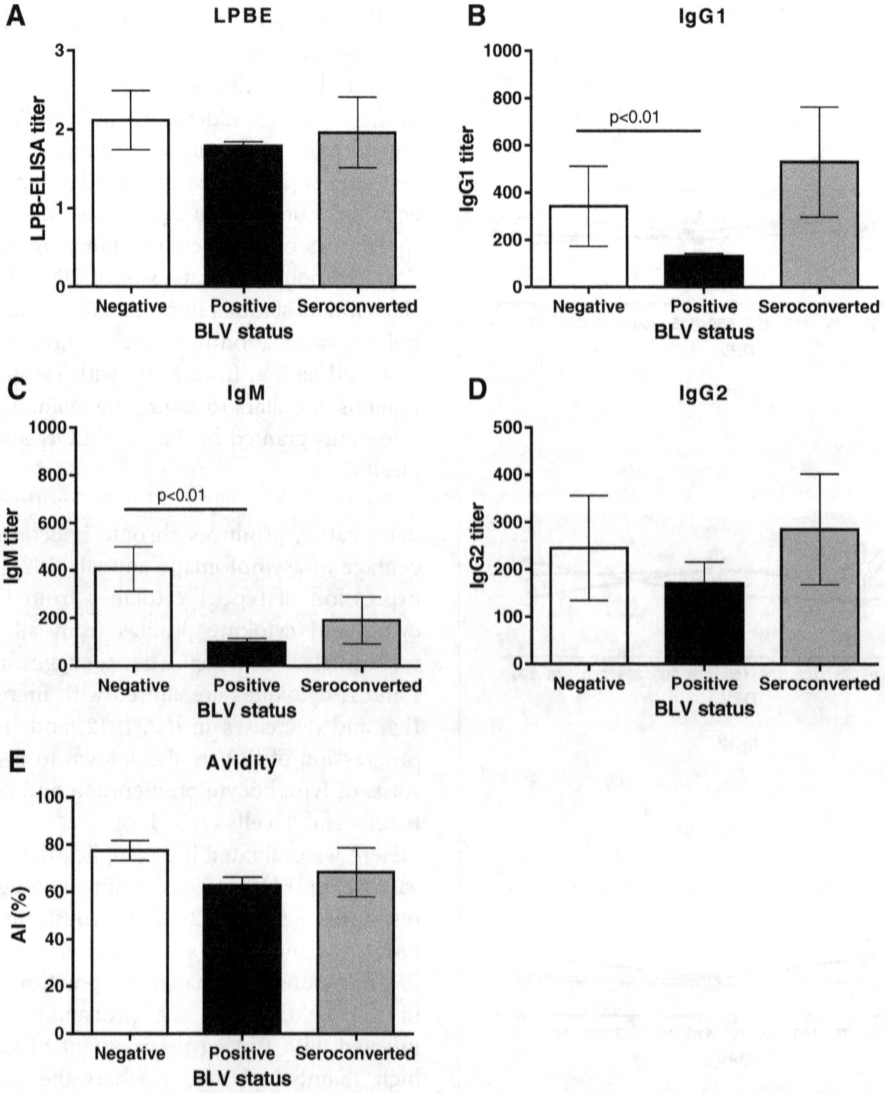

Fig. 3 Comparison of LPBE (**a**), isotypes (IgG1, (**b**) IgM, (**c**) and IgG2, (**d**) and avidity index (**e**) against A24/Cruzeiro strain for (BLV-; $n = 10$; white columns), BLV seropositive (BLV+; $n = 20$; black columns) and seroconverted groups (SC; $n = 5$; gray columns) at day 15 post vaccination. Mean titers ± standard errors (SEM) are depicted. All animals received one dose of a commercial bivalent FMD vaccine at 0 dpv. IgM and IgG1 against A24/Cruzeiro were significantly higher in BLV − compared to BLV + at 15 dpv ($p < 0.01$, Mann-Whitney test)

between groups ($p > 0.05$). After this period, a sharp decrease in antibody titers in all groups was observed at day 60, up to levels below 75 % of EPP and then remained low until the end of the experiment (Fig. 2). Based on these results and independently from BLV status of heifers, the single dose vaccination applied in this experiment was not enough to maintain animals with acceptable levels of protective antibody titers against FMD A24/Cruzeiro strain. Although an approved commercial vaccine was used and applied according to recommendations of the Uruguayan animal health authorities, the quality of this vaccine at the exact time it was applied could not be assessed by our working group, in terms of antigen payload and integrity of 140S particles, known to be essential for protection [26]. Thus, the data analyzed here correspond to the effect of a vaccine that elicits a short coverage of circulating antibodies within protective levels.

Analysis of the isotypes of the response induced against A24/Cruzeiro revealed that IgM, IgG1 and IgG2 titers increased in both BLV-and BLV+ heifers following FMD immunization, although IgM and IgG1 titers were higher in the BLV negative heifers. Levels of IgG2 can explain why the difference in antibody titers was only marginally significant when total antibodies were measured. On the other hand, while we found that the avidity index was lower in seropositive animals than that seronegative, these differences were not significant

(Fig. 3e). The avidity index and IgM titers were measured only 15 dpv because these decreases rapidly according to previous reports from some researchers from our group (Lavoria et al. [12]).

It is important to note that peak titers of both IgM and IgG1 may not reflect, however, the true course of the kinetics of the immune response, as many time points are missing. Higher IgM titers have been reported to take place about 7 to 10 dpv while IgG1 peak may be expected at 15–20 dpv [15, 18]. Thus, we cannot rule out if we had either a typical primary-secondary response, with a first boost of IgM followed by a delayed increase of IgG; or if a T-independent response was induced in both cases, though with lower magnitude in BLV-infected animals.

We hypothesize that, if we consider the first scenario, the immune-modulation exerted on the T lymphocytes in BLV-infected animals may account for the lower magnitude of the IgG1 anti FMDV-response. Alternations in cytokine expression have been shown to be correlated with disease progression in chronic retroviral infections, suggesting that cytokine imbalances may contribute to disease progressions [2]. Pyeon et al. [27] found that the production of Th1 cytokine was promoted in the first stage of the BLV infection (serologically positive without persistent lymphocytosis) than that in cattle with progressed disease stages with persistent lymphocytosis. It has also been shown that IgG1 expression is positively regulated by IL-4 and IgG2 expression is positively t regulated by IFN-gamma [28]. So, considering that the animals used in our study were young heifers that didn have persistent lymphocytosis at the beginning of the experiment and were probably in the early phase of infection (Th1 profile), we think that may have influenced immunoglobulin subclass switch. Further experiments are needed to support this hypothesis.

Animals that were infected with BLV between 15 to 60 dpv ("BLV seroconverted" group), did not show any difference with respect to BLV negative animals, indicating that only a pre-existing BLV infection modified the isotypes of antibodies against FMD induced by vaccination. This study is another contribution to the effect that BLV may have on immunization with commonly used vaccines. In this regard, Erskine et al. [1] also found differences on titer of BLV antibodies in infected cows when they were vaccinated against J5 *E. coli.*

Conclusions

Our data suggests that BLV infection in dairy cattle may modify the profile of antibody response to immunization against Foot-and-mouth disease. IgM and IgG1 titers were significantly lower in heifers infected with BLV at the 15 dpv ($p < 0.01$). More studies using vaccines of different potency are needed to dissect the role of BLV infection on the efficacy of Foot-and-mouth disease primo-vaccination.

Abbreviations

AI, Avidity Index; BLV, Bovine Leukemia Virus; dpv, days post vaccination; EPP, Expected protection percentage; FMD, Foot-and-mouth disease; FMDV, Foot-and-mouth disease virus; LPBE, Liquid phase blocking ELISA; MGAP, Ministerio de Ganadería Agricultura y Pesca; SC, Seroconverted; Th1, T helper 1 lymphocytes

Acknowledgements

We thank the personal of the "Campo de Recría La Cruz" (Florida, Uruguay) for the field activities support. We are also thankful to Dr. Mariano Perez Filgueira for helpful discussion and also Veterinarians Sebastián Di Giácomo and María Eugenia Quintana for technical assistance.

Funding

The scholarships, experimental and laboratory procedures for the study presented in this paper were funded by Fondo Sectorial Salud Animal (FSSA) de la Agencia Nacional de Investigación e Innovación - ANII (FSSA_X_2014_1_105283), Comisión Sectorial de Investigación Científica - UdelaR (INI_X_2013_1_10100), ANII (POS_NAC_2015_1_109630) and Veterinary Research Center of Instituto Nacional de Tecnología Agropecuaria (INTA) - Castelar - Argentina.

Authors' contributions

Conceived and designed the experiments: RP, LDB, AA and SL. Performed the experiments: RP, LDB, AA, VDS, GS, FM and AVC. Analyzed the data: AVC. Wrote the manuscript: RP, LDB, AA and AVC. All authors read and approved the final manuscript.

Competing interests

The authors declare that they have no competing interests.

Consent for publication

Not applicable.

Author details

[1]Immunology Area - Department of Microbiological Sciences, Faculty of Veterinary, University of the Republic (UdelaR), Montevideo, Uruguay. [2]Genetics Area, Faculty of Veterinary, University of the Republic (UdelaR), Montevideo, Uruguay. [3]Centre of Veterinary Sciences and Agronomic Investigations, INTA, Virology Institute, Buenos Aires, Argentina. [4]Independent Veterinary Practice, Florida, Uruguay. [5]CONICET – National Council of Scientific and Technological Research, Buenos Aires, Argentina.

References

1. Erskine RJ, Bartlett PC, Sabo KM, Sordillo LM. Bovine leukemia virus infection in dairy cattle: effect on serological response to immunization against J5 Escherichia coli bacterin. Vet Med Int. 2011;3:915747.
2. Kabeya H, Ohashi K, Onuma M. Host immune responses in the course of bovine leukemia virus infection. J Vet Med Sci. 2001;63(7):703–8.
3. Sordillo LM, Hicks CR, Pighetti MG. Altered interleukin-2 production by lymphocyte populations from bovine leukemia virus-infected cattle. Proc Soc Exp Biol Med. 1994;207(3):268–73.
4. Stone DM, Hof AJ, Davis WC. Up-regulation of IL-2 receptor α and MHC class II expression on lymphocyte subpopulations from bovine leukemia virus infected lymphocytotic cows. Vet Immunol Immunopathol. 1995;48(1–2):65–76.
5. Konnai S, Usui T, Ohashi K, Onuma M. The rapid quantitative analysis of bovine cytokine genes by real-time RTPCR. Vet Microbiol. 2003;94(4):283–94.

6. Tyler JW, Cullor JS, Dellinger JD. Cross-reactive affinity purification of immunoglobulin recognizing common gram-negative bacterial core antigens. J Immunol Methods. 1990;129(2):221–6.
7. Florins A, Boxus M, Vandermeers F, Verlaeten O, Bouzar AB, Defoiche J, et al. Emphasis on cell turnover in two hosts infected by bovine leukemia virus: a rationale for host susceptibility to disease. Vet Immunol Immunopathol. 2008;125(1–2):1–7.
8. Archambault D, Morin G, Elazhary MA. Possible impairment of rotavirus immune response in cattle infected with BLV. Vet Rec. 1989;124(21): 570–2.
9. Smith MT, Bennett AM, Grubman MJ, Bundy BC. Foot-and-mouth disease: technical and political challenges to eradication. Vaccine. 2014;32(31):3902–8.
10. Doel TR. FMD vaccines. Virus Res. 2003;91(1):81–99.
11. Capozzo AV, Periolo OH, Robiolo B, Seki C, La Torre JL, Grigera PR. Total and isotype humoral responses in cattle vaccinated with foot and mouth disease virus (FMDV) immunogen produced either in bovine tongue tissue or in BHK-21 cell suspension cultures. Vaccine. 1997;15(6–7):624–30.
12. Lavoria MA, Di-Giacomo S, Bucafusco D, Franco-Mahecha OL, Perez-Filgueira DM, Capozzo AV. Avidity and subtyping of specific antibodies applied to the indirect assessment of heterologous protection against foot-and-mouth disease virus in cattle. Vaccine. 2012;30(48):6845–50.
13. Brito BP, Rodriguez LL, Hammond JM, Pinto J, Perez AM. Review of the Global distribution of foot-and-mouth disease virus from 2007 to 2014. Transbound Emerg Dis. 2015. doi:10.1111/tbed.12373.
14. Pega J, Di Giacomo S, Bucafusco D, Schammas JM, Malacari D, Barrionuevo F, et al. Systemic foot-and-mouth disease vaccination in cattle promotes specific antibody-secreting cells at the respiratory tract and triggers local anamnestic responses upon aerosol infection. J Virol. 2015;89(18):9581–90.
15. Pega J, Bucafusco D, Di Giacomo S, Schammas JM, Malacari D, Capozzo AV, et al. Early adaptive immune responses in the respiratory tract of foot-and-mouth disease virus-infected cattle. J Virol. 2013;87(5):2489–95.
16. Marshak RR. Criteria for the determination of the normal and leukotic state in cattle. J Natl Cancer Inst. 1968;41:243–63.
17. Ministerio de Ganadería agricultura y Pesca (MGAP). Legislación Sanitaria Animal. Available at: http://www.mgap.gub.uy/portal/page.aspx?2,dgsg,dgsg-legislacion-sanitaria,O,es,0. Accessed 08 Dec 2015.
18. Bucafusco D, Di Giacomo S, Pega J, Juncos MS, Schammas JM, Perez-Filgueira M, et al. Influence of antibodies transferred by colostrum in the immune responses of calves to current foot-and-mouth disease vaccines. Vaccine. 2014;32(48):6576–82.
19. Maradei E, La Torre J, Robiolo B, Esteves J, Seki C, Pedemonte A, et al. Updating of the correlation between lpELISA titers and protection from virus challenge for the assessment of the potency of polyvalent aphtovirus vaccines in Argentina. Vaccine. 2008;26(51):6577–86.
20. Robiolo B, La Torre J, Duffy S, Leon E, Seki C, Torres A, et al. Quantitative single serum-dilution liquid phase competitive blocking ELISA for the assessment of herd immunity and expected protection against foot-and-mouth disease virus in vaccinated cattle. J Virol Methods. 2010;166:21–7.
21. Trotta M, Lahore J, Cardoso N, Melucci O, Catena M, et al. Simultaneous immunization of cattle with foot-and-mouth disease (FMD) and live anthrax vaccines do not interfere with FMD booster responses. Trials Vaccinol. 2015;4:38–42.
22. Amills M, Norimine J, Olmstead CA, Lewin HA. Cytokine mRNA expression in B cells from bovine leukemia virus-infected cattle with persistent lymphocytosis. Cytokine. 2004;28(1):25–8.
23. Furtado A, Rosadilla D, Franco G, Piaggio J, Puentes R. Leucosis Bovina Enzoótica en cuencas lecheras de productores familiares del Uruguay. Veterinaria. 2013;191:29–37.
24. World Organization for Animal Health (OIE). Foot and mouth disease. In: Terrestrial animal health code. Paris: OIE; 2014. Available at: http://www.oie.int/index.php?id=169&L=0&htmfile=chapitre_fmd.htm. Accessed 07 Dec 2015.
25. Patil PK, Sajjanar CM, Natarajan C, Bayry J. Neutralizing antibody responses to foot-and-mouth disease quadrivalent (type O, A, C and Asia 1) vaccines in growing calves with pre-existing maternal antibodies. Vet Microbiol. 2014;169(3–4):233–5.
26. Bucafusco D, Di Giacomo S, Pega J, Schammas JM, Cardoso N, Capozzo AV, et al. Foot-and-mouth disease vaccination induces cross-reactive IFN-γ responses in cattle that are dependent on the integrity of the 140S particles. Virology. 2015;476:11–8.
27. Pyeon D, Splitter GA. Interleukin-12 p40 mRNA expression in bovine leukemia virus-infected animals: increase in alymphocytosis but decrease in persistent lymphocytosis. J Virol. 1998;72(8):6917–21.
28. Estes DM, Brown WC. Type 1 and type 2 responses in regulation of Ig isotype expression in cattle. Vet Immunol Immunopathol. 2002;90(1–2):1–10.

7

Methodology for the assessment of brucellosis management practices and its vaccination campaign: example in two Argentine districts

M.N. Aznar[1,2*], M. Arregui[1], M.F. Humblet[3], L.E. Samartino[1] and C. Saegerman[2]

Abstract

Background: In Argentina, vaccination with *Brucella abortus* Strain 19 vaccine is mandatory. The objective of the study was to develop and test a method for evaluating, in an innovative way, some farmers' and veterinarians' management practices in relation to brucellosis and to assess the vaccination campaign and coverage. The work took place in Brandsen and Navarro districts. Four questionnaires were designed (for officials from Local Sanitary Entities, vaccinators, vet practitioners and farmers). Responses were coded as "ideal" (0) and "not ideal" (1). To assess the relative weight of each question ("item"), experts ranked the items according to their impact on management practices and vaccination. A weighted score was then calculated. A higher weighted score was assigned to the worse practices. Farmers obtaining a global weighted score above the third quartile were classified as "inappropriately managed farms", to be compared per type of production system and district. To assess the immunization coverage, female calves were sampled 30 to 50 days post vaccination; they were expected to react positively to serological diagnostic tests (DT+).

Results: There were significantly more inappropriately managed farms and higher global scores among beef farmers and in Brandsen. Eighty three percent (83%) of female calves were DT+, significantly under the ideal immunization coverage (95%). Only 48% of farms were considered well vaccinated. DT+ results were positively associated with the Brandsen district (OR = 25.94 [4.60–1146.21] and with the farms having more than 200 cow heads ((OR = 78.34 [4.09–1500.00]). On the contrary, DT+ were less associated with vaccinators being veterinary practitioners (OR = 0.07 [0.006–0.78]). Farmers are well advised by their veterinary practitioners but they should improve some management practices.

Conclusions: The vaccination campaign is globally well implemented, but the immunization coverage and some vaccinators' practices should be improved.
This study leads to a better understanding of the most common used management and control practices regarding brucellosis, which affect its epidemiology. Any vaccination campaign should be periodically assessed to highlight possible fails. The described methodology can be extrapolated to other countries and different contexts.

Keywords: Bovine brucellosis, Vaccination campaign, Management practices, Immunization coverage, Argentina

* Correspondence: aznar.maria@inta.gob.ar
[1]Instituto de Patobiología, INTA, CICVyA, Hurlingham, PC 1688 Buenos Aires, Argentina
[2]Research Unit of Epidemiology and Risk Analysis applied to veterinary sciences (UREAR-ULg), Center for Fundamental and Applied Research for Animal and Health (FARAH), Faculty of Veterinary Medicine, University of Liege, PC 4000 Liege, Belgium
Full list of author information is available at the end of the article

Background

Brucellosis is one of the most widespread zoonoses throughout the world. It is caused by various bacteria from the genus *Brucella* which mainly affects cattle, goats, pigs, sheep and also some other species. It leads to abortion, later permanently reduced fertility, and chronically lowered milk yields in affected animals. It can be transmitted to people via direct contact with livestock or through consuming unpasteurized milk and dairy products from an infected animal.

In cattle, brucellosis is predominantly caused by *Brucella abortus*; it is usually detected in aborting females [1] which may remain infected for their entire life. Prevalence of animal infections determines the incidence of human cases [2]. Therefore, the elimination of brucellosis from the animal compartments results in a substantially reduced incidence of the disease in humans [2, 3].

In cattle, the vaccination with *Brucella abortus* Strain 19 and RB 51 is the most successful method for preventing and controlling the infection, whereas eradication can only be achieved by applying the "test and slaughter" strategy, combined with effective preventive measures such as biosecurity and control of animal movements [2]. The implementation of an effective surveillance system, with an adequate laboratory support, is one of the crucial factors to achieve eradication [4].

In Argentina, bovine brucellosis is endemic. Up to the year 2002, most cattle isolates corresponded to *Brucella abortus* biovar 1 (epitope A dominant); however, *Brucella abortus* biovar 2 (epitope A dominant) was also reported [5]. The predominant biovar has remained stable in the country so far [6].

The disease is more controlled in dairy farms than in beef holdings because milk coming from holdings certified as Officially Brucellosis-Free is better valued by the industry. On the contrary, no compensation is provided to non-there is an unnecessary space Officially Brucellosis-Free beef farms [6]. Approximately 60% of the 6500 dairy farms are Officially Brucellosis-Free. Regarding beef, 12% (95% CI: 10% - 14%) of the 180,000 farms and 0.8% (95% CI: 0.5% - 1.05%) of the 46,000,000 cattle are infected (SENASA, unpublished data). Between 6 and 7 million of female calves are mandatorily vaccinated with Strain 19 every year.

Some methodology for assessing the farmers' and veterinarians' behavior concerning the disease and for evaluating its vaccination campaign should be developed to improve the surveillance system. To our knowledge, there are not many studies suggesting any methodology regarding this issue.

Therefore, the objective of this study was to develop and test a method for evaluating, in an innovative way, some farmers' and veterinarians' management practices in relation to brucellosis and for assessing the vaccination campaign and coverage in order to detect fails of the National Plan for the Control and Eradication of Bovine Brucellosis. We worked in two districts of the Buenos Aires province, Brandsen and Navarro.

Methods

National Plan for the control and eradication of bovine brucellosis in Argentina

The National Plan for the Control and Eradication of Bovine Brucellosis establishes the individual identification and mandatory sub-cutaneous vaccination of all 3 to 8 month-old females with 15–30 × 10^9 viable *Brucella abortus* Strain 19 in 2 ml-doses (SENASA, 2002). The vaccine must be controlled and approved by the National Service for Agrifood Health and Quality (SENASA). Every vaccinated female must be permanently identified (ear tags are commonly used).

SENASA entrusts the implementation of the vaccination campaign to 310 Local Sanitary Entities (LSEs). The LSEs are institutions gathering representatives of farmers and animal health institutions (including veterinarians from SENASA and other institutions playing a local role). Each district implements its own local vaccination plan, according to the SENASA general strategy, which is thus adjusted to the different regional realities. The LSEs are responsible for planning, implementing and assessing local vaccination campaigns, which must comply with the SENASA set of rules, and target a large immunization coverage within short periods of time. To achieve that goal, LSEs vaccinators (either vet practitioners or non-veterinarians) are registered and trained by the SENASA. Each entity, under the supervision of a SENASA veterinarian, manages the vaccine supply at a local level. In most cases, foot-and-mouth disease and brucellosis vaccines are administered together. The vaccines are paid by the farmers [6]. The SENASA controls the entire immunization process.

Area of study and selection of participants

This cross-sectional descriptive study covered two districts in the province of Buenos Aires, Argentina: Brandsen and Navarro (Fig. 1). Brandsen has a total of 625 bovine farms and Navarro has 648 farms (SENASA, personal communication). These districts were selected because they represent well the type of bovine production in the province and because people in charge of LSEs agreed to collaborate in the implementation of the field work. Four different types of actors (LSEs officials, vaccinators, vet practitioners and farmers) who play a key role in the immunization campaign and/or the management practices were randomly selected to be interviewed face-to-face by the corresponding author (n = 142). There was not a statistical design for computing the number of responses to be part of the study. However, 10% of farmers were expected to be interviewed. Answers were obtained upon grounds of convenience.

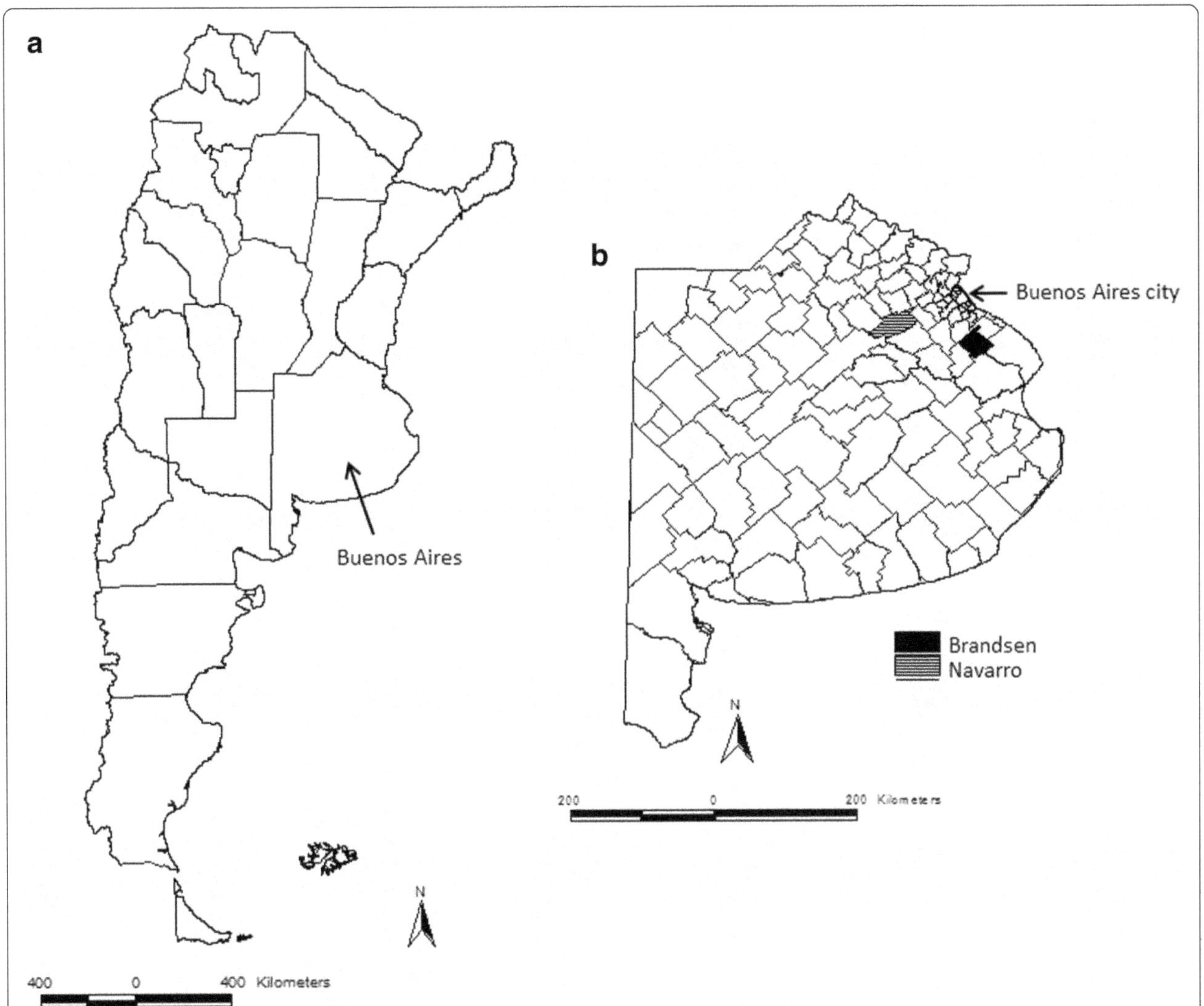

Fig. 1 Maps showing the boundaries of Argentina and its provinces (on the left) (**a**), as well as Brandsen and Navarro districts (study area), in the province of Buenos Aires (on the right) (**b**)

Questionnaires design

A questionnaire for each type of actor was designed. Questionnaires had between 6 and 18 questions ("items") with closed dichotomous answers (Tables 1, 2, 3 and 4). Possible answers for each item were coded as "ideal" (code = 0) and "not ideal" (code = 1). Besides, vet practitioners' personal opinions on vaccination aspects were recorded.

Global weighted scores

To assess the relative weight of each item, a panel of Argentine experts (n = 5) in the field of brucellosis and Sanitary Policies were consulted. They were asked to distribute a total of 100 points among the items under study, for each type of actor, on the basis of the impact they can have on the brucellosis managing practices and effectiveness of the vaccination campaign. The parameter with major impact received the maximum of points. The average of points allocated by the experts to each item was divided by the total of points (n = 100) to obtain a weighted factor. Then, a weighted score was calculated for each item through multiplying the code (1 or 0) by the weighting factor. A higher weighted score was related to worse managing and vaccinating practices. A global weighted score was obtained by adding up each weighted score per respondent.

Farmers obtaining a global weighted score above the third quartile were classified as "inappropriately-managed farms", since the authors fixed a threshold of 75% of ideal answers for the appropriate managed farms. The distribution of inappropriately-managed farms was compared per type of production (dairy vs. beef) and district (Brandsen vs. Navarro).

Some questions were used to compare both districts and production systems, but no comparison with the ideal answers (based on experts' opinion) was carried out.

Table 1 Farmers' questionnaire

Items	Answers		Experts' opinion		Weighting
	Ideal	Not ideal	Average [A]	CV	Weighted Factor [B]
Identification of all vaccinated females	Yes	No	6.4	0.699	0.064
Identification of females unvaccinated due to their age (< 3 months)	Yes	No	3.4	0.609	0.034
Coverage per farm	95%–100%	<95%	16.4	0.372	0.164
Existence of reproductive records in the farm	Yes	No	4.0	0.306	0.040
Diagnostic of abortions, placental retentions or no-pregnancy	Yes	No	8.8	0.478	0.088
Isolation of animals with reproductive disorders consistent with brucellosis	Yes	No	10.2	0.497	0.102
Sale of animals with clinical signs of brucellosis	Yes	No	12.0	0.343	0.120
Destination of the animals sold with clinical signs of brucellosis	Slaughterhouse	Other destination	3.6	1.168	0.036
Purchase of cattle from Officially Brucellosis-Free farms	Yes	No	11.0	0.497	0.110
At purchase: brucellosis serological testing of females >18 months and males 6 months	Yes	No	11.0	0.203	0.110
Isolation of purchased cattle	Yes	No	5.6	0.763	0.056
Isolation of calving cows	Yes	No	5.6	0.508	0.056
Isolation of primiparous cows	Yes	No	2.0	1.514	0.020

Legend: *CV* = coefficient of variation [A] Average of points distributed by the experts, per item. [B] Weighted factor per item. This value was obtained after dividing [A] by the total of points distributed by each expert (100 points). The sum of all weighted items equals 1

List of items, possible answers, experts' opinion and weighting

Table 2 Vet practitioners' questionnaire

Items	Answers		Experts' opinion		Weighting
	Ideal	Not ideal	Average [A]	CV	Weighted Factor [B]
The veterinarian suggests a brucellosis serological diagnostic test in case of abortions	Yes	No	105.0	0.199	0.210
The veterinarian suggests a brucellosis serological test in case of retained placenta, no-pregnancy or calf/calves born weak	Yes	No	100.0	0.176	0.200
The veterinarian suggests a brucellosis serological test in case of orchitis or epididymitis in males	Yes	No	63.0	0.407	0.126
The veterinarian suggests quarantine for purchased cattle	Yes	No	77.0	0.374	0.154
The veterinarian suggests a brucellosis serological test when purchasing females >18 months and males >6 months	Yes	No	120.0	0.093	0.240
The veterinarian performs a brucellosis serological test before selling cattle for reproductive reasons	Yes	No	35.0	0.391	0.070

Legend: *CV* = coefficient of variation [A] Average of points distributed by the experts, per item. [B] Weighted factor per item. This value was obtained after dividing [A] by the total of points distributed by each expert (100 points). The sum of all weighted items equals 1
List of items, possible answers, experts' opinion and weighting

Immunization coverage

To evaluate the compliance of vaccination field practices with SENASA regulations, serum samples of a subgroup of the farms were randomly taken from female calves, 30 to 50 days post vaccination (DPV), during the 2014-autumn brucellosis vaccination campaign. Sample size for number of female calves per farm was computed assuming a 10% relative error with a 95% confidence interval and a 95% of vaccinated cattle, which would be expected in a mandatory immunization campaign. A total of 20 female calves per farm (or all of them if less than 20 calves were vaccinated) fulfilled the previous

Table 3 Vaccinators' questionnaire

Items	Answers		Experts' opinion		Weighting
	Ideal	Not ideal	Total [A]	CV	Weighted Factor [B]
Checking of the vaccine expiration date before its use	Yes	No	38.0	0.547	0.076
A different syringe is used for Brucellosis and foot-and-mouth vaccines	Yes	No	31.0	0.447	0.062
There must be vacuum in the flask containing the lyophilized product	Yes	No	36.0	0.432	0.072
Softly shake of the vaccine flask after adding the diluent to the lyophilized product	Yes	No	34.0	0.351	0.068
Make sure there is no air in the syringe before injecting the vaccine	Yes	No	29.0	0.446	0.058
Frequency at which air verification is performed	Each time it is uploaded	Other	17.0	0.675	0.034
The needle is changed between farms	Yes	No	38.0	0.799	0.076
Syringe calibration	Yes	No	41.0	0.264	0.082
Frequency of syringe calibration	Each time it is uploaded	Other	21.0	0.547	0.042
Homogenization of the vaccine flask during vaccination	Yes	No	39.0	0.246	0.078
Frequency of vaccine homogenization	Each time it is uploaded	Other	16.0	0.978	0.032
Maximal delay for using the vaccine after adding the diluent to the lyophilized product	<5 h	Other	42.0	0.246	0.084
Vaccine storage place while vaccinating	In a cooled box, in the shade	Other	35.0	0.335	0.070
The vaccine is injected again if some of it drops after the first injection	Yes	No	23.0	0.6974	0.046
Vaccinators notice the double injections in the vaccination records	Yes	No	7.0	0.719	0.014
Future of empty vaccine flasks once vaccination is completed	LSEs	Other	10.0	0.692	0.020
The number of vaccinated females and doses used are recorded	n vaccinated females and doses used	Other	32.0	0.422	0.064
Vaccinators wear personal protective equipment (e.g. gloves, goggles, and overalls)	Yes	No	11.0	0.956	0.022

Legend: *CV* = coefficient of variation [A] Average of points distributed by the experts, per item. [B] Weighted factor per item. This value was obtained after dividing [A] by the total of points distributed by each expert (100 points). The sum of all weighted items equals 1
List of items, possible answers, experts' opinion and weighting

Table 4 Questionnaire for Local Sanitary Entities (LSE) officials

Items			Experts' opinion		Weighting
	Ideal	Not ideal	Total [A]	CV	Weighted Factor [B]
The LSE audits the vaccination process	Yes	No	51.0	0.107	0.102
Frequency of LSE audits	Twice per campaign	Other	35.0	0.484	0.070
Aspects audited by the LSE	All of them	None of them	37.0	0.377	0.074
The LSE advertises dates of the vaccination campaign beforehand	Yes	No	30.0	0.440	0.060
The LSE plans the date for vaccination with the farmers beforehand	Yes	No	36.0	0.432	0.072
The LSE controls the temperature at which the vaccine is supplied by the producing laboratories	Yes	No	50.0	0.353	0.100
Temperature at which the vaccine is stored at the LSE	2–8 ° C	Other	55.0	0.203	0.110
The LSE checks the temperature of the fridge in which the vaccines are stored	Yes	No	57.0	0.192	0.114
Frequency of temperature control	Twice a day	Other	37.0	0.454	0.074
The LSE supplies the vaccine to vaccinators in cooled boxes	Yes	No	55.0	0.240	0.110
The LSE receives the surplus of vaccine brought back by vaccinators by the end of the day	Yes	No	22.0	0.565	0.044
The LSE controls the temperature at which the vaccine surpluses are brought	Yes	No	35.0	0.404	0.070

Legend: *CV* = coefficient of variation [A] Average of points distributed by the experts, per item. [B] Weighted factor per item. This value was obtained after dividing [A] by the total of points distributed by each expert (100 points). The sum of all weighted items equals 1
List of items, possible answers, experts' opinion and weighting

assumptions and were randomly sampled per farm. The Buffered Plate Antigen Test and the Complement Fixation Test were the diagnostic tests (DT) selected to validate the exposure to vaccine.

Any female calf vaccinated 30 to 50 days before the sampling date with the commercial brucellosis vaccine approved by SENASA (2 ml-dose) was expected to react positively to the DT (DT+ = Buffered Plate Antigen Test + and/or Complement Fixation Test +) [7, 8]. We classified a farm as "well vaccinated" if the proportion of DT+ was not significantly lower than the ideal 95%. DPV on which female calves were sampled were categorized as follows: 30–35 and 35–50.

Statistical analyses

The comparison of inappropriately-managed farms and of each item per district or production system was carried out with the Fisher's exact test. The comparisons of weighted scores per respondent were performed with the Wilcoxon Rank Sum Test.

A univariate, and secondly a multivariate logistic regression using backward stepwise analysis, were applied to assess the association between the dependent "DT+/DT-" and independent variables [9]. Independent variables were categorized as dichotomous: vaccinator (vet practitioner/non-veterinarian), productive system (dairy/beef), age of female calves at the time of vaccination (4–6 months/7–8 months), individual identification of female calves (identified or not), DPV for heifer sampling (30–35 DPV/35–50 DPV), herd size (lower or higher than 200 cows, which is the median of cows per farm in both districts farms). Variables showing a significant univariate test at an initial p value < 0.2 were included in a multivariate model. In addition, a backward elimination of variables allowed assessing collinearity [10]. Any variable inducing a > 20%-variation of odds ratio (OR) was included in the final model [11]. In that final model, all pairwise interactions between variables, if biologically relevant, were examined for significance. Goodness-of-fit was assessed using the Hosmer-Lemeshow test.

Results

Responses from 113 farmers (approximately 10% of farmers of both districts, 55 from dairy and 58 from beef farms), 11 private veterinarians (which represent 80% of the veterinarians), 16 vaccinators (all of them) and the 2 LSEs officials, were collected during the years 2013 and 2014. A total of 52 (46%) surveyed farms were Officially Brucellosis-Free, out of which 12 (23%) were beef holdings.

Farmers and private vet practitioners

Almost all interviewed farmers (96%; n = 108) were advised by a private vet practitioner. Dairy and Officially Brucellosis-Free farmers kept significantly more reproductive records and tried significantly (P < 0.05) more often to diagnose causes of abortions and reproductive disorders than beef and non-Officially Brucellosis-Free farms, respectively. Although individual identification of vaccinated females is mandatory, beef farms identified significantly less animals ($P < 0.05$) than dairy holdings. The proportion of reported abortions was significantly ($P < 0.05$) higher in dairy farms. Only 14% ($n = 16$) of farmers isolated cattle with reproductive disorders consistent with brucellosis; the destination of all sold animals was the slaughterhouse. Regarding isolation of cattle suspected of brucellosis, no significant difference was observed between dairy and beef holdings on one hand, and between Officially Brucellosis-Free and non-Officially Brucellosis-Free certified farms, on the other hand ($P > 0.05$). Concerning purchase, neither the production system, nor the disease status showed a significant effect: out of 48 (42%) farmers who purchased cattle in the previous year, 18 (38%) did it from farms certified as Officially Brucellosis-Free; 13 of them (27%) resorted to a serologic diagnostic test before introducing animals into their herd (although suggested by all vet practitioners), and only 4 farmers (8%) isolated purchased cattle (although suggested by 7 veterinarians [63%]). Regarding immunization coverage of farms, 13% of farmers admitted that not 100% of females were vaccinated; such observation concerned mostly beef farms ($P < 0.05$), reporting no mating season. Calving cows were isolated from the herd by 47% of farmers ($n = 53$), and significantly ($P < 0.05$) more frequently in dairy farms. Forty-five percent (45%) of farmers ($n = 14$ dairy and 10 beef farms) isolated females at first calving.

At least one case of bovine brucellosis was reported by 4 vet practitioners (63%) for the previous year. All vet practitioners ($n = 11$) suggested to test serologically the females which aborted or showed reproductive disorders (e.g. retained placenta, no-pregnancy or delivering weak calves); 9 vets (81%) suggested serology for males with orchitis and 4 of them (36%) for epididymitis. In case of bovine brucellosis, the investigation in other domestic species (especially swine) was implemented by 6 vets (54%).

Regarding personal opinion of vet practitioners on immunization: (i) individual identification is poor, (ii) immunization coverage is incomplete, particularly in beef farms with no mating season (individual identification is not the rule, and age of calves is not reliable), (iii) vaccination is difficult to perform due to poor conditions of alleys, (iv) a 5 ml-dose would be better than a 2 ml-dose (indeed, only 1 ml is injected if the syringe is not correctly calibrated), (v) vaccine has been useful in reducing brucellosis prevalence (even in holdings where no other control measures have been implemented) and (vi) most farmers are used to vaccinate, even if it is a financial charge (few unvaccinated females are reported, only among farmers who do not immunize females under 3 months of age).

Vaccinators

In both districts, vaccinators were either vet practitioners or non-veterinarians. All of them are used to check the vaccine expiration date, the vacuum in the vaccine flask prior to dilution and to store the vaccine in coolers, in the shade, while vaccinating. Six vaccinators (38%) calibrated the syringe at the beginning of the vaccination day, 4 of them (25%) each time that they filled it, 2 of them (12%) at the beginning and each time that the vaccine is filled; 4 vaccinators (25%) never calibrate the syringe. Vaccinators (100%) do not immunize females that look older than 8 months of age, so as not to interfere with diagnostic tests. Half of them homogenize the vaccine during immunization. In case of vaccine dropping after injection, 12 vaccinators (75%) inject it again, but only 6% ($n = 10$) record the double injection in the vaccination certificate.

LSEs officials

LSEs officials audited vaccinators' performance at least once per vaccination campaign on the following topics: high immunization coverage in farms, good vaccination practices, and animal welfare.

At the LSEs, the temperature of refrigerators where vaccine flasks are stored were checked twice a day. Vaccine supply by the producing laboratories and its distribution to vaccinators in coolers were also assessed.

Comparison of practices between respondents and experts

Farmers

The 5 experts were consistent in assuming that the following items were the most susceptible to impact farmers' good management practices (low coefficient of variation [CV], as shown in Table 1): sales of cattle suspected of brucellosis, good immunization coverage per farm, purchase of cattle from Officially Brucellosis-Free holdings, and serological tests upon purchasing animals.

Considering all farmers ($n = 113$), the median global weighted score reached 0.28 [range 0–0.88; First quartile = 0.21 and Third quartile = 0.41]. For dairy farms, that score was 0.22 [range 0–0.68; First quartile = 0.16 and Third quartile = 0.31], compared to 0.36 for beef holdings [range 0.12–0.87; First quartile = 0.27 and Third quartile = 0.49]. When comparing both districts, median global weighted scores reached 0.32 [range 0–0.88; First quartile = 0.24 and Third quartile = 0.43] and 0.25 [range 0.06–0.87; First quartile = 0.16 and Third quartile = 0.39] for Brandsen and Navarro, respectively.

Twenty-three beef farms (36.7%) and 6 dairy holdings (10.9%) fell into the 'inappropriately-managed farms' category ($P < 0.05$); Brandsen district accounted for 29.3% of them, while 17.2% where located in Navarro district ($P > 0.05$; n total = 58). As illustrated in Fig. 2, the global weighted scores were significantly higher ($P < 0.05$) in beef farms and in Brandsen district.

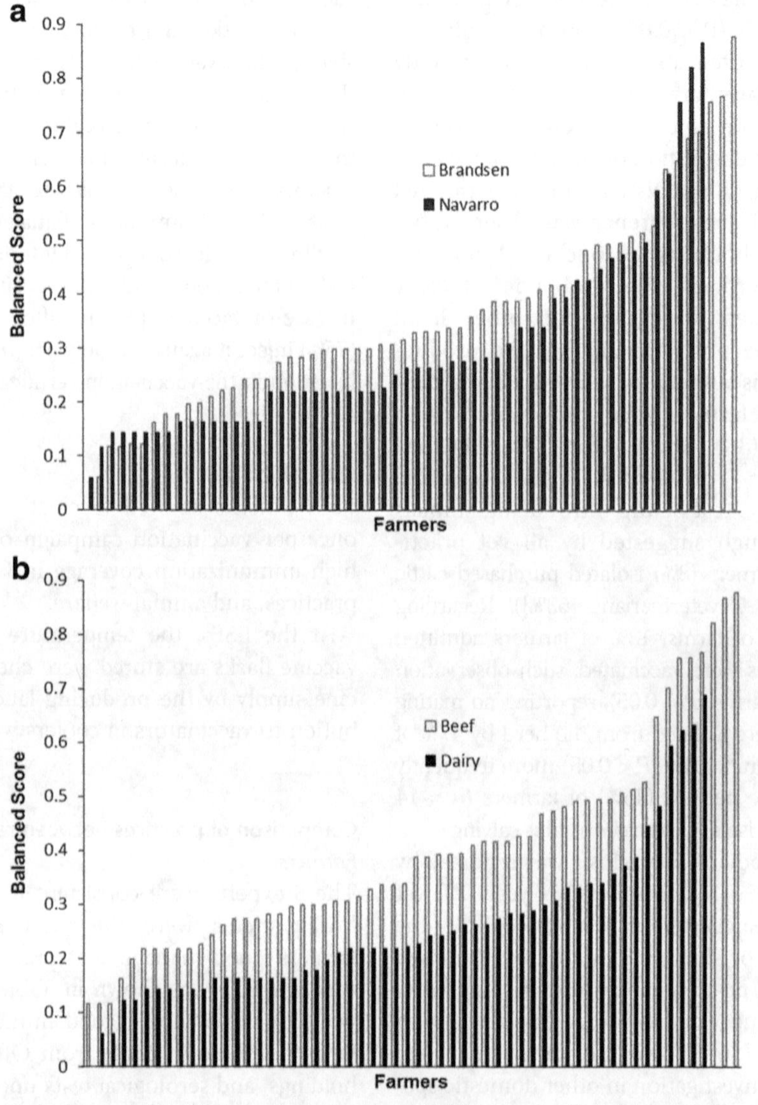

Fig. 2 Farmers' weighted scores in function of production system (**a**) and district (**b**). Legend: **a**: Dairy (First quartile = 0.16; median = 0.22; Third quartile = 0.31) and Beef (First quartile = 0.27; median = 0.36; Third quartile = 0.49). **b**: Brandsen (First quartile = 0.24; median = 0.32; Third quartile = 0.43) and Navarro (First quartile = 0.16; median = 0.25; Third quartile = 0.39)

Veterinary practitioners

For vet practitioners, the most impacting item was to suggest serological testing for females with reproductive disorders (low CV, as shown in Table 2). The median global weighted score reached 0.13 [range 0–0.48; First quartile = 0.13 and Third quartile = 0.28] and no statistical difference was observed between both districts.

Vaccinators

As shown in Table 3, the 5 experts were consistent in assuming the following items to be the most susceptible to impact the vaccinators' performance (low CV): maximal delay for using the vaccine, syringe calibration and vaccine homogenization. The median global weighted score was 0.17 [range 0.06–0.41; First quartile = 0.12 and Third quartile = 0.27].

A global weighted score above the Third quartile was obtained for 4 vaccinators (25%). No significant difference was observed between both districts. Vet practitioners obtained a higher median score compared with non-veterinarians (0.23 vs. 0.12, respectively), but that difference was not significant.

LSEs

Table 4 summarizes the items included in the questionnaires submitted to LSEs officials: experts agreed that vaccine storage at an appropriate temperature, as well as audits, had the highest impact (lowest CV).

The global weighted scores were 0.102 for Brandsen and 0.114 for Navarro.

Vaccination coverage

A total of 393 female calves (262 from Brandsen and 131 from Navarro) from 21 farms (5 dairy and 9 breeding farms from Brandsen, 3 dairy farms and 4 breeding from Navarro) were sampled. Table 5 summarizes the number of sampled farms, the number of well vaccinated and the proportion of well vaccinated per DPV category, as well as individual results of diagnostic testing. Female calves were correctly identified in 52% of farms (n = 11). A DT+ result was registered for 83% (n = 328) of sampled female calves which was significantly lower compared to an ideal 95%-immunization coverage ($P < 0.05$). Also, among all DPV categories, the proportion of well vaccinated farms was significantly lower compared to an ideal 95%-immunization coverage ($P < 0.05$).

At least one heifer was DT+ in each farm, and all tested female calves were DT+ in 33% of holdings (n = 7). Nevertheless, 48% of farms (n = 10) were assumed to be well vaccinated.

Batches of vaccines used in the sampled farms were approved by SENASA and were not beyond expiration date.

Regarding variables potentially influencing a DT+ status, no significant effect was observed for DPV, production system, Officially Brucellosis-Free vs. non- Officially Brucellosis-Free status, individual identification or age at the time of vaccination. The final multivariate logistic regression included 4 independent variables: district, vaccinator type, farm size and age at the time of vaccination. A DT+ status was significantly and positively associated with Brandsen district (OR = 25.94 [4.60–1146.21] and with farms having > 200 cows (OR = 78.34 [4.09–1500.00]). On the other side, the vaccinator being a vet practitioner was less associated with a DT+ status (OR = 0.07 [0.006–0.78]). All pairwise interactions were tested. The Hosmer-Lemeshow test showed that the final model fit the data correctly (Chi^2 = 0.26, df = 1, P = 0.96).

Table 5 Immunization coverage at farm and individual levels

A) At farm level			
DPV	nf	n WV	% WV
30–35	8	4	50[a]
35–50	13	6	46[a]
Total	21	10	48[a]
B) At individual level			
DPV	nfc	n DT+	% DT+
30–35	143	127	89
35–50	250	201	80[a]
Total	393	328	83[a]

Legend: *DPV* = days post vaccination; nf = number of farms; nWV = number of "well vaccinated" farms (farms where the proportion of DT+ was not significantly lower compared to an ideal 95%-immunization coverage); %WV = percentage of "well vaccinated" farms; nfc = number of sampled female calves; n DT + = number of female calves positive to the diagnostic tests; % DT = percentage of female calves positive to the diagnostic tests; [a]significant differences with the ideal 95%-coverage

Discussion

Although well advised by their veterinarians, farmers should improve some management practices. In particular, beef farmers should investigate abortions and reproductive disorders, and focus on individual identification of vaccinated female calves, as stated by the SENASA national regulations. Farmers should purchase cattle from Officially Brucellosis-Free farms and perform serological diagnostic tests and/or implement a quarantine procedure before introducing animals into the herd.

Vaccination is the most successful method to prevent and control brucellosis in endemic countries [4]. Increasing the immunization coverage among females is essential for animal and public health, but also for the farmers' economy [2, 3]. Besides, animal mass vaccination allows rewording money for the public health sector [12].

Although the percentage of sampled farms was small, we could identify that the vaccination campaign in the districts under study is globally well implemented, but some aspects should be improved, such as coverage and some vaccinators' practices. In fact, the relative low coverage (significantly below the 95%-expected in a mandatory vaccination campaign) is not due to the vaccine quality, which is controlled by SENASA, but rather to poor vaccination practices.

Immunization coverage (DT+ status) was better in Brandsen district, since DT+ female calves are almost 26 times more likely to be encountered. Farms having more than 200 cows seem better vaccinated, as finding DT+ female calves is 78 times more likely. Strict records and good alleys to perform the vaccination might explain such difference. Cattle vaccinated by vet practitioners are 0.07 times less likely to be DT+, but additional studies involving larger samples are needed. Beef farms should improve their recording system. In fact, the higher proportion of reported abortions in dairy farms is probably due to better records.

This original methodology, designed to monitor tuberculosis skin testing among vet practitioners, was initially performed in Belgium and in France. A scoring scale was built, based on experts' opinion, and a global score was calculated and compared with vet practitioners' responses [13, 14]. The same methodology could be adapted to evaluate farmers' and veterinarians' management practices in relation to other diseases, in different contexts and different countries.

Regular evaluation of systematic and mass vaccination campaigns is of great importance in order to quantify their effectiveness [15], detect problems, and monitor the effect of interventions aimed at correcting them. During the years 2004, 2007, 2008 and 2011, the systematic foot-and-mouth disease mass vaccination campaigns were assessed in some districts of Argentina [16], but no study had focused on brucellosis so far. In addition, the methodology applied in those surveys did not consist in questionnaires answered by the main actors, but only relied on serological tests to estimate the cattle humoral immunity level. Regarding brucellosis, the former studies estimated the disease prevalence at country level [6]; the present study is thus innovative in evaluating brucellosis vaccination practices and coverage.

As regards farmers and vaccinators, they should be informed on how to improve their management and immunization practices, respectively. Improving auditing of the whole vaccination process should be the main objective of people in charge of vaccination campaigns.

This study has been a first approach of the evaluation of brucellosis vaccination. It should be repeated in the future with more samples to obtain more precise confidence intervals for the OR. It should be repeated not only in the same districts to assess improvements among all actors, but it could also be applied in other districts. The study also allowed awareness on the campaign through evidence-based data of serology. Nevertheless, the questionnaire and the serological surveys are complementary tools; they should be implemented simultaneously: the questionnaire details the vaccination process, per actor, while the serological survey assesses the immunization coverage. Brandsen district perfectly illustrates that recommendation, even if farmers' practices were poor, vaccination was better implemented.

Conclusions

In this study, we developed and tested a method to assess the farmers' and veterinarians' behavior concerning the disease and to evaluate the vaccination campaign. It leads to a better understanding of the most common used management and control practices regarding the disease, which may affect its epidemiology. It highlights the need for policy makers to be aware of farmers' and veterinarians' practices, to detect strengths and weaknesses on diseases management in order to adapt, improve and monitor Control and Eradication Plans. It is also useful to evaluate people in charge of vaccines application, as well as the operative aspects of the whole vaccination campaigns.

Any vaccination campaign should be periodically evaluated to highlight the aspects that require improvement. The herein explored methodology, and the questionnaires combined with serologic tests are interesting to appropriately assess the subject. To our knowledge, not many studies exist on the evaluation of vaccination campaigns, being this one, though, innovative. It is not only applicable to Argentina, but also to the numerous countries that use vaccines against brucellosis or other diseases.

Our work is just a pilot study which might be the basis of a more extensive study in the rest of the country and in other countries. It can be extrapolated to other countries and different contexts.

These results were presented and discussed with the SENASA authorities. Some changes and improvements were consecutively observed during the 2015 brucellosis vaccination campaign, e.g. increased trends in animal identification and the control of vaccinators while performing their task.

Abbreviations

CV: coefficient of variation; DPV: days post vaccination; DT: diagnostic tests; LSEs: Local Sanitary Entities; OR: odds ratio; SENASA: National Service for Agrifood Health and Quality

Acknowledgments

All farmers, private vet practitioners and vaccinators who participated in the study are gratefully acknowledged. A special thank is addressed to Ms. María Celia Torlaschi (Sociedad Rural de Brandsen), Dr. Marcelo Ballerio (SENASA), Dr. Inés Irastorza (SENASA Brandsen) and Dr. Patricia Rocha (Sociedad Rural de Navarro); this study could not have been performed without their help. We also thank the experts: B. Cosentino(†), S. J. Duffy, J. Hart, E.A. León, and L.E Samartino. Ximena Velarde-Payen is acknowledged for revising the English language.

Funding

This study was founded by the INTA Project in Animal Health PNSA 1115052.

Authors' contributions

MNA, CS and LES participated in the conception and design of the study. MNA and MA performed the field work. MNA and CS analyzed the data and wrote the manuscript. MFH contributed to the analysis and helped in the manuscript discussion. All authors have read and approved the final version of the manuscript.

Ethics approval and consent to participate

The participants provided their verbal informed consent for animal blood sampling as well for the related survey questions. The participants were informed about the purpose of the study, and knew that their responses would be used in scientific research. All farmers were present at the time the blood samples were obtained, helping to work with the animals. In this way, cattle were less nervous. The INTA IACUC local ethics committee (Institutional Animal Care and Use Committee) ruled that no formal ethics approval was required in this case. Nonetheless, collection of blood samples was carried out by professional veterinarians according to the IACUC standardized procedures. Blood collection was performed by means of jugular puncture, after minimal restraining and without anesthesia. Sera were used for the purpose of this study and also for testing other diseases, as part of the routine sanitary diagnose regularly performed in the farms.

Consent for publication

Not applicable.

Competing interests

The authors declare that they have no competing interests.

Author details
[1]Instituto de Patobiología, INTA, CICVyA, Hurlingham, PC 1688 Buenos Aires, Argentina. [2]Research Unit of Epidemiology and Risk Analysis applied to veterinary sciences (UREAR-ULg), Center for Fundamental and Applied Research for Animal and Health (FARAH), Faculty of Veterinary Medicine, University of Liege, PC 4000 Liege, Belgium. [3]Department for Occupational Safety and Health, Biosafety and Biosecurity Unit, University of Liege, PC 4000 Liege, Belgium.

References

1. England T, Kelly L, Jones RD, MacMillan A, Wooldridge MA. Simulation model of brucellosis spread in British cattle under several testing regimes. Prev Vet Med. 2004;63:63–73.
2. Saegerman C, Berkvens D, Godfroid J, Walravens K. Bovine brucellosis. Infectious and parasitic disease of livestock , Editions Tec et Doc. Lavoisier, France, 2010;991–1011.
3. Godfroid J, Nielsen K, Saegerman C. Diagnosis of brucellosis in livestock and wildlife. Croat Med J. 2010;51:296–305.
4. Corbel MJ. Brucellosis in humans and animals. World Health Organization, Food and Agriculture Organization and World Organization for Animal Health. WHO Library Cataloguing-in-Publication Data; 2006.
5. Samartino LE. Brucellosis in Argentina. Vet Microbiol. 2002;90:71–80.
6. Aznar MN, Samartino LE, Humblet M-F, Saegerman C. Bovine brucellosis in Argentina and bordering countries: update. Transbound Emerg Dis. 2014;61:121–33.
7. Sutherland SS, Le Cras DV, Robertson AG, Johnston JM, Evans RJ. Serological response of cattle after vaccination and challenge with Brucella abortus. Vet Microbiol. 1982;7:165–75.
8. Aguirre NP, Vanzini VR, Torioni de Echaide S, Valentini BS, De Lucca G, Aufranc C, Canal A, Vigliocco A, Nielsen K. Antibody dynamics in Holstein Friesian heifers vaccinated with *Brucella abortus* strain 19, using seven serological tests. J Immunoassay Immunochem. 2002;23:471–8.
9. Petrie A, Watson P. Statistics for veterinary and animal science. Oxford: Blackwell Publishing; 2006.
10. Preux PM, Odermatt P, Perna A, Marin B, Vergnenègre AQ. est-ce qu'une régression logistique ? Rev Mal Respir. 2005;22:159–62.
11. Hosmer D, Lemeshow S. Applied logistic regression. New York: Wiley; 2000.
12. Zinstaag J, Schelling E, Roth F, Bonfoh B, de Savigny D, Tanner M. Human benefits of animal interventions for zoonosis control. Emerg Infect Dis. 2007;13:527–31.
13. Humblet M-F, Moyen J-L, Bardoux P, Boschiroli ML, Saegerman C. The importance of awareness for veterinarians involved in cattle tuberculosis skin testing. Transbound Emerg Dis. 2011;58:531–6.
14. Humblet M-F, Walravens K, Salandre O, Boschiroli ML, Gilbert M, Berkvens D, Fauville-Dufaux M, Godfroid J, Dufey J, Raskin A, Vanholme L, Saegerman C. Monitoring of the intra-dermal tuberculosis skin test performed by Belgian field practitioners. Res Vet Sci. 2011;91:199–207.
15. Roth F, Zinsstag J, Orkhon D, Chimed-Ochir G, Hutton G, Cosivi O, Carrin G, Otte J. Human health benefits from livestock vaccination for brucellosis: case study. Bull World Health Organ. 2003;81:867–76.
16. León EA, Perez AM, Stevenson MA, Robiolo B, Mattion N, Seki C, La Torre J, Torres A, Cosentino B, Duffy SJ. Effectiveness of systematic foot and mouth disease mass vaccination campaigns in Argentina. Rev Sci Tech. 2014;33:917–26.

Preparation and evaluation of goose reovirus inactivated vaccine

Xiaoyu Niu†, Bingqian Zhang†, Xianglong Yu, Xin Zhang, Yanguo Dou, Yi Tang* and Youxiang Diao*

Abstract

Background: Infection with Goose Reovirus (GRV) can cause serious economic losses in the goose breeding industry. In this study, the GRV allantoic fluid was concentrated and used as an antigen in a formalin-inactivated oil-emulsion vaccine.

Results: When 6 day-old geese were inoculated, antibodies against GRV became detectable at 6 days post-vaccination, their concentration peaked at 3 weeks. These antibodies were maintained for longer than 2 weeks. As the most susceptible age for GRV infection is birds under 2 weeks of age this vaccine should provide adequate cover for the most at risk birds. When geese were exposed to reovirus at different time intervals after immunization, the data revealed that the vaccine can provide a protection rate of 80%. The developed vaccine has good stability and could be stored at 4 °C for at least 12 months.

Conclusion: These results indicate that the developed GRV vaccine is safe, effectively absorbed, efficacious in inducing a rapid immune response, and effective in controlling GRV infection. Our results should be useful for the application of vaccines for controlling GRV in different goose flocks.

Keywords: Reovirus, Goose, Inactivated vaccine

Background

Avian reovirus (ARV) belongs to the genus *Orthoreovirus* within the family *Reoviridae* [1, 2]. Avian reovirus was first isolated from the respiratory tract of a chicken with chronic respiratory disease, liver necrosis, and arthritis by Fahey and Crawley in 1954 [3]. In 1972, Walke et al. confirmed the virus as a "reovirus" [4]. Researchers subsequently identified ARV infection in South Africa, France, Israel, Italy, China, and many other countries [5–7]. In 1997, the main Muscovy duck breeding region in China was affected by an outbreak of duck reovirus (DRV) disease, which resulted in white spots on the liver. Then, the duck reovirus was isolated from ducks in other breeding regions. Previous research has shown that the degree of identity at the sigma C protein level between the deduced amino acid sequence of the DRV and ARV was only 21–22% [8] and serological data showed that the DRV was antigenically different from the Avian Reoviruses present in chickens [9, 10]. All these above suggest that the DRV is very different from ARV and should be classified separately.

It has been reported that GRV can cause viral arthritis in geese, and infected geese often exhibited spleen inflammation, while those with subacute or chronic onset showed pericarditis, arthritis, and/or tenosynovitis [7]. The GRV induced clinical symptoms appeared at 2–3 weeks of age, and the disease course lasted 3–6 weeks [11]. GRV has been isolated from various organs/tissues of infected geese [7]. A previous experiment showed that the virus strains from ducks and geese shared high homology in the S1 genome segment and [12] physico-chemical, clinical and biological characteristics and molecular properties were also identical to each other [7]. Based on sequence data currently available and on criteria established for demarcation of reovirus species, previous reports [7] believe that GRVs and DRVs should be classified into a common species.

ARVs do not have a capsule membrane; instead, they have a double-capsid structure and spherical symmetry of 20 bodies. The virus particle diameter is approximately 60–80 nm. Its buoyant density in cesium chloride (CsCl) is 1.36 g/mL [13–15]. It does not aggregate red blood cells of the chicken, turkey, duck, goose, rat, or mouse [12, 16]. The virus also has the capacity to survive at low temperatures [17]. The viral genome is linear double-stranded RNA, which is composed of 10 genome segments. The

* Correspondence: tyck288@163.com; yxdiao@126.com
†Equal contributors
College of Animal Science and Technology, Shandong Agricultural University, Daizong Road 61, Tai'an, Shandong 271018, China

genome segments were divided into three groups according to the different electrophoretic mobility of the fragments. There are three large gene segments (L1, L2, L3), three medium-sized gene segments (M1, M2, M3), and four small gene segments (S1, S2, S3, S4) [18–21]. The virus recombination rate is as high as 3%–5% [22].

GRV can replicate upon inoculation into goose embryos in the yolk sack, allantoic cavity, and allantoic membrane, the most effective option of which is inoculation in the yolk sac. Embryos inoculated with the virus generally die within 7 days [23–25]. The dead embryos show systemic bleeding, allantoic membrane thickening, and clear allantoic fluid [26, 27]. Those embryos that do survive more than seven days exhibit necrosis of the liver and spleen. Reovirus can cause significant inhibition of growth in birds, the age group of birds between one day and 9 weeks of age [28]. Reovirus transmission can be classified into two types: horizontal and vertical. The presence of the virus in the cloaca of injected hens has been confirmed, but the rate of vertical transmission in this context is low [29].

GRV disease has become common in many provinces of China. The reovirus can also occur as a co-infection with other pathogenic microorganisms, making the GRV infection more serious [20]. The most effective way to prevent the disease is vaccination. However, there are no vaccines available for GRV prevention. To bridge this gap, in this study, an oil emulsion inactivated vaccine for GRV was developed. The antibody responses in immunized geese were detected by an indirect ELISA method that was established in our laboratory. The results of challenge experiments demonstrated the efficacy of the inactivated GRV vaccine. The success of this study lays the foundations for the prevention and control of the disease, which should have major significance for the vitality of the goose industry.

Methods

Virus and animals

The SPF chicken embryos were purchased from the Poultry Research Institute of Shandong Academy of Agricultural Sciences. The geese and goose eggs were purchased from a company in Jinan, Shandong. The geese used in the study were allowed to acclimatize to their new surroundings and were healthy at the start of the experiment. Serum samples were collected from geese prior to challenge or immunization to confirm that these animals were free of GRV antibody via the ELISA assay.

Goose reovirus was isolated at our laboratory from the liver and spleen of infected geese from Jiangsu province in China, after several passages via the chorioallantoic membrane (CAM) of GRV antibody-negative goose eggs. The strain was named JS-01, the sigma C gene sequence of which has been deposited with the Genbank accession number MF139036. The virus was titrated on fertile SPF chicken eggs. The GRV liquid was subjected to a series of tenfold dilutions from 10^{-1} to 10^{-5}, and each dilution was inoculated in 9-day-old SPF chick embryos. The egg lethal dose 50 (ELD50) was calculated by the method of Reed and Muench (1938).

Pathogenicity of the JS-01 strain

The experimental geese were housed in SPF animal isolators that were ventilated under negative pressure, and were provided with feed and water ad libitum. Inoculations of 6 day-old geese were performed intramuscularly with 0.2 ml JS-01 strain, which contained $10^{-3.75}$ ELD50. 20 geese were infected to investigate the pathogenicity of JS-01, and another 15 birds were left uninoculated as controls. Goslings in each group were inspected daily for signs of disease. Three birds per group were killed and necropsied on days 4, 6, 8,10 and 14 post injection.

Preparation of oil-adjuvant inactivated GRV vaccine

The GRV JS-01 strain was propagated via the CAM of GRV antibody-negative goose eggs. Eggs that died within 24 h were abandoned. Allantoic fluid of the remaining eggs was collected at 120 h post inoculation as the virus fluid. The allantoic fluid was inactivated by adding 0.2% formalin (*v*/v) and kept at 37 °C for 36 h, shaken every 8 h. The formalin-treated virus fluid was inoculated into SPF chicken embryos, and the harvested allantoic fluid, after three passages, was used to perform reverse transcriptase PCR (RT-PCR) for GRV detection to determine whether the virus was inactivated totally or not.

Firstly, 184 ml sterilized mineral, 12 ml span-80 (Sorbitan (Z)-mono-9-octadecenoate, ThermoFisher, USA) and 4 ml stearic acid aluminum were mixed uniformly as the oil phase. Then the oil phase and 200 ml inactivated virus fluid, which contains sterilized 4% tween-80 (Polysorbate-80) were churned at 3000 round per minute (rpm) for 30 min with homogenizer (voshin, Jiangsu China).

Purity of vaccine

Tests for microbial contaminants included mycoplasma examination and virus RT-PCR. The vaccine was innoculated onto Thiolglycollate medium (T.G) and Soybean-Casein Digest Agar Medium (TSA) cultivated at 37 °C and examined for microbial colony formation.

The vaccine was subcultured in modified Frey's medium to perform the mycoplasma testing [30, 31].

RT-PCR assay was carried out to detect the presence of Avian Influenza virus and Newcastle disease Virus (Table 1).

Immunization and challenge procedures

Ninety geese were randomly divided into three groups (A, B and C) and kept in SPF animal isolators that were ventilated under negative pressure with consistent conditions (Table 2). Geese from group A and B were injected intramuscularly with GRV vaccine preparations at a volume of 0.2

Table 1 Primes used in the RT-PCR assay to detect the presence of virus

Virus		Sequence
GRV	GRV-F	TGAGACGCCTGACTACGATT
	GRV-R	ATGCTTGGAGTGAGACGACT
AIV	AIV-F	GGAGGTTGGTCAGGATTAGTTG
	AIV-R	ACAAGAGATGAGGCGACAGT
NDV	NDV-F	AGGGACTGAAGAGGAGGATT
	NDV-R	TGAGTGTGATTGTATTAGGTGG

($5.9276 \times 10^{-5}ELD_{50}$) or 0.5 ($1.4819 \times 10^{-4}ELD_{50}$) mL, while group C were injected with 0.5 mL of PBS via the same route as challenge group. All geese were challenged intramuscularly with 0.2 ml of the JS-01 strain, which contained $10^{-3.75}ELD_{50}$ at 7, 12, and 27 days after vaccination, five geese each time. After challenge, the birds were kept separately. Cloacal and oropharynx swabs were taken from each group on days 3, 7, and 12 days post injection, and viral shedding was tested by virus isolation and the RT-PCR assay. All geese including those died during the observation period were weighed twice a week and examined for gross lesions.

Sample collection, RNA extraction and nucleotide sequencing

Samples of liver and spleen were collected from the dead animals in each group and processed for the microscopic examination of lesions. Oropharyngeal and cloacal swabs were collected on days 3, 7, and 12 post-challenge (p.c.) for virus isolation and testing for viral shedding, and geese were observed for disease signs and death for 2 weeks p.c.. The swabs were immediately placed in 0.5 mL PBS (pH 7.2) and extensively vortexed. The swab fluids were freeze thawed three times, sterilized by passage through a 0.22 mm filter and stored at −20 °C for further virus isolation via injecting goose embryos. Viral RNA was extracted from the allantoic fluid harvested from the goose embryos used for virus isolation or homogenate using the Tranzol RNA Extraction Kit (TransGen Biotech, Beijing, China) according to the manufacturer's instructions. The first-strand cDNA was generated from extracted RNA solution extracted using the Reverse Transcriptase M-MLV (Takara, Dalian, China) with Random Primer (pd(N)6, Takara, Dalian, China). The PCR mix containing 0.25 μL EX Taq polymerase (5 U/mL), 5 μl of 10× EX Taq Buffer (Mg^{2+} Plus), 4 μL of dNTP mixture (2.5 mM each dNTP) and 1 μL of each of the two primers (20 μM) was brought to 50 μL with RNase-free water. The reaction conditions were as follows: initial denaturation at 94 °C for 5 min, followed by 35 cycles of denaturation at 94 °C for 1 min, annealing at 54 °C for 30 s and extension at 72 °C for 2 min, with a final extension for 7 min at 72 °C. The RT-PCR products were purified, cloned into pMD18-T vector (TaKaRa, Dalian, China) and sequenced by BGI (Shenzhen, PR China).

Table 2 90 birds divided into three groups (A, B and C) were used to test protective efficacy of vaccine. A4, B4 and C4 were kept to collect serum for antibody detecting without challenging. All groups were kept in different SPF animal isolator

Group		Immunisation dose (intramuscularly)	Challenge at (days post immunisation)
A	A1	0.2 ml vaccine	7
	A2	0.2 ml vaccine	12
	A3	0.2 ml vaccine	27
	A4	0.2 ml vaccine	none
B	B1	0.5 ml vaccine	7
	B2	0.5 ml vaccine	12
	B3	0.5 ml vaccine	27
	B4	0.5 ml vaccine	none
C	C1	0.5 ml PBS	7
	C2	0.5 ml PBS	12
	C3	0.5 ml PBS	27
	C4	0.5 ml PBS	none

A separate set of samples from tissues, such as liver and spleen were fixed in 10% neutral buffered formalin and embedded in paraffin wax, then cut into 4 mm thick sections. Sections were stained with hematoxylin and eosin for microscopic examination.

Before the challenge, sera were obtained from 10 geese from the control and vaccinated groups. After the challenge, five serum samples were also collected from the three groups. The serum samples were collected every three days in each week and evaluated for the development of an immune response against GRV using indirect ELISA. All serum samples were stored at −20 °C.

Alignment of JS-01 strain oC gene with selected reference sequences was performed using Clustal W method of MegAlign program of DNAStar software (version 7.10). A phylogenetic tree was assembled using the neighbor-joining method of the MEGA program (version 5.0) with absolute distances following 1000 bootstrap replicates [32].

The procedure for detecting GRV antibody by ELISA

A total of 100 μL of GRV fluid, harvested from goose eggs and concentrated by PEG20000, in 0.05 M carbonate buffer (pH 9.6) was coated onto the wells of an ELISA plate (Greiner Bio-One, Germany), which was incubated at 37 °C for 2 h. These plates were blocked by phosphate-buffered saline (PBS) containing 0.5% Polyoxyethy-lene(20)Sorbaitan Monolaurate (Tween-20, ThermoFisher, USA) and 5% powdered milk (solarbio, Beijing, China, *w*/*v*) and incubated at 37 °C for 1 h. After blocking, diluted goose serum (1: 10) was added into wells (200 μl/well) and incubated at 37 °C for 1 h. Afterward, the plates were washed three times with PBS and incubated with rabbit anti-goose IgG (1: 800) conjugated to horseradish peroxidase (HRP, Sigma-Aldrich) at 100 μl/well. The plates were, again, incubated at 37 °C for 1 h, washed three times with PBS, and 3′, 3′, 5′, 5′-tetramethylbenzidine substrate solution (TransGen, Beijing, China) was added into each well (100 μl/well). 50 μl of 3 M H_2SO_4 (Wuxi JINGKE Chemical CO., LTD.) was added to stop the reaction, and the optical density (OD) values were observed at 450 nm using an automated ELISA plate reader (Thermo, Waltham, MA, USA). The cut off value of the ELISA assay was an OD of 0.37 at 450 nm.

The rabbit anti-goose IgG was prepared by our lab. In order to isolate IgG from the goose egg yolk, we used the method of chloroform extraction, salt precipitation and DEAE chromatography. Sodium sulphate polyacrylamide gel electrophoresis indicates that we derived relative pure IgG. Rabbits were inoculated with the purified IgG 4 times in all. Serum from the rabbits was collected and purified IgG precipitated with saturated ammonium sulphate. Finally, the purified rabbit IgG was labeled with HRP.

Statistical evaluation

The data were analyzed by GraphPad Prism version 5.0 software (GraphPad Software Inc., San Diego, CA). To investigate the differences of the antibody titre among three groups, the data was analyzed using ANOVA via the method of Bonferroni. The p values <0.025 were considered to be statistically significant (SPSS Statistics 17.0, IBM, USA).

Results

Alignment and phylogenetic tree

The virus strain used in the study was sequenced for the σC gene, which shared homology of 94.8% ~ 96.5% with the waterfowl reovirus (Fig. 1). The σC gene of JS-01 (GenBank accession: MF139036) isolated in the study has been clustered, and it9 was in the same clade with other goose reovirus strains isolated from China. Among them, the YY10G strain (Genebank accession: KF729971.1) isolated in China shared the closest relationship with JS-01 strain (Fig. 2).

Pathogenicity of the JS-01 strain

The experimental infection of goslings resulted in mortality of 85% (17/20). Acute deaths occurred at the 2nd and 3rd day post injection. Those birds still alive showed general malaise and exhibited lameness during the whole period of observation. Splenomegaly and necrotic foci in the liver and spleen were obvious on post mortem. Virus was detected from the inoculated birds, dead and alive, from homogenate of liver and spleen via RT-PCR assay.

Response to challenge

To investigate the protective efficacy of the vaccine developed in the study, geese were challenged at different time points post vaccination. The results of these experiments are summarized in Table 3. At post-mortem examination, geese that died in the period of observation showed swelling of the kidneys, liver and spleen; necrotic foci were present in the last two organs (Fig. 3 and Fig. 4).

Antibody response of vaccinated geese

Before the vaccination, GRV antibody was measured by the ELISA assay. The antibody level began to rise markedly at 6 d.p.v., and peaked after 3 weeks (Fig. 3). During the next two weeks, the ELISA values fell slowly, but still remained in the positive range and were much higher than the cut-off value (Fig. 5). The age of the highest susceptibility to GRV infection is from 1 to 4 weeks old, therefore the results demonstrate that the vaccine can provide protection rate over 80% in susceptible birds.

The results showed that, the group immunized with 0.5 ml of vaccine acquired protection rate of 80% against GRV (Table 4). Taking the titer of antibody into consideration, (Table 4), when the ELISA values of serum antibody increased to 0.60 or higher, the geese were

Percent Identity

Divergence	1	2	3	4	5	6	7	8	9	10	11		
1		97.7	96.2	95.8	94.8	41.2	50.7	40.0	41.4	40.2	51.3	1	JX826587.1 DRV strain TH11 CHINA 2015.
2	2.3		97.3	97.1	95.8	40.8	50.7	40.1	41.8	40.3	51.7	2	KJ879930.1 DRV SD-12 CHINA 2014.seq
3	4.0	2.8		96.9	95.7	40.8	51.4	40.8	42.3	41.1	52.0	3	JX145334.1 GRV strain 03G CHINA 2012.
4	4.4	3.0	3.2		96.5	40.6	51.3	40.6	41.9	40.8	52.2	4	KF729971.1 GRV strain YY10G cell CHINA
5	5.4	4.3	4.4	3.6		40.7	49.3	39.9	40.0	39.9	50.5	5	JS-01.seq
6	115.5	117.0	116.9	117.8	117.6		37.8	54.0	54.1	54.3	36.9	6	L07069.1 ARV 1994.seq
7	81.7	82.0	79.5	79.9	86.4	132.5		36.6	38.3	36.9	91.2	7	KF809668.1 ARV strain D20 99 HUNGAR
8	121.3	120.8	116.8	117.9	121.9	71.5	144.8		75.9	99.1	38.6	8	L39002.1 ARV 1995 .seq
9	113.8	112.4	109.9	111.9	120.9	71.4	130.7	30.4		76.4	39.9	9	HE985301.1 ARV AUSTRILIA 2012 .seq
10	120.1	119.6	115.7	116.8	121.8	70.7	141.8	0.9	29.6		38.7	10	AF330703.1 ARV-S1133 SPAIN 2000.seq
11	80.1	79.1	77.9	77.5	82.7	137.9	9.5	130.2	121.2	129.5		11	AJ310525.1 MDRV strain 89026 FRANCE
	1	2	3	4	5	6	7	8	9	10	11		

Fig. 1 Alignment of the σC gene sequence among JS-01 and other avian reovirus strain

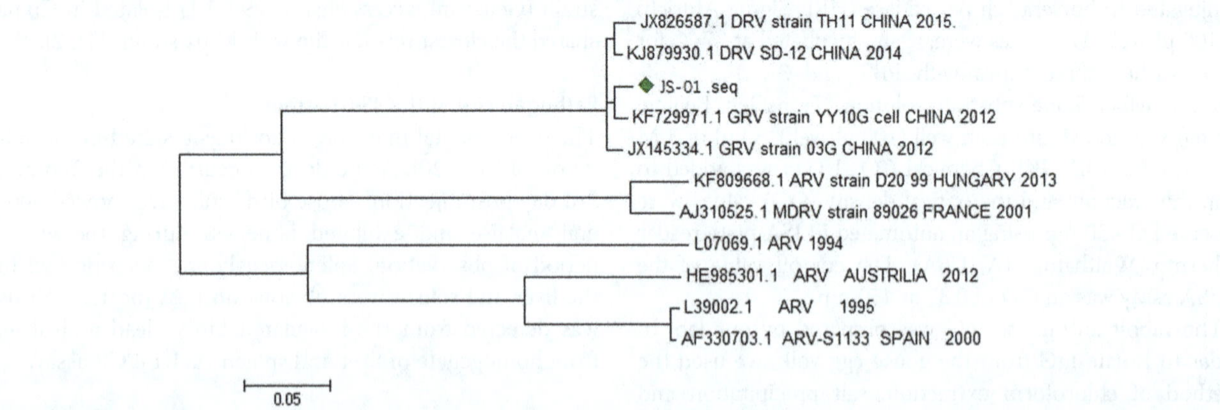

Fig. 2 Phylogenetic tree constructed using the neighbor-joining method, based on the sequence of the σC gene of virus strains isolated in the study and other waterfowl reovirus isolates available in GenBank database

completely protected. These results also demonstrate that geese were protected from the viral challenge for at least 1 month after inoculation, which is sufficient to cover the whole of the highly infectious period.

Viral shedding and virus isolation after challenge

To test for viral shedding, oropharyngeal and cloacal swabs were collected for virus isolation via goose embryos. Harvested allantoic fluid was detected by RT-PCR. Positive results in the RT-PCR indicated that the geese were shedding virus. (dates are shown in Table 4).

Discussion

In this experiment, we developed a GRV inactivated vaccine and evaluated its safety and efficacy in protecting goslings from GRV infection. The ELISA results showed that the antibody level in innoculated birds increased to OD0.6 or higher, and the vaccine exhibited a strong protective effect in geese.

When inoculated with 0.5 ml vaccine at 7 dpi, it can provide 80% protection. However, innoculation at 12 dpi with 0.5 ml vaccine can providing 100% protection. (Table 4).

Inactivated vaccines are used to control many infectious diseases in the poultry, due to their readily availability. In addition, inactivated whole-virus vaccines has been confirmed to be safe and high efficacy [33, 34]. However there has been little research into the protective immune response to GRV vaccines, possibly as the disease is newly emergent and largely present in China.

Compared with the live virus vaccines, the inactivated vaccine preparation does not appear to be toxic to goslings and produces a protective antibody response in inoculated birds for a length of time that would protect from natural disease. Selection of the inactivation agent is the most important factor in the production of an inactivated vaccine. Ideally, inactivation involves the virus completely losing its activity while maintaining good immunogenicity; therefore, there is a strong

Table 3 Description of waterfowl parvovirus isolates involved in this study

Strain	GenBank accession	Host	Separatum	Year
JS-01	MF139036	Goose	China	2016
TH11	JX826587.1	Duck	China	2015
SD-12	KJ879930.1	Duck	China	2014
03G	JX145334.1	Goose	China	2012
YY10G	KF729971.1	Goose	China	2012
Somerville 4	L07069.1	Chicken	Australia	1994
D20/99	KF809668.1	Chicken	Hungary	2013
S1133	L39002.1	Chicken	Australia	1994
12–1167	HE985301.1	Chicken	Australia	2012
S1133	AF330703.1	Chicken	Spain	2000
89,026	AJ310525.1	Muscovy duck	France	2001

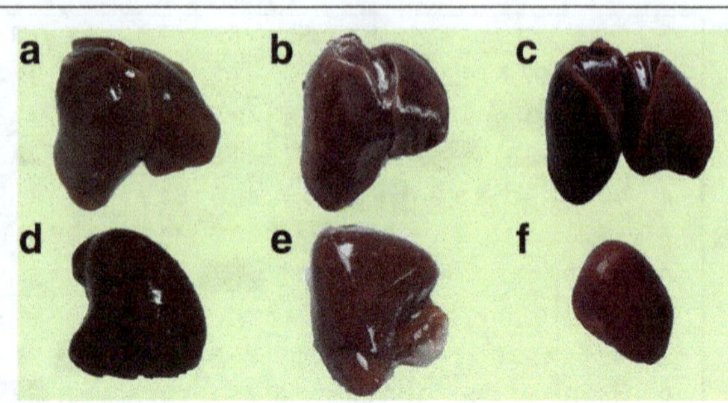

Fig. 3 Necropsy of geese infected with JS-01 strain. **a** and **b** Liver hemorrhage and the appearance of white necrotic spots. **d** and **e** Spleen sclerosis, with a large number of necrotic spots appearing in the spleen. **c** liver of healthy a goose from vaccinated group. **f**: spleen of a healthy goose from vaccinated group

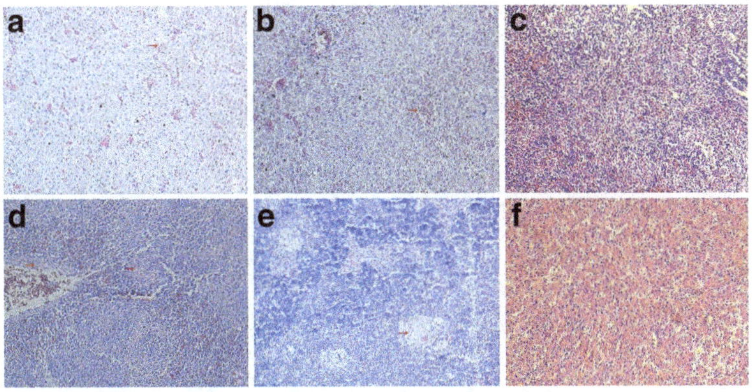

Fig. 4 The histopathological changes of geese infected with JS-01 strain. **a** Punctate hemorrhage of liver cells, atrophy of hepatic acini, and necrosis. Inflammatory cell infiltration. **b** Necrosis of liver cells and vacuolization. **c** Intact structures of hepatic lobules, no degeneration and infiltration of lymphocytes. **d** Spleen cell necrosis and cellular hyperplasia. **e** Spleen cell hemorrhage. **f** Arranged densely lymphocytes, no necrosis

relationship between the effect of inactivation and the choice of the inactivated agent. Formaldehyde is the most commonly used inactivation agent for RNA viruses. Considering that ARV is resistant to low temperatures and a low concentration of formaldehyde solution, in this study, we chose reaction conditions of 0.2% formaldehyde and incubation at 37 °C.

An indirect ELISA was developed using concentrated virus as the antigen. Serological responses following vaccination, as measured by this ELISA, were effective in most birds and correlate closely with protection. Over the whole observation after vaccination, the antibody titre of the control group against GRV was significantly lower when compared with vaccinated groups (p value <0.025, Fig. 6).

Previous study has confirmed the efficacy of oil-emulsion inactivated vaccines for protecting ducks from DRV [35]. Efficacy evaluations have been based on a challenge study performed a few weeks after vaccination, when the antibody titers reach or are around their peak. Our study has indicated that the vaccinated geese could be completely protected from GRV challenge when the antibody titers to the challenge virus equaled or were greater than OD0.6, a titer that can be easily induced by inactivated vaccine immunization.

Horizontal transmission is a major route of infection for GRV. The elimination time of GRV from the intestinal and respiratory tracts is long, especially in the intestines, which means that fecal pollution is a major source of infection [36, 37]. Specifically,

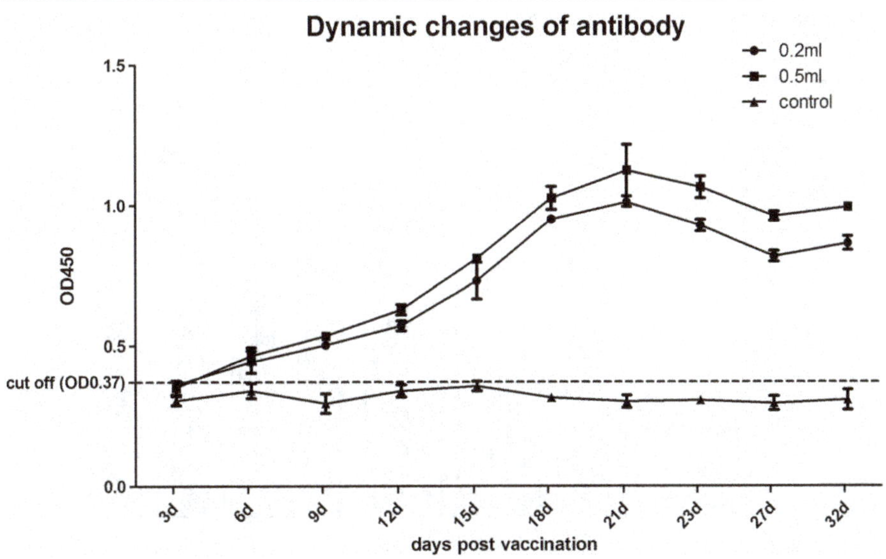

Fig. 5 The dynamic changes in antibodies induced by the inactivated vaccine in geese. One-week-old geese were injected intramuscularly (i.m.) with 0.2 or 0.5 mL of formalin-inactivated vaccine, and sera were collected randomly from six geese every three days for GRV antibody detection. The bars indicate the standard deviation

Table 4 Results of viral shedding after the challenge Results showed that birds vaccinated with 0.5 ml of vaccine at 12 dpi can be completely protected from GRV. While vaccinating with 0.2 ml and 0.5 ml of vaccine can also provide complete protection

Challenge time (dpv)	Group	Virus isolation from the swabs collected on different days after challenge: positive/total						Survival rate	Protection rate	OD value
		Day 3		Day 7		Day 12				
		Oropharyngeal	Cloacal	Oropharyngeal	Cloacal	Oropharyngeal	Cloacal			
7	0.2 mL	1/5	1/5	0/4[a]	0/4[a]	0/4[a]	1/4[a]	80%	60%	OD 0.45
	0.5 mL	0/5	0/5	0/5	0/5	0/5	1/5	100%	80%	OD 0.47
	Control	0/5	5/5	0/3[a]	3/3[a]	0/1[a]	1/1[a]	20%	0%	OD 0.34
12	0.2 mL	0/5	1/5	0/4[a]	0/4[a]	0/4[a]	0/4[a]	80%	80%	OD 0.57
	0.5 mL	0/5	0/5	0/5	0/5	0/5	0/5	100%	100%	OD 0.60
	Control	0/5	5/5	0/2[a]	1/2 [a]	0/2[a]	1/2 [a]	40%	20%	OD 0.29
27	0.2 mL	0/5	0/5	0/5	0/5	0/5	0/5	100%	100%	OD 0.82
	0.5 mL	0/5	0/5	0/5	0/5	0/5	0/5	100%	100%	OD 0.96
	Control	0/5	4/5	0/3[a]	0/3 [a]	0/3[a]	0/3 [a]	60%	60%	OD 0.30

[a] The sample number was less than 5 because geese had died. Complete protection: no viral shedding and death in the group; partial protection: viral shedding or/and death in the group

infection can quickly spread through feces in the same house. In this study, young geese immunized by the inactivated vaccine showed a high protection rate, which is over 80%, against viral challenging. Thus, we believe that the vaccine can aid in preventing the disease from spreading.

The data indicate that the inactivated GRV vaccine may represent an effective method for controlling GRV infection in the goose industry. However, vertical transmission is also an important route of GRV infection. Vertically transmitted GRV causes great economic losses due to mortality of the affected offspring, although infected breeding geese do not show clinical signs. It could thus have significant economic benefits for the industry if immunizing laying breeders could prevent vertical transmission [38]. In chickens the immune effect is generally better for breeding hens if inoculation with a living vaccine is performed before that with an inactivated vaccine [29]. We plan to study the immune effect of this vaccine in breeding geese in future work.

In this context, it has yet to be studied whether our vaccine would interfere with other vaccines for goose diseases, but this is worthy of investigation in future studies. We also need to develop and improve immunization programs for geese field use. Nonetheless, this study has provided a useful foundation by showing that the inactivated GRV vaccine could control and prevent infection.

Conclusion

The present work demonstrated that immunization with the new inactivated vaccine provides protective

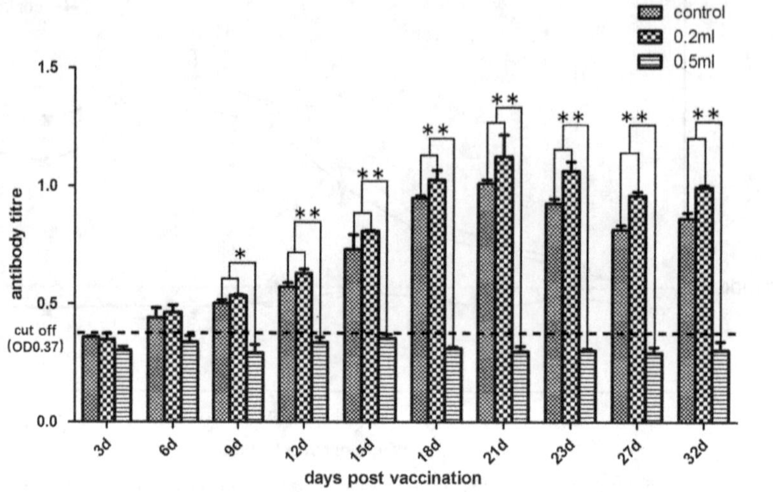

Fig. 6 Statistical significance of antibody titre between vaccinated group and control group. The data was analyzed via ANOVA (method of Bonferroni). * $p < 0.025$; ** $p < 0.001$

immunity to goslings, thereby reducing mortality, morbidity, and fecal shedding through challenge-exposure with virulent GRV. Since the advent of new, effective, and safe GRV vaccines on the market is in urgent in the near future to combat GRV. We should bear in mind that full biosecurity and husbandry management in the field can maximize vaccine effectiveness for prevention and control of GRV.

Abbreviations

ANOVA: Analysis of variance; ARV: Avian reovirus; CAM: Chorioallantoic membrane; DRV: Duck reovirus; ELD50: Egg lethal dose 50; ELISA: Enzyme linked immunosorbent assay; GRV: Goose reovirus; HRP: Horseradish peroxidase; OD: Optical density; p.c.: Post-challenge; PBS: Phosphate buffered saline; PCR: Polymerase chain reaction; PEG: Polyethylene glyco; RNA: Ribonucleic acid; RT-PCR: Reverse transcriptase PCR; SPF: Specific pathogen free; T.G: Thiolglycollate medium; TSA: Soybean-Casein Digest Agar Medium

Acknowledgements

The work was done at Research Institute of Poultry Disease, Agricultural University of Shan Dong Province.

Funding

This study was supported by the China Agriculture Research System (grant number: CARS-43-10) and the Shandong Science and Technology Development Program (grant number: 2014GNC111023).

Authors' contributions

YD and YT made substantial contributions to conception and design, and had the initial idea, was partially guiding the experiments and contributed substantially to the manuscript. XN performed the experiment and statistical analysis and drafted the manuscript. BZ made substantial contributions to conception and design, was actively involved in the planning and conduction of the experiment, and revised the manuscript critically. XY, YD and XZ performed measurements in the interpretation of the results as well as in the statistics. All authors have read and approved the final version of the manuscript.

Consent for publication

Not applicable.

Competing of interest

The authors declare that they have no competing interests.

References

1. Kawamura H, Tsubahara H. Common antigenicity of avian reoviruses. Natl Inst Anim Health Q (Tokyo). 1966;6(4):187–93.
2. van der Heide L. The history of avian reovirus. Avian Dis. 2000;44(3):638–41.
3. Fahey JE, Crawley JF. Studies on chronic respiratory disease of chickens II. Isolation of a virus. Can J Comp Med Vet Sci. 1954;18(1):13–21.
4. Walker ER, Friedman MH, Olson NO. Electron microscopic study of an avian reovirus that causes arthritis. J Ultrastruct Res. 1972;41(1):67–79.
5. Adair BM, Burns K, McKillop ER. Serological studies with reoviruses in chickens, turkeys and ducks. J Comp Pathol. 1987;97(5):495–501.
6. Dandar E, et al. The complete genome sequence of a European goose reovirus strain. Arch Virol. 2014;159(8):2165–9.
7. Palya V, et al. Reovirus identified as cause of disease in young geese. Avian Pathol. 2003;32(2):129–38.
8. Zhang Y, et al. Characterization of the sigmaB-encoding genes of muscovy duck reovirus: sigmaC-sigmaB-ELISA for antibodies against duck reovirus in ducks. Vet Microbiol. 2007;121(3–4):231–41.
9. Kuntz-Simon G, et al. Muscovy duck reovirus sigmaC protein is atypically encoded by the smallest genome segment. J Gen Virol. 2002;83(Pt 5):1189–200.
10. Bassel-Duby R, et al. Sequence of reovirus haemagglutinin predicts a coiled-coil structure. Nature. 1985;315(6018):421–3.
11. Gouvea V, Schnitzer TJ. Pathogenicity of avian reoviruses: examination of six isolates and a vaccine strain. Infect Immun. 1982;38(2):731–8.
12. Banyai K, et al. The goose reovirus genome segment encoding the minor outer capsid protein, sigma1/sigmaC, is bicistronic and shares structural similarities with its counterpart in Muscovy duck reovirus. Virus Genes. 2005;31(3):285–91.
13. Glass SE, et al. Isolation and characterization of a virus associated with arthritis of chickens. Avian Dis. 1973;17(2):415–24.
14. Schnitzer TJ, Ramos T, Gouvea V. Avian reovirus polypeptides: analysis of intracellular virus-specified products, virions, top component, and cores. J Virol. 1982;43(3):1006–14.
15. Spandidos DA, Graham AF. Physical and chemical characterization of an avian reovirus. J Virol. 1976;19(3):968–76.
16. Kawamura H, Shimizu F, Tsubahara H. Avian Adenovirus: Its Properties and Serological Classification. Natl Inst Anim Health Q (Tokyo). 1964;4:183–93.
17. Gouvea, V.S. and Schnitzer TJ, Polymorphism of the genomic RNAs among the avian reoviruses. J Gen Virol, 1982. 61 (Pt I): p. 87–91.
18. Schwartz LD, et al. Infectious tenosynovitis in commercial white leghorn chickens. Avian Dis. 1976;20(4):769–73.
19. Varela R, Benavente J. Protein coding assignment of avian reovirus strain S1133. J Virol. 1994;68(10):6775–7.
20. Cook ME, et al. Severity of tenosynovitis in reovirus-infected chickens fed various dietary levels of choline, folic acid, manganese, biotin, or niacin. Avian Dis. 1984;28(3):562–73.
21. Benavente J, Martinez-Costas J. Avian reovirus: structure and biology. Virus Res. 2007;123(2):105–19.
22. Xu, Y., Molecular virology. 2000: Hubei Science & Technology Press.
23. Jones RC, Jordan TW, Lioupis S. Characteristics of reovirus isolated from ruptured gastrocnemius tendons of chickens. Vet Rec. 1975;96(7):153–4.
24. Guneratne JR, Jones RC, Georgiou K. Some observations on the isolation and cultivation of avian reoviruses. Avian Pathol. 1982;11(3):453–62.
25. Barta V, Springer WT, Millar DL. A comparison of avian and mammalian cell cultures for the propagation of avian reovirus WVU 2937. Avian Dis. 1984;28(1):216–23.
26. Van Der Heide L. Viral arthritis/tenosynovitis: a review. Avian Pathol. 1977;6(4):271–84.
27. Al-Muffarej SI, Savage CE, Jones RC. Egg transmission of avian reoviruses in chickens: comparison of a trypsin-sensitive and a trypsin-resistant strain. Avian Pathol. 1996;25(3):469–80.
28. van Loon AA, et al. Isolation of a new serotype of avian reovirus associated with malabsorption syndrome in chickens. Vet Q. 2001;23(3):129–33.
29. Wood GW, Muskett JC, Thornton DH. Observations on the ability of avian reovirus vaccination of hens to protect their progeny against the effects of challenge with homologous and heterologous strains. J Comp Pathol. 1986;96(2):125–9.
30. Ansari AA, Taylor RF, Chang TS. Application of enzyme-linked immunosorbent assay for detecting antibody to mycoplasma gallisepticum infections in poultry. Avian Dis. 1983;27(1):21–35.
31. Frey ML, Hanson RP, Andrson DP. A medium for the isolation of avian mycoplasmas. Am J Vet Res. 1968;29(11):2163–71.
32. Felsenstein J. Confidence limits on phylogenies: an approach using the bootstrap. Evolution. 1985:783–91.
33. Couch RB, et al. A randomized clinical trial of an inactivated avian influenza a (H7N7) vaccine. PLoS One. 2012;7(12):e49704.
34. Liu L, et al. Study of the integrated immune response induced by an inactivated EV71 vaccine. PLoS One. 2013;8(1):e54451.
35. Liu SJ, Wang FY, Cheng ZQ, et al. Development of the proplis-adjuvant inactivated vaccine of reovirus disease in muscovy duck. Chinese Journal of Preventive Veterinary Medicine. 2006;2:027.
36. Jones RC, Onunkwo O. Studies on experimental tenosynovitis in light hybrid chickens. Avian Pathol. 1978;7(1):171–81.
37. Macdonald JW, et al. Observations on viral tenosynovitis (viral arthritis) in Scotland. Avian Pathol. 1978;7(4):471–82.

Comparative efficacy of the Leucofeligen™ FeLV/RCP and Purevax™ RCP FeLV vaccines against infection with circulating feline Calicivirus

T. Almeras, P. Schreiber, S. Fournel, V. Martin, C. S. Nicolas, C. Fontaine*, C. Lesbros and S. Gueguen

Abstract

Background: Feline calicivirus (FCV) is a common virus, found worldwide, mainly responsible for chronic ulceroproliferative faucitis and periodontitis. This virus has a high mutation rate, leading to the presence of numerous FCV strains in the field. The objectives of this study was to evaluate and compare the efficacy of two vaccines (Leucofeligen™ FeLV/RCP and Purevax™ RCP FeLV), which differ by their nature (live vs. inactivated) and the vaccinal strains, against circulating FCV strains. Thirty 9-week-old specific pathogen free (SPF) kittens were thus randomised into 3 groups and were either not vaccinated (control) or vaccinated (2 injections, 3 weeks apart) with one of the vaccines. Four weeks after the second injection of primary vaccination, the cats were inoculated with a pathogenic strain representative of the ones circulating in Europe (FCV-FR4_01) and followed for 2 weeks.

Results: After challenge, significant differences ($p < 0.05$) between control cats and cats vaccinated with Leucofeligen™ FeLV/RCP or Purevax™ RCP FeLV were observed for body weight variation, rectal temperature rise and maximum clinical scores, reflecting the intensity of the signs (83% and 67% lower in the respective vaccinated groups than in the control group). Significant differences were observed between the vaccinated groups, as cats vaccinated with Leucofeligen™ FeLV/RCP had a lower temperature rise ($p < 0.05$ at days post-challenge 3 to 5) and lower virus shedding titres ($p < 0.05$ at days post-challenge 8, 9 and 11) than cats vaccinated with Purevax™ RCP FeLV. Finally, only cats vaccinated with Leucofeligen™ FeLV/RCP had a significantly lower cumulative score, reflecting the intensity and duration of calicivirosis clinical signs, than the control cats (77% lower vs. 62% lower for cats vaccinated with Purevax™ RCP FeLV).

Conclusions: Both vaccines, Leucofeligen™ FeLV/RCP and Purevax™ RCP FeLV, were found to be efficacious in reducing clinical signs induced by FCV-FR4_01, a FCV strain representative of the circulating ones. However, cats vaccinated with Leucofeligen™ FeLV/RCP were able to control the infection more efficiently than those vaccinated with Purevax™ RCP FeLV, as evidenced by the shorter duration of clinical signs and lower viral titre in excretions.

Keywords: Calicivirus, Coryza, Cat, Vaccine, Efficacy, Live, Leucofeligen, Feligen, Purevax

* Correspondence: christelle.fontaine@virbac.com
Virbac, 13ème rue, LID, 06511 Carros, France

Background

Feline calicivirus (FCV) is a RNA virus which can cause various symptoms that affect mainly the oral cavity and, occasionally, the upper respiratory tract [1, 2]. It is one of the main pathogens responsible for coryza (cat flu), a very common disease in cats. Symptoms possibly induced by FCV include oral ulcerations, salivation, gingivitis, stomatitis, conjunctivitis, sneezing and nasal discharge. Some atypical FCV can cause lameness or skin ulcerations while some hypervirulent strains can lead to systemic diseases [1, 2].

Feline calicivirus shows a high antigen variability and can evolve quickly [3, 4]. In a recent study conducted in Europe, 46 strains (pairwise genetic distance >20%) were identified from 72 FCV isolates [3]. However, the phylogenetic analysis of partial variable regions of polymerase or capsid sequences showed that the different strains found in the field had a median uncorrected nucleotide distance of around 40% when compared pairwise or when compared with the F9 strain, currently used in some live vaccines [3].

Vaccines against FCV are available and widely used. They contain one or two FCV strains that are either live attenuated or inactivated. Although regulatory agency approved vaccines should trigger protective immunity, their efficacy can differ according to the type of immunity stimulated [5, 6]. Inactivated vaccines are known to elicit the production of neutralising antibodies (NAb) directed against specific extracellular antigens (humoral immunity). Live vaccines, however, mimic the natural infection and stimulate the cellular component of the immune system (cell-mediated immunity) in addition to the humoral response [5, 6]. Since live attenuated viruses can replicate, live vaccines generally induce a quicker, longer lasting and more efficient immune response than inactivated vaccines [6, 7].

The first aim of this study was to confirm that currently commercialised vaccines against FCV are still efficacious against circulating strains. The second aim was to compare the efficacy of two vaccines containing either the live attenuated strain FCV-F9 (Leucofeligen™ FeLV/RCP, Virbac, France) or two inactivated strains of FCV (431 and G1 [8]; Purevax™ RCP FeLV, Merial, France).

Methods

This controlled, randomised, not blinded, experimental study was carried out under the supervision of the Ethical Committee of Virbac, in accordance with the recommendations issued in the European Pharmacopoeia [9].

Animals and study protocols

Thirty specific-pathogen free European kittens (9 weeks old; average ± SD body weight of 1.1 ± 0.12 kg, ranging from 0.87 to 1.34 kg) obtained from a commercial supplier (Liberty Research, USA), were randomly assigned to 3 groups: group 1 (vaccinated with Leucofeligen™ FeLV/RCP), group 2 (vaccinated with Purevax™ RCP FeLV) and group 3 (not vaccinated). Cats were acclimatised for 7 days to the animal housing conditions (12 h light/dark cycle, 18 ± 3 °C, 55 ± 10% humidity with free access to water and commercial dried food daily feeding). During the acclimation and post-challenge phases, a commercial humid food was proposed in addition to ease the acclimation and limit the effect of oral-ulcer-related anorexia.

Cats included in groups 1 and 2 were vaccinated twice, 3 weeks apart (day 0 and day 21), by subcutaneous injection according to the recommendations of the manufacturers. Cats in group 3 did not receive any vaccine.

Four weeks after the second injection of primary vaccination, on day 49, equivalent to day post-challenge (DPC) 0, all cats were inoculated with a virulent heterologous strain of calicivirus (FCV-FR4_01) and observed for 14 days. All cats of each group were housed together but the groups were separated to avoid contaminations.

Vaccines

Leucofeligen™ FeLV/RCP was granted a pan-European marketing authorisation (centralised procedure) in 2009. It is packaged as a freeze-dried fraction containing the live attenuated viruses, that is, FCV (F9 strain), Feline Herpes Virus-1 (FHV-1; F2 strain), and Feline Panleukopenia Virus (FPV; LR72 strain), and a liquid fraction containing the recombinant FeLV-envelope antigen p45 (derived from FeLV gp70) with aluminium hydroxide and QA-21 adjuvants. Purevax™ RCP FeLV is presented as a freeze-dried fraction containing inactivated strains of FCV (431 and G1) and attenuated strains of FHV (F2) and FPV (PLI IV), and a liquid fraction containing a recombinant virus canarypox FeLV (vCP97).

The vaccine vials were stored between +2 °C and +8 °C and were reconstituted immediately prior to use by rehydrating the freeze-dried fraction with the liquid fraction.

Challenge

The FCV-FR4_01 strain (Genbank accession number MF882991) was isolated during the field epidemiology study performed by Hou et al. [3]. This strain was chosen for the challenge since it was identified as a single isolate (unique sequence) with a high titration from a single cat presenting various clinical signs typical of a calicivirus infection. The strain was amplified through two passages on CRFK cells and controlled in order to ensure the absence of any interfering pathogens. Regulatory compliant reproducible experimental infections were developed (internal data). The same clinical signs, identical to the ones observed in the original cat, were constantly reproduced: a marked weight loss in the first week, hyperthermia, a depression of the general status and apparition of oral and nasal ulcers, typical of FCV infections. Minor nasal and ocular discharge could also be observed. The FCV-FR4_01 challenge strain was therefore considered as representative of the initial FCV-FR4_01 isolate and thus representative also of the FCV circulating strains.

Further analyses of the sequence identities, performed on partial capside sequences, showed that the FCV-FR4_01 strain had 73% homology with FCV-F9, 75% with FCV-G1 and 76% with FCV-431 while the three vaccination strains shared between 70% and 74% identities. These levels of homology were in accordance with the homology found between circulating strains [3]. None of the vaccine strains clustered with the FCV-FR4_01 challenge strain (pairwise genetic distance >20%, Fig. 1) [10, 11].

The challenge was performed on anesthetised cats inoculated intranasally with $10^{7.5}$ cell culture infecting dose, 50% endpoint ($CCID_{50}$) per cat of FCV-FR4_01 suspension using a volume of 0.25 mL/nostril.

Monitoring

During the vaccination phase, cats were checked daily for appearance of any clinical signs. The animals were examined and weighed weekly. In the post-challenge phase, clinical examinations were performed daily, starting with Group 2 then 1 and ending with Group 3 to avoid contamination between groups, and included rectal temperature measurement and observation of clinical signs (general status, nasal and ocular discharge, ulcers) until DPC 14. Weighing was performed twice a week.

Scoring

The clinical status was evaluated according to a scoring system based on that specified in the pharmacopoeia monograph [9] (see Table 1). A score was given for each parameter, each cat, on every assessment day. For

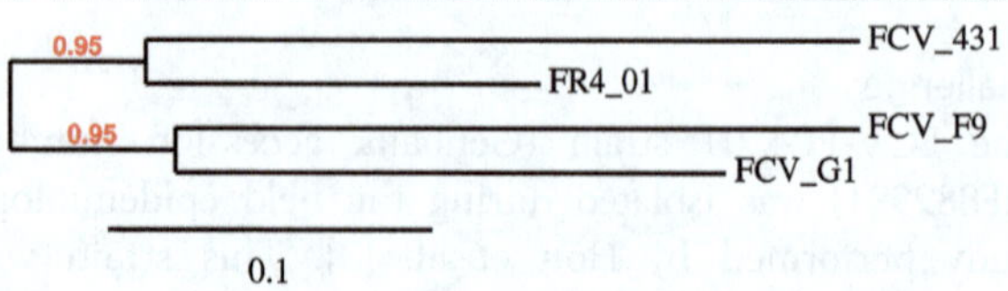

Fig. 1 Unrooted tree of the partial capsid sequences of 4 feline calicivirus (FCV) strains, the FCV-FR4_01 challenge strain (GenBank accession No. MF882991) and the 3 vaccine strains FCV-F9 (GenBank accession No. M86379), FCV 431 (National French patent registration number 00 01761), FCV G1 (National French patent registration number 00 01761). This phylogenetic tree was reconstructed using the maximum likelihood method implemented in the PhyML program (v3.1/3.0 aLRT). The percentage of replicate trees in which the associated taxa clustered together in bootstrap tests (1000 replicates) is shown newt to the branches. Only bootstrap values >95 are shown. Distances are drown to scale and relate to the distance bar

Table 1 Scoring system for the different signs observed, based on the European Pharmacopoeia monograph 1102 [9]

Observed signs	Description	Score
Death		10
Depressed state		2
Temperature	≥39.5 °C	1
	≤37 °C	2
Ulcer (nasal or oral)	Small and few in number	1
	Large and numerous	3
Nasal discharge	slight	1
	copious	2
Ocular discharge		1
Weight loss ≥3%		2

comparison of scores between groups, two methods were used. The first method, the cumulative score, consisted of adding up all daily scores recorded for each cat and for each parameter (cumulative score per cat for parameter x = sum of scores recorded from DPC 0 to DPC 14). The median of the cumulative scores per parameter was then calculated in each group as well as the median of the total cumulative scores recorded per cat, taking into account all parameters.

For the second method, the maximum score recorded per cat and per parameter during the period was taken as a reference to calculate the median maximum scores for each parameter and the total of maximum scores recorded for each cat. The median of the total of maximum scores was used to assess differences in the severity of the clinical picture while the median of the total cumulative scores was used to evaluate the severity and duration of each sign. For both methods, scores for general status, nasal discharge, ocular discharge, ulcers and rectal temperature were included. The score for weight loss (scored once on DPC 7 to evaluate the loss over the first week) was also taken into account for the calculation of the maximum scores.

Efficacy assessment

A vaccine was judged to be efficacious if the median of the total maximum scores was significantly lower in the vaccinated group than in the control group.

Viral shedding

Viral shedding was assessed from nasal washings performed daily from DPC 2. Successive dilutions (10-fold steps) of samples were mixed with plated CRFK cells and incubated for one hour at 37 °C before adding more medium. They were then further incubated for 6 days and the cytopathogenic effect of FCV viruses was assessed microscopically. Cats were considered negative when the titre was $<10^{0.3}$ $DICC_{50}$/mL, which was the detection threshold.

Serological assessments

The serological assessments included evaluation of the titres of total immunoglobulin G (IgG) and of neutralising antibodies (NAb) directed against the FCV-FR4_01 strain. Blood samples were collected on days 0, 21, 35, 49 (DPC 0), 56 (DPC 7) and 63 (DPC 14).

Total IgG

Titres of IgG reactive to FCV antigens were assessed using an immunofluorescent antibody assay. Briefly, two-fold dilutions of each serum (from 1/8 to 1/8192) were added to a 96-well plate containing acetone-fixed CRFK cells infected with FCV-FR4_01. Positive and negative sera were diluted the same way and used as controls. They were incubated for 1 h at 37 °C and revealed with a fluorescein-conjugated anti-feline IgG antibody and a solution of Evans Blue. The positivity threshold was 1/128 (equivalent to a dilution of $10^{2.1}$).

Neutralising Ab

Titres of NAb were determined by serum neutralisation (SN) of the FCV-FR4_01 strain. Briefly, each serum was diluted to provide six 2-fold dilution steps (1/8 to 1/256). Diluted sera were incubated for 1 h with FCV-FR4_01 suspension (100–502 $DICC_{50}$/test) to allow viral neutralisation. Each mixture was then added to six 96-well plates containing 70% confluent CRFK cells. After 6 days of incubation, the characteristic cytopathic effect was assessed. The titre was determined by the Spearman and Karber method [12] and considered negative when inferior to $10^{0.9}$ which was the detection threshold.

Statistical tests

All statistical analyses were performed using SAS 9.3 software. For the comparison of parameters with repeated measures (antibody titration, rectal temperature, body weight, and viral shedding), a mixed model analysis of variance was used to compare the 3 groups over time. For weight and temperature, the baseline values were used as covariates. In case of significant interaction, adjusted group comparisons (Tukey-Kramer) at each significant time point were performed. Assumptions of normality and homogeneity of variances of residuals were checked. If the Levene's test of homogeneity of variances was significant, an ANOVA model allowing for different variances in each group using Kenward & Roger method was used to compute the denominator degree of freedom for the tests involving fixed effects.

For other parameters (scores, days of hyperthermia, area under the hyperthermia curve and weight change between DPC 0 and DPC 7), a Kruskal-Wallis test was performed to compare groups, followed in case of a significant *p*-value by a Dunn's test for multiple comparisons. The area under the hyperthermia (≥39.5 °C) curve was calculated using the trapezoidal rule (using NCSS 2004 software).

A p value <0.05 was considered significant.

Results

Vaccination phase (day 0 – day 49)

Clinical monitoring and safety

During the vaccination phase, one control cat was found dead while all other cats remained healthy. Weight gain was similar between groups and rectal temperature remained stable in all groups (mean temperatures between 38.5 °C and 39 °C in all groups). No abnormal general or local reaction was observed with any vaccine.

Immune response

The presence of FCV antibodies was assessed using immunofluorescence (IF) or SN against the FCV-FR4_01 challenge strain. Titration of total FCV antibodies (IgGs) assessed by IF showed a detectable seroconversion from day 21 in 10/10 (100%) cats in group 1 (Leucofeligen™ FeLV/RCP) but only in 5/10 (50%) cats in group 2 (Purevax™ RCP FeLV). Mean FCV-FR4_01 IgGs titre was significantly higher in group 1 (Leucofeligen™ FeLV/RCP) than in group 2 (Purevax™ RCP FeLV) 3 weeks after the first injection of primary vaccination: mean log10 (± SD) of 2.9 ± 0.2 vs. 1.1 ± 1.1 (p < 0.001, n = 10 in each group, Fig. 2a). Mean titration was similar in both vaccinated groups 3 weeks after the second injection of primary vaccination. All vaccinated cats (20/20) had seroconverted at that time. No antibodies were found in the serum of cats in the control group before inoculating cats with the FCV-FR4_01 strain (n = 10). During the vaccination phase, neutralising antibodies were not present in any group or at a very low level on days 21 and 42 (Fig. 2b).

Post-challenge phase
(day 49 – day 63 or DPC 0 - DPC 14)

Clinical monitoring

Weight Before challenge on DPC 0, mean (± SD) body weights were not significantly different between groups: 2.11 ± 0.20 kg in the control group; 1.98 ± 0.25 kg in cats vaccinated with Purevax™ RCP FeLV and 1.92 ± 0.29 kg in cats vaccinated with Leucofeligen™ FeLV/RC. A decrease in mean body weight was observed during the first week of the challenge phase in the control group but not in the vaccinated groups (Fig. 3a). Indeed, all kittens (9/9) in the control group lost more than 3% of their body weight (a loss considered significant at this age and taken as a reference for severity [13]) between DPC 0 and DPC 7 compared to only 2 cats in each vaccinated group. Mean weight (± SD) in the control group went from 2.11 ± 0.20 kg to

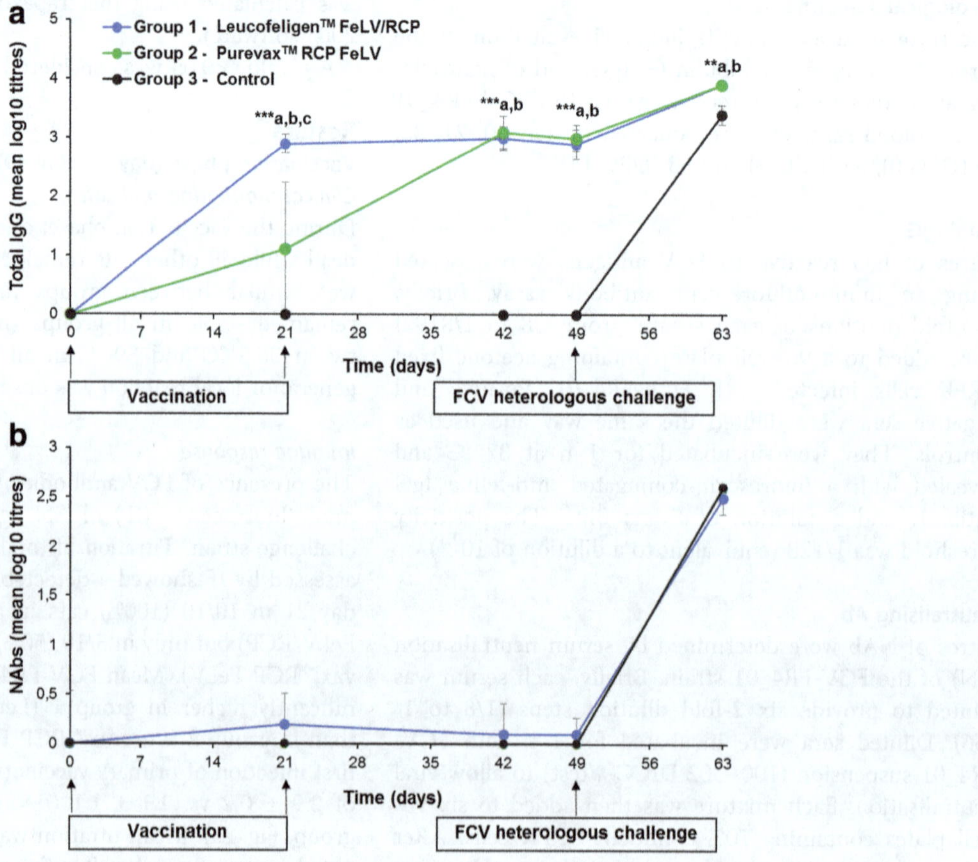

Fig. 2 Titration of total IgG and neutralising antibodies directed against the FCV-FR4_01 strain, during the course of the study. Titration of total IgG was assessed by immunofluorescence (IF; **a**) while neutralising antibodies were assessed by a SN assay (**b**). Titrations were performed from samples collected on days 0, 21, 42, 49 (DCP 0) and 63 (DCP 14) in group 1 (Leucofeligen™ FeLV/RCP, *blue*, *n* = 10), group 2 (Purevax™ RCP FeLV, *green*, n = 10) and group 3 (control, *black*, *n* = 9). Mean values (and SD as error bars) are reported. **a** A value of 0 was attributed to titration <2.1 log 10 (positive threshold) and 3.9 log 10 was the maximum value which could be measured. In the vaccinated groups, all values from day 21 were significantly different from day 0 and from values in control group ($p < 0.05$, Tukey adjusted multiple comparisons). **a**, **b** and **c**: statistically significant difference between group 1 (Leucofeligen™ FeLV/RCP) and control (a); between group 2 (Purevax™ RCP FeLV) and control (**b**); and between group 1 (Leucofeligen™ FeLV/RCP) and group 2 (Purevax™ RCP FeLV) (**c**). * $p < 0.05$; ** $p < 0.01$; *** $p < 0.001$. **b** A value of 0 was attributed to titration <0.9 log 10 (positive threshold) and 2.56 log 10 was the maximum value. No difference between groups was observed

1.96 ± 0.19 kg and 1.86 ± 0.21 kg from DPC 0 to DPC 4 ($p < 0.001$) and DPC 7 ($p < 0.001$), respectively, and was of 2.09 ± 0.24 kg at DPC 14 (NS).

Temperature An increase in rectal temperature was observed in all groups with a peak of hyperthermia (≥39.5 °C) on days 3 to 5 after challenge (Fig. 3b). However, compared to DPC 0, cats in the control group had, on average, a higher increase in temperature ($p < 0.05$) than cats in the vaccinated group 1 (Leucofeligen™ FeLV/RCP) on DPC 2 to 6, and than cats in the vaccinated group 2 (Purevax™ RCP FeLV) on DPC 2, 3 and 6 (Fig. 3c). A greater mean increase in rectal temperature was also observed in cats vaccinated with Purevax™ RCP FeLV than in cats vaccinated with Leucofeligen™ FeLV/RCP, on DPC 3, 4 and 5 ($p < 0.05$, Fig. 3c). The number (%) of cats with severe hyperthermia (>40 °C) was of 5/10 (50%), 8/10 (80%) and 9/9 (100%) in group 1, 2 and 3 (control), respectively. Furthermore, cats in the control group remained, on average ± SD, longer in hyperthermia than those in vaccinated groups 1 and 2 (5.2 ± 1.6 vs. 2.1 ± 1.3 and 3 ± 1.4 days, respectively, $p < 0.05$). Cats vaccinated with Purevax™ RCP FeLV remained longer, on average ± SD, in severe hyperthermia than cats vaccinated with Leucofeligen™ FeLV/RCP (3.2 ± 1.2 vs. 0.8 ± 1.0 days, $p < 0.05$). Overall, by comparing the areas under the hyperthermia curves (>39.5 °C), the cats in group 1 (Leucofeligen™ FeLV/RCP), unlike those in group 2 (Purevax™ RCP FeLV), responded differently than the cats in the control group (1.10 ± 1.01; 2.26 ± 1.37 and 3.77 ± 1.29 °C.day, mean ± SD respectively, $p < 0.05$). These data suggest that control cats had a more severe and longer lasting hyperthermia than cats vaccinated with Leucofeligen™ FeLV/RCP.

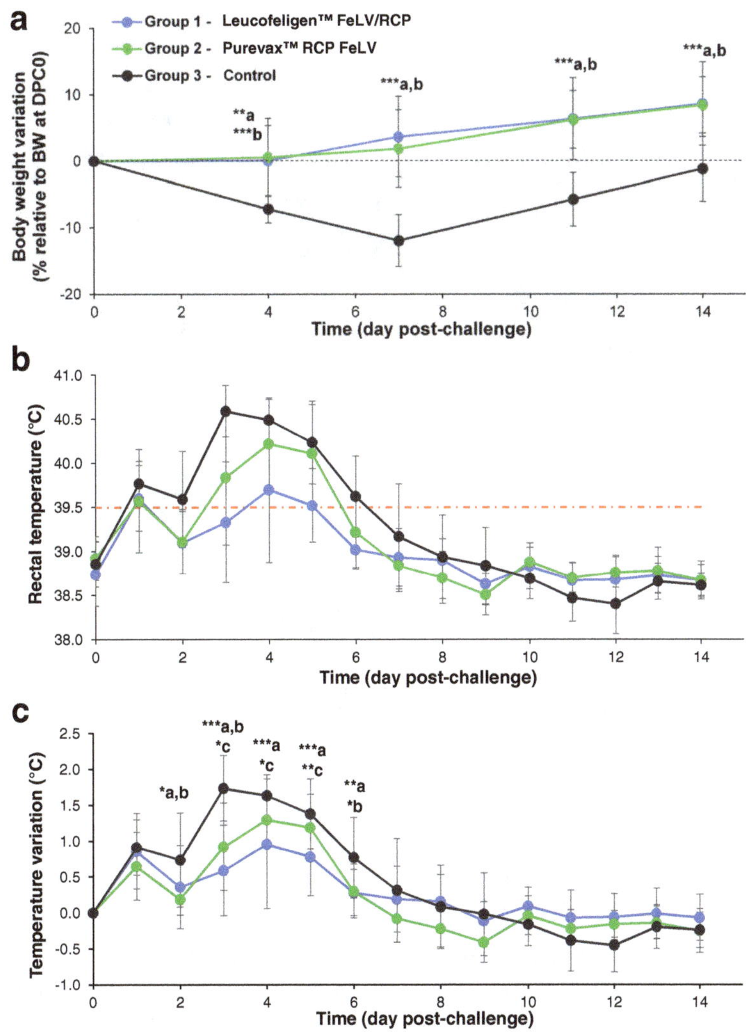

Fig. 3 Variations in weight and rectal temperature after challenging cats with the FCV-FR4_01 strain (DPC 0). Weight was assessed on DCP 0, 4, 7, 11 and 14 in group 1 (Leucofeligen™ FeLV/RCP, *blue*, *n* = 10), group 2 (Purevax™ RCP FeLV, *green*, n = 10) and group 3 (control, *black*, *n* = 9) and mean body weight variation (in % from initial body weight at DPC 0) are reported in **a**. Rectal temperature was assessed daily and mean temperatures are reported in **b**. Mean temperature variations (difference from value at DPC 0) are reported in **c**. All data are presented as mean and SD (error bars). Statistically significant differences in variation between groups were observed and are annotated as in Fig. 1

Clinical signs Concerning general status, 7/9 (78%) cats in the control group showed apathy or depression while the cats in the vaccinated groups 1 and 2 showed no general signs. Rare, minor and transient ocular and nasal discharges were observed in very few cats, in groups 1 (Leucofeligen™ FeLV/RCP, 1 cat with ocular discharge for 1 day) and 3 (control, 1 cat with ocular discharge and 1 with nasal discharge for 1 day each). Fewer cats vaccinated with Leucofeligen™ FeLV/RCP had buccal and nasal ulcers (3/10: 30%) than cats in the other groups (7/10: 70% of cats vaccinated with Purevax™ RCP FeLV and 7/9: 78% of control cats). Large ulcers (≥5 mm) were found in 0/10 (0%), 1/10 (10%) and 2/9 (22%) cats in groups 1, 2 and 3, respectively. Ulcers lasted for up to 3 days in group 1 but up to 10 days in groups 2 and 3.

Scores

Cumulative clinical scores take into account the scores recorded daily for each parameter (general status, nasal discharge, ocular discharge, ulcers and rectal temperature). The median (inter-quartile range or IQR) of the total cumulative clinical scores, indicative of the clinical severity and duration of signs, was significantly higher in the control group [13.0 (11.0–14.0); $n = 9$] than in the group vaccinated with Leucofeligen™ FeLV/RCP [3.0 (1.0–5.0); $n = 10$; $p < 0.05$] but was not significantly different than in the group vaccinated with Purevax™ RCP FeLV [5.0 (5.0–8.8); $n = 10$, Fig. 4a]. Compared to unvaccinated cats, the median of the total cumulative clinical scores was 77% lower in cats vaccinated with Leucofeligen™ FeLV/RCP and was 62% lower in those vaccinated with Purevax™ RCP FeLV.

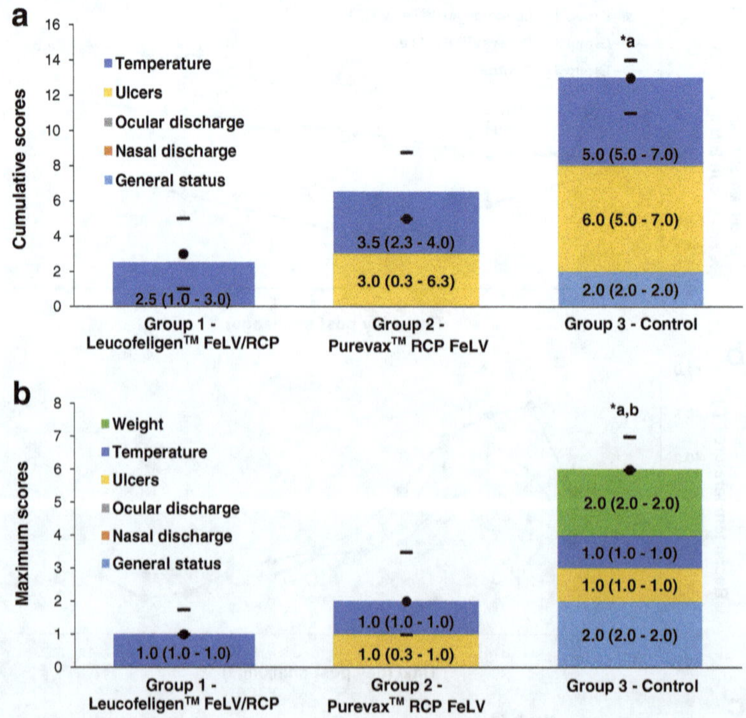

Fig. 4 Clinical scores in the post-challenge phase. **a**: Median (IQR in brackets) of cumulative clinical scores for temperature, ulcers, ocular discharge, nasal discharge and general status, in each group. The *black circle* indicates the median of total cumulative scores recorded in each cat and the dashes the 1nd and 3rd quartiles. **b**: Median (IQR in brackets) of maximum scores observed for each sign. The 6 parameters assessed are represented (weight, temperature, ulcers, ocular discharge, nasal discharge and general status). The *black circle* indicates the median of total maximum scores recorded in each cat and the dashes the 1nd and 3rd quartiles. Statistically significant differences between groups were observed on the median of the total scores per cat and are annotated as in Fig. 1. Leucofeligen™ FeLV/RCP: n = 10; Purevax™ RCP FeLV: n = 10 and control: n = 9

The median (IQR) of the total maximum scores (all parameters/cat: general status, nasal discharge, ocular discharge, ulcers, rectal temperature and weight) was significantly higher ($p < 0.05$) in the control group [6.0 (6.0–7.0); $n = 9$] than in the group vaccinated with Leucofeligen™ FeLV/RCP [1.0 (1.0–1.8); 83% lower; $n = 10$] and the group vaccinated with Purevax™ RCP FeLV [2.0 (1.0–3.5); 67% lower; n = 10; Fig. 4b).

Viral shedding

A peak of viral shedding was observed in all groups between DPC 2 and DPC 5 (Fig. 5). However, viral elimination seemed to occur earlier and faster in some animals vaccinated with Leucofeligen™ FeLV/RCP than in the control group or the group of cats vaccinated with Purevax™ RCP FeLV. Indeed, viral titres were significantly lower in cats vaccinated with Leucofeligen™ FeLV/RCP than in the control group on DPC 7 to 11 ($p < 0.05$, n = 10 and 9, respectively, Fig. 5) and significantly lower than in group 2 on DCP 8, 9 and 11 ($p < 0.05$, n = 10 in each group, Fig. 5). No statistical differences were observed between groups 2 (Purevax™ RCP FeLV) and 3 (control).

Immune response

As shown in Fig. 2, all cats had seroconverted at the end of the study. The titre of total IgG was, however, significantly lower in the control group than in both vaccinated groups ($p < 0.01$, Fig. 2a).

Discussion

The feline calicivirus has the propensity to evolve quickly, so that different strains can be found in the field [3,4]. Because of the heterogeneity between strains [3], it was of importance to verify that vaccines formulated with strains isolated a few years ago were still efficacious against circulating strains.

In this study, cats were inoculated with one of the strains (FCV-FR4_01) isolated during a field epidemiology study conducted in Europe and published in 2016 [3]. This strain was chosen as it was genetically representative of the circulating classical FCV pathogenic strains. This statement is based on the lack of evidence for FCV sub-species clustering or serotypes except for viruses sharing immediate temporal or spatial links [3]. Moreover, the clinical signs induced by the FCV-FR4_01 challenge strain were also representatives of a classical feline calicivirosis [2]. In all cats (10/10) in the control

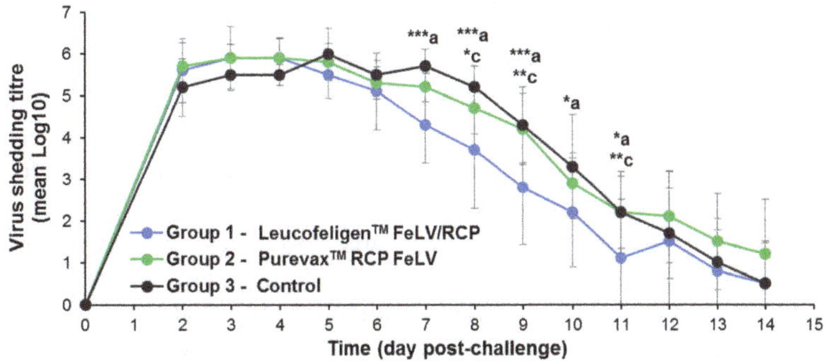

Fig. 5 Viral shedding during the post-challenge phase. Viral shedding was assessed from nasal washings performed daily in the different groups (*blue*: group 1 – Leucofeligen™ FeLV/RCP, n = 10; *green*: group 2 – Purevax™ RCP FeLV, n = 10 and *black*: group 3 – control, n = 9). Data are presented as mean and SD (error bars). Statistically significant differences between groups were observed and are annotated as in Fig. 1

group, the dose and route of administration used for the experimental infection induced one or several typical signs of feline calicivirosis, ie a marked weight loss in the first week, hyperthermia, a depression of the general status and apparition of oral and nasal ulcers. These signs were similar to those presented by the initial cat [3] and cats previously challenged with this strain (internal data). This percentage of unvaccinated cats showing notable clinical signs of feline calicivirosis (hyperthermia, bucal ulcers and respiratory signs) is higher than the minimum of 80% required by the European pharmacopeia to validate a FCV experimental infection. This result suggests that the experimental FCV-FR4_01 infection performed was particularly severe and that this strain can be an excellent candidate to test FCV vaccines efficacy in the future.

The efficacy evaluations of the Leucofeligen™ FeLV/RCP and of the Purevax™ RCP FeLV vaccines against this heterologous strain were based on the scores obtained for different parameters. Their efficacy against FCV heterologous strains has been reported in the past [13–15] but not against circulating ones. Consistently with the results obtained in these previous studies [13, 15], the median of the total of maximum clinical scores obtained in the vaccinated groups were significantly lower than the one obtained in the control group (83% and 67% lower for the Leucofeligen™ FeLV/RCP and Purevax™ RCP FeLV vaccines, respectively). The maintenance of the protection conferred by the commercial vaccines against circulating FCV strains supports the idea that the observed inter-strain genetic difference [3] may not induce a significant change in the FCV capsid amino acid sequence and/or configuration. These data also show that the clinical cross-protection triggered by a FCV vaccine is independent of the number of strains it contains. Indeed, the Leucofeligen™ FeLV/RCP vaccine, containing one FCV strain (FCV-F9), brings a similar (or even better under the experimental conditions of this study) clinical cross-protection than the Purevax™ RCP FeLV vaccine which contains two FCV stains (FCV-G1 and FCV-431) [8, 15].

Interestingly, vaccinated cats were protected despite the lack of detectable SN during the vaccination phase (Fig. 2). This observation is in agreement with previous studies showing that the absence of seroneutralising FCV antibodies is not correlated with an absence of protection [13, 15] and in terms of antibody protection, the levels of IgA mucosal antibodies, if available, would be a more appropriate marker of the efficacy of the mucosal defense and ultimate shedding [13]. Indeed, despite a certain level of cross-neutralisation, NAbs are quite specific of the strain used to induce them [13, 16, 17]. The protection against heterologous strains is also and sometimes mainly induced by the cell-mediated immune response triggered by the vaccine and the IgGs, not necessarily neutralising, directed against various viral or infected-cell antigens (total IgGs) [5–7, 18]. Therefore, it would be more relevant to analyse the cell-mediated immune response to evaluate a FCV vaccine efficacy rather than evaluating the level of Nabs in vitro [15–17]. However, since no technique can be routinely used to assess, in vitro, the cell-mediated immune response, experimental infection in vivo remains the only reliable way to assess FCV vaccines efficacy.

Both vaccines were deemed efficacious. However, some differences were observed between the cats vaccinated with Purevax™ RCP FeLV and those vaccinated with Leucofeligen™ FeLV/RCP. First, the cats vaccinated with Leucofeligen™ FeLV/RCP could seroconvert faster (within the 3 weeks after the first primary injection) than some cats vaccinated with Purevax™ RCP FeLV (two injections of primary vaccination required for seroconversion of all cats) (Fig. 2a). The difference in the types of vaccine used, live versus killed, may provide a partial explanation for this result [5, 6]. For example, live organisms induce a greater up-regulation of activation molecules and granulocyte-macrophage colony-stimulating factors than do killed organisms [19]. This difference may explain both, the delay in producing IgGs and the requirement for two injection of primary vaccination for the cats vaccinated with Purevax™ RCP FeLV [5–7]. On the contrary, the Leucofeligen™ FeLV/RCP vaccine may require only one injection as a primary vaccination since IgGs were detected after the first injection. Further tests are required to confirm this. Similar findings regarding the speed of onset of immunity, number of injections for primary vaccination and clinical efficacy properties of vaccines depending on their nature, live or killed, might also be observed in other mammals including humans.

The severity and duration of symptoms such as temperature rise or ulcerations also differed between groups. The median of the total cumulative scores was lower in cats vaccinated with Leucofeligen™ FeLV/RCP than in cats vaccinated with Purevax™ RCP FeLV. Although this difference was not statistically significant, only the group of cats vaccinated with Leucofeligen™ FeLV/RCP had a significantly lower score than the control group (77% lower vs. 62% lower for the group vaccinated with Purevax™ RCP FeLV). These data suggest that the Leucofeligen™ FeLV/RCP vaccine would bring a better protection against the heterologous FCV-FR4_01 strain than the Purevax™ RCP FeLV vaccine. Indeed, when assessing the viral shedding, it was found that the titres of viruses eliminated by cats vaccinated with Leucofeligen™ FeLV/RCP was lower than in cats vaccinated with Purevax™ RCP FeLV on DPC 8, 9 and 11. No difference was found between this latter group and the control group, though. These results are consistent with previous studies and the general knowledge that live attenuated vaccines provide a quicker and more efficient protection than inactivated vaccines [6, 20, 21]. They further confirm that a vaccine with a combination of several FCV strains (e.g. Purevax™ RCP FeLV) is not more efficient against heterologous strains than a vaccine with one FCV valence (e.g. Leucofeligen™ FeLV/RCP) and does not seem to broaden the protection against antigenically distant strains, as previously mentioned [15].

In this study, an FCV strain representative of the circulating ones was used for the challenge [3] to ensure that currently commercialised FCV vaccines were efficacious against heterologous circulating strains. Due to the comparable level of genetic difference between FCV strains, similar clinical results are expected if another FCV circulating strain is used for the challenge, as shown previously [13, 15]. However, the results may differ if a highly virulent strain is chosen for challenge and further analyses are required to assess the efficacy of vaccines against this type of strains [4].

Conclusion

In this study, we compared the ability of two vaccines (Leucofeligen™ FeLV/RCP and Purevax™ RCP FeLV) directed against FCV and other viruses to protect against a heterologous FCV strain circulating in the field (FCV-FR4_01). Both vaccines were found to be efficacious in reducing the clinical signs induced by this strain, compared to an unvaccinated group. However, some differences concerning the rapidity of seroconversion, the duration of clinical signs, and the reduction in viral titre in excretions were found, in favor of the Leucofeligen™ FeLV/RCP vaccine. This study therefore showed that both vaccines still have a good efficacy against circulating strains but that Leucofeligen™ FeLV/RCP may bring a better protection than Purevax™ RCP FeLV against a heterologous strain.

Abbreviations

Ab: Antibodies; $CCID_{50}$: Cell culture infecting dose, 50% endpoint; CRFK: Crandell Rees feline kidney; DPC: Day post-challenge; FCV: Feline calicivirus; FeLV: Feline leukemia virus; FHV: Feline herpesvirus; FPV: Feline panleukopenia virus; IgG: Immunoglobulin G; IQR: Inter-quartile range; NAb: Neutralising antibodies; RCP: Feline rhinotracheitis virus, calicivirus and panleukopenia virus; SD: Standard deviation

Acknowledgements

Not applicable.

Funding

This study was funded by Virbac.

Authors' contributions

CL and TA conceived of and designed the study. TA, and PS participated in its coordination and in the data acquisition. SF performed the statistical analysis. VM participated in the data acquisition. SG helped to conceive and to design the study. CSN and CF participated in the data analysis and drafted the manuscript. All the authors read and approved the final version.

Consent for publication

Not applicable.

Competing interests

All the authors of this paper were employed by Virbac.

References

1. Radford AD, Coyne KP, Dawson S, Porter CJ, Gaskell RM. Feline calicivirus. Vet Res. 2007;38(2):319–35.
2. Radford AD, Addie D, Belák S, Boucraut-Baralon C, Egberink H, Frymus T, Gruffydd-Jones T, Hartmann K, Hosie MJ, Lloret A, Lutz H, Marsilio F, Pennisi MG, Thiry E, Truyen U, Horzinek MC. Feline calicivirus infection. ABCD guidelines on prevention and management. J Feline Med Surg. 2009;11(7): 556–64.
3. Hou J, Sánchez-Vizcaíno F, McGahie D, Lesbros C, Almeras T, Howarth D, O'Hara V, Dawson S, Radford AD. European molecular epidemiology and strain diversity of feline calicivirus. Vet Rec. 2016;178(5):114–5.
4. Radford AD, Dawson S, Coyne KP, Porter CJ, Gaskell RM. The challenge for the next generation of feline calicivirus vaccines. Vet Microbiol. 2006;117(1):14–8.

5. Saalmüller A. New understanding of immunological mechanisms. Vet Microbiol. 2006;117(1):32–8.
6. Greene CE, Schultz RD. Immunoprophylaxis. In: Greene CE, editor. Infectious diseases of the dog and cat. 3rd ed. St Louis: Saunders Elsevier; 2006. p. 1069–119.
7. Day MJ, Horzinek MC, Schultz RD, Squires RA, Vaccination Guidelines Group (VGG) of the World Small Animal Veterinary Association (WSAVA). WSAVA guidelines for the vaccination of dogs and cats. J Small Anim Pract. 2016; 57(1):E1–E45.
8. Poulet H, Jas D, Lemeter C, Coupier C, Brunet S. Efficacy of a bivalent inactivated non-adjuvanted feline calicivirus vaccine: relation between in vitro cross-neutralization and heterologous protection in vivo. Vaccine. 2008; 26(29–30):3647–54.
9. "Feline calicivirosis vaccine (live)" European pharmacopoeia monograph 04/ 2013:1102, p 5350–5351.
10. Dereeper A, Guignon V, Blanc G, Audic S, Buffet S, Chevenet F, Dufayard JF, Guindon S, Lefort V, Lescot M, Claverie JM, Gascuel O. Phylogeny.Fr: robust phylogenetic analysis for the non-specialist. Nucleic Acids Res. 2008; 10. 1093/nar/gkn180.
11. Dereeper A, Audic S, Claverie JM, Blanc G. BLAST-EXPLORER helps you building datasets for phylogenetic analysis. BMC Evol Biol. 2010; 10.1186/ 1471-2148-10-8.
12. Lorenz RJ, Bögel K. Laboratory techniques in rabies: methods of calculation. Monogr Ser World Health Organ. 1973;23:321–35.
13. Lesbros C, Martin V, Najbar W, Sanquer A, McGahie D, Eun HM, Gueguen S. Protective efficacy of the Calicivirus Valency of the Leucofeligen™ FeLV/RCP vaccine against a virulent Heterologous challenge in kittens. Vet Med Int. 2013;2013:232397.
14. Jas D, Frances-Duvert V, Vernes D, Guigal PM, Poulet H. Three-year duration of immunity for feline herpesvirus and calicivirus evaluated in a controlled vaccination-challenge laboratory trial. Vet Microbiol. 2015;177(1–2):123–31.
15. Poulet H, Brunet S, Leroy V, Chappuis G. Immunisation with a combination of two complementary feline calicivirus strains induces a broad cross-protection against heterologous challenges. Vet Microbiol. 2005;106(1–2): 17–31.
16. Wensman JJ, Samman A, Lindhe A, Thibault JC, Berndtsson LT, Hosie MJ. Ability of vaccine strain induced antibodies to neutralize field isolates of caliciviruses from Swedish cats. Acta Vet Scand. 2015;57:86.
17. Addie D, Poulet H, Golder MC, McDonald M, Brunet S, Thibault JC, Hosie MJ. Ability of antibodies to two new caliciviral vaccine strains to neutralise feline calicivirus isolates from the UK. Vet Rec. 2008;163(12):355–7.
18. Tizard IR. Veterinary Immunolgy: an introduction. 8th ed. Philadelphia: W.B. Saunders Company; 2008. p. 302–3.
19. Tizard IR. Veterinary Immunolgy: an introduction. 8th ed. Philadelphia: W.B. Saunders Company; 2008. p. 258–9.
20. Shewen PE, Povey RC, Wilson MR. A comparison of the efficacy of a live and four inactivated vaccine preparations for the protection of cats against experimental challenge with Chlamydia psittaci. Can J Comp Med. 1980; 44(3):244–51.
21. Gambaryan AS, Lomakina NF, Boravleva EY, Kropotkina EA, Mashin VV, Krasilnikov IV, Klimov AI, Rudenko LG. Comparative safety, immunogenicity, and efficacy of several anti-H5N1 influenza experimental vaccines in a mouse and chicken models (testing of killed and live H5 vaccine). Influenza Other Respir Viruses. 2012;6(3):188–95.

10

Nitric oxide-generating compound GSNO suppresses porcine circovirus type 2 infection in vitro and in vivo

Chuanmin Liu[1,2,3,4], Libin Wen[1,2,3,4], Qi Xiao[1,2,3,4] and Kongwang He[1,2,3,4*]

Abstract

Background: Nitric oxide (NO), an important signaling molecule with biological functions, has antimicrobial activity against a variety of pathogens including viruses. To our knowledge, little information is available about the regulatory effect of NO on porcine circovirus type 2 (PCV2) infection. This study was conducted to investigate the antiviral activity of NO generated from S-nitrosoglutathione (GSNO), during PCV2 infection of PK-15 cells and BALB/c mice.

Results: GSNO released considerable NO in the culture medium of PK-15 cells, and NO was scavenged by its scavenger hemoglobin (Hb) in a dose-dependent manner. NO strongly inhibited PCV2 replication in PK-15 cells, and the antiviral effect was reversed by Hb. An in vivo assay indicated that GSNO treatment reduced the progression of PCV2 infection in mice, evident as reductions in the percentages of PCV2-positive sera and tissue samples and in the viral DNA copies in serum samples. GSNO also improved the growth performance and immune organs (spleens and thymuses) of the PCV2-infected mice to some degree.

Conclusions: Our data demonstrate that the NO-generating compound GSNO suppresses PCV2 infection in PK-15 cells and BALB/c mice, indicating that NO and its donor, GSNO, have potential value as antiviral drugs against PCV2 infection.

Keywords: Nitric oxide, GSNO, PCV2, PK-15 cells, BALB/c mice

Background

Porcine circovirus type 2 (PCV2), which belongs to the family *Circoviridae*, is a small, non-enveloped virus with a circular, single-stranded DNA genome [1]. PCV2 is the primary causative agent of porcine circovirus-associated disease (PCVAD) [2], a globally emerging disease, currently causing great economic losses in the global swine industry today [3]. The most significant pathological conditions considered to be PCVADs are post-weaning multisystemic wasting syndrome, porcine dermatitis and nephropathy syndrome, and PCV2-reproductive disease [4, 5]. PCV2-infected piglets are readily contract concomitant infections, including porcine respiratory and reproductive syndrome virus, porcine parvovirus and *Haemophilus parasuis*, suggesting that PCVAD is actually an immunosuppressive disease [6]. Besides piglets, mice and calves are also found to be able to infect this virus [7, 8]. The control of PCVD is based on management strategies, control of coinfections, and vaccination [9]. Vaccination is traditionally considered the most effective method for preventing viral diseases, but the period of protection afforded by a vaccine is limited and the virus cannot be eradicated by vaccination [10]. Furthermore, no effective vaccines are available for preventing multifactorial diseases such as PCVAD [11]. Therefore, alternative effective measures to control the disease are urgently required.

NO is an important molecule with key roles in a broad range of biological processes including neurotransmission, vasodilatation and immune responses [12]. NO is generated by mammalian cells from the guanidino nitrogen of L-arginine in a reaction catalyzed by a family of NO synthase enzymes [13]. NO can also be released from exogenous donors, such as sodium nitroprusside (SNP), S-nitroso-acetylpenicillamine (SNAP) and GSNO [14]. Previous studies have presented considerable evidence that NO can prevent viral infections [15–20]. However,

* Correspondence: kwh2003@263.net
[1]Institute of Veterinary Medicine, Jiangsu Academy of Agricultural Sciences, 50 Zhong-ling Street, Xuanwu District, Nanjing 210014, China
[2]Key laboratory of Veterinary Biological Engineering and Technology, Ministry of Agriculture, 50 Zhong-ling Street, Xuanwu District, Nanjing 210014, China
Full list of author information is available at the end of the article

the antiviral effects of NO against PCV2 infection are so far poorly studied.

In this study, the NO-generating compound GSNO was used to analyze the kinetics of NO production in the culture supernatant of PK-15 cells. The antiviral activity mediated by GSNO during PCV2 infection was also investigated in PK-15 cells and BALB/c mice.

Methods

Cells and virus

PCV-free PK-15 cells, purchased from the China Institute of Veterinary Drug Control (Beijing, China), were grown at 37 °C in an atmosphere of 5% CO_2 in Dulbecco's modified Eagle's medium (DMEM; Sigma, USA) supplemented with 10% fetal bovine serum (GIBCO, USA) and 1% penicillin-streptomycin antibiotics (Sangon, China). The PCV2-Haian strain (GenBank accession number: FJ712216.1) is maintained by Institute of Veterinary Medicine, Jiangsu Academy Agricultural Sciences, Jiangsu, China. PCV2 was propagated in PK-15 cells, harvested after incubation for 72 h, and stored at −70 °C until use.

Experimental design

In vitro

The safe concentrations of the drugs were determined in PK-15 cells with a 3-(4,5-dimethylthiazol-2-yl)-2,5-diphenyltetrazolium bromide (MTT) assay, and the kinetics of NO production in the culture supernatant were assessed from 0 to 96 h after drug treatment. To investigate the antiviral activity of the NO-generating compound GSNO during PCV2 infection in vitro, 80% confluent PK-15 cells in 24-well cell culture plates were pretreated with GSNO or GSNO plus hemoglobin (Hb) for 6 h, and then infected with PCV2 (multiplicity of infection (MOI) of 1) in the presence of the drugs for an additional 72 h. Untreated cells, cultured in medium alone, were used as the mock control, and cells infected with PCV2 alone (MOI = 1) were used as the PCV2-infected control. The antiviral activity of GSNO was determined from the appearance of PCV2-infected cells, viral titers, and PCV2 DNA copy numbers. The NO levels in the various groups were also determined.

In vivo

Seventy-eight 4-week-old specific-pathogen-free BALB/c mice were purchased from the Comparative Medicine Centre, Yangzhou University, Jiangsu, China. The mice were maintained in isolation rooms, in which the temperature was maintained at 25 °C under a 12-h light cycle. The experimental animals were allowed to acclimatize for 7 days. The protocols for the care and use of animals in this study were approved by the Committee on the Ethics of Animal Experiments of Jiangsu Academy of Agricultural Sciences. The mice were randomly divided into three groups, each containing 26 animals. The mice in group I were injected intraperitoneally with 0.2 ml of phosphate-buffered saline (PBS) and intranasally with 0.02 ml of PBS, and used as negative control(NC). Mice in group II were inoculated intraperitoneally with 0.2 ml of PCV2 (10^5 $TCID_{50}$/ml) and intranasally with 0.02 ml of PCV2 (10^5 $TCID_{50}$/ml), and used as the PCV2-infected control. The mice in group III were inoculated intraperitoneally with 0.2 ml of PCV2 (10^5 $TCID_{50}$/ml) and intranasally with 0.02 ml of PCV2 (10^5 $TCID_{50}$/ml), and injected intraperitoneally with 0.1 ml of GSNO (10 mM) once daily from 0 to 6 days postinoculation (DPI). To exclude the stress induced by the injection, the mice in groups I and II were also injected intraperitoneally with 0.1 ml of PBS once daily at 0–6 DPI. At -1, 12, 17, 22, 27, and 32 DPI, all the mice were weighed, and necropsies were performed on four mice from each group. At 6 DPI, blood samples were withdrawn from the orbital venous plexus of each mouse to isolate serum for the detection of NO. At the time of necropsy, serum samples and tissue samples were collected and stored at −70 °C for PCV2 polymerase chain reaction (PCR) or real-time PCR. The spleen and thymus from each killed mouse were weighed to calculate the organ indexes. The mice were monitored daily and evaluated for clinical signs throughout the trial.

Cytotoxicity assay

In this study, we used GSNO (Sigma, USA) as the exogenous NO donor; Hb (Sigma, USA), as the NO scavenger to scavenge the NO released from GSNO. The cytotoxicity of the drugs was evaluated with a MTT assay. In brief, PK-15 cells were seeded in 96-well cell culture plates at a density of 5×10^4 cells/well. When the cells in each well reached 80% confluence, they were washed twice with PBS and treated with different concentrations of the drugs as serial two-fold dilutions, with eight wells for each concentration. After incubation for 72 h, the viability of PK-15 cells was evaluated with a colorimetric MTT assay, as reported previously [11]. The absorbance at 570 nm (A_{570}) of each well was measured with a microliter enzyme-linked immunosorbent assay reader (Sunrise, TECAN Co., Switzerland).

Measurement of NO

NO production was measured with a colorimetric assay using the Griess reaction [21]. Briefly, at various time points during cell culture, the supernatants (100 μl/well) were harvested, and incubated with an equal volume of Griess solution (1% sulfanilamide, and 0.1% naphthyl ethylene diamine dihydrochloride in 5% phosphoric acid) (Sigma, USA) for 10 min at room temperature. The absorbance was read at 540 nm, and the concentrations of

NO were determined from a least squares linear regression analysis of a standard curve for sodium nitrite.

Indirect fluorescence assay (IFA)

PCV2-based IFA was performed according to previously described procedures [22]. In brief, cells were fixed in frozen methanol at 4 °C for 10–15 min. The fixed cells were washed with PBS, and incubated with porcine anti-PCV2 antibody (VMRD, USA) at 37 °C for 1 h. The cells were washed with PBS again, incubated with FITC-conjugated goat anti-pig antibody (Abcam, UK) at 37 °C for 45 min, washed again with PBS, and examined under a fluorescence microscope (Olympus, Japan). The cells positive for PCV2 viral antigens were counted in six fields of view.

Viral titers

Samples collected from the cell culture plates were frozen and thawed three times, then serially diluted 10-fold in DMEM (1:10 to 1:10^6). PK-15 cells were seeded in 96-well plates, and when the cells in each well reached 40%–50% confluence, they were inoculated with the diluted samples, with eight wells used for each dilution. After incubation for 48 h, the PCV2-positive samples were detected by IFA, as mentioned above, and the viral titers were calculated by Reed-Muench method [23].

DNA extraction, PCR and TaqMan-based real-time PCR

DNA was extracted by using the Column Viral DNAout Kit (TIANDZ, Beijing, China), according to the manufacturer's instructions. The total DNA was stored at –70 °C until use.

To evaluate PCV2 viremia or viral loading in the PCV2-infected tissues of mice, a pair of primers was designed based on the published sequences of PCV2 (forward primer 5′-TTACCGGCGCACTTCGGCAG-3′, reverse primer 5′-ACTCCGTTGTCCCTGAGAT-3′), and PCR was performed with the thermal cycling parameters: 94 °C for 5 min followed by 30 cycles of 94 °C for 1 min, 58 °C for 1 min, and 72 °C for 1.5 min, with a final extension step for at 72 °C for 7 min. The PCR products were subjected to electrophoresis on a 1% agarose gel.

To analyze the viral DNA copy numbers in the cell and serum samples, primers and a TaqMan probe specific for the PCV2 sequence were designed: forward primer 5′-TAAATCTCATCATGTCCACATTCCA-3′, reverse primer 5′-CGTTACCGCTGGAGAAGGAA-3′ and TaqMan probe 5′-[6-FAM]AATGGCATCTTCAACACCCGCC TCT[TAMRA]-3′. Taqman-based real-time PCR was performed on the 7500 Real-Time PCR System (Applied Biosystems, USA) using the thermal cycling parameters: 95 °C for 30 s, 40 cycles of 95 °C for 5 s and 60 °C for 34 s.

Statistical analysis

The differences among different treatment groups were analyzed and compared by one-way analysis of variance (ANOVA), followed by a least-significant difference test, using the statistical package SPSS ver. 17.0 for Windows. A value of $P < 0.05$ was considered statistically significant.

Results

Antiviral activity of GSNO in PK-15 cells

As shown in Fig. 1a, the A_{570} value of PK-15 cells treated with 125 μM GSNO did not differ significantly from that of the control cells in the MTT assay ($P > 0.05$). Therefore, 125 μM GSNO was used as a safe

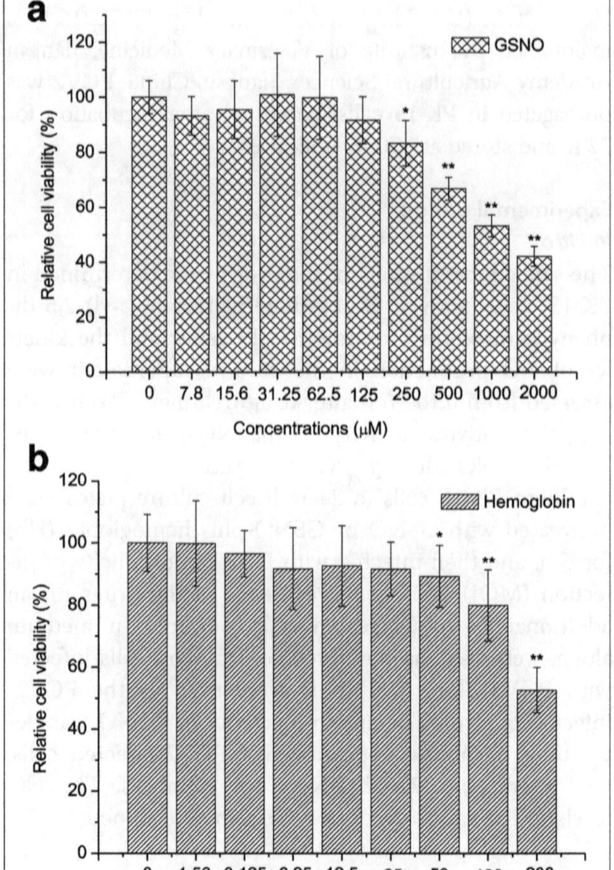

Fig. 1 Cytotoxicity of GSNO and Hb on PK-15 cells tested by MTT assay. After incubation with the drugs for 72 h, MTT was added into each well. The cells were cultured for another 4 h, and 200 μl DMSO was added into each well for dissolving formazan, then A_{570} of the samples were determined by a microplate reader. Relative viability was calculated according to the equation: Relative viability (%) = A_{570} of the drug-treated sample / A_{570} of the untreated sample × 100. Data shown were means ± SD from three independent experiments. **a** Cytotoxicity of GSNO on PK-15 cells. **b** Cytotoxicity of Hb on PK-15 cells. $^*P < 0.05$, $^{**}P < 0.01$ vs untreated control group

concentration for the cells in this study. The safe concentration of Hb for PK-15 cells was determined to be 25 μM (Fig. 1b).

To determine the kinetics of NO production, the supernatants of the samples from 24-well cell culture plates was collected at different time points after drug treatment, and the NO levels were assayed by the Griess reaction. The NO production was significantly higher in GSNO-treated groups, with or without PVC2 infection, than the control group ($P < 0.01$; Figs. 2 and 3b). The NO levels tended to increase in the GSNO-treated groups at 0–72 h after drug treatment, reaching a plateau at around 72 h (Fig. 2). However, the NO generated from GSNO was effectively and dose-dependently scavenged by the NOscavenger Hb (Fig. 3b).

The inhibitory effect of the NO-generating compound GSNO on PCV2 replication was shown in Fig. 3. The PCV2-positive cells detected by IFA indicated that treatment with GSNO reduced the progression of PCV2 infection (Fig. 3a). The percentage of PCV2-infected cells decreased to 69.5% after treatment with 125 μM GSNO relative to the infected control ($P < 0.05$; Fig. 3c), whereas the percentage of PCV2-infected cells in the groups incubated with 125 μM GSNO plus 5, 10, or 15 μM Hb was 73.3%, 85.5% or 89.7% respectively (Fig. 3c). The viral titers and viral DNA copy numbers in the PCV2-infected groups decreased significantly after GSNO treatment relative to those in the PCV2-infected control ($P < 0.01$ or $P <$ 0.05; Fig. 3d, e). However, the reductions in the viral titers and viral DNA copy numbers induced by GSNO were dose-dependently reversed by the NO scavenger Hb (Fig. 3d, e).

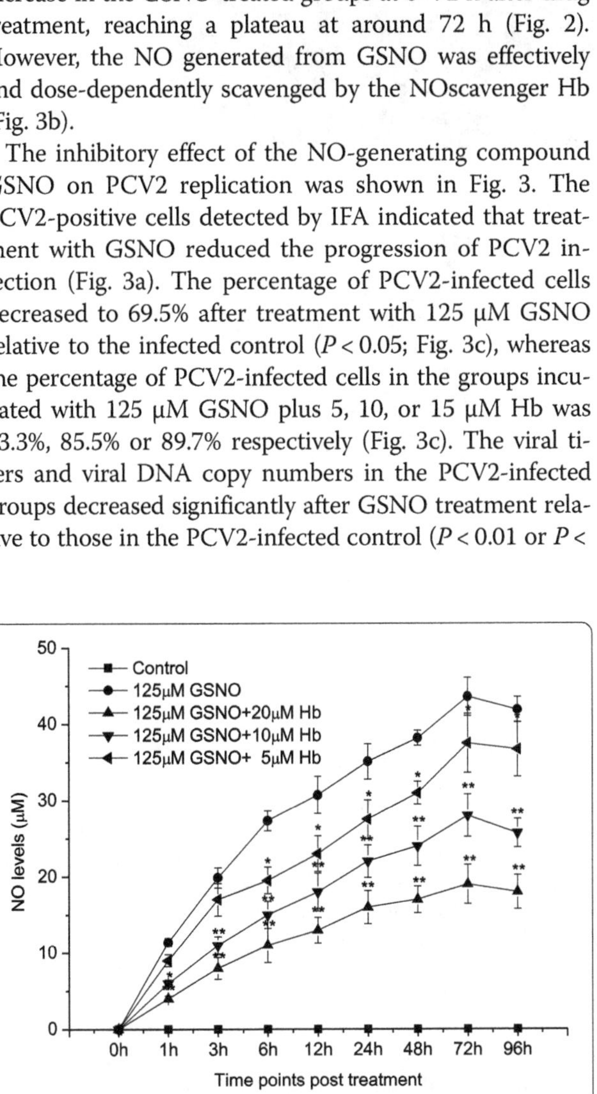

Fig. 2 Kinetics of NO production in the culture supernatants of PK-15 cells. When 80% confluent monolayers formed, 125 μM GSNO or 125 μM GSNO plus Hb (5, 10, 20 μM) were added into 96-well cell culture plates, with four wells for each concentration, and untreated cells served as the control. The supernatant from each sample was collected at different time points, and the NO levels were determined by Griess reaction with a microplate reader at 540 nm according to a standard curve made from sodium nitrite. Data were presented as means ± SD from three independent experiments. *$P < 0.05$, **$P < 0.01$ vs 125 μM GSNO-treated group

Antiviral activity of GSNO in BALB/c mice

All the mice survived PCV2 inoculation with or without GSNO treatment and none of the mice were clinically affected during the study. There were no obvious gross lesions in the tissues of the experimental animals.

GSNO treatment caused a significant increase in serum NO levels in the mice during PCV2 infection ($P < 0.05$; Fig. 4). As shown in Fig. 5a, the average daily weight gain (ADWG) tended to decrease in the PCV2-inoculated control mice at 12–32 DPI, and was lower than that in the NC mice ($P > 0.05$). However, the ADWG of the PCV2-inoculated mice treated with GSNO was significantly higher than that of PCV2-inoculated control mice ($P <$ 0.05) at 22 and 32 DPI. An analysis of the kinetics of spleen index (SI) and thymus index (TI) demonstrated some GSNO-induced improvement in the mouse spleens and thymuses during PCV2 infection from −1 to 32 DPI. As shown in Fig. 5b and c, SI and TI were significantly higher in the GSNO-treated mice at 12 DPI than that in the untreated mice during PCV2 infection ($P < 0.05$ or $P < 0.01$). SI of the PCV2-inoculated control mice also decreased significantly at 12, 22 and 27 DPI compared with that of the NC mice ($P < 0.05$ or $P < 0.01$) (Fig. 5b), whereas TI decreased significantly in the PCV2-inoculated control mice at 17 DPI ($P < 0.05$; Fig. 5c). However, there were no significant differences in the SI and TI of the GSNO-treated mice and NC mice at −1—32 DPI ($P > 0.05$).

Throughout the experiment, all the serum samples obtained from the NC mice were negative for PCV2-specific nucleic acids when analyzed by gel-based PCR and quantitative real-time PCR assays. In the PCV2-inoculated mice, PCV2 DNA was detected by gel-based PCR in the pooled tissue samples and serum samples, and PCV2 DNA was determined in 75% (15/20) of the tissue samples and in 70% (14/20) of the serum samples from the PCV2-inoculated control mice between 12 and 32 DPI (Tables 1 and 2). However, the percentages of PCV2-positive tissue samples and serum samples from the GSNO-treated mice infected with PCV2decreased to 45% (9/20) and 40% (8/20) respectively (Tables 1 and 2). Significant differences were also noted in the PCV2-positive tissue samples ($P = 0.012$) and PCV2-positive serum samples ($P = 0.005$) from the PCV2-inoculated control mice and PCV2-inoculated mice treated with GSNO (Tables 1 and 2). As described in Fig. 6, the number of PCV2 DNA copies reached a plateau at 12 DPI, but declined to some extent between 12 and 32 DPI in the PCV2-inoculated mice treated with or without GSNO.

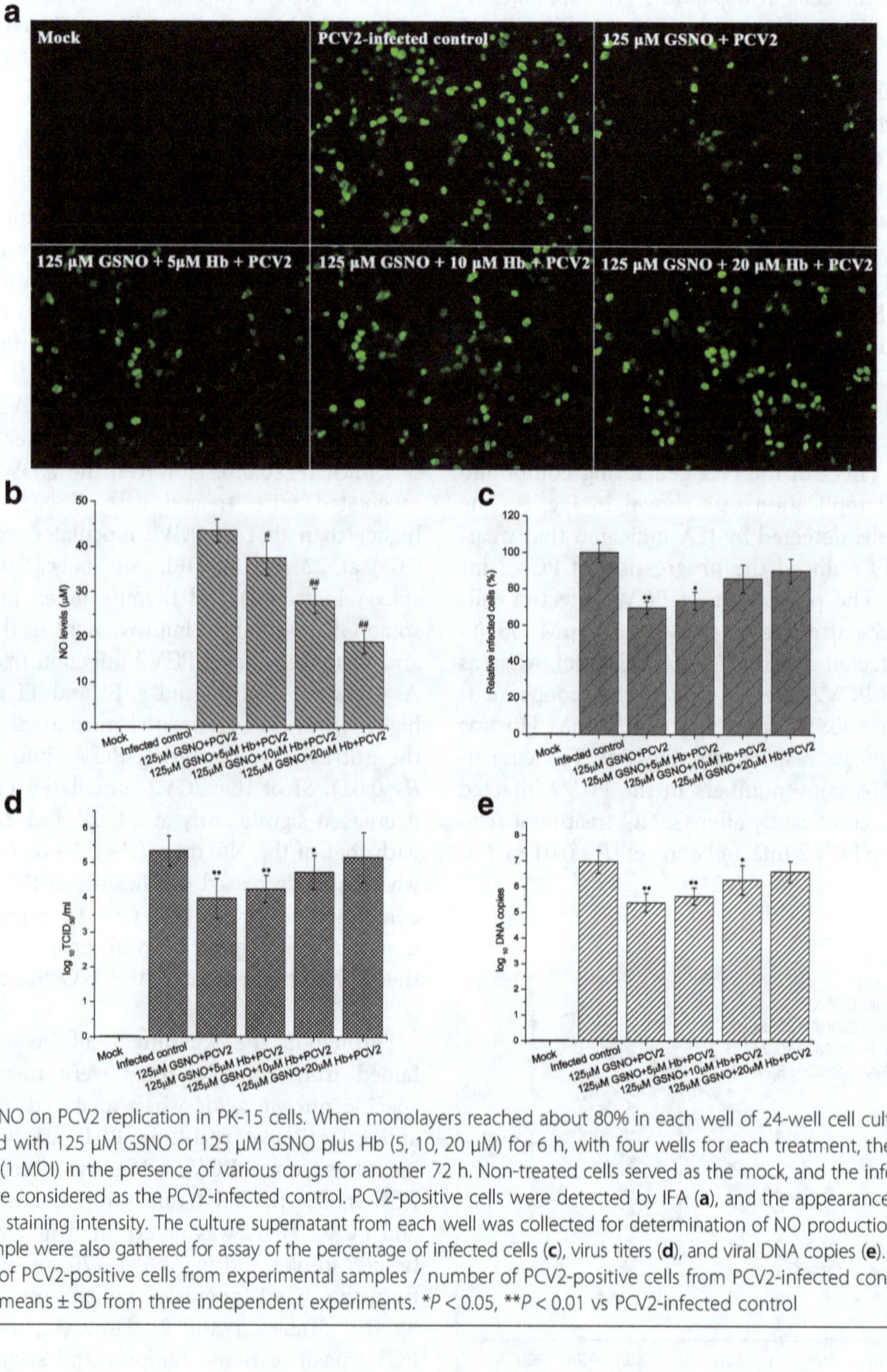

Fig. 3 Effects of GSNO on PCV2 replication in PK-15 cells. When monolayers reached about 80% in each well of 24-well cell culture plates, the cells were incubated with 125 μM GSNO or 125 μM GSNO plus Hb (5, 10, 20 μM) for 6 h, with four wells for each treatment, then the cells were infected with PCV2 (1 MOI) in the presence of various drugs for another 72 h. Non-treated cells served as the mock, and the infected cells without drug treatment were considered as the PCV2-infected control. PCV2-positive cells were detected by IFA (**a**), and the appearance of infected cells was judged by FITC staining intensity. The culture supernatant from each well was collected for determination of NO production (**b**), in addition, the cells in each sample were also gathered for assay of the percentage of infected cells (**c**), virus titers (**d**), and viral DNA copies (**e**). Relative infected cells (%) = number of PCV2-positive cells from experimental samples / number of PCV2-positive cells from PCV2-infected control × 100. Data were presented as means ± SD from three independent experiments. $^{*}P < 0.05$, $^{**}P < 0.01$ vs PCV2-infected control

However, at 12–32 DPI, the number of PCV2 DNA copies xwas significantly lower in the PCV2-inoculated mice treated with GSNO at each time point compared with those in the PCV2-inoculated control mice ($P < 0.01$; Fig. 6).

Discussion

NO, an important cellular messenger, is involved in complex and diverse functions in various physiological and pathological processes, displaying a broad spectrum of antimicrobial activities in vitro and in vivo [24]. In this study, we verified the antiviral activity of the NO-generating compound GSNO during PCV2 infection in PK-15 cells and BALB/c mice.

The in vitro experiment showed that treatment with GSNO induced significant declines in PCV2-infected cells, viral titers and viral DNA copy numbers compared with those of the PCV2-infected samples, whereas the effect of GSNO was dose-dependently reversed by the NO scavenger Hb. These results demonstrate that the

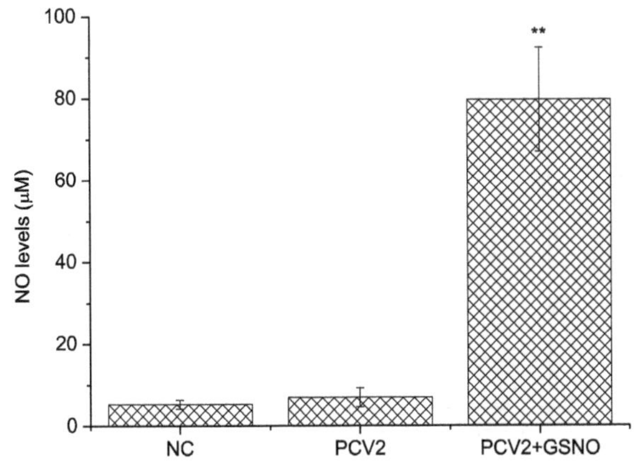

Fig. 4 NO production in serum from the experimental mice. At 6 DPI, serum samples were obtained from six mice in each group for NO detection by Griess reaction. Data were presented as means ± SD. $^{**}P < 0.01$ vs infected control

NO donor GSNO exerts significant antiviral activity against PCV2 replication in PK-15 cells. Similarly, in previous studies, the NO donor SNAP has been shown to block the replication of severe acute respiratory syndrome coronavirus (SARS coronavirus) [16], porcine parvovirus [25] and porcine respiratory coronavirus [26]. Although the inhibition of PCV2 by NO was clearly demonstrated here, it is unclear whether the antiviral effect of the NO donor GSNO was actually attributable to other factors. To address this question, convincing evidence has been presented in this study. First, the data from a MTT assay clearly excluded the possibility that antiviral effects of the NO donor GSNO on PCV2 replication might have resulted from its toxicity to the cells. Second, GSNO generated NO in the culture supernatant of PK-15 cells and NO dose-dependently suppressed PCV2 replication. Finally, the inhibitory effect of GSNO on PCV2 replication was reversed by the NO scavenger, Hb. Overall, these results strongly suggest that NO, generated from the donor GSNO, inhibits the replication of PCV2 in PK-15 cells.

The mechanisms involved in the antiviral properties of NO have partly been clarified in previous studies, which have suggested that NO plays important roles in the regulation of a viral protease [27], the innate immunity of the host [15], and the synthesis of viral proteins and nucleic acids [12]. Depending on its concentration, NO exerts its antimicrobial effects in two ways: At low concentrations, NO acts as a signaling molecule that promotes the growth and activity of immune cells, whereas at high concentrations, NO covalently binds DNA, proteins and lipids, thereby inhibiting or killing the target

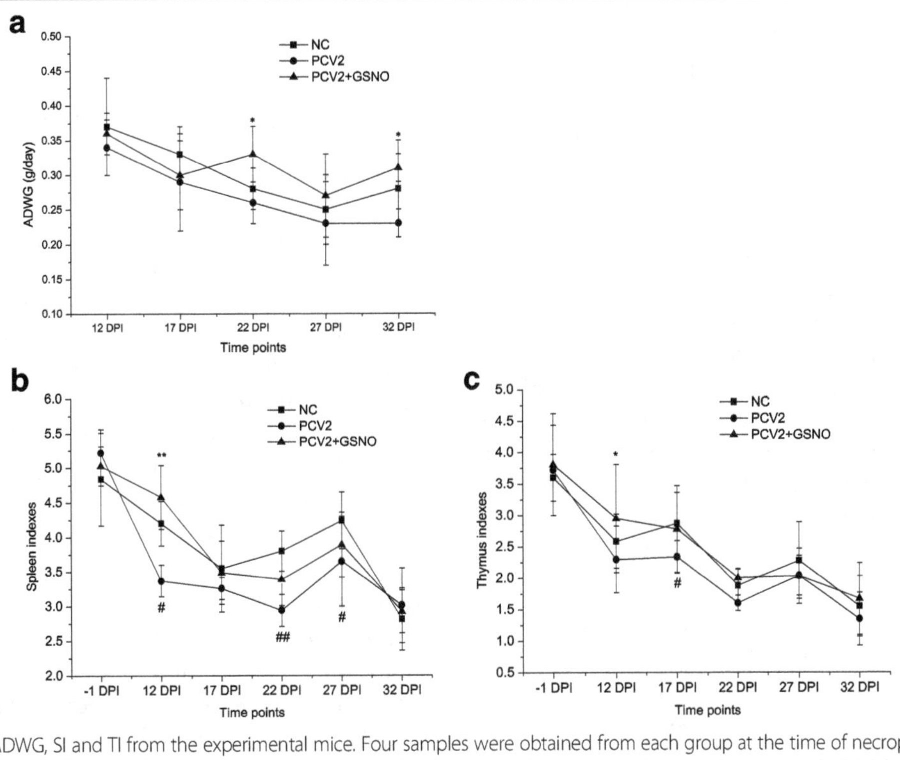

Fig. 5 Kinetics of ADWG, SI and TI from the experimental mice. Four samples were obtained from each group at the time of necropsy. **a** ADWG (g/day) = (final weight − initial weight) / days; **b** SI =spleen weight (g) / the weight of mice (g) × 1000. **c** TI =thymus weight (g) / the weight of mice (g) × 1000. Kinetics of ADWG, SI and TI demonstrated that, to some extent, GSNO improved growth performance and protected the immune organs (spleens and thymuses) of the mice during PCV2 infection. Data were presented as means ± SD. $^{*}P < 0.05$, $^{**}P < 0.01$ vs PV2-inoculated control; $^{\#}P < 0.05$, $^{\#\#}P < 0.05$ vs NC

Table 1 Incidence of PCV2-positive tissue pool from the experimental mice detected by gel-based PCR analysis

Groups	12 DPI	17 DPI	22 DPI	27 DPI	32 DPI	Total
NC	0/4	0/4	0/4	0/4	0/4	0/20
PCV2	4/4	3/4	3/4	2/4	3/4	15/20
PCV2 + GSNO	2/4	2/4	2/4	1/4	2/4	9/20

The tissue pools consisted of liver, thymus, lung and spleen. Data were presented as number of PCV2 PCR positive tissue pools/total number tissue pools analyzed

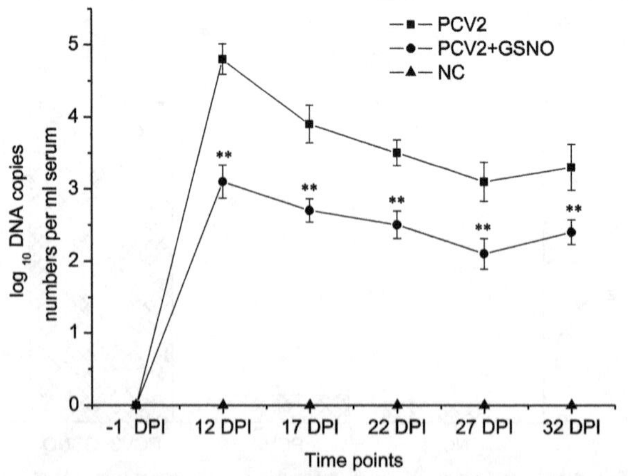

Fig. 6 PCV2 DNA copies, detected by Taqman real-time PCR, in the sera samples from the mice with different treatments. Four sera samples were collected from each group at the time of necropsy. Data were presented as means ± SD. ** $p < 0.01$ vs PCV2-inoculated control

pathogen [28]. The antiviral activity of NO against PCV2 was demonstrated in vitro by its reduction of the numbers of virus-infected cells, viral titers and DNA copy numbers. The decline in the number of virally infected cells is probably attributable to the blockage of viral penetration to the cytoplasm or to the suppression of transcriptional steps mediated by NO [29], whereas the reduced viral titers and viral DNA copy numbers are probably attributable to the inhibition of viral protein and nucleic acid synthesis by NO [12]. However, the binding, cell entry and transcription characteristics of PCV2 that are influenced by NO were not investigated in this study. Therefore, the mechanisms underlying the inhibition of PCV2 replication by NO remain to be evaluated in future studies.

Although the antiviral activity of GSNO was clearly demonstrated in vitro, in vivo studies are also essential to confirm the effects of GSNO on PCV2 infection under clinical conditions. Mice, including BALB/c, C57BL/6, C3H/HeJ and Kunming mice, are susceptible to PCV2, although susceptibility to PCV2 is limited among the above-mentioned mouse lines [30–32]. Therefore, the mouse is important in the epidemiology of PCV2 and can be used as an experimental model of PCV2. In this study, BALB/c mice were artificially inoculated with PCV2 and treated with or without GSNO. Our data showed that GSNO treatment released a large amount of NO, which contributed to the effective inhibition of PCV2 replication in the mice. The poor growth performance and immune organ (spleen and thymus) dysfunction induced by PCV2 infection were also improved to some extent by GSNO. Previous reports have demonstrated that dietary L-arginine supplementation induces significant increase in serum NO production and suppresses PCV2 infection in mice [33, 34], suggesting that the antiviral effects of L-arginine are predominantly mediated by NO because L-arginine is the sole substrate for NO synthesis [35]. This hypothesis was confirmed in our in vivo study, because GSNO was the exogenous NO donor and released NO in mice. Although no weight loss or wasting was observed in the PCV2-inoculated mice, as has been described previously, the ADWG of the mice infected with PCV2 decreased to some extent in the present study, which might be be attributable to the different mouse line used there. Since Kiupel et al. (2005) demonstrated that PCV2 induces apoptosis by activating caspases 8 and 3 in the spleens of infected mice [36]. Therefore, the impaired immune organs detected in the PCV2-inoculated control mice in our study might be attributable to the apoptosis induced by PCV2. Interestingly, the GSNO treatment improved growth performance and protected the immune organs (spleen and thymus) of the PCV2-inoculated mice. As we know, NO acts as a key molecule in inflammation and the immune response [37, 38], so the NO-generating compound GSNO may play a critical role in the regulation of inflammation and immunity during PCV2 infection, as well as inhibiting PCV2 replication, in mice. More research is required to confirm this hypothesis.

Table 2 Incidence of PCV2 positive serum sample from the experimental mice as detected by gel-based PCR analysis

Groups	12 DPI	17 DPI	22 DPI	27 DPI	32 DPI	Total
NC	0/4	0/4	0/4	0/4	0/4	0/20
PCV2	3/4	3/4	3/4	2/4	3/4	14/20
PCV2 + GSNO	2/4	2/4	1/4	1/4	2/4	8/20

Data were presented as number of PCV2 PCR positive serum samples/number of mice sampled

Conclusions

GSNO, an exogenous NO donor, released NO into the culture supernatants of PK-15 cells and the sera of BALB/c mice. The antiviral effects of GSNO on PCV2 were also demonstrated in both PK-15 cells and BALB/c mice. As well as the significant inhibition of PCV2, GSNO also positively regulated the growth performance and immune organs of the PCV2-infected mice. Therefore, NO and its donor GSNO have potential valve as antiviral reagents during PCV2 infection. However, the mechanisms underlying the antiviral activity of GSNO remain to be investigated in our future studies. The effects of GSNO on PCV2 infection in the target animal, the pig, must also be evaluated.

Abbreviations

ADWG: average daily weight gain; DPI: days post inoculation; GSNO: S-Nitrosoglutathione; Hb: hemoglobin; IFA: indirect fluorescence assay; MOI: multiplicity of infection; MTT: 3-(4,5-Dimethylthiazol-2-yl)-2,5-diphenyltetrazolium bromide; NC: negative control; NO: nitric oxide; PCR: polymerase chain reaction; PCV2: porcine circovirus type 2; PCVAD: porcine circovirus-associated disease; PDNS: porcine dermatitis and nephropathy syndrome; PMWS: post-weaning multisystemic wasting syndrome; PPV: porcine parvovirus; PRRSV: porcine respiratory and reproductive syndrome virus; SI: spleen index; SNAP: S-nitroso-acetylpenicillamine; SNP: sodium nitroprusside; TI: thymus index

Acknowledgments

The authors thanked Song Gao, Ph.D. (College of Veterinary Medicine, Yangzhou University) for his positive advice on experimental design. The authors also thanked Yiyi Hu, Ph.D. and Wei Wang, M.S. (Institute of Veterinary Medicine, Jiangsu Academy of Agricultural Sciences) for their great help throughout the study.

Funding

This work was supported by grants from the National Natural Science Foundation of China (NFSC) (Grant number 31502099), China Postdoctoral Science Foundation (Grant number 2015 M581755) and Postdoctoral Foundation of Jiangsu Province (Grant number 1501161B).

Authors' contributions

KWH directed the research, reviewed the data and manuscript; and directed revisions. CML conducted research, compiled data, and wrote paper. LBW provided clinical diagnostics and participated in drafting the manuscript. QX was involved in data analysis and participated in drafting the manuscript. All authors have read and approved the manuscript.

Competing interests

The authors declare that they have no competing interest.

Consent for publication

Not applicable.

Author details

[1]Institute of Veterinary Medicine, Jiangsu Academy of Agricultural Sciences, 50 Zhong-ling Street, Xuanwu District, Nanjing 210014, China. [2]Key laboratory of Veterinary Biological Engineering and Technology, Ministry of Agriculture, 50 Zhong-ling Street, Xuanwu District, Nanjing 210014, China. [3]National Center for Engineering Research of Veterinary Bio-products, 50 Zhong-ling Street, Xuanwu District, Nanjing 210014, China. [4]Jiangsu Co-innovation Center for Prevention and Control of Important Animal Infectious Diseases and Zoonoses, 12 Wen-Hui East Road, Hanjiang District, Yangzhou 225009, China.

References

1. Tischer I, Gelderblom H, Vettermann W, Koch MA. A very small porcine virus with circular single-stranded DNA. Nature. 1982;295:64–6.
2. Opriessnig T, Meng XJ, Halbur PG. Porcine circovirus type 2 associated disease: Update on current terminology, clinical manifestations, pathogenesis, diagnosis, and intervention strategies. J Vet Diagn Invest. 2007;19:591–615.
3. Gillespie J, Opriessnig T, Meng XJ, Pelzer K, Buechner-Maxwell V. Porcine circovirus type 2 and porcine circovirus-associated disease. J Vet Intern Med. 2009;23:1151–63.
4. Rose N, Opriessnig T, Grasland B, Jestin A. Epidemiology and transmission of Porcine circovirus type 2 (PCV2). Virus Res. 2012;164:78–89.
5. Segalés J. Porcine circovirus type 2 (PCV2) infections: clinical signs, pathology and laboratory diagnosis. Virus Res. 2012;164:10–9.
6. Du Q, Huang Y, Wang TT, Zhang XJ, Chen Y, Cui BB, Li DL, Zhao XM, Zhang WL, Chang LL, Tong DW. Porcine circovirus type 2 activates PI3K/Akt and p38 MAPK pathways to promote interleukin-10 production in macrophages via Cap interaction of gC1qR. Oncotarget. 2016;7:17492–507.
7. Deng ZB, Wang ND, Xu DJ, Yuan AW, Ge M, Luo W, Xue LQ, Yu XL. Viral distribution and lesions in Kunming mice experimentally infected with porcine circovirus type 2b. Vet Res Commun. 2011;35:181–92.
8. Halami MY, Freick M, Shehata AA, Muller H, Vahlenkamp TW. Susceptibility of calves to porcine circovirus-2 (PCV2). Vet Microbiol. 2014;173:125–31.
9. Grau-Roma L, Fraile L, Segalés J. Recent advances in the epidemiology, diagnosis and control of diseases caused by porcine circovirus type 2. Vet J. 2011;187:23–32.
10. Feng H, Blanco G, Segalés J, Sibila M. Can Porcine circovirus type 2 (PCV2) infection be eradicated by mass vaccination? Vet Microbiol. 2014;172:92–9.
11. Sun N, Sun PP, Lv HP, Sun YG, Guo JH, Wang ZR, Luo TT, Wang SY, Li HQ. Matrine displayed antiviral activity in porcine alveolar macrophages co-infected by porcine reproductive and respiratory syndrome virus and porcine circovirus type 2. Sci Rep. 2016;6:24401.
12. Akerström S, Gunalan V, Keng CT, Tan YJ, Mirazimi A. Dual effect of nitric oxide on SARS-CoV replication: Viral RNA production and palmitoylation of the S protein are affected. Virology. 2009;395:1–9.
13. Treuer AV, Gonzalez DR. Nitric oxide synthases, S-nitrosylation and cardiovascular health: From molecular mechanisms to therapeutic opportunities (Review). Mol Med Rep. 2015;11:1555–65.
14. Taylor EL, Megson IL, Haslett C, Rossi AG. Nitric oxide: a key regulator of myeloid inflammatory cell apoptosis. Cell Death Differ. 2003;10:418–30.
15. Koci MD, Kelley LA, Larsen D, Schultz-Cherry S. Astrovirus-induced synthesis of nitric oxide contributes to virus control during infection. J Virol. 2004;78:1564–74.
16. Akerstrom S, Mousavi-Jazi M, Klingstrom J, Leijon M, Lundkvist A, Mirazimi A. Nitric oxide inhibits the replication cycle of severe acute respiratory syndrome coronavirus. J Virol. 2005;79:1966–9.
17. Klingstrom J, Akerstrom S, Hardestam J, Stoltz M, Simon M, Falk KI, Mirazimi A, Rottenberg M, Lundkvist A. Nitric oxide and peroxynitrite have different antiviral effects against hantavirus replication and free mature virions. Eur J Immunol. 2006;36:2649–57.
18. Fagundes CT, Costa VV, Cisalpino D, Amaral FA, Souza PRS, Souza RS, Ryffel B, Vieira LQ, Silva TA, Atrasheuskaya A, Ignatyev G, Sousa LP, Souza DG, Teixeira MM. IFN-γ production depends on IL-12 and IL-18 combined action and mediates host resistance to dengue virus infection in a nitric oxide-dependent manner. PLoS Negl Trop Dis. 2011;5, e1449.
19. Mehta DR, Ashkar AA, Mossman KL. The nitric oxide pathway provides innate antiviral protection in conjunction with the type I interferon pathway in Fibroblasts. PLoS One. 2012;7, e31688.
20. Moore TC, Bush KL, Cody L, Brown DM, Petro TM. Control of early Theiler's murine encephalomyelitis virus replication in macrophages by interleukin-6 occurs in conjunction with STAT1 activation and nitric oxide production. J Virol. 2012;86:10841–51.
21. Legorreta-Herrera M, Rivas-Contreras S, Ventura-Gallegos JL, Zentella-Dehesa A. Nitric oxide is involved in the upregulation of IFN-γ and IL-10 mRNA expression by CD8+ T cells during the blood stages of *P. chabaudi* AS infection in CBA/Ca mice. Inter J Biol Sci. 2011;7:1401–11.
22. Liu XJ, Wang XB, Song Y, Fan J, Gao S, Liu XF. A candidate inactivated chimeric vaccine PCV1-2 constructed based on PCV1 and PCV2 isolates originating in China and its evaluation in conventional pigs in regard to protective efficacy against PCV2 infection. Microbiol Immunol. 2011;55:254–66.
23. Reed LJ, Muench H. A simple method of estimating fifty percent endpoints. Am J Hyg. 1938;27:493–7.
24. Akaike T, Maeda H. Nitric oxide and virus infection. Immunology. 2000;101:300–8.
25. Wei ZY, Wang XB, Ning XD, Wang YB, Zhang HY, Wang DF, Chen HY, Cui BA. Nitric oxide inhibits the replication cycle of porcine parvovirus in vitro. Arch Virol. 2009;154:999–1003.
26. Jung K, Gurnani A, Renukaradhya GJ, Saif LJ. Nitric oxide is elicited and inhibits viral replication in pigs infected with porcine respiratory coronavirus

but not porcine reproductive and respiratory syndrome virus. Vet Immunol Immunopathol. 2010;136:335–9.

27. Saura M, Zaragoza C, McMillan A, Quick RA, Hohenadl C, Lowenstein JM, Lowenstein CJ. An antiviral mechanism of nitric oxide: inhibition of a viral protease. Immunity. 1999;10:21–8.
28. Schairer DO, Chouake JS, Nosanchuk JD, Friedman AJ. The potential of nitric oxide releasing therapies as antimicrobial agents. Virulence. 2012;3:271–9.
29. Ubol S, Hiriote W, Anuntagool N, Utaisincharoen P. A radical form of nitric oxide suppresses RNA synthesis of rabies virus. Virus Res. 2001;81:125–32.
30. Kiupel M, Stevenson GW, Choi J, Latimer KS, Kanitz CL, Mittal SK. Viral replication and lesions in BALB/c mice experimentally inoculated with porcine circovirus isolated from a pig with postweaning multisystemic wasting disease. Vet Pathol. 2001;38:74–82.
31. Opriessnig T, Patterson AR, Jones DE, Juhan NM, Meng XJ, Halbur PG. Limited susceptibility of three different mouse (*Mus musculus*) lines to Porcine circovirus-2 infection and associated lesions. Can J Vet Res. 2009;73:81–6.
32. Li J, Yuan X, Zhang C, Miao L, Wu J, Shi J, Xu S, Cui S, Wang J, Ai H. A mouse model to study infection against porcine circovirus type 2: viral distribution and lesions in mouse. Virol J. 2010;7:158.
33. Liu G, Ren WK, Su DD, Wu MM, Li YH, Luo W, Yu XL, Li TJ, Fang J. Dietary L-arginine supplementation improves the immune responses in mouse model infected porcine circovirus types 2. J Anim Vet Adv. 2012;11:2980–5.
34. Ren W, Yin Y, Liu G, Yu X, Li Y, Yang G, Li T, Wu G. Effect of dietary arginine supplementation on reproductive performance of mice with porcine circovirus type 2 infection. Amino Acids. 2012;42:2089–94.
35. Baecker N, Boese A, Schoenau E, Gerzer R, Heer M. L-arginine, the natural precursor of NO, is not effective for preventing bone loss in postmenopausal women. J Bone Miner Res. 2005;20:471–9.
36. Kiupel M, Stevenson GW, Galbreath EJ, North A, Hogenesch H, Mittal S. Porcine Circovirus type 2 (PCV2) causes apoptosis in experimentally inoculated BALB/c mice. BMC Vet Res. 2005;1:7.
37. Coleman JW. Nitric oxide in immunity and inflammation. Int Immunopharmacol. 2001;1:1397–406.
38. Predonzani A, Cali B, Agnellini AHR, Molon B. Spotlights on immunological effects of reactive nitrogen species: When inflammation says nitric oxide. World J Exp Med. 2015;5:64–76.

11

Evaluation of ELISA for the detection of rabies virus antibodies from the thoracic liquid and muscle extract samples in the monitoring of fox oral vaccination campaigns

Tomislav Bedeković[1*], Ivana Šimić[1], Nina Krešić[1], Ivana Lojkić[1], Željko Mihaljević[1], Ivica Sučec[3], Ivana Lohman Janković[3] and Peter Hostnik[2]

Abstract

Background: The main goal of oral vaccination of foxes is eradication of rabies in the red fox population as rabies reservoirs. To evaluate the success of vaccination a serological testing is conducted as a part of monitoring program. Two different methods are used regarding rabies serology: virus neutralisation test and ELISA.

Methods: In this study the reliability of BioPro ELISA was evaluated for testing haemolytic thoracic liquids and muscle extracts originated from 147 foxes in comparison to mFAVN. Also, the influence of heat treatment of samples on test results was investigated.

Results: The specificity of the test for not-heat treated samples was 92.98 % and sensitivity 79.20 %. Diagnostic validity of the ELISA compared to the mFAVN test when not-heat treated samples were used was 89.16 %. The specificity of the test for heat treated samples was 79.10 % and sensitivity 96.36 %. Diagnostic validity of the BioPro ELISA compared to the mFAVN test for heat treated samples was 94.30 %.

Conclusion: According to this study, the BioPro ELISA is reliable tool for detection of rabies specific antibodies in the context of evaluation of oral vaccination of foxes from poor quality samples as a substitution for virus neutralisation tests.

Keywords: BioPro ELISA, Muscle extract, Thoracic liquid, Evaluation

Background

In Europe, the main goal of oral vaccination (ORV) is eradication of rabies in wildlife [1]. To achieve this objective, oral vaccine baits (vaccine Lysvulpen, Bioveta, Czech Republic) containing live attenuated rabies virus is used in Croatia. The ORV of foxes in Croatia was carried out simultaneously with similar programs in the neighbouring countries as a part of control and eradication of rabies in Western Balkan countries co-financed by European Commission [2]. As a part of monitoring, vaccination efficacy is evaluated considering the rabies incidence, bait uptake and humoral immune response [1]. This approach showed very good results in effectiveness of elimination of terrestrial rabies in Europe [3].

Considering the assessment of vaccination efficiency the main obstacle in evaluation of humoral response is the low quality of the samples. The quality of the samples depends on the sampling procedure. In some countries the sampling is organised immediately after killing of foxes, but in most countries the carcasses of foxes are frozen before sampling. Time between shooting and sampling in the lab can be extended (up to 10 days). In such case it is difficult to collect serum from the foxes. Consequently, it is not possible to perform serological test and evaluate humoral immunological response. As a substitution for the serum, the liquid from thoracic cavity or extracts of the muscles can be used as samples [4].

* Correspondence: bedekovic@veinst.hr
[1]Croatian Veterinary Institute, Savska cesta 143, 10000 Zagreb, Croatia
Full list of author information is available at the end of the article

Currently two different methods are used regarding rabies serology: virus neutralisation test and ELISA. Neutralisation tests: fluorescent antibody virus neutralisation (FAVN) test and rapid fluorescent focus inhibition test (RFFIT) are known to be the most reliable tests for evaluation of successful vaccination [5–8]. However, the neutralisation tests are time consuming, expensive and require live rabies virus [9]. Also, sometimes the results cannot be read off due to cytotoxic effect on the cells [10]. In order to overcome that problem the ELISA has been developed. Currently two ELISAs for detection of rabies specific antibodies existed on the European Union market: Bio-Rad (Platelia Rabies II - Biorad, Marnes-La-Coquette, France) and BioPro (Prague, Czech Republic). BioPro ELISA is recently developed test especially designed for the detection of rabies virus antibodies in the monitoring of the fox ORV campaigns [9]. This test was evaluated on fresh foxes samples and also on dogs and cats samples [9, 11] and showed to be a reliable tool for serological testing. Until now, muscle extracts and poor quality thoracic liquid samples were not used as samples for serological testing with virus neutralisation tests. The main reason for that was cytotoxic effect caused by quality of the samples. Because of the same reason it was also impossible to evaluate ELISA on those samples. Recently, the new test – modified fluorescent virus neutralisation test (mFAVN) was developed and problem with cytotoxicity has been eliminated [4]. Furthermore, according to that study, very good agreement between antibody titre in dog sera, thoracic liquids and muscle extracts were recorded. Those findings allow evaluation of ELISA for the detection of rabies virus antibodies from the thoracic liquid and muscle extract samples in the monitoring of fox ORV campaigns.

This paper evaluates the specificity and sensitivity of commercial BioPro ELISA kit for the detection of rabies virus antibodies from the haemolytic thoracic liquid and muscle extract samples in the monitoring of fox ORV campaigns. Furthermore, the possibility to improve diagnostic validity of the ELISA by heat treatment of the samples was investigated.

Methods

Ethics statement

All samples were collected by hunters in compliance with national regulations according to "Order on oral vaccination of foxes on territory of Republic of Croatia" [12]. Sampling was performed strictly as a part of program "Control and eradication of rabies in Croatia" cofinanced by IPA project (number of project: 2008-0303-0804). Sampling was approved by ethics committee of Croatian Veterinary Institute (decision number: Z-VI-4-2261-1/12).

Samples

The samples were collected from the 147 foxes during the monitoring of fourth ORV campaign (autumn 2012). The first choice for sampling was thoracic liquid. However, in the case that thoracic liquid could not be collected the piece of *m. femoralis* was taken in order to obtain muscle extract. So, the muscle and thoracic liquid samples were never taken from the same animal. Therefore, from the 55 foxes the fluid from the thoracic cavity was taken and from 92 foxes the piece of *m. femoralis* (approximately 5 × 7 cm) was taken. The carcasses of foxes were not frozen before sampling. The carcasses were placed at ambient temperature and sampled 3–4 days post mortem.

The collected haemolytic liquid samples from the thoracic cavity were centrifuged at 220 × g for 10 min and the separated liquid was placed in two sterile tubes and stored at −20 °C until testing. In order to collect muscle extracts, the muscles in sterile flasks were frozen at - 20 °C for 4 days and then placed at 4 °C for 3–5 days. From each piece of muscle, a sample approximately 200–300 µl of the muscle extract was collected, centrifuged at 220 × g for 10 min, placed in two sterile tubes and stored at −20 °C prior to analysis. On the day of testing, from each sample one tube was heat-treated at 56 °C for 30 min and centrifuged (220 × g). Before testing, all samples were centrifuged one more time.

The heat treated samples were tested using the both tests: mFAVN test and BioPro ELISA. The not-heat treated samples were tested only using the BioPro ELISA. The not-heat treated samples were not tested with mFAVN test because in that case unspecific reactions could be observed [13].

Virus neutralisation test

Rabies neutralising antibodies were detected in thoracic liquids and muscle extracts with the mFAVN as described previously [4]. In that paper mFAVN test was evaluated using the dog samples with the cut off 0.5 IU/ml. However, in this paper instead of the term "positive" (0.5 IU/ml) the term "threshold of detection" (0.1 IU/ml) in the context of evaluation of fox ORV was adopted. Because of that, for the purpose of this study the mFAVN test was compared with FAVN test on the dog samples as described previously [4] and evaluated using the cut of 0.1 IU/ml.

ELISA

The rabies antibodies were detected in thoracic liquids and muscles extracts with the BioPro Rabies ELISA kit according to the manufacturer instructions. The BioPro ELISA is blocking ELISA for detection of rabies virus antibodies in serum or plasma. The wells of microplates are coated with rabies antigen. Diluted samples are incubated in the wells. After washing biotinylated anti-rabies antibody is added to wells. In the case of positive samples specific antibodies will block binding of biotynylated anti-rabies antibodies with coated rabies antigen. The conditions of validation described by the manufacturer were implemented to interpret the results obtained for the samples. The percentage of blocking was calculated for each sample according to the manufacturer's specifications. For checking the effectiveness of ORV campaigns, the manufacturer was established the threshold of positivity to 40 %.

Statistical analysis

The true positive and true negative test results were determined by the mFAVN. Evaluation of ELISA and results were interpreted according to previous studies [14, 15]. The validity or degree to which the test measures what it claims to measure is assessed by area under ROC curve using STATA 10 (Stata Press, College station, Texas, USA). The agreement beyond chance level between the two diagnostic tests (kappa value), and measurements of the test performance area under the ROC curve were calculated using STATA 10 (Stata Press, College station, Texas, USA).

Results

Virus neutralisation test

In this paper complete neutralization at serum dilution above of 1:4 was corresponding to titer 0.1 IU/ml. The validation of mFAVN test for difference cut-off was performed using the results from the previous study [4]. The sensitivity and specificity of the mFAVN test compared to FAVN test for difference cut-off are recorded in Table 1. Diagnostic agreement (when cut-off was set on 0.1 IU/ml in both test) between FAVN and mFAVN tests of serum was perfect.

BioPro ELISA

To establish the specificity and sensitivity of the ELISA, 147 samples (thoracic liquids and muscle extracts) were tested in parallel with the mFAVN and ELISA (Table 2). No cytotoxicity was observed for either type of samples when mFAVN were used.

The results regarding sensitivity, specificity, diagnostic agreement and diagnostic validity for either type of samples are recorded in Table 3. Correlation between titres of antibodies titrated by mFAVN test and percent of blocking obtained with BioPro ELISA are recorded in Figs. 1, 2 and 3.

Discussion

The most effective method for evaluation of ORV campaign success is monitoring program. [1]. Main parts of program are control of bait uptake (tetracycline detection) and evaluation of immunological response (detection of specific antibodies) [16]. The specific rabies antibodies in the monitoring of fox ORV campaigns can be detected by using two different methods: virus neutralisation test and ELISA [16]. ELISA is simpler and faster method but the virus neutralization test is still considered as a golden standard. Although the principle of ELISA is different compared to virus neutralization test for the validation purpose the ELISA is usually compared with the virus neutralisation test. However, the possibility of evaluation depends on quality of samples. The poor quality samples may prevent the successful performance of virus neutralisation test. Because of that ELISA has never been evaluated for detection of antibodies against rabies in muscle extracts. Recently, the ELISA was evaluated on fresh collected thoracic liquid samples of foxes [11] and on sera samples of dogs and cats [9].

In this study ELISA was evaluated in the part of ORV campaigns monitoring as a tool for detection of specific rabies antibodies in poor quality hemolytic thoracic liquids and muscle extract samples. For that purpose the term "threshold of detection" (0.1 IU/ml) was applied instead of generally accepted adequate immunological response after vaccination (0.5 IU/ml). As is mentioned previously [17], because no specific rabies virus neutralisation antibodies level can been identified as absolute protection under all circumstances and in all hosts against all rabies virus variant infections, antibodies level attained by the majority of subjects in vaccine clinical trials formed the basis for the levels currently recognized as the minimal adequate response in vaccinated humans. According to World Health Organisation (WHO) that minimal adequate response is 0.5 [18]. This level was also adopted from World Organisation for Animal Health (OIE) as a minimal adequate response in vaccinated animals [13]. However, according to United States Advisory Committee on Immunization Practices (US ACIP) the adequate response is if no nonspecific inhibition reactions

Table 1 The sensitivity and specificity for the mFAVN test compared to FAVN test for different cut-offs

	Cut-off value	Sensitivity	Specificity	Correctly classified	Cumulative AUC
1.	0.100	1.0000	1.0000		
2.	0.200	1.0000	1.0000		
3.	0.300	1.0000	0.9655	99.0000	0.9976
4.	0.400	0.9706	0.8750	94.0000	0.9910
5.	0.500	0.9440	0.8880	94.0000	0.9900

Table 2 Results of testing for muscle extracts and thoracic liquids

	mFAVN test		ELISA		ELISA	
			Not-heat-treated		Heat-treated	
	Positive	Negative	Positive	Negative	Positive	Negative
Thoracic liquid	38	17	36	19	40	15
Muscle extract	15	77	5	87	23	69
Total	53	94	41	106	63	84

The cut -off for mFAVN test was set on 0.1 IU/ml
The cut -off for BioPro ELISA was set on 40 %

were found in serum dilutions above 1:5 [19]. The level described in the US ACIP is approximately 0.1 IU/ml in the RFFIT as originally described [20]. Furthermore, the main point regarding ORV serological monitoring is that for the purpose of detection of immunological response, a lower level is better suited than the globally recognized 0.5 IU/ml level for proof of adequate response to vaccination. Also, according to the previous study [17] the titer 0.1 IU/ml corresponding to a complete neutralisation at 1:5 serum dilution in the RFFIT. However, according to the same authors this can represent different titers and IU/ml values in laboratories that perform modified RFFIT which is the case with the mFAVN test described in this paper. In addition, United States Department of Agriculture considers an even lower cut-off >50 % neutralization at the 1:5 serum dilution when evaluating oral vaccination (~0.05 IU/ml) [21]. Also, according to manufacturer's instructions in the context of evaluation of fox ORV results the threshold of positivity of ELISA is decreased from the 70 to 40 %. According to manufacturer's instructions the percentage of blocking of 70 % is equivalent to 0.5 IU/ml obtained with virus neutralisation test. According to that, the percent of blocking 40 % in ELISA is lower than 0.5 IU/ml obtained with virus neutralisation test. In this study the purpose of detection of rabies virus antibodies in the monitoring of fox ORV campaigns was to detect immunological response on vaccination but not to consider the WHO or OIE minimal adequate response (0.5 IU/ml) [11]. Also, according to previous study the level of antibodies in muscle extracts and haemolytic thoracic liquids was lower compared to serum samples [4]. Because of the all above mentioned facts, the threshold of detection of virus neutralisation test as a part of monitoring of ORV campaigns was decreased to 0.1 IU/ml in order to establish the adequate immunological response to vaccination which can be the proof of seroconversion [20]. However, before the testing the mFAVN test was validated in comparison to FAVN test using difference cut-offs. As are recorded in Table 1 the sensitivity and specificity of the mFAVN compared with FAVN test were even higher for cut-off 0.1 IU/ml compared to cut off 0.5 IU/ml and show perfect agreement.

According to results in this study, the agreement between BioPro ELISA and mFAVN was 89.12 % for not-heat treated samples, and 87.76 % for heat treated samples. This means that heat treatment of the samples has not influence on kappa value of the BioPro ELISA test. Also, heat treatment of the samples just slightly increases a diagnostic validity of the test. However, if we compare an agreement of BioPro ELISA and mFAVN for thoracic liquids and muscle extracts separately, results are different.

According to previous study performed on foxes [11] the agreement between the BioPro ELISA and virus neutralisation test was 95.10 %. In that study thoracic liquid from the carcasses of the fresh foxes were used as a sample. In our study samples were not collect from the fresh foxes and because of that extremely haemolytic thoracic liquid samples were used for testing. The agreement between the BioPro ELISA and the mFAVN test was 89.09 % for not-heat treated and 92.73 % for heat treated samples. So, according to results in our study the quality

Table 3 Results of sensitivity, specificity, diagnostic agreement and diagnostic validity for BioPro ELISA

	All samples		Muscle extracts		Thoracic liquids	
	Not-heat treated treated	Heat	Not-heat treated treated	Heat	Not-heat treated treated	Heat
Specificity	92.98 %	79.10 %	100 %	87.50 %	89.47 %	85.00 %
Sensitivity	79.20 %	96.36 %	60 %	83.33 %	90.00 %	97.43 %
Diagnostic agreement	89.12 %	87.76 %	89.13 %	84.78 %	89.09 %	92.73 %
Diagnostic validity	89.16 %	94.3 %	70.30 %	88.70 %	95.98 %	94.90 %
Confidential interval	0.825–0.958	0.906–0.979	0.519–0.886	0.801–0.973	0.912–1.00	0.888–1.00
Kappa $p < 0.001$	0.7517	0.7449	0.4560	0.5410	0.7526	0.8240

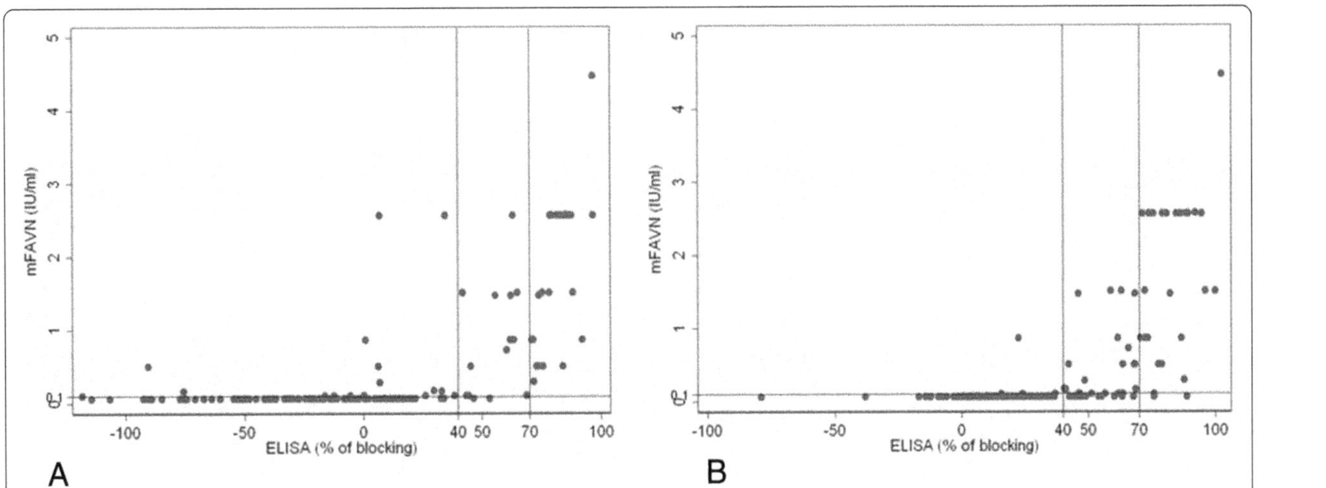

Fig. 1 a Correlation between titres of antibodies (IU/ml) in not-heat treated samples titrated by mFAVN test (cut off was set on 0.1 IU/ml) and percent of blocking obtained with BioPro ELISA (cut off was set on 40 %). **b** Correlation between titres of antibodies (IU/ml) in heat treated samples titrated by mFAVN test (cut off was set on 0.1 IU/ml) and percent of blocking obtained with BioPro ELISA (cut off was set on 40 %)

of thoracic liquid samples does not have influence on results obtained with BioPro ELISA or it insignificantly decreases the agreement between tests. Also, when thoracic liquids were used, heat treatment does not increase the validity of the test.

The opposite situation was recorded when muscle extracts were used as a sample. Even though diagnostic agreement between ELISA and mFAVN for heat treated samples is slightly decreased (4 %) the validity of the test is significantly increased (18 %). The reason for that is that according to this study heat treatment of the muscle extracts causes increase in sensitivity of the test but also causes decrease in test specificity. This finding is expected because in general, the higher the sensitivity, the lower the specificity, and vice versa. However, in this study the improvement in sensitivity was significantly higher compared to specificity decreasing which result in increase of the test validity. The lower sensitivity when not-heat treated muscle extracts were used as samples is very important; in that case a lot of false negative results could be obtained with ELISA. The reason for different influence of heat treatment on thoracic liquids and muscle extracts can be explained in different chemical composition of muscle (enzymes, proteins) compared to blood. Also, the reason for decreasing of the test specificity can be due to influence of heat treatment on specific antibody structure (proteins) or antibody activity. However, the influence of heat treatment on test specificity and sensitivity should be further investigated.

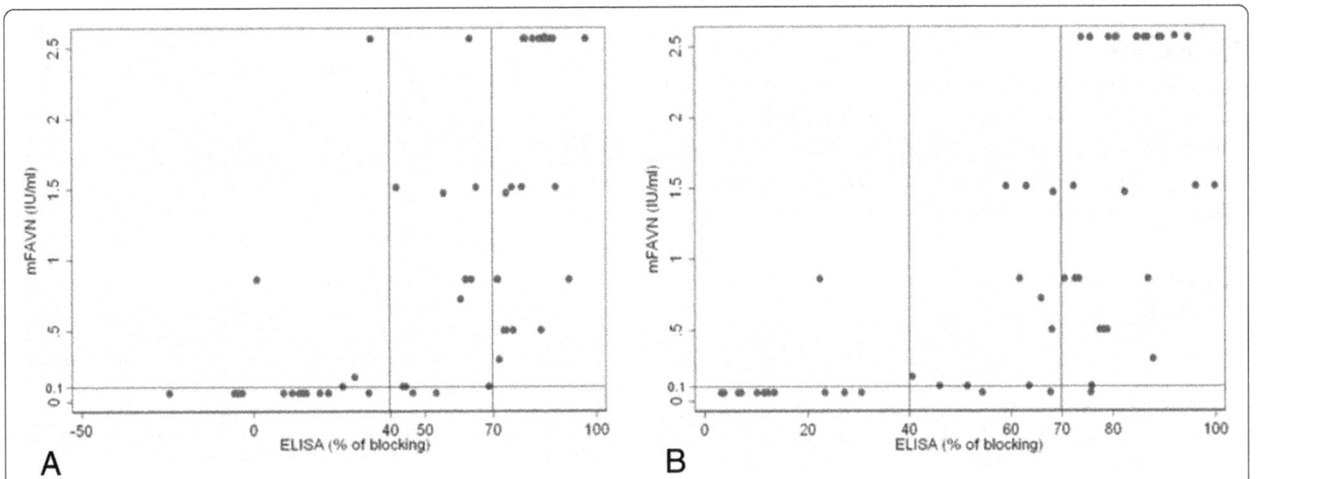

Fig. 2 a Correlation between titres of antibodies (IU/ml) in not-heat treated thoracic liquids samples titrated by mFAVN test (cut off was set on 0.1 IU/ml) and percent of blocking obtained with BioPro ELISA (cut off was set on 40 %). **b** Correlation between titres of antibodies (IU/ml) in heat treated thoracic liquids samples titrated by mFAVN test (cut off was set on 0.1 IU/ml) and percent of blocking obtained with BioPro ELISA (cut off was set on 40 %)

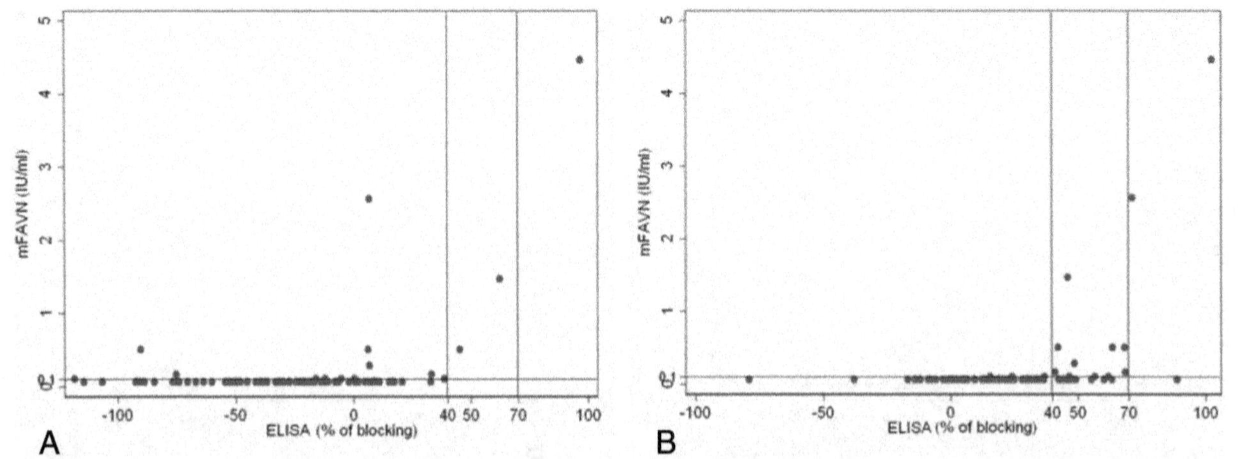

Fig. 3 a Correlation between titres of antibodies (IU/ml) in not-heat treated muscle extracts samples titrated by mFAVN test (cut off was set on 0.1 IU/ml) and percent of blocking obtained with BioPro ELISA (cut off was set on 40 %). **b** Correlation between titres of antibodies (IU/ml) in heat treated muscle extracts samples titrated by mFAVN (cut off was set on 0.1 IU/ml) and percent of blocking obtained with BioPro ELISA (cut off was set on 40 %)

According to this study the kappa value ranged between 0.4560 for not-heat treated muscle extract samples to 0.8240 for thoracic liquids heat treated samples. Overall, the kappa value was significantly lower for muscle extracts compared to thoracic liquids and indicated only moderate agreement of the test when muscle extracts were used as samples. However, the more relevant measure is the test validity or degree to which the test measures what it claims to measure. The kappa value only considers the cut offs but the diagnostic validity considers all results and provides better overview of test. According to our study the diagnostic validity for all samples except not-heat treated muscle extracts was very high (88.70 95.98 %) and indicated very good reliability of the BioPro ELISA test.

Conclusions

According to this study haemolytic thoracic liquids and muscle extracts can be used as samples for detection of specific rabies antibodies with BioPro ELISA. Muscle extracts samples should be heat treated before testing in order to increase the validity of the test.

Consent to publish

Not applicable.

Abbreviations

ACIP: Advisory Committee on Immunization Practices; ELISA: enzyme linked immunosorbent assay; FAVN test: fluorescent antibody virus neutralisation test; IU/ml: international unit/millilitre; mFAVN test: modified fluorescent antibody virus neutralisation test; RFFIT: rapid fluorescent focus inhibition test; WHO: World Health Organisation.

Competing interests

The authors declare that they have no competing interests.

Authors' contributions

TB and PH conceived the study, designed the experiments, performed all the experiments and drafted the manuscript. IŠ, NK and IL participated in writing the manuscript. IS and ILJ helped in study design, study implementation and manuscript revision. ŽM analyzed the data (statistical analysis) and helped in manuscript revision. All the authors have read and approved the final manuscript.

Acknowledgements

The Ministry of Science, Education and Sports, Republic of Croatia is acknowledged for they support in this study.

Funding

No funding was obtained for this study.

Author details

[1]Croatian Veterinary Institute, Savska cesta 143, 10000 Zagreb, Croatia. [2]University of Ljubljana, Veterinary Faculty, Gerbičeva 60, 1115 Ljubljana, Slovenia. [3]Veterinary Directorate, Planinska 2a, 10000 Zagreb, Croatia.

References

1. Freuling MC, Hampson K, Selhorst T, Schroder R, Meslin XF, Mettenleiter CT, Müller T. The elimination of fox rabies from Europe: determinants of success and lessons for the future. Phil Trans R Soc B. 2013; 368. http://rstb.royalsociety publishing.org/content/368/1623/20120142.full.html#ref-list-1
2. Blas Rico A, Panayiotis D. Status of EU support of CSF and rabies eradication, control and monitoring programmes in the EU-MS and neighbouring countries. Budapest: 1st Veterinary Forum for South East Europe; 2011. http://www.fao.org/fileadmin/user_upload/Europe/documents/Events_2011/1stvetforum/1CSF-Rabies_EC_en.pdf.
3. Cliquet F, Freuling C, Smreczak M, van der Poel WHM, Horton D, Fooks AD, Robardet E, Picard-Meyer E, Müller T. Development of harmonised schemes for monitoring and reporting of rabies in animals in the European Union. 2010. 60 EFSA Scientific report. http://www.efsa.europa.eu/sites/default/files/scientific_output/files/main_documents/67e.pdf
4. Bedekovic T, Lemo N, Lojkic I, Mihaljevic Z, Jungic A, Cvetnic Z, Cac Z, Hostnik P. Modification of the fluorescent antibody virus neutralisation test-elimination of the cytotoxic effect for the detection of rabies virus neutralising antibodies. J Virol Methods. 2013;189:204–8.
5. Cliquet F, Aubert M, Sagne L. Development of a fluorescent antibody virus neutralisation test (FAVN test) for the quantitation of rabies-neutralising antibody. J Immunol Methods. 1998;212:79–87.
6. Johnson N, Cunningham AF, Fooks AR. The immune response to rabies virus infection and vaccination. Vaccine. 2010;28:3896–901.

7. Moore SM, Ricke TA, Davis RD, Briggs DJ. The influence of homologous vs. heterologous challenge virus strains on the serological test results of rabies virus neutralizing assays. Biologicals. 2005;33:269–76.
8. Smith JS, Yager PA, Baer GM. A rapid reproducible test for determining rabies neutralizing antibody. Bull World Health Organ. 1973;5:902.
9. Wasniewski M, Cliquet F. Evaluation of ELISA for detection of rabies antibodies in domestic carnivores. J Virol Methods. 2012;179:166–75.
10. Shiraishi R, Nishimura M, Nakashima R, Enta C, Hirayama N. Determination of critical factors causing cytotoxicity in the virus neutralization test. J Virol Methods. 2014;199:46–52.
11. Wasniewski M, Guiot AL, Scherrefer JL, Tribout L, Mähar K, Cliquet F. Evaluation of an ELISA to detect rabies antibodies in orally vaccinated foxes and raccoon dogs sampled in the field. J Virol Methods. 2013;187:264–70.
12. Official gazette, number 47, 2012, Croatia. http://narodne-novine.nn.hr/
13. OIE/Office Internationale des Epizooties. Rabies. In: Manual for diagnostic tests and vaccines for terrestrial animals. Paris: OIE; 2011. http://www.oie.int/fileadmin/Home/eng/Health_standards/tahm/2.01.13_RABIES.pdf.
14. Greiner M, Gardner IA. Epidemiologic issues in the validation of veterinary diagnostic tests. Prev Vet Med. 2000;45:3–22.
15. Drobatz KJ. Measures of accuracy and performance of diagnostic tests. J Vet Card. 2009;11:33–40.
16. Servat A, Wasniewski M, Cliquet F. Tools for rabies serology to monitor the effectiveness of rabies vaccination in domestic and wild carnivores. Dev Biol. 2006;125:91–4.
17. Moore MS, Gordon RC, Hanlon AC. Measures of Rabies Immunity. In: Jackson CA, editor. Rabies, scientific basis of the disease and its management. San Diego: Academic Press; 2013. p. 461–96.
18. World Health Organization. WHO expert committee on rabies. World Health Organ Tech Rep Ser. 2005;931:1–121.
19. Advisory Committee on Imunization Practices. Human rabies prevention-United States. Morb Mortal Wkly Rep. 1999;48:1–17.
20. Moore SM, Hanlon CA. Rabies-specific antibodies: measuring surrogates of protection against a fatal disease. PloS Neg Trop Dis. 2010;4:e595. doi:10.1371/journal.pntd.0000595.
21. Fry TL, Vandalen KK, Shriner SA, Moore SM, Hanlon CA, Vercauteren KC. Humoral immune response to oral rabies vaccination in raccoon kits: Problems and implications. Vaccine. 2013;31(26):2811–5.

12

Evaluation of spray and oral delivery of Newcastle disease I2 vaccine in chicken reared by smallholder farmers in central Ethiopia

Kibrom Mebrahtu[1*], S. Teshale[2*], Wendimeneh Esatu[3], Tadios Habte[3] and Esayas Gelaye[4]

Abstract

Background: Newcastle disease (ND) is a highly infectious disease causing considerable economic losses to poultry farmers worldwide. Conventional vaccine delivery methods are not suitable for smallholder and rural poultry producers, and thus appropriate vaccination methods need to be sought. This study was carried out with the main objective of evaluating the efficacy of ND I2 vaccine delivered via drinking water and spray under smallholder farmers' condition in Minjar-Shenkora district, central Ethiopia. Twenty households were randomly assigned to intervention and control groups. Chickens owned by the selected households were randomly assigned to one of the three intervention groups. Blood samples were collected regularly for antibody assay from individual chicken vaccinated with ND I2 vaccine using different routes.

Results: At baseline, there was no difference in antibody titer among the experimental groups. After the first and booster vaccinations, the three vaccinated groups had significantly higher antibody titer ($P < 0.001$) than the unvaccinated control group. Interestingly, there was no statistically significant difference in antibody titer among the vaccinated groups. Out of the 40 chicken in the unvaccinated control only 14 had antibody titter≥ $\log_2^3$. Similarly 19/37 of chicken in the drinking water group, 19/37 of chicken in the eye drop group and 20/40 chicken in the spray group had antibody titer ≥ $\log_2^3$. Two weeks after the first vaccination the proportion of chicken with antibody titer ≥ $\log_2^3$ rose to 23/37, 30/37 and 29/40 in the group vaccinated via drinking water, eye drop and spray, respectively. The proportion remained low in unvaccinated group. Hundred percent of the vaccinated chicken survived after infection with the virulent ND virus (Alemaya strain); whereas only 40% survived from the unvaccinated control group.

Conclusion: The results of this study showed that ND I2 vaccine administered via drinking water and spray under smallholder farmers' situation provoked protective antibody level similar to the eye drop method. The use of ND I2 vaccine could contribute to food security if used by rural poultry farmers properly.

Keywords: Newcastle disease, I2 vaccine, Smallholder, Village, Chicken

* Correspondence: kibrommebrahtu@gmail.com; teshalesori2002@yahoo.com
[1]Jinka Agricultural Research Center, Department of Animal Health, Southern Ethiopian Nations, Nationalities and People's Regional State, Jinka, Ethiopia
[2]Addis Ababa University College of Veterinary Medicine and Agriculture, Bishoftu Ethiopia, Department of Clinical Studies, P.O. Box 34 Bishoftu, Ethiopia
Full list of author information is available at the end of the article

Background

Chicken production is considered an important source of quality animal proteins and can break the vicious cycle of poverty and malnutrition in developing countries. They particularly play important role in the well-being of women and children [1]. In Ethiopia, locally produced chickens are genetically diverse [2] with low production [3], which may be attributed to ND.

Increasing productivity and financial return from backyard chicken requires better knowledge of diseases such as ND. Newcastle disease can intercept the expansion of small scale poultry farms in the rural Ethiopia unless its incidence is reduced. Distribution of various breeds and uncontrolled marketing can aid the spread of ND between and within poultry farms. For example, more than 15 outbreaks of ND were confirmed in 2016 whereas as hundreds of outbreaks were confirmed in 2015 in the country. This shows that ND is continuing to impact the livelihood of poultry farmers. To improve productivity and financial return from backyard flocks, improvements to education and biosecurity measures are required.

Effective control of ND is needed to improve the livelihood of smallholder farmers particularly women in developing countries [4]. Vaccination has been considered effective and affordable control option in several countries [4–8]. It has been widely used in commercial poultry farms. The demand for vaccine against ND has grown in smallholder and village poultry producers. However, the conventional vaccine application methods are not suitable for smallholder and village poultry production systems [6]. An innovative alternative for smallholder and village poultry producers was developed in Australia using heat stable ND I2 virus [7]. It has been proven to be suitable for village poultry in Asian and some African countries in the absence of cold chain [9] and is cheaper than conventional ND vaccines [8]. Despite expansion of smallholder poultry production, information on the use of ND I2 vaccine and route of vaccine delivery with optimal protection level has not been sufficiently explored in Ethiopia. Suitable vaccine delivery route that can be used by the farmers could contribute to food security. The main objective of this study is, therefore, to evaluate the efficacy of ND I2 vaccine delivered via drinking water and spray.

Methods

Study area

This study was conducted in Minjar-Shenkora district, North Shoa Zone, Amhara Regional State, central Ethiopia. It is located between 90°6′ and 90°5′ N and 39°46′ and 39°26′ East 135 km south east of Addis Ababa (Fig. 1). The altitude of the area ranges from 1400 to 2400 m.a.s.l. The average annual rainfall of the district ranges from 62.8 mm – 1028 mm in bimodal pattern. The mean annual temperature of the last 10 years ranges from 7.3 °C – 20 °C. Agriculture is the main stay of the economy of people inhabiting the district in which livestock production plays key role. The livestock population of the district comprises cattle (95270), sheep (57603), goats (74049), poultry (168,702) and equines (3826). Exotic poultry such as Sasso, Kockock and White leghorn are widely reared in the district although the majority is made of indigenous chicken (Chefe ecotype) [10]. Chickens in the study area have never been vaccinated against ND.

Study methods

Minjar-Shenkora district was purposively selected for this study. It has several peasant associations, which are the smallest administrative units within the district. The peasant associations were selected purposively considering the presence of higher chicken population per household, the accessibility of the peasant association to the road and the consent of the farmers to participate in the study. The selection of peasant association was facilitated by livestock experts and extension staff of the district. Households from the selected peasant associations were selected purposively based on the number of indigenous and exotic chickens they own. This was facilitated by community leaders and extension staffs. Accordingly 20 households who owned ten or more chicken (indigenous and exotic) per household were selected and included in the experiment. A total of 154 4 weeks old chickens, 82 indigenous and 72 exotic breeds owned by the 20 selected households were selected and individually identified using numbered wing tags. The farmers are smallholder farmers who use open housing and small areas enclosed with fence. The feed resources for the chickens are household refuse, homestead pickings, crop residues and seeds offered by the flock owners. This study was submitted to the Animal Research Ethics Review Committee and approved.

Experimental design

The selected households were randomly assigned to either intervention or control groups. The chicken owned by the households assigned to intervention were randomly assigned to one of the three intervention groups: the first group comprises of chicken which received ND I2 vaccine via drinking water, the second group comprises of chicken which received ND I2 vaccine via spray and the last group comprises of chicken which received ND I2 vaccines via eye drop (positive control). The chickens were stratified by their breeds. Randomization of households was carried out using

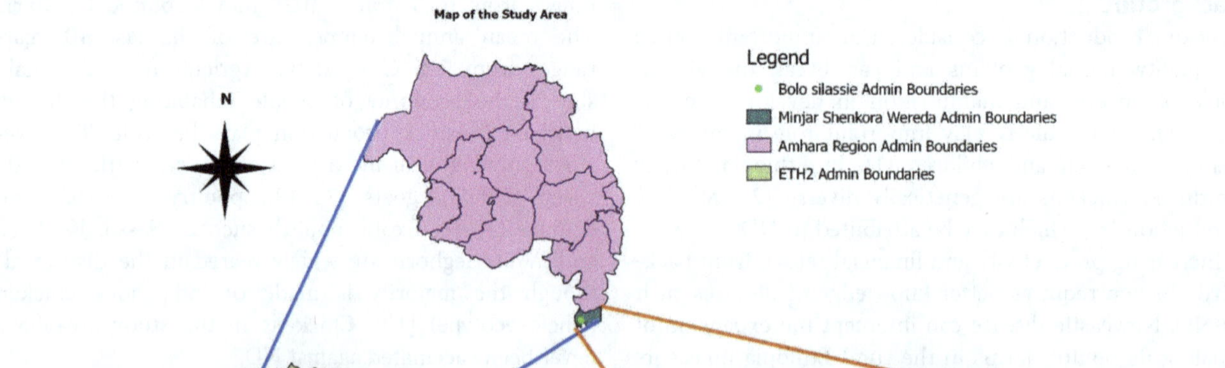

Fig. 1 Map of the study area (Quantum Geographic Information System (QGIS) software Version 2.0.1)

lottery systems whereas that of chickens was carried out by random sampling method using R statistical software. The unvaccinated control group and the group that received ND I2 via spray comprise 40 chickens each (22 indigenous and 18 exotic chicken per group) whereas the other two groups had 37 chickens each (19 indigenous and 18 exotic chickens per group). Blood sample was collected to estimate the baseline antibody level against ND virus.

Vaccination and follow up

Vials of 400 and 200 doses of freeze dried ND I2 vaccine (batch number NVI-4/16 and 1/17, respectively) containing 10^6 EID_{50} viruses were purchased from the National Veterinary Institute (NVI), Bishoftu, Ethiopia. The vaccine was reconstituted with non-chlorinated distilled water (manufacturer's instruction) and given to experimental chickens except the unvaccinated group. Booster vaccination was given 15 days after the first vaccination using the same vaccine. Blood samples were collected 15 days after the first and booster vaccinations. The chickens were followed for 3 months after which they were infected with virulent ND virus. The vaccine delivery was carried out by veterinary technicians in the district who were not aware of the experiment.

For oral delivery via drinking water a vial of the freeze-dried ND I2 vaccine containing 400 doses was reconstituted in 4000 mL of distilled water following the manufacturer's instructions (1 dose per 10 mL of distilled water). Each chicken per group received 10 mL of the reconstituted vaccine. Prior to vaccination farmers were informed to withhold water for few hours. The chickens were provided with reconstituted vaccine individually. For ocular administration a vial of the freeze-dried ND I2 vaccine containing 200 doses was reconstituted in 10 mL of saline solution as recommended by the manufacturer. Individual chicken in the group was provided with one drop of the reconstituted vaccine using sterile pipette. For the group receiving ND I2 vaccine by spray a spray bottle was used to spray the vaccine in saline water. In this group hundred mL of saline water was used to reconstitute 100 dose of the vaccine as per the recommendation of the manufacturer. Therefore, one vial of the freeze-dried ND I2 vaccine containing 400 doses was reconstituted in 400 mL of saline water. That is, the dose of the vaccine was adjusted at 1 mL of vaccine per chicken in a cage and the chickens were kept in closed cage for 30 min after spray.

Blood collection

Blood samples (1–1.5 mL) per bird were collected using 3 mL sterile disposable syringe from the wing vein following the standard methods described by Alders and Spradbrow [6]. The collected blood samples were labeled with individual chicken number and allowed to clot overnight at room temperature to facilitate serum separation. The sera were harvested in to labeled cryovials and stored at −20 °C until HI was carried out.

Collection of the blood for serological testing was carried out by the district veterinary technicians.

Hemagglutination inhibition (HI) assay

HI assay was conducted in the serology laboratory of the NVI, Bishoftu, Ethiopia by personnel who were not aware of the groups of chickens. The sera samples were heat inactivated at 56 °C for 30 min before assay. The level of anti-ND virus antibodies in the sera was estimated using the HI test as described by OIE [11]. The antigen used was reconstituted commercial NDV La Sota vaccine (TAD, Cuxhaven, Germany). Two-fold serial dilutions of serum samples were used to estimate the anti-NDV antibody titers as logarithms to the base two. In this study, we used the published cut off value for the protective HI antibody titer (HI titer ≥ $\log_2^3$ i.e. GM ≥ 3) for ND vaccination in chickens [9, 11, 12].

Challenge infection with virulent virus

Four weeks after booster vaccination was provided 40 chickens (10 from each treatment group) were randomly selected, purchased and brought to the College of Veterinary Medicine Addis Ababa University, Bishoftu, Ethiopia. The chickens were housed in experimental poultry house. They were infected with local virulent NDV strain designated Alemaya strain obtained from the NVI, Bishoftu, Ethiopia. It has a mean embryonic death time of 51.1 h, an intracerebral pathogenicity index of 1.84 and an intravenous pathogenicity index of 2.51 [13]. Each bird was inoculated with 1 mL of the viral suspension containing 10^7 EID_{50}/mL via breast muscle as described by Reta et al. [14]. The chickens from each treatment group were kept separately and followed daily for morbidity and mortality for 1 month. The birds were kept in experimental poultry house that is isolated from poultry and other livestock farms under the auspice of the National Veterinary Institute, Bishoftu, Ethiopia. The experimental house is equipped with necessary containment facility.

Data analysis

Sample size calculation was done taking into account 5% error, 80% power and the expected difference among the group to be 0.75 units. Accordingly at least 28 chickens were needed per group. The data collected during this study were analyzed using STATA version 13. The variation in mean antibody titres among the four experimental groups was analyzed using one way ANOVA at each sampling time. When difference was observed among the groups, Bonferroni multiple pair-wise comparison was used and significance is reported at $P < 0.05$. For all analysis intention-to-treat analysis was used.

Results

Results of Hemaglutination inhibition assay

At baseline the overall mean ($\log_2 \pm$ SE) antibody titer against NDV was 3.9 ± 0.21, which was slightly higher than the protective level in all the treatment groups (Table 1). At this time there was no statistically significant difference in antibody titer among chicken in all the experimental groups. There was no statistically significant difference in mean antibody titers between indigenous and exotic chickens. However, the mean antibody titer was higher in exotic breeds than the indigenous chickens.

Two weeks after the first vaccination the three vaccinated groups had significantly higher ($P < 0.001$) mean ($\log_2 \pm$ SE) antibody titer than the unvaccinated ones (Table 2). However, there was no statistically significant difference in antibody titer among the vaccinated groups although the group that received the ND I2 vaccine via spray had highest titer followed by the eye drop group. Similarly, after booster vaccination was provided the vaccinated groups had significantly higher antibody titer than the unvaccinated groups whereas there was no statistically significant difference among the vaccinated groups (Table 3). Highest antibody titer was observed in chickens vaccinated by spray followed by those that received the vaccine via drinking water.

Proportion of chickens with protective (Log_2^3) HI titer

At baseline 14/40 of the chicken in the unvaccinated control, 19/37 of chicken in the drinking water group, 19/37 of chicken in the eye drop group and 20/40 chicken in the spray group had antibody titer ≥ $\log_2^3$. Two weeks after the first vaccination the proportion of chicken with antibody titer ≥ $\log_2^3$ rose to 23/37, 30/37 and 29/40 in the group vaccinated via drinking water, eye drop and spray, respectively (Table 4). At this time the proportion of chicken with antibody titer ≥ $\log_2^3$ in the unvaccinated control group was 16/40. Two weeks after booster vaccination the proportion of chicken with antibody titer ≥ $\log_2^3$ slightly increased in the group vaccinated via drinking water and spray. The proportion of chickens with antibody titer ≥ $\log_2^3$ remained low in the unvaccinated control group.

Survival of chicken after challenge infection

After infection with virulent virus, chicken in the vaccinated group showed 100% survival while 60% of the unvaccinated controls died after showing typical clinical signs of ND. Two chicken from the group vaccinated via drinking water had shown mild clinical signs of ND but both recovered well after a week. The number of chicken owned by farmers in the study area showed decreased

Table 1 The baseline and post-vaccination mean ± SE antibody titer of chicken in all experimental groups

Treatment Group	M ± SE HI antibody titer (log2) of chickens vaccinated by different methods			
	N	Day 0	Day 15	Day 31
Unvaccinated	40	3 ± 0.41	4.45 ± 0.58	4.4 ± 0.60
Drinking water	37	4.7 ± 0.39	7 ± 0.51	7.6 ± 0.38
Eye drop	37	4.1 ± 0.38	7.2 ± 0.41	7.1 ± 0.41
Spray	40	3.7 ± 0.46	8.05 ± 0.43	7.7 ± 0.41

mortality for household who vaccinate their chicken. At the beginning of this experiment 12 households owning a total of 151 chickens were registered of which 4 household were willing to participate in the study. In these households the average number of chicken per household dropped from 12.58 to 4.08 at the end of the study. In contrast 16 households owning 337 chickens (21.06 chickens per household) who got their chicken vaccinated had 296 (18.5 chickens per household) at the end of the study showing the impact of vaccination (Table 5).

Discussion

Newcastle Disease is a highly virulent disease of poultry which can devastate the entire flock in short period of time. This was evident from frequent outbreaks affecting several farms in many areas during this study. Besides, the higher proportion of chickens with mean antibody titer greater than the protective level at the baseline shows exposure of the chickens to the virus as there is no vaccination in the study area. The antibody titer declines through time in unvaccinated group suggesting the need for vaccination. That means control of ND needs to be a priority issue in the achievement of food security and reduction of poverty in Ethiopia. Vaccine delivery that is suitable for smallholder farmers is important since biosecurity issues are difficult to achieve in rural settings. In this study, oral delivery of ND I2 vaccine via drinking water and spray were compared with the recommended route of vaccination (eye drop method).

The results showed that chickens vaccinated with ND I2 via drinking water and spray elicited anti-NDV antibody level sufficiently higher than the protective level (log_2^3), against virulent field virus [9, 12]. That is, the level of protection as shown by the antibody titer conferred by these routes of vaccination is comparable to the antibody level elicited by the eye drop method. This shows that smallholder farmers can choose among the methods of vaccination that suits their particular farming systems and needs. Elsewhere, it was shown that chickens vaccinated via oral route elicited good protection level even though booster vaccination was needed 2–4 weeks later [6, 15].

The proportion of chickens having antibody titer $\geq log_2^3$ after the first and booster vaccinations in the group vaccinated via drinking water and spray is comparable to that of chickens vaccinated using eye drop method. Particularly the proportion of chickens with antibody titers greater than log_2^3 after the booster vaccinations was greater than 70%, the level of herd immunity to ensure control of outbreaks. This observation is in consent with the earlier reports of Nassir et al. [13] and Reta et al. [14] in Ethiopia. Similarly, it agrees with the reports made elsewhere in the world such as the findings of Wegdan et al. [16] who used eye drop method and drinking water to deliver ND I2 vaccines in chicken. The protection level observed in chickens vaccinated by spray is also in agreement with earlier reports of Tadios et al. [17]. The high level of protection offered by vaccination via spray could be due to higher chance of getting the vaccine virus through natural routes of infection such as the eye and nostrils. Our observation shows that oral delivery of ND I2 vaccine via drinking water, which can be carried out by farmers themselves and spray with locally available materials can provoke sufficient immunity comparable to eye drop method. Literature shows that oral administration of ND vaccines primarily

Table 2 Results of multiple pair-wise comparison of log_2 HI antibody titer in experimental chicken at day 15 after primary vaccination

Treatment Group-1	Treatment Group-2	MD	SE	P- value	95% CI
D. water[b]	Control[a]	2.55	0.705	0.002	0.66–4.43
Eye drop[b]	Control[a]	2.82	0.705	0.001	0.93–4.70
Spray[b]	Control[a]	3.6	0.691	0.000	1.75–5.44
Eye drop[b]	D. water[b]	0.27	0.718	1.000	−1.65 - 2.19
Spray[b]	D. water[b]	1.05	0.705	0.831	−0.83 - 2.93
Spray[b]	Eye drop[b]	0.77	0.705	1.000	−1.10 - 2.66

Groups with different letters significantly differ from each other; MD = mean difference; SE = standard error; D. water = drinking water

Table 3 Results of multiple pair-wise comparison of log_2 HI antibody titer in experimental chicken at day 15 after booster vaccination

Treatment Group-1	Treatment Group-2	MD	SE	*P*-value	95% CI
D. water[b]	Control[c]	3.22	0.662	0.000	1.45–4.99
Eye drop[b]	Control[c]	2.73	0.662	0.000	0.96–4.50
Spray[b]	Control[c]	3.32	0.649	0.000	1.58–5.06
Eye drop[b]	D. water[d]	−0.48	0.675	1.000	−2.29 - 1.31
Spray[b]	D. water[d]	0.10	0.662	1.000	−1.66 - 1.87
Spray[b]	Eye drop[d]	0.66	0.662	1.000	−1.18 - 2.36

Groups with different letter significantly differ from each other; MD: mean difference; D. water = drinking water

provokes mucosal immunity [18]. This is important to confer protection against NDV, which is often acquired either by inhalation or ingestion or both [19].

The 100% survival observed in chickens vaccinated via drinking water, spray and eye drop methods compared to the control group after challenge infection indicates that vaccination with ND I2 vaccine can reduce mortality significantly. It reduces mortality at least by 60% in vaccinated chicken. This has important implication in terms of food security and financial revenue for smallholder chicken farmers. This is further evident from the drop in average number of chickens per household from 12.5 to 4.08 in farmers who did not vaccinate their flock. In all households who got their chicken vaccinated whether they were involved in the experiment or not the average number of chicken per households only dropped from 21.06 to 18.5. This implies that vaccination against ND with ND I2 vaccine via suitable delivery route can significantly reduce mortality and maintain flock size and ultimately contribute to household income. In consent to our observation previous authors showed that vaccination significantly increased chicken number and egg consumption per household in vaccinated village compared to control villages [4]. Women and children can particularly benefit from such vaccinations. In agreement with our findings Nasser et al. [13] and Musa et al. [20] reported 100% protection in chickens vaccinated via drinking water and eye drop following challenge with virulent virus. Reta et al. [14] also reported 100% protection in chickens vaccinated with ND I2 via drinking water after infection with the same strain of virus used in this study. Tadios et al. [17] also reported 100% survival after challenge infection with the same strain of virus in chickens vaccinated by spray. In Vietnam, after extensive laboratory and field trials in village chickens, ND I2 has been officially recognized as the ND vaccine for village chickens [8]. In Tanzania, it has been shown to offer protection for at least 2 months after vaccination [21]. Field records in Mozambique indicated that ND I2 vaccine provides approximately 80% protections in the face of outbreaks [6].

Table 4 The proportion of chickens with HI titer ≥ log_2^3 among the four experimental groups

Treatment Group	Number of chickens (%) with HI $log2^3 \geq 3.0$			
	N	Day 15	N	Day 31
Control	40	17(42.5%)	40	16(40%)
Drinking water	37	23(62.16%)	37	27(72.97%)
Eye drop	37	30(81.08%)	37	30(81.08%)
Spray	40	29(72.5%)	40	31(77.5%)

Notwithstanding the small number of households and chickens included in this study, the results showed that ND I2 vaccine provoke similar level of antibody production in indigenous and exotic chickens. In consent to our observation Nega et al. [22] reported similar level of protection in indigenous and exotic chickens after vaccination with ND I2 vaccine. This is important finding for poultry producers and veterinary personnel since information on the efficacy of ND vaccines in indigenous chicken is scarce. Regular vaccination of village chickens with ND I2 vaccine is suggested to reduce the circulation of virulent ND viruses and their spill over to commercial farms.

Conclusions

In conclusion, ND I2 vaccine administered via drinking water and spray provoked protective antibody level and survival after infection with virulent virus similar to the eye drop method under smallholder farmers' situation. The level protection conferred was similar in indigenous and exotic chickens

Table 5 Number of chicken owned and survived at the end of the study period in Minjar-Shenkora district

	No. owned	No. died	No. alive	Survival
Unvaccinated				
Total	151	102	49	32.45%
Average/household	12.58	7.75	4.08	
Vaccinated group				
Total	337	41	296	87.83%
Average/household	21.06	2.56	18.5	

reared by smallholder farmers in the area. Therefore, smallholder farmers can choose the suitable vaccine delivery routes to prevent outbreaks of ND. Vaccination can make a vital contribution to the improvement of household food and financial security in smallholder farmers.

Abbreviations
EID: Embryo Infective Dose; HI: hemaglutination Inhibition; ND: Newcastle Disease; NVI: National Veterinary Institute

Acknowledgements
The Ethiopian Institute of Agricultural Research, Debre Zeit Agricultural Research Center is appreciated for supporting sample collection and execution of field trials. The National Veterinary Institute of Ethiopia also acknowledge for providing laboratory facilities for challenge virus propagation. Dr. Teferi Degefa is highly acknowledged for his involvement in the preparation of the challenge virus. The authors would also like to acknowledge the collaboration of poultry farmers during field trials.

Funding
Seed fund was obtained from the Ethiopian Institute of Agricultural Research to carry out this study.

Authors' contributions
KM and TS conceived and carried out field trials and collected clinical samples for molecular analysis. WE and TH obtained fund from EIAR for this study and coordinated the field experiments and were involved in the conception, design and acquisition of data. EG provided the virulent virus used for challenge infection. KM and TS analyzed the data. TS, EG and KM wrote the paper. All authors read and approved the final manuscript.

Consent for publication
Not applicable

Competing interests
The authors declare that they have no competing interests.

Author details
[1]Jinka Agricultural Research Center, Department of Animal Health, Southern Ethiopian Nations, Nationalities and People's Regional State, Jinka, Ethiopia. [2]Addis Ababa University College of Veterinary Medicine and Agriculture, Bishoftu Ethiopia, Department of Clinical Studies, P.O. Box 34 Bishoftu, Ethiopia. [3]Ethiopian Institute of Agriculture, Debre Zeit Agricultural Research Center, Bishoftu, Ethiopia. [4]National Veterinary Institute, Bishoftu, Ethiopia.

References
1. Hailemichael A, Gebremedhin B, Gizaw S, Tegegne A. Analysis of village poultry value chain in Ethiopia: implications for action research and development, International livestock research institute (ILRI); 2016. p. 1–15.
2. Reta D. Understanding the role of indigenous chicken during the long walk to food security in Ethiopia. LRRD. 2009; 21(116): http://www.lrrd.org/lrrd21/8/dugu21116.htm. Accessed 2 Feb 2017.
3. Reta D. Phenotypic characterization of some indigenous chicken ecotypes of Ethiopia. LRRD. 2006; 18(131): http://www.lrrd.org/lrrd18/9/dugu18131.htm. Accessed 2 Feb 2017.
4. Knueppel D, Cardona C, Msoffe P, Demment M, Kaiser L. Impact of vaccination against chicken Newcastle disease on food intake and food security in rural households in Tanzania. Food Nutr Bull. 2010;31:436–45.
5. Palya V. Manual for the production of Marek's disease, Gumboro disease and inactivated Newcastle disease vaccines, Technical Centre for Agricultural and Rural Cooperation. FAO animal production and health; 1991. p. 1–25.
6. Alders R, Spradbrow P. Controlling ND in village chickens. ACIAR Monograph. 2001;82:112.
7. Spradbrow PB, Ibrahim AC, Mustaffa-Bajee A, Kim SJ. Use of an avirulent Australian strain of Newcastle disease virus (NDV) as a vaccine. Avian Dis. 1977;22(2):329–35.
8. Tu TD, Phuc KV, Dinh NTK, Quoc DN, Spradbrow PB. Vietnamese trials with a thermostable Newcastle disease vaccine (strain I2) in experimental and village chickens. Prev. Vet. Med. 1998;34:205–14.
9. Spradbrow PB. Newcastle disease in village chickens. Poultry Scie Rev. 1993; 5:57–96.
10. MSWARDO. Minjar Shenkora Wereda agriculture and rural development office. Annu Rep. 2016:1-79. Report number 11.
11. OIE. Newcastle disease. In: OIE manual for diagnostic tests and vaccines for terrestrial animals, vol. 1. 5th ed; 2004. p. 270–83.
12. van Boven M, Bouma A, Fabri THF, Katsma E, Hartog L, Koch G. Herd immunity to Newcastle disease virus in poultry by vaccination. Avian Pathol. 2008;37:1–5.
13. Nassir M, Lohr JE, Mebratu GY, Zessin KH, Baumann MPO, Ademe Z. Oral Newcastle disease vaccination trials in Ethiopia. Avian Pathol. 2000;29:27–34.
14. Reta D. A., Kasahun A., Olana M., Yilkal A., Esayas G., Marta Y. and Teshale S. Serological response and protection level evaluation in chickens exposed to grains coated with I2 Newcastle disease virus for effective oral vaccination of village chickens. BMC Vet Res 2016;12:150. DOI https://doi.org/10.1186/s12917-016-0785-6.
15. Bell JG, Fotzo TM, Amara A, Agbebe G. A field trial of the heat resistant V4 vaccine against Newcastle disease by eye-drop inoculation in village poultry in Cameroon. Prev. Vet. Med. 1995;25:19–25.
16. Wegdan H, Mahasin E, Khalafalla AI. The effect of route of administration and dose on the immunogenicity and protective efficacy of Newcastle disease Thermostable vaccine I2 strain. Int J Prev Med Res. 2015;5:276–81.
17. Tsegaw F, Kara D, Tesfu K, Mesfin S, Giovanni C. Effect of vaccination on transmission characteristics of highly virulent Newcastle disease virus in experimentally infected chickens. Avian Pathol. 2014;43(5):420–6.
18. Jayawardane GWL, Spradbrow PB. Cell mediated immunity in chickens vaccinated with the V4 strain of Newcastle disease virus. Vet Microbiol. 1995;46:37–41.
19. Alexander DJ. Newcastle disease and other avian paramyxoviruses. A laboratory manual for the isolation, identification and characterization of avian pathogens. In: Swayne DE, Glisson JR, Jackwood MW, editors. American Association of Avian Pathologists, Kenneth Square. 4th ed; 1998. p. 156–63.
20. Musa U, Abdu PA, Mera UM, Emmenna PE, Ahmed MS. Vaccination with Newcastle disease vaccines strain I_2 and Lasota in commercial and local chickens in plateau state Nigeria. Nigerian Vet J. 2010;31(1):6–55.
21. Wambura PN, Kapaga AM, Hyera JMK. Experimental trials with thermostable Newcastle disease virus (strain I-2) in commercial and village chickens in Tanzania. Prev Vet Med. 2000;43(2):75–83.
22. Nega M, Moges F, Mazengia H, Zeleke G, Tamir S. Evaluation of I2 thermostable Newcastle disease vaccine on local chickens in selected districts of western Amhara. Online J Anim Feed Res. 2012;2(3):244–8.

13

A randomized controlled study on the efficacy of a novel combination vaccine against enzootic pneumonia (*Mycoplasma hyopneumoniae*) and porcine Circovirus type 2 (PCV2) in the presence of strong maternally derived PCV2 immunity in pigs

Panagiotis D. Tassis[1*], Ioannis Tsakmakidis[1], Vassileios G. Papatsiros[2], Dimitrios Koulialis[1], Tom Nell[3], Georgia Brellou[4] and Eleni D. Tzika[1]

Abstract

Background: *Mycoplasma hyopneumoniae* (M. hyo) and Porcine Circovirus Type 2 (PCV2) are major pathogens that cause significant health problems in swine worldwide. Maternal derived immunity (MDI) has been suggested as a significant immediate defence factor for newborn piglets and may interfere with piglet's vaccination-induced immunity. The study aimed to assess the efficacy of a novel combination vaccine (consisting of PCV2 subunits and inactivated M. hyo strain J), against PCV2 and M. hyo natural infection [Porcilis® PCV M Hyo (MSD Animal Health, Boxmeer, the Netherlands)], in the presence of strong maternally derived PCV2 immunity (antibody titre averaged 11.08 $\log_2$), under field conditions. The study was performed according to a controlled, randomized and blinded design in a Greek swine unit with Enzootic Pneumonia (EP) and subclinical PCV2 infection. In total, 600 healthy three-week-old suckling piglets were allocated randomly, either to treatment (vaccinated with the test product) or control group (injected with sterile buffered saline).

Results: Vaccination significantly reduced the severity of lung lesions at slaughter (lesions of cranio-ventral pulmonary consolidation) ($P < 0.001$). The overall mean lung lesion score (LLS) was 9.6 in the vaccinated group and 12.2 in controls. The level of PCV2 viraemia was significantly reduced in vaccinated pigs. Furthermore, 25 g higher average daily weight gain (ADWG) was observed during the finishing phase ($P < 0.001$) and 18 g greater ADWG overall ($P < 0.001$).

Conclusions: Results of LLS, PCV2 viremia and ADWG support the test product's efficacy in the face of strong maternally derived PCV2 immunity.

Keywords: Porcilis PCV M Hyo, Enzootic pneumonia, *Mycoplasma hyopneumoniae*, Porcine circovirus type 2, Pigs

* Correspondence: ptassis@vet.auth.gr
[1]Farm Animals Clinic, School of Veterinary Medicine, Aristotle University of Thessaloniki, St. Voutyra 11, 54627 Thessaloniki, Greece
Full list of author information is available at the end of the article

Background

Mycoplasma hyopneumoniae (M. hyo) and Porcine Circovirus Type 2 (PCV-2) are two major pathogens of ubiquitous nature that cause critical health disorders in swine worldwide. M. hyo is part of the aetiology of a chronic insidious bronchopneumonia, also described as enzootic pneumonia (EP) which causes severe economic losses in the global pig industry [1]. Other bacterial agents usually coexist in cases of EP along with M. hyo. The EP clinical manifestations include a dry, non-productive cough, variable reduction of feed intake and growth retardation [2]. Moreover, viral pathogens such as Porcine Reproductive and Respiratory Syndrome virus (PRRSv) and PCV2 have been suggested as agents that contribute further in converting EP into the more complex Porcine Respiratory Disease Complex [2, 3].

PCV-2, with four genotypes documented up to today (PCV2a, PCV2b, PCV2c, PCV2d-mPCV2b), has been etiologically associated with certain Porcine Circovirus Diseases (PCVD) [4]. Those include disorders such as PCV2 - Systemic Disease (PCV2-SD) (formerly known as postweaning multisystemic wasting syndrome) which is characterised by growth retardation - wasting, anaemia, possible respiratory problems and diarrhoea, as well as lymphocyte depletion and immune suppression. Moreover, PCV2 is present in the aetiology of porcine dermatitis and nephropathy syndrome, and clinical manifestations of pneumonia, reproductive failure or intestinal disorders [5–7]. However, subclinical PCV2 infection occurs frequently and although clinically "silent", gradually results in significant economic losses due to growth retardation [8].

Vaccination of piglets is the main control method against clinical disease associated with M. hyo (eg. more than 85% of US farms vaccinate against M. hyo) [1, 3]. For almost a decade (since 2007), control of PCVD has been also based on vaccination of sows and/or piglets [3, 9]. Nevertheless, those two pathogens persist, circulate and interact with other pathogens in the host, making their clearance extremely difficult [7, 10].

The double edged sword case of maternal derived immunity (MDI) as a significant immediate defence factor for newborn piglets and its possible interference on piglet's active immunity is a point of controversy. So far, it seems that MDI [including cell-mediated (CMI) and antibody-mediated immunity (AMI)] through colostrum and milk may interfere to some extent with the induction of AMI and CMI responses in piglets after vaccination [11–13]. Previous studies suggested that high MDI levels at the moment of vaccination could affect vaccine-induced seroconversion [5, 14–17].

The objective of this study was to assess the efficacy of a ready-to-use combination vaccine [Porcilis® PCV M Hyo (MSD Animal Health, Boxmeer, The Netherlands)] against concurrent clinical M. hyo and subclinical PCV2 infection under field conditions, in the face of strong maternally derived PCV2 immunity in piglets at the time of vaccination.

Methods

Trial design

Farm selection was performed after pre-trial scoring of lung lesions according to the method of Goodwin and Whittlestone [18], along with PCV2 serology. Pre-trial results suggested an existing EP with typical lung lesions (cranio-ventral pulmonary consolidation) in >90% of tested lungs, along with high maternally derived PCV2 antibody titres at three weeks of piglets' age. In addition, PCV2 antibodies were also measured after the 16th week of age and further increased until the pigs' slaughter age (22nd week). Thus, the trial farm was considered as clinically affected with EP and subclinically affected by PCV-2. The farrow-to-finish farm was in Northern Greece with approximately 800 sows under production.

The test product is a new combination vaccine that induces immunity against PCV2 and M. hyo, and consists of Baculovirus expressed PCV2 subunits and inactivated M hyo strain J in Emunade adjuvant (Porcilis® PCV M Hyo, MSD Animal Health, Boxmeer, The Netherlands). The test product evaluated in this study is registered in the European Union [19].

The efficacy evaluation of the test product was set as a placebo controlled, randomized and blinded study. Piglets were assigned individually (within litters) to the treatment groups. At admission, the animals were ear tagged as they came to hand and were allocated with the use of a computer-generated randomisation list (only known to EDT) to one of the two treatment groups, until the required number of piglets had been reached. In total, 600 three-week-old suckling piglets from three production batches (equal number of male and female) were allocated randomly to one of two groups (day 0 of the trial - December 2010). Each group consisted of 300 animals at day 0 of the study. Only clinically healthy piglets were included in the study. Diseased piglets, runts and animals with abnormalities (e.g. hernia) were excluded. On day 0 of the trial, treatment group pigs were vaccinated intramuscularly (neck area) with 2 ml of the combination vaccine and control group animals were injected in a similar way with Unisol (sterile phosphate buffered saline and sucrose). In total, 285 pigs from the treatment group and 277 control animals reached the end of the study.

Allocation sequence was concealed until administration of the test product or Unisol to the trial animals. Enrollment, administration of products to the trial animals and assignment to each group was performed by two members (namely, P. Tassis and E. Tzika) of the research group. Animals of both groups were commingled throughout the study and they received feed and water according to the farm's schedule. Although the test and control product were visibly different (only relevant at the time of administration), the study was blinded. After vaccination, all farm and laboratory, or other personnel involved, either carrying out observations or measurements, could not identify the vaccination status of the pigs, as it was not possible to differentiate piglets by treatment without unblinding the ear tag number. A detailed study flow diagram is presented in Fig. 1. Furthermore, the sows from which study piglets originated had been routinely vaccinated against major pathogens (PCV-2, Aujeszky's disease virus, PRRSv, porcine parvovirus, *Erysipelothrix rhusiopathiae*, atrophic rhinitis and *Escherichia coli*).

Recorded parameters

Each individual pig was weighed at admission, at transfer to the finishing unit (week five post-vaccination) and shortly before the first animals of each batch were transferred to the slaughterhouse [week 20 post-vaccination (end of study)]. Medication was recorded and pigs that died during the study were examined post-mortem to establish the cause of death based on gross lesions, with the exception of cases where the cause was clear and unrelated to PCV2, or M. hyo infection, or vaccination (e.g. cases of severe post-traumatic lameness). The lungs of trial animals were examined individually by the same pathologist at slaughter to score the severity of typical M. hyo lesions according to the same methodology as in the pre-trial screening [18]. The lesions of cranio-ventral pulmonary consolidation (expressed as lung lesions score - LLS) of each tested lung was the addition of the proportion of each lobe surface with signs of typical M. hyo associated inflammation (consolidated, grey to purple coloured), multiplied with the weighting factor of each lobe [20]. The LLS score ranged from 0 to 55 at maximum. Also pleuritis lesions were scored as Grade 0 - no pleuritis lesions, Grade 1 - topical adhesions (spots) and Grade 2 - larger adhesions. Due to a minor data recording error, weighing data from 282 animals (out of 285) from the treatment group and 274 control pigs (out of 277) were analyzed at slaughter. Similarly, pleuritic lesions were evaluated from 279 vaccinated and 269 control pigs. Technical issues during lung extraction at slaughter, led to the evaluation of LLS data from a total of 266 treated animals and 257 controls.

The LLS, average daily weight gain (ADWG) in the finishing period and PCV2 viraemia results, were considered primary parameters for the assessment of vaccine efficacy. Additionally, overall ADWG (from vaccination until slaughter), mortality, morbidity (referring to the number of pigs that received individual medication) and the pleuritis lesions score, were also evaluated as secondary parameters. All procedures during this clinical study were carried out according to the Guidelines on Good Clinical Practices [21] and the

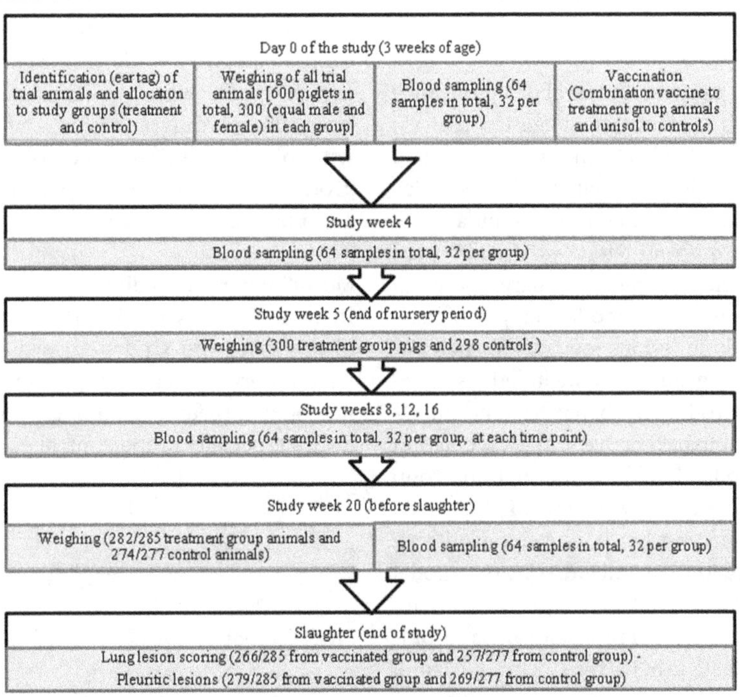

Fig. 1 Study flow diagram

animals were maintained in accordance with National and European Animal Welfare Requirements [22].

Blood sampling and serology

Thirty-two piglets per vaccination group were bled for serum samples every four weeks, starting from day 0. To monitor field infections and to assess serological response to vaccination, the sera were tested with PCV2 ELISA [23] and M. hyo ELISA (Swine HerdChek M. Hyo IDEXX) as per manufacturer instructions. The PCV2 titres were expressed as the reciprocal of the serum dilution with a calculated maximum extinction value of 50%. For calculation of the mean and standard deviation of antibody titres, samples that were negative at the lowest dilution (<4) were set at three. Similarly, samples that were positive at the highest dilution (>14) were set at 15.

The M. hyo test results were expressed as sample to positive (S/P) ratio and scored as 'positive', 'inconclusive' or 'negative'. Based on serology, natural PCV2 infection and relative seroconversion occurred during early finishing (12–20 weeks post vaccination), thus PCV2 levels in serum were measured by qPCR [23] during that period. The qPCR results were expressed as log10 copies/μl DNA extract. If the viral load was below the detection limit of 2 log10 copies/μl DNA extract, the result was considered negative and set at zero (0). The serum samples taken on study week 20 were also tested for antibodies to Actinobacillus pleuropneumoniae with APP OMP ELISA [24], swine influenza virus (H1N1, H1N2 and H3N2) with haemagglutination inhibition tests and PRRSv with ELISA (IDEXX PRRS X3 Ab Test).

Statistical analysis

The pig was the statistical unit and the level of significance was set at 0.05. Sample size calculation suggested that inclusion of approximately 300 piglets in each group had 80% power to detect a difference in means of 25 g a day between groups, assuming that the common standard deviation was 100 g in a two group t-test with a 0.05 two-sided significance level. The LLS were compared between the vaccination groups using mixed model analysis of variance (ANOVA) with the lung lesions log transformed before analysis. Vaccination group was included as fixed effect and the sow and production batch as random effects. The ADWG was compared between the vaccination groups using a mixed model ANOVA. Vaccination group and gender with their interaction were included as fixed effects and sow and production batch as random effects. The bodyweight at admission was included in the model as a covariate. The proportions of pigs with pleuritis lesions (absent or present), as well as mortality and morbidity were compared between groups by Cochran Mantel Haenszel method with production batch as classification variable. The mean individual qPCR results for PCV2 viraemia were compared between groups with Wilcoxon's rank sum test.

Results

Weight gain

The ADWG in the vaccinated group significantly increased by 25.3 g per day during the finishing period (Mixed model ANOVA: $P < 0.001$). Moreover, ADWG during the total study period was also significantly greater by 18.0 g per day in vaccinated pigs than controls (Mixed model ANOVA: $P < 0.001$). Results of ADWG are presented in Table 1.

PCV2 viraemia

A total of 101 samples were tested by qPCR for PCV2 viral DNA. The mean viral load was significantly (Rank Sum test: $P = 0.0004$) lower in the vaccinated pigs than the controls. The results, expressed as the mean $\log_{10}$ DNA copies per μl DNA extract, are summarised in Fig. 2. Presented data refer only to the period when results were above the detection limits.

Lung and pleuritis lesions score

The primary parameter of LLS was significantly reduced in the vaccinated group when compared with the controls (Mixed model ANOVA $P < 0.001$). Table 2 summarizes results of LLS and pleuritis lesions among groups. The LLS was further "separated" into four categories [i.e. score = 0 (absent), score= > 0–5 (mild), score= > 5–10 (moderate), score > 10 (severe)]. The evaluation of this distribution showed that more than half of the control group cases were categorized in the fourth category, while less than 40% of the vaccinated group cases were in the same category (Fig. 3). Insignificant differences in the proportion of animals with pleuritis lesions were observed between the trial groups ($P = 0.0759$). Representative findings of lung and pleuritis lesions are presented in Fig. 4.

Mortality and morbidity

In total, 38 pigs (6.3%), 15 vaccinated and 23 controls, died during the study. According to gross lesions that were reported after necropsy, respiratory disease (fibrinonecrotizing pleuropneumonia) was an important cause of death, especially in the control group (12 cases), compared

Table 1 Mean average daily weight gain (standard error of the mean) by vaccination group and period

Period	Vaccinated group (g/day)	Control group (g/day)
Nursery period	341 (5)	349 (5)
Finishing period	770^{a}(8)	745^{b}(8)
Overall	665^{c}(6)	647^{d}(6)

^{a,b,c,d}Mean values with different superscripts in the same row are significantly different. Pairwise comparison (Mixed model ANOVA): **ab**: $P < 0.0001$, **cd**: $P < 0.0001$

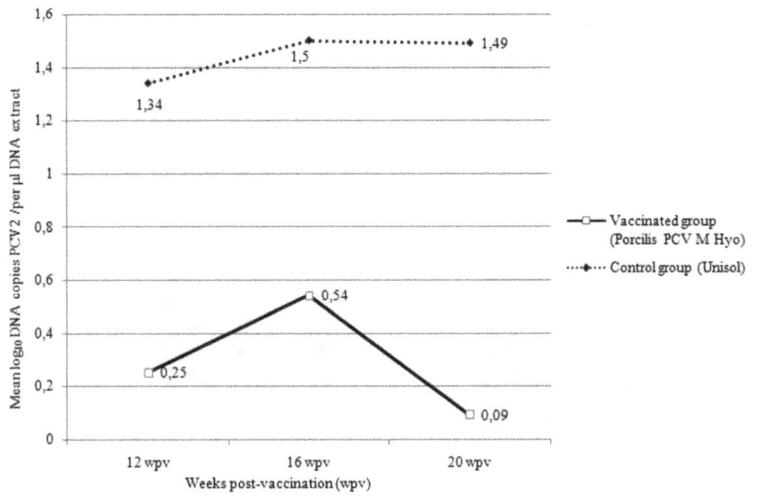

Fig. 2 Mean $\log_{10}$ DNA copies PCV2 /per µl DNA extract, by vaccination group and weeks post-vaccination. Presented data refer only to the period when results were above the detection limits

with only three cases in the vaccinated group. On the other hand, gastrointestinal disease (enteritis) was the cause of death in two cases from the vaccinated group and five cases from the control group. The remaining animals died of other causes (mainly post-traumatic). Mortality between the groups was not statistically significant ($P = 0.1799$).

Fifty two vaccinated animals and 54 control piglets received individual medication, mostly for gastro-intestinal (diarrhoea) or respiratory problems. The number of treatments for respiratory signs (18) was lower than for gastro-intestinal disease (25) in the vaccinated group, while the opposite was observed in the control group (28 v 25). Morbidity between groups was not statistically significant ($P = 0.8307$).

Serology

At the beginning of the study (day 0), approximately 45% of piglets were seropositive for M hyo. Towards the end of the study, the percentage of seropositive pigs increased to 100% in the vaccinated group and approximately 75% in the controls (Fig. 5). On the day of vaccination, PCV2 maternally derived antibody titre averaged 11.2 $\log_2$ in the vaccinated group and 10.9 $\log_2$ in the control group (average 11.08 $\log_2$ for all trial animals), which is considered high [5]. The mean PCV2 antibody titres in both treatment groups increased between 12 and 20 weeks after vaccination (Fig. 6). The maximum mean titre in the control group remained below 8 $\log_2$, which is considered low. At the end of the study, all pigs were seropositive for PRRSv and had moderate to high antibody titres to the outer membrane protein of *Actinobacillus pleuropneumoniae*. Low antibody titres were measured for swine influenza types H1N1 and H2N3, while the titres against type H1N2 were all below the detection limit (4 $\log_2$).

Table 2 Results of LLS and pleuritis lesions among trial groups

Lung lesions score (Mean score ± SD)		
Vaccinated group ($n = 266$)	Control group ($n = 257$)	
$9.6^a \pm 6.6$	$12.2^b \pm 7.8$	
Pleuritis lesions score (% of total cases examined)		
	Vaccinated group ($n = 279$)	Control group ($n = 269$)
No pleurisy lesions*	77%	70%
Topical lesions /spots	21%	25%
More extended lesions	3%	5%

[a,b]Mean values with different superscripts in the same row are significantly different
Pairwise comparison (Mixed model ANOVA): ab: $P < 0.0001$
*Cochran Mantel Haenszel method: $P = 0.0759$

Discussion

The current study demonstrates efficacy of the M hyo and PCV2 combination vaccine in 3 week old piglets in the presence of high PCV2 MDI level. Results of this study are in agreement with previous findings regarding the efficacy of the combination vaccine in the face of average PCV2 MDI levels (9.38 $\log_2$) [25].

Definitive diagnosis of EP is based on the demonstration of typical lung lesions [3]. The mean LLS in this study were significantly reduced in the vaccinated pigs, indicating the test product's efficacy against M. hyo. In addition, lung lesions were also less severe in vaccinated pigs as nearly two thirds of vaccinated animals had a score < 10 compared to more than half of the controls with a score > 10. This finding further supports the vaccine's efficacy against EP.

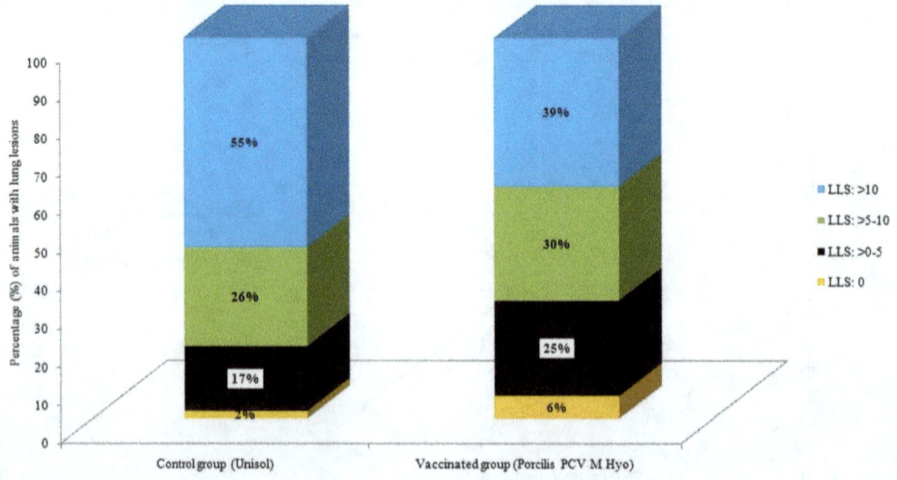

Fig. 3 Distribution of lung lesion scores among value-range categories per group

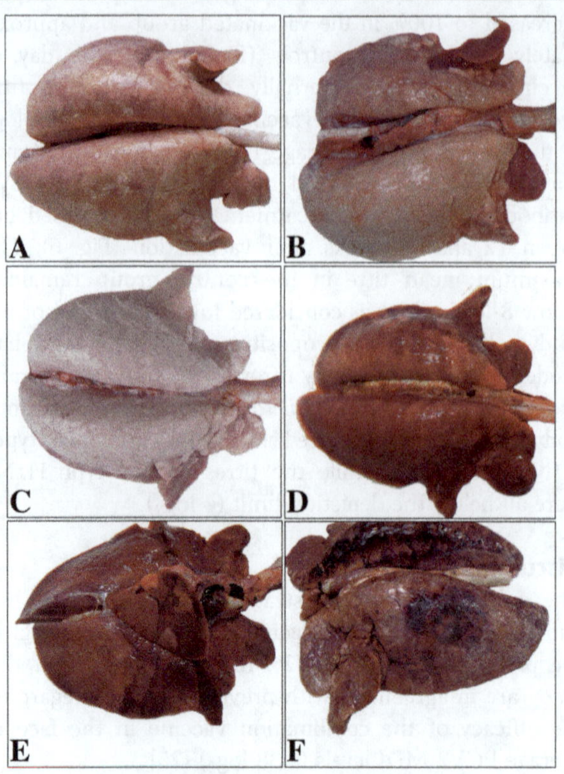

Fig. 4 Representative findings of lung and pleuritis lesions in trial animals. Figure **a**: lung has normal appearance. Figures **b** and **c**: *purple* (**b**) and *grey* (**c**) consolidation located in cranial and middle lobes. In Fig. **c** the caudal lobes are also affected. Figure **d**: lung shows intense purple consolidation of the cranial, middle and caudal lobes. Figure **e**: in ventral view of the previous lung (**d**), lesions of bronchopneumonia are distributed in all lobes. Figure **f**: enzootic pneumonia complicated with *Actinobacillus pleuropneumoniae* infection accompanied by localized fibrous pleurisy (*left* caudal lobe). [**a** - **c**: Vaccinated group (Porcilis PCV M Hyo)] [**d** - **f**: Control group (Unisol)]

Moreover, during the finishing period, vaccinated pigs had a significantly better ADWG and the overall gain was 18 g per day greater than in the control pigs. The ADWG results were also in agreement with several previous studies with monovalent intramuscular M. hyo vaccination in piglets [2, 26, 27]. Since serology results suggested a subclinical PCV2 farm infection, alterations of ADWG probably can also be attributed to some extent to the control of PCV-2. The reduced viraemia after the 16th week in comparison with controls can be considered as the main factor that contributed to the PCV-2-control-related improvement of ADWG.

The M. hyo serology results on Study day 0 suggest a natural farm infection with M. hyo. Therefore, most likely maternally derived M. hyo antibodies were detected in suckling piglets on day 0, due to pathogen circulation in breeding animals. Differences in antibody titres among groups on Day 0, can be attributed to natural M. hyo infection dynamics. Differences in M. hyo circulation, and the consequent seroconversion in sows, along with the effect of serum half-life of maternally derived M. hyo antibodies, resulted in variation of their relative levels in colostrum and blood of suckling piglets. Furthermore, during the progress of the study, seroconversion and relative differences in M. hyo antibody levels between groups were observed in the last two samplings. Those differences were mainly attributed to the beneficial immune-boosting effect of vaccination. Thus, a strong immune response was observed in animals that received the test product and counteracted natural M. hyo infection with significant antibody production. On the contrary, control animals had a weaker humoral response. Similar immune response of piglets against natural M. hyo infection after administration of the combination vaccine has been previously reported [25].

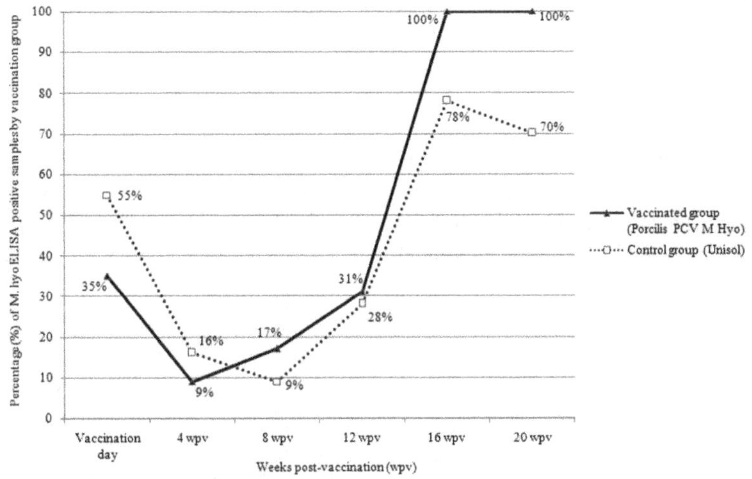

Fig. 5 Percentage (%) of M. hyo ELISA positive samples, by vaccination group and weeks post-vaccination

Previous studies suggest that PCV2 persists in swine tissues and seroconversion has been shown in both subclinical and PCV2-SD clinically affected pigs under field conditions. In contrast, weaker immune responses have been associated with PCV2-SD clinical cases [28–30]. The trial farm was a subclinical PCV2 infected farm and a probable enhancement of PCV2 replication around the 12th week of age occurred possibly due to animal movement and/or introduction of a different PCV2 genotype [20, 31]. PCV2 serology results suggested an increased antibody response in vaccinated pigs in comparison with controls, throughout the course of the study. More important, after the time of natural infection, the humoral immune response of vaccinated animals was greater than control pigs, thus demonstrating a strong protective effect of the test product to a subclinical PCV2infection. Furthermore, qPCR results provided evidence that the mean PCV2 viral load was lower in vaccinated pigs than in controls, while viral circulation after PCV2 seroconversion was also reduced during the period when the virus was detectable.

Maternal derived immunity transfer to piglets is very important for the neonate's immune response and survival during the first days of life. Moreover, it has been suggested that MDI is a factor that may have a significant impact on the success of vaccination under field conditions [32]. In this subclinically infected PCV2 trial farm, the level of maternally derived PCV2 antibodies on the day of vaccination was high, thus a significant negative interference with piglets immune priming could be anticipated. However, our results do not support such a negative MDI effect, considering that primary vaccine

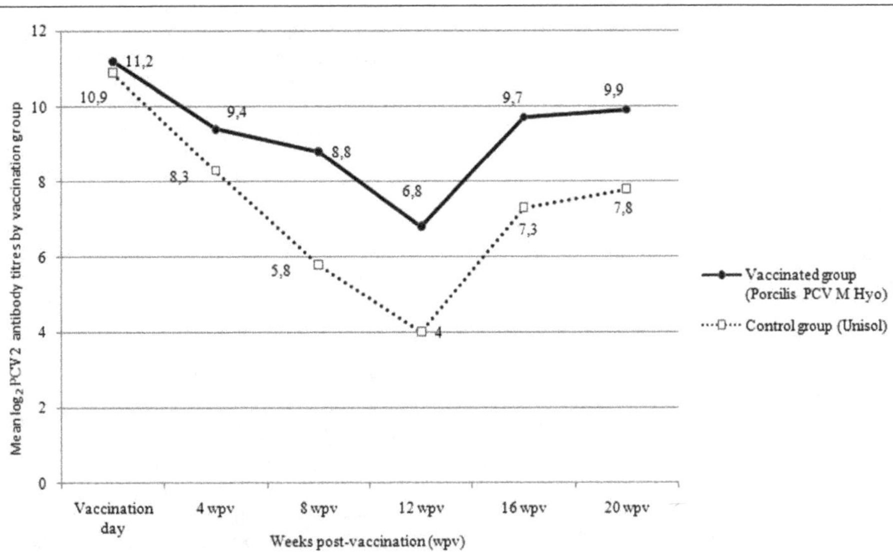

Fig. 6 Mean $\log_2$ PCV2 antibody titres, by vaccination group and weeks post-vaccination

efficacy parameters such as LLS, ADWG, viraemia were all significantly improved/promoted in the vaccinated versus control animals.

Conclusions

According to the results of the present field study, vaccination with a ready to use PCV2/M hyo combination vaccine of three-week-old piglets with high MDI was effective against concurrent clinical M. hyo and subclinical PCV-2 infection based on reduced LLS severity and PCV2 viraemia, as well as improved ADWG.

Abbreviations

ADWG: Average daily weight gain; AMI: Antibody-mediated immunity; CMI: Cell-mediated immunity; EP: Enzootic pneumonia; LLS: lung lesion score; M. hyo: *Mycoplasma hyopneumoniae*; MDI: Maternal derived immunity; PCV2: Porcine circovirus type 2; PCV2-SD: PCV2 - Systemic disease; PCVD: Porcine circovirus diseases; PRRSv: Porcine reproductive and respiratory syndrome virus; SD: Standard deviation

Acknowledgements

The authors would like to acknowledge the support of the personnel of the Laboratory of Pathology, School of Veterinary Medicine Aristotle University of Thessaloniki, Greece, for lung lesion scoring and post mortem examinations. Also, we would like to thank the personnel of the laboratories of MSD Animal Health, Boxmeer, The Netherlands, for performing serological tests.

Funding

The test product and the control group solution for injection were supplied by MSD Animal Health, Boxmeer, The Netherlands, who also funded the trial.

Authors'contributions

PDT, TN, EDT: Conception of protocol, trial interventions, data analysis and interpretation, manuscript preparation. IT, VGP, DK: trial interventions, data recording, manuscript corrections. GB: Pathological evaluation, interpretation of results and data evaluation. All authors read and approved the final manuscript.

Competing interests

One of the authors (TN) is an employee of the funding body.

Consent for publication

Not applicable.

Author details

[1]Farm Animals Clinic, School of Veterinary Medicine, Aristotle University of Thessaloniki, St. Voutyra 11, 54627 Thessaloniki, Greece. [2]Clinic of Medicine, Faculty of Veterinary Science, University of Thessaly, P.O. Box 199Trikalon 224, Karditsa, Greece. [3]Animal Health, Clinical Study Team Biologicals, P.O. Box 31, Boxmeer 5830 AA, the Netherlands. [4]Laboratory of Pathology, School of Veterinary Medicine, Aristotle University of Thessaloniki, University Campus, 54124 Thessaloniki, Greece.

References

1. Simionatto S, Marchioro SB, Maes D, Dellagostin OA. Mycoplasma hyopneumoniae: from disease to vaccine development. Vet Microbiol. 2013;165:234–42.
2. Maes D, Segales J, Meyns T, Sibila M, Pieters M, Haesebrouck F. Control of Mycoplasma hyopneumoniae infections in pigs. Vet Microbiol. 2008;126:297–309.
3. Thacker E, Minion F. (2012) Mycoplasmosis. In: Zimmerman J, Karriker L, Ramirez A, Schwartz K, Stevenson G, editors. Diseases of swine. 10th ed. Chichester: Wiley and Sons Inc; 2012. p. 779–788.
4. Franzo G, Cortey M, Olvera A, Novosel D, De Castro AMMG, Biagini P, et al. Revisiting the taxonomical classification of porcine Circovirus type 2 (PCV-2): still a real challenge. Virol J. 2015;12:131.
5. Fort M, Sibila M, Pérez-Martín E, Nofrarías M, Mateu E, Segalés J. One dose of a porcine circovirus 2 (PCV-2) sub-unit vaccine administered to 3-week-old conventional piglets elicits cell-mediated immunity and significantly reduces PCV2 viremia in an experimental model. Vaccine. 2009;27:4031–7.
6. Segalés J. Porcine circovirus type 2 (PCV-2) infections: clinical signs, pathology and laboratory diagnosis. Virus Res. 2012;164:10–9.
7. Kekarainen T, Segalés J. Porcine circovirus 2 immunology and viral evolution. PHM. 2015;1:17.
8. Alarcon P, Rushton J, Nathues H, Wieland B. Economic efficiency analysis of different strategies to control post-weaning multi-systemic wasting syndrome and porcine circovirus type 2 subclinical infection in 3-weekly batch system farms. Prev Vet Med. 2013;110:103–18.
9. Beach NM, Meng XJ. Efficacy and future prospects of commercially available and experimental vaccines against porcine circovirus type 2 (PCV-2). Virus Res. 2012;164:33–42.
10. Del Pozo Sancristan R. Treatment and control of Mycoplasma hyopneumoniae infections. PhD thesis. Ghent University, Belgium. 2014. https://www.google.gr/url?sa=t&rct=j&q=&esrc=s&source=web&cd=2&ved=0ahUKEwiZnMaK5__MAhXBWCwKHS5XD5oQFggqMAE&url=http%3A%2F%2Fwww.rohh.ugent.be%2Fv3%2Fresearch%2Fphd%2F2014%2FdelPozoSacristan_R.pdf&usg=AFQjCNG8samqgw9cOzJBtZ0kiY6gQiKFcQ&sig2=otgb8s3KbqQJgXWGLQ7Qcg&cad=rja. Accessed 1 Apr 2017.
11. Bandrick M, Theis K, Molitor TW. Maternal immunity enhances Mycoplasma hyopneumoniae vaccination induced cell-mediated immune responses in piglets. BMC Vet Res. 2014;10:124.
12. Bandrick M, Ariza-Nieto C, Baidoo SK, Molitor TW. Colostral antibody-mediated and cell-mediated immunity contributes to innate and antigen-specific immunity in piglets. Dev Comp Immunol. 2014;43:114–20.
13. Martelli P, Saleri S, Ferrarini G, De Angelis E, Cavalli V, Benetti M, et al. Impact of maternally derived immunity on piglets' immune response and protection against porcine circovirus type 2 (PCV-2) after vaccination against PCV2 at different age. BMC Vet Res. 2016;12:77.
14. Fraile L, Sibila M, Nofrarías M, López-Jimenez R, Huerta E, Llorens A, et al. Effect of sow and piglet porcine circovirus type 2 (PCV-2) vaccination on piglet mortality, viraemia, antibody titre and production parameters. Vet Microbiol. 2012;161:229–34.
15. Fraile L, Grau-Roma L, Sarasola P, Sinovas N, Nofrarías M, López-Jimenez R, et al. Inactivated PCV2 one shot vaccine applied in 3-week-old piglets: improvement of production parameters and interaction with maternally derived immunity. Vaccine. 2012;30:1986–92.
16. Oh Y, Seo HW, Park C, Chae C. Comparison of sow and/or piglet vaccination of 3 commercial porcine circovirus type 2 (PCV-2) single-dose vaccines on pigs under experimental PCV2 challenge. Vet Microbiol. 2014;172:371–80.
17. Feng H, Segalés J, Fraile L, López-Soria S, Sibila M. Effect of high and low levels of maternally derived antibodies on porcine circovirus type 2 (PCV-2) infection dynamics and production parameters in PCV2 vaccinated pigs under field conditions. Vaccine. 2016;34:3044–50.
18. Goodwin RFW, Whittlestone P. Enzootic pneumonia of pigs: immunisation attempts inoculating M. Suipneumoniae antigen by various routes and with different adjuvants. Brit Vet J. 1973;129:456–62.
19. EMA - European Medicines Agency Summary of opinion (initial authorisation) - Porcilis PCV M Hyo. 2014. https://www.google.gr/url?sa=t&rct=j&q=&esrc=s&source=web&cd=1&ved=0ahUKEwj4k7-TpufNAhUKuBQKHbG-BzkQFggcMAA&url=http%3A%2F%2Fwww.ema.europa.eu%2Fdocs%2Fen_GB%2Fdocument_library%2FSummary_of_opinion_-_Initial_authorisation%2Fveterinary%2F003796%2FWC500172824.pdf&usg=AFQjCNE_BXqRlhpiohL76tJi35WOxKF1uQ&sig2=syyvEBH39F1yCrV4Q9qbiQ&cad=rja. Accessed 1 Apr 2017.
20. Segales J, Allan GM, Domingo M. Porcine circoviruses. In: Zimmerman J, Karriker L, Ramirez A, Schwartz K, Stevenson G, editors. Diseases of swine. 10th ed. Chichester: Wiley and Sons Inc; 2012. p. 405–15.
21. EMEA - European Agency for the evaluation of Medicinal Products. Guidelines on Good Clinical Practices. 2000. https://www.google.gr/url?sa=t&rct=j&q=&esrc=s&source=web&cd=1&ved=0ahUKEwjugPGfp-fNAhVKnRQKHTIbAgAQFggcMAA&url=http%3A%2F%2Fwww.ema.europa.eu%2Fdocs%2Fen_GB%2Fdocument_library%2FScientific_guideline%2F2009%2F10%2FWC500004343.pdf&usg=AFQjCNHdT6MARc1-9X1EYk38DRejsRv84w&sig2=sa5T4DNjk53xkX86DxjmmQ&cad=rja. Accessed 1 Apr 2017.

22. FVE - Federation of Veterinarians of Europe. European Veterinary Ethics and Principles of Conduct. 2002. https://www.google.gr/url?sa=t&rct=j&q=&esrc=s&source=web&cd=1&ved=0ahUKEwjU_vS8p-fNAhVDwBQKHacFDy0QFggcMAA&url=http%3A%2F%2Fwww.fve.org%2Fnews%2Fpublications%2Fpdf%2Fgvp.pdf&usg=AFQjCNFK2kfzkfn79clPB5rxnukovW2Cuw&sig2=gf32byTepVL4kr7muUjUWg&cad=rja. Accessed 1 Apr 2017.
23. Haake M, Palzer A, Weissenbacher-Lang C, Fachinger V, Eggen A, Ritzmann M, et al. Influence of age on the effectiveness of PCV2 vaccination in piglets with high levels of maternally derived antibodies. Vet Microbiol. 2014;168:272–80.
24. Van den Bosch H, Frey J. Interference of outer membrane protein PalA with protective immunity against Actinobacillus pleuropneumoniae infection in vaccinated pigs. Vaccine. 2003;21:3601–7.
25. Tzika ED, Tassis PD, Koulialis D, Papatsiros VG, Nell T, Brellou G, Tsakmakidis I. Field efficacy study of a novel ready-to-use vaccine against mycoplasma hyopneumoniae and porcine circovirus type 2 in a Greek farm. PHM. 2015;1:15.
26. Maes D, Deluyker H, Verdonck M, Castryck F, Miry C, Lein A, et al. Effect of vaccination against Mycoplasma hyopneumoniae in pig herds with a continuous production system. J Veterinary Med Ser B. 1998;45:495–505.
27. Maes D, Deluyker H, Verdonck M, Castryck F, Miry C, Vrijens B, et al. Effect of vaccination against Mycoplasma hyopneumoniae in pig herds with an all-in/all-out production system. Vaccine. 1999;17:1024–34.
28. Larochelle R, Magar R, D'allaire S. Comparative serologic and virologic study of commercial swine herds with and without postweaning multisystemic wasting syndrome. Can J Vet Res. 2003;67:114–20.
29. Meerts P, Misinzo G, Lefebvre D, Nielsen J, Bøtner A, Kristensen CS, et al. Correlation between the presence of neutralizing antibodies against porcine circovirus 2 (PCV-2) and protection against replication of the virus and development of PCV-2-associated disease. BMC Vet Res. 2006;2:6.
30. Grau-Roma L, Hjulsager CK, Sibila M, Kristensen CS, Lopez-Soria S, Enøe C, et al. Infection, excretion and seroconversion dynamics of porcine circovirus type 2 (PCV-2) in pigs from post-weaning multisystemic wasting syndrome (PMWS) affected farms in Spain and Denmark. Vet Microbiol. 2009;135:272–82.
31. Rose N, Opriessnig T, Grasland B, Jestin A. Epidemiology and transmission of porcine circovirus type 2 (PCV-2). Virus Res. 2012;164:78–89.
32. Maes D. Vaccination against Mycoplasma hyopneumoniae infection in pigs: room for improvement. Vet J. 2014;200:214–5.

14

Comparative innocuity and efficacy of live and inactivated sheeppox vaccines

Zineb Boumart[1*], Samira Daouam[1], Imane Belkourati[2], Lamya Rafi[1], Eeva Tuppurainen[2], Khalid Omari Tadlaoui[1] and Mehdi El Harrak[1]

Abstract

Background: Sheeppox (SPP) is one of the priorities, high-impact animal diseases in many developing countries, where live attenuated vaccines are routinely used against sheeppox virus (SPPV). In an event of an SPP outbreak, historically disease-free countries would hesitate to use of live vaccines against SPPVdue to the safety and trade reasons. Currently no killed SPPV vaccines are commercially available. In this study, we developed an inactivated Romanian SPPVvaccine and assessed its efficacy and potency in comparison with a live attenuated Romanian SPPV vaccine. Four naïve sheep were vaccinated once with the Romanian SPPV live attenuated vaccine and16 sheep were vaccinated twice with the inactivated vaccine. All sheep in the live vaccine group were included in the challenge trial, which was conducted using a highly virulent Moroccan SPPV field strain. Eight sheep of the inactivated vaccine group were challenged and the remaining sheep were monitored for seroconversion. Experimental animals were closely monitored for the appearance of clinical signs, body temperature and inflammation at the injection site. Two naïve sheep were used as unvaccinated controls.

Results: The inactivated Romanian SPPV vaccine was found to be safe and confer a good protection, similar to the live vaccine. Specific antibodies appeared from seven days post vaccination and remained up to nine months.

Conclusion: This study showed that the developed inactivated Romanian SPPV vaccine has a potential to replace attenuated vaccine to control and prevent sheep pox in disease-free or endemic countries.

Keywords: Sheeppox, Romanian strain, Inactivated vaccine, Efficacy, Potency

Background

Sheeppox virus (SPPV), the etiological agent of sheeppox (SPP), is a member of the genus *Capripoxvirus* within the family *Poxviridae*. SPP is a transboundary disease which is notifiable to the World Organization of Animal Health (OIE) [1]. The disease can be mild in indigenous sheep breeds, but usually causes severe or fatal infection in newly introduced, fully susceptible animals. In naïve animals, morbidity and mortality may be as high as 100 % [2]. SPPV affects all ages of sheep but the clinical signs are more severe in young lambs [3]. The disease is characterized by fever, generalized papules or nodules in the skin, respiratory distress, pox lesions in the respiratory and gastrointestinal tracts, and sometimes death. SPP is endemic in Central and North Africa, the Middle East, Central Asia and the Indian subcontinent. Recently, SPP has also reached southern Europe [4].

In endemic countries, vaccination is considered the only economically feasible way to control the disease and improve small ruminant productivity. Numerous live vaccines have been developed and worldwide used, while inactivated vaccines are considered less effective and have only been tested at the laboratory level [5]. Despite the high efficacy of live vaccines, SPP is still endemic in those regions where vaccination is routinely practiced. In North Africa where SPPV has a strict sheep tropism, after decades of vaccination using a live attenuated vaccine, SPP is still causing significant economic losses for sheep farming industry [6]. In Greece, SPP re-occurred in 2013 and in 2015 the outbreak is still continuing, despite extensive stamping-out of infected and in-contact animals, movement restrictions and other supportive control and eradication measures (OIE Wahid database). The use of SPPV live vaccine is not

* Correspondence: Z.Boumart@mci-santeanimale.com
[1]Research and Development Virology, Multi-Chemical Industry, Lot. 157, Z I, Sud-Ouest (ERAC) B.P.: 278, Mohammedia 28810, Morocco
Full list of author information is available at the end of the article

permitted within the European Union (EU) member states. However, in a situation like in Greece, a safe non-replicating, effective and cheap inactivated emergency vaccine could provide a more efficient tool to limit the spread of the disease without a need for culling a large number of animals which is expensive and highly stressful for the farmers, destroying decades of work for the genetic improvement of a flock.

According to current OIE trade recommendations and EU directive (90/425/EEC of 26 June 1990), both SPP outbreak and use of any SPPV vaccines would inflict immediate restrictions to the export of live animals and their products from affected to disease-free countries. In addition, three years after the last SPP case or last vaccination, are required to re-gain the disease-free status. The lack of DIVA component in currently available vaccines would hamper the retrospective serological surveys, although it is unlikely that the antibody levels in vaccinated animals would remain on the detectable level for three years.

In another hand, it has been reported that some attenuated live vaccines induced severe pock reactions at the injection site or even mild disease in vaccinated animals [7]. Poor quality live vaccines (low vaccine titre) may also serve as vehicles for extraneous virus contaminants such as Border Disease virus (BDV). In the past, outbreak of BDV occurred inTunisia after vaccination by a BDVcontaminated SPPV vaccine and in France abovine viral diarrhea (BVD) contaminated Aujeszky disease live vaccine [8, 9]. In addition, theoretically there is a possibility that an attenuated vaccine virus could revert back to virulent, although such an occurrence has never been reported in SPPV vaccines.

Thus, an inactivated SPPV vaccine would provide a safe and valuable tool to protect livestock against SPPV, particularly during the first incursion of the virus in the previously disease-free country. In this study, we developed an inactivated vaccine against SPPV and tested its efficacy and potency by serology and challenge experiment in comparison with a live attenuated SPPV vaccine.

Methods

Vaccine preparation

The SPPV Romanian strain was propagated on Vero cells [10] and maintained in Dulbecco's Modified Eagle's Medium (DMEM) with 10 % irradiated fetal calf serum. The inoculation was carried out using an M.O.I (Multiplicity of Infection) of 0.01.

The live vaccine was prepared from the virus suspension by the addition of stabilizer (4 % peptone, 8 % sucrose and 2 % glutamate) followed by lyophilization. The inactivated vaccine was prepared from the same virus suspension by inactivating the virus with β-propiolactone. The complete inactivation of the vaccine virus and sterility of the product was confirmed before vaccine formulation. The aluminum hydroxide adjuvant was added at 2.1 mg/ml. The final product was distributed in 50 ml vials and stored at 4 °C before use.

Sheep vaccination

Eighteen healthy sheep, six to eight months of age, representing the Timehdit breed of the Atlas mountains, were tested SPPV seronegative by virus neutralization (VN) test. Group 1 (G1) comprised 16 sheep which were vaccinated subcutaneously in the groin area with a volume of 2 ml of the inactivated SPPV vaccine representing a dose of $10^{5.5}$ $TCID_{50}$. Two sheep were kept as unvaccinated controls. Group 2 (G2) comprised four animals which were vaccinated with 0.5 ml of the live attenuated vaccine, representing a dose of $10^{3.0}$ $TCID_{50}$. All immunized animals were daily monitored for 14 days for rise in body temperature, appearance of clinical signs typical for SPP and inflammation at the injection site. Animals in G1, received a booster vaccination at D21 in the same conditions. Serum samples were collected from the vaccinated sheep weekly until 2 months, then at one month interval for the remaining unchallenged eight sheep up to 9 months.

Experimental challenge infection

Vaccine potency testing was carried out by a challenge trial, using a virulent field SPPV strain (Hd2012) at the BSL3 laboratory. In the inactivated vaccine group G1, eight sheep out of 16 were challenged on D35 and in live vaccine group G2 four sheep were challenged on D28 after vaccination. Two naïve sheep were challenged as unvaccinated controls.

The challenge was conducted using a local Moroccan highly virulent SPPV field strain. The virus was administered by intra-dermal (ID) route in the flank of the animals at ten fold dilutions (10^{-1} to 10^{-6}) to perform a virus titration comparatively on vaccinated and control animals.

Sheep were monitored daily for clinical signs, rectal temperature and the development of inflammation in each of the injection site. The presence of any inflammation was considered positive for the virus titration. The average virus titres of G1 and G2 were compared with the titre obtained in the unvaccinated animals and the difference between the two titres, expressed in log_{10}, represented the protection index [11].

Serological response

Serum samples were tested for the development of specific SPPV antibodies using VN test as described in the OIE Terrestrial Manual (OIE Chapters 2.7.11 and 2.7.14). This test is based on a serial ¼ dilutions of heat inactivated sera and a set amount of infectious virus

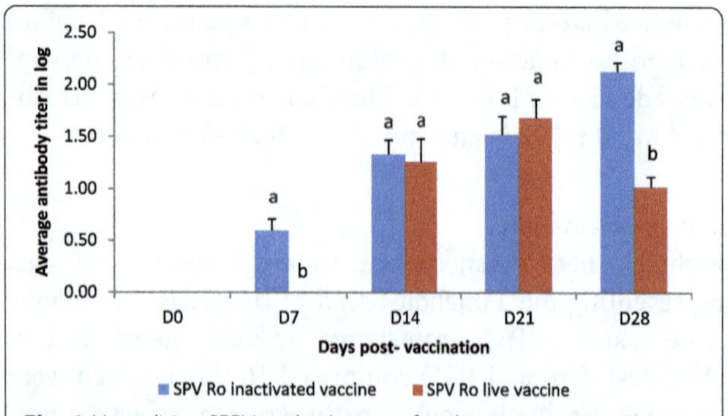

Fig. 1 Neutralizing SPPV antibody titers after sheep vaccination. The results correspond to the mean antibody titers ± SEM of 16 sheep vaccinated with the inactivated Romanian SPPV vaccine strain (G1) and 4 sheep vaccinated with the live attenuated Romanian SPPV vaccine (G2). (a–b) indicate a significant difference in means antibody titers between animals of G1 and G2 at the 0.05 level

(100 $TCID_{50}$). The neutralizing antibody titer was calculated in accordance to Reed and Muench method [12].

Statistical analyses

Differences between antibody titers obtained with live and inactivated vaccines, and between virus titers in vaccinated and unvaccinated animals, were determined using a one-way analysis of variance (ANOVA) followed by a student t-test. Values of $P \leq 0.05$ were considered significant.

Results

Sheep vaccination

Three weeks following vaccination, the body temperature of vaccinated sheep in G1 remained within normal limits and no clinical signs typical for SPP were observed. At the vaccination site, transitory inflammation 1 cm to 2 cm in diameter was observed in some animals, disappearing in few days. In G2, slight increase in body temperature was observed six to eight days after vaccination and in some animals a local reaction was observed atthe vaccination site, persisting in some cases up to 20 days.

In G1, anti SPPV antibodies appeared as early as D7 post-vaccination. Compared to live vaccine, they registered similar values at D14 and D21, but reached a significantly higher value of antibody neutralizing titer (2.1 $\log_{10}$) on D28 ($P \leq 0.05$). In G2, the rise of anti SPPV antibodies was noted later on D14 post-vaccination, and showed a slight decrease on D28 to reach a value of 1 $\log_{10}$ (Fig. 1).

Most vaccinated sheep in G1showed an increase of antibody titre following the booster. In eight unchallenged vaccinated sheep, the immunity persisted for at least 9 months. The antibody neutralizing titre seemed to stabilize at 1 to 2.1 $\log_{10}$ (Fig. 2).

Experimental infection

On the challenge, the two unvaccinated control animals exhibited a rise in body temperature between D4 and D11 (Fig. 3). Local reactions at the injection sites were observed from D3, increasing in size the following days. Typical SPPV skin nodules (not associated with injection sites) appeared between D10 and D11 (Fig. 4). The obtained virus titres on the flank of the two unvaccinated control animals were 5.5 $\log_{10}$ ID50/ml and 5.9 $\log_{10}$ ID50/ml, significantly higher than that obtained with vaccinated animals ($P \leq 0.05$) (Table 1).

After the challenge, the vaccinated sheep of G1 and G2 showed a transient two days increase in temperature between 39.6 °C and 39.7 °C at D6 and D7(Fig. 3) and a hypersensitivity reaction at the injection site two days after the challenge, generally in the first dilutions.

None of the immunized animals showed clinical signsof SPP during the observation period. Inflammations due to the virus replication were observed in dilutions 10^{-1} and 10^{-2} between D4 and D12. There was no significant difference in the titer and the protection index between G1 and G2 ($P \geq 0.05$). The obtained infectious titre was 1.4 log10 ID_{50}/ml for the inactivated vaccine G1 and 0.75 $\log_{10}$ ID_{50}/ml for the live vaccine G2 (Table 1). The protection index was estimated to 4 for G1 and 4.6 for G2.

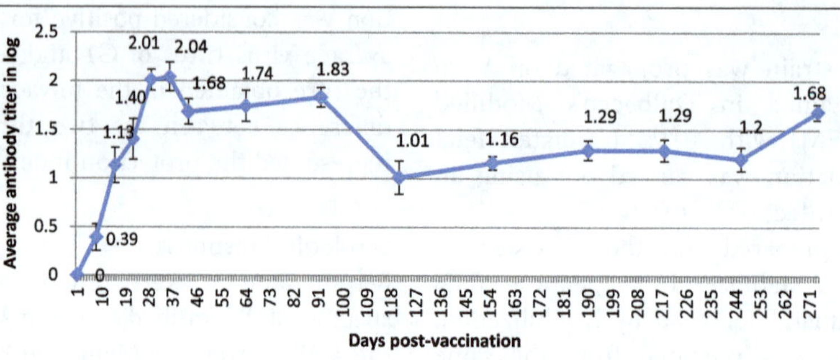

Fig. 2 Neutralizing SPPV antibody titers after vaccination of sheep with the inactivated Romanian SPPV vaccine strain. The results correspond to the mean of antibody titer of eight vaccinated sheep ± SEM

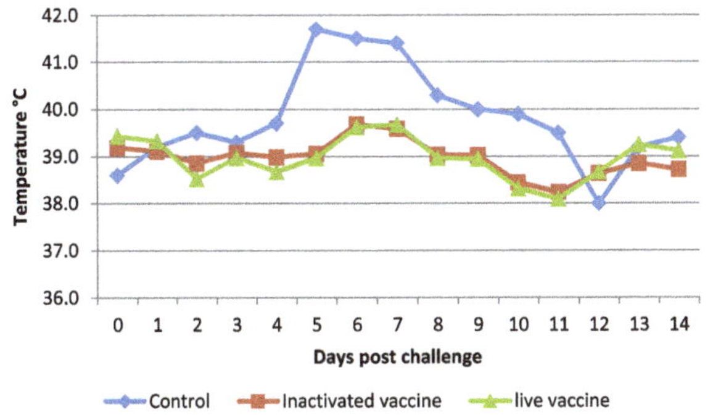

Fig. 3 Temperature monitoring of unvaccinated and vaccinated (G1 and G2) sheep during 14 days post-challenge

All vaccinated animals of G1 and G2 showed ananti-body response that increased after the challenge.

Discussion

In endemic countries a variety of attenuated live vaccines have been used against SPPV. Live attenuated vaccine protection is mediated by both cellular and humoral immunity. While, inactivated vaccines are believed to be less effective in stimulating the cell mediated immune response, which is the predominant protective response to poxvirus infection. In addition, in vaccinated sheep a poor correlation between antibody levels and immune status of animals has been reported [5], suggesting that live replicating vaccines are required for the development of effective immunity against pox disease [13, 14].

Nevertheless, in many countries, live vaccines use was banished because of its potential to induce mild diseases in animals and the risk of contamination by extraneous pathogens. The use of inactivated vaccines would be, thus, an alternative to protect livestock against pox diseases. In the present study, an inactivated and live attenuated SPPV vaccines, were compared in terms of their safety and potency. Romanian strain has been selected for vaccine preparation because it proved to be effective for protection against SPP infection [10, 15].

Sheep were observed for three weeks following immunization. The inactivated vaccine was safe to use, as all vaccinated animals remained healthy, no increase in body temperature after vaccination was detected and only a small inflammation at the injection site was observed. A serological response was detected one week earlier for the inactivated vaccine group than for the live attenuated vaccine. This is in agreement with the previous studies, showing an increase in antibody titres between D7 and D21 post-vaccination and a boost of the immune response following a challenge [16, 17]. Nevertheless, the need of a booster for inactivated vaccines is usually a constraint compared to live attenuated vaccine that need only one shot. Thus, it will be interesting, in a further study, to assess the vaccine protection using a single vaccination with killed vaccine.

The kinetic of antibody response in vaccinated sheep showed that inactivated vaccine provide detectable antibody levels for more than nine months, suggesting that an annual booster with this vaccine is enough to maintain a good protection at the population level. The long term duration of the protection needs to be confirmed using a challenge experiment. The findings of the present study are in agreement with other studies, demonstrating the efficacy of the inactivated SPP vaccines to protect sheep against challenge [17, 18].

The challenge was conducted according to the protocol defined by Fassi-Fehri and co-workers [11]. This method allows quantitative assessment of the conferred immunity and it is based on the obtained titres of the challenge virus in vaccinated and control animals. The difference of 2 log titers is used to determine the protection threshold. The method provides a protection index that is high as the immune response is strong and durable. Despite the high titres of the virulent challenge virus, both inactivated and live SPPV vaccines protected experimental animals against generalization of the disease observed in unvaccinated sheep. A short increase in body temperature in both vaccinated groups was observed for two days, which can be a physiological response triggered by any antigen. In contrast, unvaccinated sheep exhibited characteristic

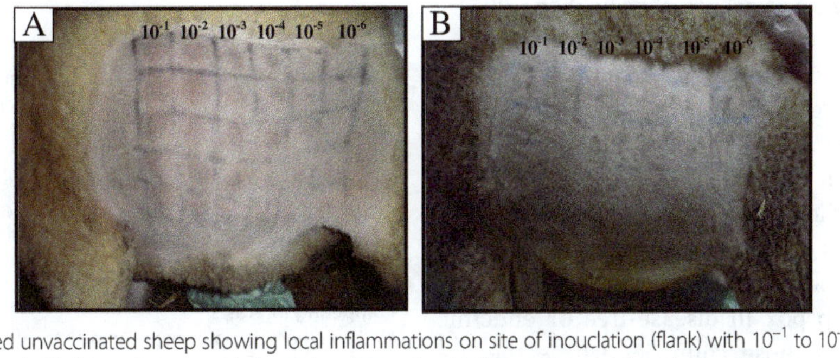

Fig. 4 a Figure of challenged unvaccinated sheep showing local inflammations on site of inouclation (flank) with 10^{-1} to 10^{-6} dilutions (left to right) of virulent SPPV in five replica. **b** Challenged vaccinated sheep showing no local inflammations on the injection sites

Table 1 Challenge results in control and vaccinated sheep with live and inactivated Romanian SPPV vaccine. Antibody neutralizing titers of vaccinated sheep obtained before challenge. The infectious titer represents the maximum value obtained between day 6 and 8 post challenge

Vaccine	Animals	Hypersensitivity titer in $TCID_{50}$		Antibody neutralizing titers in log_{10}		Infectious titer (ID_{50}/ml)		Protection value	
		Per animal	Group average	Per animal	Group average	Per animal	Group average	Per animal	Group average
Control animals	299	0	0	0	0	5.2	5,4[(a)]	0	0[(a)]
	277	0		0		5.6		0	
Live SPPV vaccine	977	1,6	1,6	1,9	1,7	1,5	0,75[(b)]	3,9	4,6[(b)]
	928	1,6		1,26		0,5		4,9	
	934	1,4		1,98		0,5		4,9	
	999	1,8		1,5		0,5		4,9	
Inactivated SPPV vaccine	948	2,7	2,2	1,98	2,2	2,1	1,4 [(b)]	3,3	4 [(b)]
	941	0		2,22		2,5		2,9	
	949	4,5		2,46		0,5		4,9	
	397	1,1		1,98		0,5		4,9	
	398	2,5		2,46		0,5		4,9	
	998	0,9		1,74		0,5		4,9	
	973	4,5		2,46		0,5		4,9	
	969	1,5		2,7		4,1		1,3	

(a–b) indicate a significant difference in means of infectious titers and protection values between vaccinated and unvaccinated animals and between G1 and G2 at the 0.05 level

clinical signs, primary and secondary pox lesions with high fever between D4 and D11 post-infection with the challenge virus. The obtained virus titre in unvaccinated control animals reached $10^{5.7}$ID50/mlwhich is the normal titre of the virulent strain in sheep.

Inflammation due to the virus replication was observed only in low dilutions for both groups with lower infectious titres if compared to control animals, giving evidence of the virulent virus neutralization by the conferred immunity. There was no significant difference between live and inactivated vaccines after the challenge as indicated by the protection index values (4.6 versus 4.0). These values are comparable to those normally obtained with other live vaccines [19] and are in compliance with the OIE procedure of testing the vaccine potency taking a difference of log_{10} titre > 2.5 as evidence of protection [20].

Conclusion

There are only limited studies on inactivated SPP vaccines and very few reports comparing the efficacy of live and attenuated vaccines [17, 18]. The current study showed that the developed inactivated Romanian SPPV vaccine is as potent as live vaccine and has a potential to replace attenuated vaccine to control and prevent sheep pox in disease-free or endemic countries, especially in those countries where the use of live vaccine is unauthorized. Inactivated vaccine is completely safe in all animals, does not present any risk of diffusion, reversion or extraneous pathogens spread.

Abbreviations

SPP, sheeppox; SPPV, sheeppox virus; DIVA, differentiating infected from vaccinated animals; $TCID_{50}$, tissue culture infective dose; MOI, Multiplicity of Infection; VN, virus neutralization

Acknowledgements

All the authors have seen and approved the content and have contributed significantly to the work. The authors gratefully acknowledge the support for this study by MCI (Multi-Chemical Industry) Santé animale.

Funding

No funding was obtained for this study.

Authors' contributions

ZB carried out the seroneutralisation and drafted the manuscript, SD participated in the vaccine pilot batch production, IB performed the safety testing, LR carried out the protency testing, ET conceived of the study and reviewed the manuscript, KT participated in the design and the follow up of the study, ME member of the ethic committee participated in the design of the study, manuscript drafting and data analysis and interpretation. All authors read and approved the final manuscript.

Competing interests

All the authors do not have a commercial or other association that might pose a conflict of interest. None of them participated to the ethic committee meeting to make decision on the project.

Consent to publish
Not applicable.

Author details
[1]Research and Development Virology, Multi-Chemical Industry, Lot. 157, Z I, Sud-Ouest (ERAC) B.P.: 278, Mohammedia 28810, Morocco. [2]Capripoxvirus Reference Laboratory, The Pirbright Institute, Ash Road, Pirbright, Woking, Surrey GU24 0NF, United Kingdom.

References

1. Anonymous: Sheeppox and goat pox. In: Manual of diagnostic tests and vaccines for terrestrial animals (mammals, birds and bees). 6th ed. Pa. Edited by Office F, Manual I des E.; 2008:1058–1068.
2. Bhanuprakash V, Indrani BK, Hosamani M, Singh RK. The current status of sheep pox disease, Comparative Immunology, Microbiology and Infectious Diseases. 2006. p. 27–60.
3. Zhu XL, Yang F, Li HX, Dou XY, Meng XL, Li H, Luo X, Cai X. Identification and phylogenetic analysis of a sheep pox virus isolated from the Ningxia Hui Autonomous Region of China. Genet Mol Res. 2013;14:1670–8.
4. Yogisharadhya R, Bhanuprakash V, Hosamani M, Venkatesan G, Balamurugan V, Bora DP, Bhanot V, Prabhu M, Singh RK. Comparative efficacy of live replicating sheeppox vaccine strains in Ovines. Biologicals. 2011;39:417–23.
5. Kitching RP. The control of sheep and goat pox. Rev Sci Tech. 1986;5:503–11.
6. Zro K, Zakham F, Melloul M, El Fahime E, Ennaji MM. A sheeppox outbreak in Morocco: isolation and identification of virus responsible for the new clinical form of disease. BMC Vet Res. 2014;10:31.
7. Rao TV, Bandyopadhyay SK. A comprehensive review of goat pox and sheep pox and their diagnosis. Anim Health Res Rev. 2000;1:127–36.
8. Thabti F, Fronzaroli L, Dlissi E, Guibert JM, Hammami S, Pepin M, Russo P. Experimental model of Border Disease virus infection in lambs: Comparative pathogenicity of pestiviruses isolated in France and Tunisia. Vet Res. 2002;33:35–45.
9. Vannier P, Leforban Y, Carnero R, Cariolet R. Contamination of a live virus vaccine against Pseudorabies (Aujeszky's disease) by an ovine pestivirus pathogenfor the pig. Ann Rech Vet. 1988;19:283–90.
10. Precausta P, Kato F, Vellut G. A new freeze-dried living virus vaccine against sheep-pox. Comp Immunol Microbiol Infect Dis. 1979;1:305–19.
11. Fassi-Fehri M, El-Harrak M, Johnson D, Abbadi M, El-Idrissi AH. Experimental study of postvaccinal immunity to sheep-pox. Ann Rech Vet. 1984;15:59–64.
12. Saganuwan S. A modified arithmetical method of Reed and Muench for determination of a relatively ideal median lethal dose (LD50). African J Pharm. 2011;5:1543–6.
13. Perenlei L, Solyom F. Study of the duration of immunity of sheep vaccinated against sheep pox with a live virus vaccine. Acta Vet Hung. 1983;31:131–4.
14. Ramani K, Sundarajan S. Comparative efficacy of different sheep pox vaccines. Indian Vet J. 1976;53:313–8.
15. Achour HA, Bouguedour R, Bouhbal A, Guechtouli A, Aouissat M. Comparative study of the immunizing ability of some attenuated strains of sheep pox virus and of a sensitizing vaccine. Rev Sci Tech. 2000;19:773–83.
16. Bhanuprakash V, Indrani BK, Hegde R, Kumar MM, Moorthy ARS. A classical live attenuated vaccine for sheep pox. Trop Anim Health Prod. 2004;36:307–20.
17. Awad M, Michael A, Soliman SM, Samir SS, Daoud AM. Trials for preparation of inactivated sheep pox vaccine using binary ethyleneimine. Egypt J Immunol. 2003;10:67–72.
18. Sólyom F, Perenlei L, Roith J. Sheep-pox vaccine prepared from formaldehyde inactivated virus adsorbed to aluminium hydroxide gel. Acta Microbiol Acad Sci Hung. 1982;29:69–75.
19. Fakri F, Ghzal F, Daouam S, Elarkam A, Douieb L, Zouheir Y, Tadlaoui K, Fassi-Fihri O. Development and field application of a new combined vaccine against Peste des Petits Ruminants and Sheep Pox. Trials Vaccinol. 2015;4:33–7.
20. OIE: Sheep pox and Goat Pox. *OIE Terr Man* 2010, Chapter 2.:1–12.

15

The immune mechanism of *Mycoplasma hyopneumoniae* 168 vaccine strain through dendritic cells

Yumeng Shen[1], Weiwei Hu[1], Yanna Wei[2], Zhixin Feng[2] and Qian Yang[1*]

Abstract

Background: *Mycoplasma hyopneumoniae* (*Mhp*) causes porcine enzootic pneumonia, a disease that cause major economic losses in the pig industry. Dendritic cells (DCs), the most effective antigen-presenting cells, are widely distributed beneath respiratory epithelium, DCs uptake and present antigens to T cells, to initiate protective immune responses in different infections. In this study, we investigated the role of porcine DCs in vaccine *Mhp*-168 exposure.

Results: The antigen presenting ability of DCs were improved by vaccine *Mhp*-168 exposure. DCs could activate T-cell proliferation by up-regulating the antigen presenting molecule MHCII expression and co-stimulatory molecule CD80/86. However, the up-regulation of IL-10 and accompany with down-regulation of IFN-γ gene level may account for the limitation of attenuated *Mhp-168* strain use as vaccine alone.

Conclusion: These findings are benefit for exploring the protection mechanisms and the possible limitations of this attenuated *Mhp-168* vaccine.

Keywords: Vaccine *Mhp*-168 strain, Dendritic cells, Immune protection

Background

Mycoplasma hyopneumoniae (Mhp) causes porcine enzootic pneumonia (EP) and causes tremendous economic losses all over the swine industry [1]. *Mhp* infection is difficult to eradicate and it will long term existence in most herds by direct sow-to-pig exposure [2]. *Mhp* infection causes physical damage on the respiratory tract and modulates the host immune response [3], the primary *Mhp* infection often becomes complicated by secondary bacterial and viral infections [4]. *Mhp* infection causes the release of inflammatory cytokines, such as interleukin (IL)-1β, IL-18 both in vivo and in vitro [5]. In healthy animal, the lower respiratory tract (trachea and lung) is essentially sterile, pathogenic microorganisms have the opportunity to colonize and invade the host when the cilia clearance ability is impaired [6]. *Mhp*-derived lipid-associated membrane proteins (LAMPs) result in either necrosis or apoptosis in macrophages and porcine peripheral blood mononuclear cells (PBMCs) in vitro [7]. Accordingly, cilia clearance loss, macrophages and PBMC dysfunction are responsible for immunosuppression and predisposes pigs to secondary infections. Some drugs and antibiotics are effective against *Mhp*,but they can't completely clear the infection of *Mhp*. In addition, drug resistance and antibiotic residues are important issues. Vaccination is another essential strategy in controlling *Mhp* infection. Some commercially available vaccines are the inactivated whole cells of *Mhp*, however, inactivated vaccine only provide the partly protection for Mycoplasmal pneumonia of swine (MPS) [8]. Shao et al. have identified that the attenuated *Mhp* 168 strain vaccine developed an effective protection against MPS [9]. However, the exact immunologic mechanism of this attenuated vaccine still has not been researched detailedly.

Dendritic cells (DCs), the most professional antigen-presenting cells (APCs) [10], are widely distributed in the mucosal tissue, preparing for monitor the invasion of pathogens [11]. By extending trans-epithelial dendrites, DCs sample incoming pathogens and migrate to the T-cell region of the mucosa-associated lymphoid tissue (MALT) to trigger an effective immune response [12]. The nasal mucosa barrier is a key impediment for

* Correspondence: zxbyq@njau.edu.cn
[1]Veterinary College, Nanjing Agricultural University, Weigang 1, Nanjing, Jiangsu 210095, People's Republic of China
Full list of author information is available at the end of the article

Mhp up-take and subsequent antigen-specific adaptive immune responses. The interactions between *Mhp* and DCs have not been investigated. Whether DCs result in the generation of beneficial immune responses during attenuated *Mhp* immune process still unclear.

The vaccine *Mhp*-168 has been used in some Chinese farms with good immune-protection against *Mhp*. Our study aimed to gain a better understanding of the immunologic mechanism of this attenuated vaccine. We have characterized the immune responses of porcine DCs after exposure with vaccine *Mhp*-168 and their capacity to induce T cell responses in vitro.

Methods

Animals

A total of 20 five weeks old, Yorkshire, Landrace, and Large White cross-bred pigs were bred and maintained under specific pathogen-free conditions (e.g. Transmissible Gastroenteritis Virus, Porcine Epidemic Diarrhoea Virus, Porcine Circovirus Type 2, Porcine Reproductive and Respiratory Syndrome Virus, *Mhp*). All animal experiments were approved by the Institutional Animal Care and Use Committee of Nanjing Agricultural University (Nanjing, China) and followed National Institutes of Health guidelines.

Reagents

Antibodies PE-conjugated co-stimulatory molecules cluster of differentiation (CD) 80/86 (ab69778), PE-conjugated CD1a(ab25599), FITC-conjugated Workshop Cluster 3a (SWC3a, ab24885) were obtained from Abcam (New Territories, Hong Kong). FITC-conjugated histocompatibility leukocyte Ag II-DR (MHCII, LS-C129867) was obtained from LifeSpan BioSciences (Seattle, WA, USA). PE-conjugated SWC3a (74-22-15A) was obtained from BD Biosciences (USA). Recombinant swine interleukin 4 (IL-4), was bought from BioSource (USA). Recombinant swine granulocyte-macrophage colony-stimulating factor (GM-CSF), was bought from Invitrogen (USA). Lipopolysaccharide (LPS) was bought from Sigma (Japan). RPMI 1640 medium and 4,6-diamidino-2-phenylindole (DAPI) solution were bought from Invitrogen (Grand Island, NY, USA). Fetal bovine serum (FBS) was bought from MULTI-Cell (Canada). SABC-POD (rabbit IgG) Kit and Peroxidase Substrate Kit were bought from BOSTER (Wuhan, China). RNA extraction kit was bought from TianGen Biotech (Beijing, China).

Mycoplasma pneumonia 168

Vaccine *M. hyopneumoniae strain 168* (vaccine *Mhp*-168) was an attenuated vaccine strain, which cultured from continuous passage of *Mhp* wild strain [13]. The wild strain was completely attenuated by more than 300 passages in KM_2 media. The 340th passage of M. *hyopneumoniae* 168 strain was confirmed safety for cross-bred pigs and 360th passage of M. *hyopneumoniae* 168 strain could developed the effective protection against MPS [9]. We obtained vaccine *Mhp*-168 from Jiangsu Academy of Agricultural Sciences,Key Laboratory of Veterinary Biological Engineering and Technology and the 360 th passage of M. *hyopneumoniae* 168 strain was used in our experiment. This vaccine *Mhp*-168 was cultured in KM_2 medium until the beginning of the stationary phase. Then it was collected after centrifugation at 12,000 × g for 20 min and washed twice with PBS.

Generation of bone marrow-derived DCs (BMDCs)

BMDCs were isolated and cultured using our advanced method [14]. Briefly, bone marrow was extracted from the femurs of 1.5 months old piglets and treated with red blood cell lysing buffer. The bone marrow cells were differentiated into DCs by suspending the cells in complete medium (RPMI 1640 medium supplemented with 10% foetal bovine serum (FBS), 1% penicillin-streptomycin, and 10 ng/ml GM-CSF and IL-4). After 60 h of culture, non-adherent granulocytes were removed gently by discarding the medium, and fresh medium was added. Non-adherent and loosely adherent cells were harvested on day 6 and sub-cultured overnight in complete medium. On day 7, immature DCs were collected for further experiments.

Exposure of BMDCs to vaccine *Mhp*-168

On day 7 of the culture, immature DCs were collected and seeded into 24-well plates (5×10^5 cells/well). RPMI 1640 medium (negative control), 10 ng/ml of LPS (positive control) or vaccine *Mhp*-168 (40/dendritic cell) were added for 8 h, 12 h and 24 h incubation period respectively. Both the Mock and the stimulated DCs were collected after 24 h for flow cytometry analysis. Both the Mock and the stimulated DCs were collected at 8 h, 12 h and 24 h respectively for total RNA extraction.

Flow cytometry

In order to determine the modulation of surface markers on DCs treated with LPS or vaccine *Mhp*-168 in particular time point, treated DCs samples were washed with cold PBS twice and stained with fluorescent mAbs specific for swine or human SWC3a, CD80/86, CD1a and MHCII at 4 °C for 0.5 h as per manufacturer's guidelines. After washed three times with PBS, FACS was used to detect phenotype of DCs.

Real-time quantitative PCR analysis of the cytokine secretion by DCs

The total RNA of Mock DCs and stimulation DCs were obtained using TRIzol Reagent (Invitrogen) according to the manufacturer's instructions. The cDNA was generated by reverse transcription using HiScript TM QRT SuperMix for qPCR (Vazyme) according to the manufacturer's instructions. Gene expression data were collected using 7500 Real-Time PCR System (Applied Biosystems, Hercules, CA) and analyzed by the $\Delta\Delta$Ct methods. The relative IL-10/IL-12/IFN-γ mRNA was normalized with glyceraldehyde 3-phosphate dehydrogenase (GAPDH). The specific primers were shown in Table 1.

Mixed leukocyte reaction (MLR) assay

To analyze the capacity of DCs to activate T lymphocytes, Pig was anaesthetized before exsanguinated. Inguinal lymph nodes were collected for lymphocytes separation. Purified T cells were stained with CFSE following the instruction. CFSE-labelled T-lymphocytes (5×10^5) were co-cultured with Mph-DCs or Mock-DCs at a ratio of 1:1; 1:5 (DCs: lymphocytes). Co-cultures were incubated for five days. Finally, the cells were harvested, and the fluorescence intensity of the CFSE was determined by flow cytometry analysis.

Statistical analysis

Each of the experiments was performed at least three individual times. Data was performed using Statistical Product and Services Solutions (SPSS) package. Statistical difference was determined by one-way ANOVA followed by Dunnett's test. P values < 0.05 were considered statistically significant.

Results

Morphology of BMDCs after 6 days culture

Bone marrow-derived cells were cultured for 6 days by using RPMI 1640 media with GM-CSF and rpIL-4 to allow them to differentiate into immature BMDCs. Cell phenotypes were then evaluated by using microscopy. BMDCs formed clusters until the day 5 (Fig. 1a), and dendritic processes could be observed on the day 6 (Fig. 1b). When porcine monocytes were cultured without adding GM-CSF and IL-4, only a few live cells were left and no cell aggregates were observed in the plates by day 6 (Fig. 1c).

Table 1 Primers used for RT-qPCR

Gene	Sequence (5′ to 3′)
IL-10 forwardIL-10 forward	TCTGAGAACAGCTGCATCCAC
IL-10 reverse	CGCCCATCTGGTCCTTCGTT
IL-12 forward	TCAGAAGGCCAAACAAACCCT
IL-12 reverse	GGCAACTCTCATTCGTGGCTA
INF-γ forward	CGCAAAGCCATCAGTGAACTCA
INF-γ reverse	TCTGGCCTTGGAACATAGTCT
GAPDH forward	TCATCATCTCTGCCCCTTCT
GAPDH reverse	GTCATGAGTCCCTCCACGAT

Phenotypic alteration of BMDCs stimulated by vaccine *Mhp*-168 in vitro

DCs phenotypic maturation is essential for T cells activation and immune response. DCs up-regulate the expression of co-stimulatory and antigen presentation associated factors at the mature stage [15]. We used flow cytometry and the antibodies described earlier to detect surface expression of CD80/86, MHCII and CD1a to determine whether vaccine *Mhp*-168 affects the maturation and activation of DCs. By gating on untreated BMDCs, we compared the variation of phenotype between the untreated BMDCs and vaccine *Mhp*-168 treated-BMDCs in the same culture condition. Comparing with untreated immature Mo-DCs, immature Mo-DCs showed changes in surface marker expression characteristic of DC maturation (up-regulation of SWC3a + CD80/86+ and SWC3a + MHCII+), after being stimulated by the vaccine Mhp-168 or LPS (Fig. 2b and c). There is no significant change of SWC3a$^+$CD1a$^+$ co-stimulatory molecule expression after being exposed to vaccine *Mhp*-168 (Fig. 2a and b). These results suggest that stimulation of immature Mo-DCs triggers maturation.

Vaccine *Mhp*-168 stimulation modulates the expression of cytokines

Cytokines production by DCs also play an important role in immunomodulation besides the expression of surface molecules [16]. Therefore, we investigated whether vaccine *Mhp*-168 was able to modulate cytokine production by monitoring the mRNA expression level of IL-10, IL-12, INF-γ in vaccine *Mhp*-168 stimulated BMDCs lysis. Immature Mo-DCs stimulated with vaccine *Mhp*-168 show up-regulation of IL-10 and IL-12 mRNA expression level at 8 h incubation and increased at a steady-state level, with maximal production at 24 h incubation (Fig. 3a and b). While down-regulation expression of cytokines was observed in INF-γ at 8 h incubation and at a steady-state level, with maximal production at 24 h incubation (Fig. 3c). All LPS stimulated immature Mo-DCs showed increasing in IL-12, IFN-γ and IL-10 mRNA expression level. These results indicated that immature Mo-DCs have the capacity to activate an immune response to vaccine *Mhp*-168 by up-regulation IL-12 and IL-10 mRNA expression level.

Vaccine *Mhp*-168 treated-BMDCs promote T cells proliferation

The immune stimulatory properties of DCs to T cells are essential for adaptive immune responses. Here, allogenic mixed lymphocyte reaction (MLR) was performed to determine whether the ability of BMDCs induced T cells proliferation have changed after being

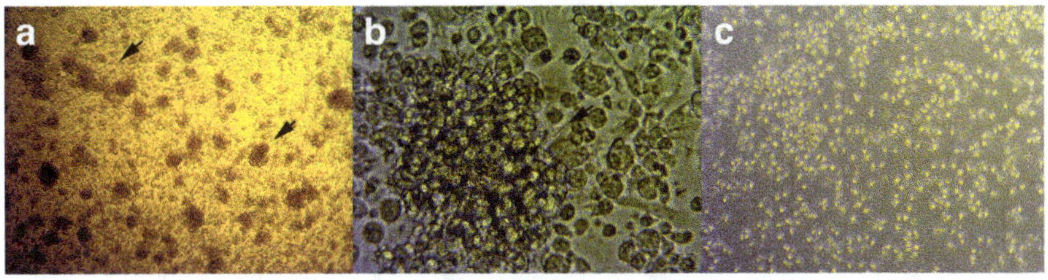

Fig. 1 Generation of BMDCs. Porcine BMDCs were cultured in RPMI 1640 medium supplemented with GM-CSF and IL-4. **a** The clusters of BMDCs on day 5, as viewed by optical microscopy at 100 ×magnification. **b** Morphology of cells after 6 days of culture, dendritic processes could be observed using optical microscopy at 400 × magnification. **c** Porcine BMDCs were cultured in RPMI 1640 medium supplemented without GM-CSF and IL-4 as control

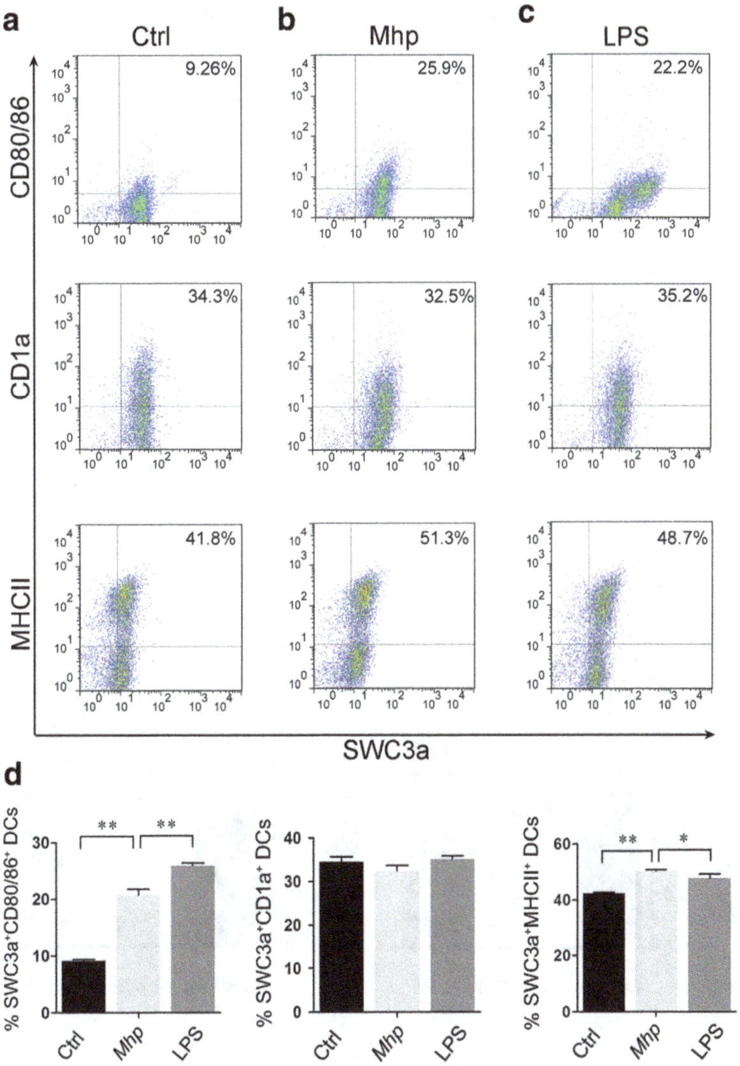

Fig. 2 Expression of antigen presenting molecules and co-stimulatory molecules on DCs after vaccine *Mhp*-168 exposure at 24 h.p.i. Immature BMDCs were exposed to vaccine *Mhp*-168 (40/dendritic cell) or LPS (10 ng/ml) as positive control for 24 h. Dot plots show the percentage of $CD1a^+SWC3a^+$DCs, $CD80/86^+SWC3a^+$ DCs and $MCHII^+SWC3a^+$ DCs. **a** Untreated BMDCs. **b** *Mhp* 168 treated DCs. **c** LPS treated DCs. **d** Bar graphs show the percentage of $CD1a^+SWC3a^+$, $CD80/86^+SWC3a^+$, $MHCII^+SWC3a^+$ cells in BMDCs populations after vaccine *Mhp*-168 exposure. Data show the means ± SEM ($n = 3$ per group). All experiments were performed independently three times. Statistical significance was assessed by Student's *t*-test. Differences were considered significant at (*) $0.01 < p < 0.05$, (**) $p < 0.01$

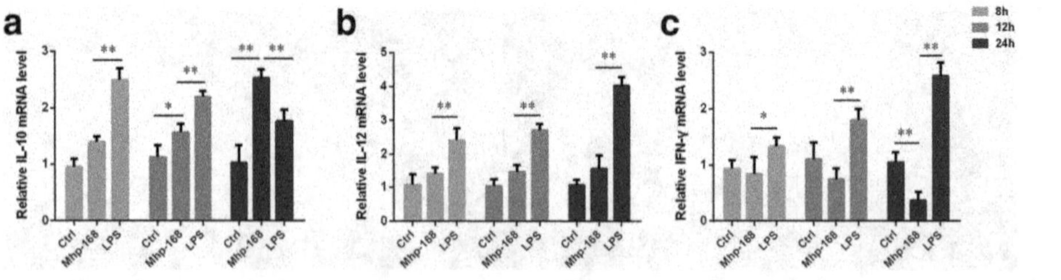

Fig. 3 Cytokines mRNA expression levels of DCs after vaccine *Mhp*-168 exposure. **a** IL-10; **b** IL-12; **c** IFN-γ. BMDCs were treated with vaccine *Mhp*-168 or LPS (10 ng/mL) for 8 h, 12 h and 24 h. The mRNA expression levels of IL-10, IL-12, IFN-γ were detected by real-time quantitative PCR (RT-qPCR). Data are expressed as means ± SD (n = 3 per group). All experiments were performed independently three times. Statistical significance was assessed by Student's t-test. Differences were considered significant at (*) $0.01 < p < 0.05$, (**) $p < 0.01$

treated with vaccine *Mhp*-168. As shown in Fig. 4, mature BMDCs stimulated by LPS up-regulate the ability of T cells proliferation at a DC/T cell ratio of 1:1 and 1:5. The proliferation capacity of T cells were promoted after being stimulated by *Mhp-168* both at a DC/T cell ratio of 1:1 and 1:5.

Discussion

Mhp is the primary etiological agent responsible for swine enzootic pneumonia (EP), which cause tremendous economic losses all over the swine industry [17]. There are many strategies to prevent *Mycoplasma* infection, such as drugs and antibiotics. However, they have not been proved effective inhibition of this pathogens in vivo, and still have problems of resistance and antibiotics residue [18]. Until now, vaccination is one of the essential strategy in controlling EP. Clinical study shows vaccine *Mhp*-168 activated the systemic cellular immunity and local mucosal immunity, which is benefit for prevention and control of EP [9]. Dendritic cells (DCs), the most effective antigen-presenting cells, are widely distributed beneath respiratory epithelium. DCs have the ability to capture antigens and then present to T cells, initiating protective immune responses during infection [19]. In the present study, we examined whether vaccine *Mhp*-168 could affect DCs generated from porcine monocytes in the presence of GM-CSF and IL-4 [14]. The function of antigen presentation of DCs is related to surface molecules [20]. In this study, we demonstrated that exposure of immature BMDCs to vaccine *Mhp*-168 results in the up-regulation of MHCII and CD80/86, which stimulates immature BMDCs to develop antigen presentation functions. Generally, DCs present antigen with CD1a or MHCII as the first signal and CD80/86 as the second co-stimulatory signal to activate T cells [20]. CD1a is a member of the MHCI family which involves in the presentation of intracellular and lipid antigens [21]. Many pathogenic microorganisms, such as porcine epidemic diarrhea virus (PEDV) and Mycobacterium tuberculosis, can be presented by CD1a [22, 23].

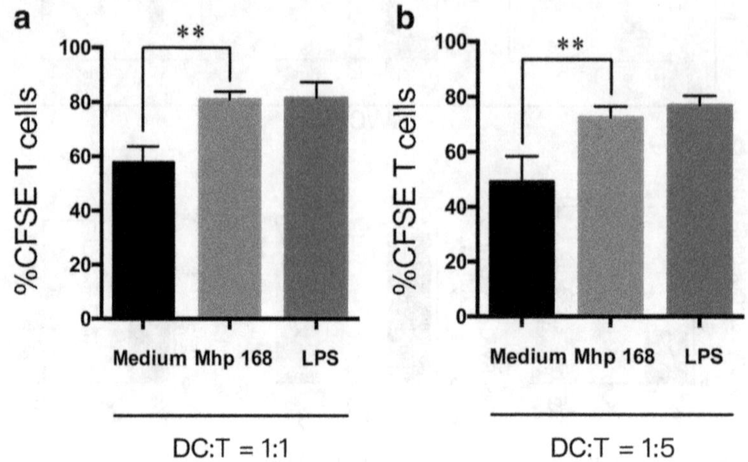

Fig. 4 Vaccine *Mhp*-168 treated DCs increased the capacity of T lymphocytes stimulation. Pretreatment DCs with vaccine *Mhp*-168 for 24 h. Vaccine *Mhp*-168-treated DCs were co-cultured with T lymphocytes (ratios 1:1, 1:5) for another 5 days (**a**, **b**). DCs were stimulated with LPS or remained unstimulated then co-cultured with T lymphocytes as positive or control group. T lymphocytes proliferation was evaluated using CFSE. Data are presented as mean ± SEM (n = 3 per group). All experiments were performed independently three times. Statistical significance was assessed by Student's t-test. Differences were considered significant at (*) $0.01 < p < 0.05$, (**) $p < 0.01$

However, surface molecule CD1a has no significant difference between vaccine *Mhp*-168 treated group and control group. This results indicate that DCs present *Mhp-168* to T cells do not via CD1a. These results indicate that vaccine *Mhp*-168 exposure causes the maturation of immature BMDCs. Up-regulating the expression of surface molecules and co-stimulatory molecules such as CD80/86, mature BMDCs present antigen information to T cells.

In addition to antigen recognition and presentation, DCs provide different cytokine microenvironments that leading differentiation of T cells into effector cells [24]. IL-10 is an anti-inflammatory cytokine, which can both impede pathogen clearance and ameliorate immunopathology [25]. Autocrine IL-10 signaling in DC can inhibit chemokine production and prevent their homing to lymph nodes, leading to the failure to recruit and induce TH1 differentiation of naïve T cells [26]. Many bacterial infections induce overexpression of IL-10, which is leading to uncontrolled pathogen growth [27]. Studies have shown that the systemic and local immune levels were not effectively activated after intranasal vaccination with the attenuated *Mhp-168* strain alone [28]. IFN-γ secretion by DCs is a crucial cytokine for the control of infectious diseases [29]. IFN-γ production were negatively regulated by IL-10 [30]. Our results demonstrate that exposure of vaccine *Mhp-168* to DCs induces significant increase in IL-10 production. The increase indicated that although *Mhp-168* exposure would induce maturation of DCs, it also promotes massive secretion of IL-10. Our study also found a down-regulation of IFN-γ produced by DCs. Overexpression of IL-10 and accompany with down-regulation of IFN-γ level may be one of the reasons why vaccination with the *Mhp-168* strain alone could not achieve productive immune effect in practical application.

Stimulation of T cell proliferation is one of the important functions of dendritic cells. We used mixed leukocyte reaction (MLR) assay to evaluate the ability of DCs to induce T cell proliferation [31]. We found that vaccine *Mhp*-168 treated BMDCs increase the proliferation of T cells both at DC/T cell ratio of 1:1 and 1:5. The stimulation level at a DC/T cell ratio of 1:1 exhibited a stronger stimulatory effect. This results indicate that primary T cells is activated by presentation of BMDCs though surface molecule MHCII and CD80/86. This results are also correlated with the highest expression of CD80/86 and MHCII in Mhp-168 treated immature BMDCs.

Conclusions

In conclusion, this study is the first description of the interaction between vaccine *Mhp*-168 and porcine BMDCs. Our data indicates that *Mhp-168* enhances the ability of BMDCs to present and induce the proliferation of T lymphocytes. However, vaccine *Mhp-168* exposure induce significant increase in IL-10 and accompany with decrease in INF-γ expression by DCs, which indicate the possibility of immune failure in practical application with vaccine *Mhp-168* alone.

Abbreviations

APC: Antigen-presenting cells; BMDCs: Bone marrow-derived DCs; DCs: Dendritic cells; EP: Porcine enzootic pneumonia; LAMPs: Lipid-associated membrane protein; MALT: Mucosa-associated lymphoid tissue; *Mhp*: *Mycoplasma hyopneumoniae*; PBMCs: Peripheral blood mononuclear cells

Acknowledgments

We thank Prof. Guoqing Shao and Prof. Zhixin Feng for providing us with the *Mycoplasma hyopneumoniae* strains as well as his laboratory space and for the experiments.

Funding

This work was supported by National Science Grant of PR China (No. 31372465) and a project funded by the Priority Academic Program Development of Jiangsu Higher Education Institutions (PAPD).

Authors' contributions

YMS contributed to study design, collected and analyzed data and wrote the first draft of the paper. WWH analyzed data and revised the manuscript. YNW analyzed data and revised the manuscript. ZXF revised the manuscript. QY conceived the study, contributed to study design and revised the manuscript. All authors read and approved the final manuscript.

Consent for publication

Not applicable.

Competing interests

The authors declare that they have no competing interests.

Author details

[1]Veterinary College, Nanjing Agricultural University, Weigang 1, Nanjing, Jiangsu 210095, People's Republic of China. [2]Institute of Veterinary Medicine, Jiangsu Academy of Agricultural Sciences, Key Laboratory of Veterinary Biological Engineering and Technology, Ministry of Agriculture, National Center for Engineering Research of Veterinary Bio-products, Nanjing 210014, People's Republic of China.

References

1. DeBey M, Jacobson C, Ross R. Histochemical and morphologic changes of porcine airway epithelial cells in response to infection with Mycoplasma hyopneumoniae. Am J Vet Res. 1992;53(9):1705–10.
2. Rautiainen E, Wallgren P. Aspects of the transmission of protection against Mycoplasma hyopneumoniae from sow to offspring. J Veterinary Med Ser B. 2001;48(1):55–65.
3. Opriessnig T, Thacker E, Yu S, Fenaux M, Meng X-J, Halbur P. Experimental reproduction of postweaning multisystemic wasting syndrome in pigs by dual infection with Mycoplasma hyopneumoniae and porcine circovirus type 2. Vet Pathol Online. 2004;41(6):624–40.
4. Maes D, Segales J, Meyns T, Sibila M, Pieters M, Haesebrouck F. Control of Mycoplasma hyopneumoniae infections in pigs. Vet Microbiol. 2008;126(4):297–309.
5. Woolley LK, Fell SA, Djordjevic SP, Eamens GJ, Jenkins C. Plasmin activity in the porcine airways is enhanced during experimental infection with Mycoplasma hyopneumoniae, is positively correlated with proinflammatory cytokine levels and is ameliorated by vaccination. Vet Microbiol. 2013;164(1):60–6.
6. Mizgerd JP. Acute lower respiratory tract infection. N Engl J Med. 2008;358(7):716–27.

7. Bai F, Ni B, Liu M, Feng Z, Xiong Q, Shao G. Mycoplasma hyopneumoniae-derived lipid-associated membrane proteins induce inflammation and apoptosis in porcine peripheral blood mononuclear cells in vitro. Vet Microbiol. 2015;175(1):58–67.
8. Thacker EL, Thacker BJ, Boettcher TB, Jayappa H. Comparison of antibody production, lymphocyte stimulation, and protection induced by four commercial Mycoplasma hyopneumoniae bacterins. J Swine Health Prod. 1998;6(3):107–12.
9. Feng Z-X, Shao G-Q, Liu M-J, Wu X-S, Zhou Y-Q, Yuan G. Immune responses to the attenuated Mycoplasma hyopneumoniae 168 strain vaccine by intrapulmonic immunization in piglets. Agric Sci China. 2010;9(3):423–31.
10. Harman AN, Bye CR, Nasr N, Sandgren KJ, Kim M, Mercier SK, Botting RA, Lewin SR, Cunningham AL, Cameron PU. Identification of lineage relationships and novel markers of blood and skin human dendritic cells. J Immunol. 2013;190(1):66–79.
11. Lee H, Ruane D, Law K, Ho Y, Garg A, Rahman A, Esterházy D, Cheong C, Goljo E, Sikora A. Phenotype and function of nasal dendritic cells. Mucosal Immunol. 2015;8(5):1083–98.
12. von Garnier C, Nicod LP. Immunology taught by lung dendritic cells. Swiss Med Wkly. 2009;139(13–14):186–92.
13. Jing H, Mao H. Diagnosis and prevention for mycoplasmal pneumonia of swine. Nanjing: Jiangsu Science and Technology Publications; 1993. p. 4–6. (in Chinese).
14. Chen X, Tu C, Qin T, Zhu L, Yin Y, Yang Q. Retinoic acid facilitates inactivated transmissible gastroenteritis virus induction of cd8+ t-cell migration to the porcine gut. Sci Rep. 2016;6:24152.
15. Banchereau J, Steinman RM. Dendritic cells and the control of immunity. Nature. 1998;392(6673):245–52.
16. Steinman RM. The dendritic cell system and its role in immunogenicity. Annu Rev Immunol. 1991;9(1):271–96.
17. Sørensen V, Ahrens P, Barfod K, Feenstra AA, Feld NC, Friis NF, Bille-Hansen V, Jensen NE, Pedersen MW. Mycoplasma hyopneumoniae infection in pigs: duration of the disease and evaluation of four diagnostic assays. Vet Microbiol. 1997;54(1):23–34.
18. Hannan P, Windsor H, Ripley P. In vitro susceptibilities of recent field isolates of Mycoplasma hyopneumoniae and Mycoplasma hyosynoviae to valnemulin (Econor®), tiamulin and enrofloxacin and the in vitro development of resistance to certain antimicrobial agents in Mycoplasma hyopneumoniae. Res Vet Sci. 1997;63(2):157–60.
19. Farache J, Koren I, Milo I, Gurevich I, Kim K-W, Zigmond E, Furtado GC, Lira SA, Shakhar G. Luminal bacteria recruit CD103+ dendritic cells into the intestinal epithelium to sample bacterial antigens for presentation. Immunity. 2013;38(3):581–95.
20. Mellman I, Steinman RM. Dendritic cells: specialized and regulated antigen processing machines. Cell. 2001;106(3):255–8.
21. Barral DC, Brenner MB. CD1 antigen presentation: how it works. Nat Rev Immunol. 2007;7(12):929–41.
22. Spada FM, Grant EP, Peters PJ, Sugita M, Melián A, Leslie DS, Lee HK, Van Donselaar E, Hanson DA, Krensky AM. Self-Recognition of Cd1 by γ/δ T Cells. J Exp Med. 2000;191(6):937–48.
23. Gao Q, Zhao S, Qin T, Yin Y, Yu Q, Yang Q. Effects of inactivated porcine epidemic diarrhea virus on porcine monocyte-derived dendritic cells and intestinal dendritic cells. Res Vet Sci. 2016;106:149–58.
24. Merad M, Sathe P, Helft J, Miller J, Mortha A. The Dendritic Cell Lineage: Ontogeny and Function of Dendritic Cells and Their Subsets in the Steady State and the Inflamed Setting. Annu Rev Immunol. 2013;31(5):563.
25. Couper KN, Blount DG, Riley EM. IL-10: the master regulator of immunity to infection. J Immunol. 2008;180(9):5771.
26. Demangel C, Bertolino P, Britton WJ. Autocrine IL-10 impairs dendritic cell (DC)-derived immune responses to mycobacterial infection by suppressing DC trafficking to draining lymph nodes and local IL-12 production. Eur J Immunol. 2002;32(4):994–1002.
27. Groux H, Cottrez F, Rouleau M, Mauze S, Antonenko S, Hurst S, Mcneil T, Bigler M, Roncarolo MG, Coffman RL. A transgenic model to analyze the immunoregulatory role of IL-10 secreted by antigen-presenting cells. J Immunol. 1999;162(3):1723.
28. Li Y, Li P, Wang X, Yu Q, Yang Q. Co-administration of attenuated Mycoplasma hyopneumoniae 168 strain with bacterial DNA enhances the local and systemic immune response after intranasal vaccination in pigs. Vaccine. 2012;30(12):2153–8.
29. Suzue K, Asai T, Takeuchi T, Koyasu S. In vivo role of IFN-γ produced by antigen-presenting cells in early host defense against intracellular pathogens. Eur J Immunol. 2003;33(10):2666–75.
30. Fukao T, Matsuda S, Koyasu S. Synergistic effects of IL-4 and IL-18 on IL-12-dependent IFN-γ production by dendritic cells. J Immunol. 2000;164(1):64–71.
31. Sallusto F, Lanzavecchia A. Efficient presentation of soluble antigen by cultured human dendritic cells is maintained by granulocyte/macrophage colony-stimulating factor plus interleukin 4 and downregulated by tumor necrosis factor. J Exp Med. 1994;179(4):1109–18.

16

Safety and immunogenecity of a live attenuated Rift Valley fever vaccine (CL13T) in camels

S. Daouam[1,2*], F. Ghzal[1], Y. Naouli[1], K. O. Tadlaoui[1], M. M. Ennaji[2], C. Oura[3] and M. EL Harrak[1]

Abstract

Background: Rift Valley fever is an emerging zoonotic viral disease, enzootic and endemic in Africa and the Arabian Peninsula, which poses a significant threat to both human and animal health. The disease is most severe in ruminants causing abortions in pregnant animals, especially sheep animals and high mortality in young populations. High mortality rates and severe clinical manifestation have also been reported among camel populations in Africa, to attend however none of the currently available live vaccines against RVF have been tested for safety and efficacy in this species. In this study, the safety and efficacy (through a neutralizing antibody response) of the thermostable live attenuated RVF CL13T vaccine were evaluated in camels in two different preliminary experiments involving 16 camels, (that 12 camels and 4 pregnant camels).

Results: The study revealed that the CL13T vaccine was safe to use in camels and no abortions or teratogenic effects were observed. The single dose of the vaccine stimulated a strong and long-lasting neutralizing antibody response for up to 12 months.

Conclusion: The presence of neutralization antibodies is likely to correlate with protection; however protection would need to be confirmed by challenge experiments using the virulent RVF virus.

Keywords: Rift Valley fever, Thermostable, Clone 13T vaccine, Camels

Background

Rift Valley fever (RVF) is a zoonotic viral disease caused by Rift Valley fever virus (RVFV), which is a virus within the genus *Phlebovirus* and family *Bunyaviridae*. RVF is enzootic and endemic in Africa, Saudi Arabia and Yemen and poses a significant threat to both human and animal health [1–3]. The disease is most severe in sheep, goats and cattle, causing abortions in pregnant females and high mortality in young animals [4–8].

Vaccination is considered to be the most effective way to prevent and control the expansion of the disease. However, the available attenuated vaccines for RVF cause abortions and teratogenic effects (Smithburn strain vaccine) or are thermolabile (CL13 strain vaccine) [6, 9, 10]. An evaluation of efficacy and safety of the CL13 vaccine in ewes at different stages of pregnancy indicated that the vaccine did not induce clinical manifestation of RVF, such as abortion in pregnant ewes, teratogeny in their offspring or pyrexia in vaccinated animals [11]. Vaccination with CL13 vaccine also prevented clinical RVF following virulent challenge. A recent study carried out by Daouam et al. [12] revealed that the CL13 vaccine strain was unstable in both lyophilized and liquid forms at 22–25 °C and at 37 °C, which highlight the importance of cold chain when using the CL13 vaccine in endemic tropical countries. In response to this need, the CL13 vaccine strain was made thermostable through three cycles of heating (56 °C) and selection of thermostable particles (12). The thermostable vaccine clone (CL13T) was found to be safe when tested on sheep, goats and cattle with no clinical signs or side effects observed. Neutralizing antibodies were detected in vaccinated animals for a minimum of one year in sheep

* Correspondence: s.daouam@mci-santeanimale.com
[1]Research and Development Virology, Multi-Chemical Industry, Lot. 157, Z I, Sud-Ouest (ERAC) B.P: 278, Mohammedia 28810, Morocco
[2]Laboratory of Virology, Hygiene & Microbiology, Faculty of Sciences & Technics, University Hassan II Mohammedia-Casablanca, 20650 Mohammedia, Morocco
Full list of author information is available at the end of the article

and goats, and for at least 4 months in cattle indicating that the vaccine also provide a good protection [12].

Recent outbreaks of RVF in western Africa have resulted in high mortality and severe clinical signs among dromedary camel populations [13]. Serological surveys in northern and eastern Africa have revealed high percentages of seropositive camels after the occurrence of an outbreak [14, 15]. Camels are therefore susceptible to RVFV, and are likely to play a role in the epidemiology of the disease and should be included in any vaccination program. There have been no previous reports of camels being vaccinated against RVF, and no RVF vaccines including a thermostablized vaccine have been tested for safety and efficacy in this species. This study therefore was conducted to evaluate the safety and efficacy of the thermostable live attenuated CL13T vaccine in camels.

Methods

Vaccine (CL13T) production and titration

The CL13T attenuated virus was propagated and titrated on African Green monkey kidney cells (Vero, ATCC) [9]. The vaccine was formulated by mixing V/V the viral suspension with a stabilizer of lyophilisation (4 % peptone, 8 % sucrose and 2 % glutamate). The viral suspension titre is fixed to have a minimum of 10^6 $DICT_{50}$ per dose. The RVF CL13T vaccine was distributed in glass vials and freeze dried. Before administration, the vaccine was reconstituted by adding a saline solution.

Safety and efficacy testing of the CL13T candidate vaccine in camels

All experiments involving camels (*Camelus Dromedarius*) were carried out in accordance with guidelines for the care and handling of experimental animals these animals are dedicated to research and maintained an experimental farm. The animal experiments were approved by the MCI ethics committee in charge of the control and supervision of experiments on animals and the experiments were conducted in high containment level 3 facilities. Sixteen dromedary's camels 2–3 year old, negative for RVFV antibody by the neutralization test were divided in two groups of six and one group of 4.

In experiment 1: Two groups of 6 camels were vaccinated subcutaneously (SC) with a dose of 10^6 $TCID_{50}$ of the CL13T vaccine. Camels in group 1 received a single dose of the vaccine and camels of group 2 received a booster dose, four weeks after the first vaccination. The general behavior and rectal temperature of the camels were recorded daily for two weeks after each vaccination as well as observation for local inflammation at the injection site. Sera samples were obtained daily for the first 15 days post-vaccination (PV) and tested for RVFV RNA and infectious virus by quantitative real-time PCR [16] and virus isolation in Vero cells, respectively. Antibody titers were monitored over a 12 months period by virus-neutralization (VN) on Vero cell culture as described in the OIE manual (OIE, 2012). VN was performed on 96 wells plates using 100 DL_{50} of the RVFV (CL13) per well with a serial 3 fold dilution of the serum in a 4 wells replicate foe each dilution. After 60 mn of neutralization at 37 °C, the cells suspension was added and the plate incubated 5 days before reading. The neutralizing titre is determined by Reed et Muench method and expressed in log10/ml. Sera were also tested for IgG detection by a competitive ELISA (ID-VET RIFTC-4P).

In experiment 2: a group of 4 pregnant she camels were vaccinated via the SC route with a 10X the normal dose (10^7 $TCID_{50}$) of the CL13T vaccine. Rectal temperatures, appetite and behavior of each animal were documented daily for 1 month and then every month during five months after vaccination until calving for a potential abortions effect and teratogenicity.

Statistical analysis

The antibody titers detected in the first and second group of camels were compared using the Student *t* test; with a significance level of $p = 0.05$.

Results

Safety testing of CL13T candidate vaccine in camels

The C13T vaccine was found to be safe, with no evidence of abortions or teratogenicity among the offsprings of the vaccinated pregnant camels. All camels were healthy and did not have any sign of illness. Normal body temperatures were recorded in the pregnant as well as among the camels in Group 1 and 2 before vaccination and no local reactions were recorded at the injection sites. In the 15 days after vaccination no abnormal behavior was observed in any of the vaccinated animals and their body temperatures remained in the normal range. Very low levels of viral RNA (Cycle Threshold values from 37.6 to 38.6 among a total of 40 cycles) were detected in the blood of 7 of the camels in Groups 1 and 2 during the first 2 weeks following vaccination. However, no infectious virus was isolated from the samples after 2 blind passages on Vero cells. The absence of RVFV in the inoculated cells was confirmed by qPCR.

Serological responses in camels vaccinated with the CL13T candidate vaccine virus

Neutralizing antibody were recorded in all the vaccinated camels by day 12 PV, with peak neutralizing titers of 2.5 log DN_{50} (equivalent to a serum dilution of 1:500) being observed on day 28 (PV) (Fig. 1). High titers of neutralizing antibody were maintained for a period of 6 months PV, at which time the titers started to wane over the next 6 months, reaching at titer of 0.92 log DN_{50} (equivalent to a serum dilution of 1:10) at twelve

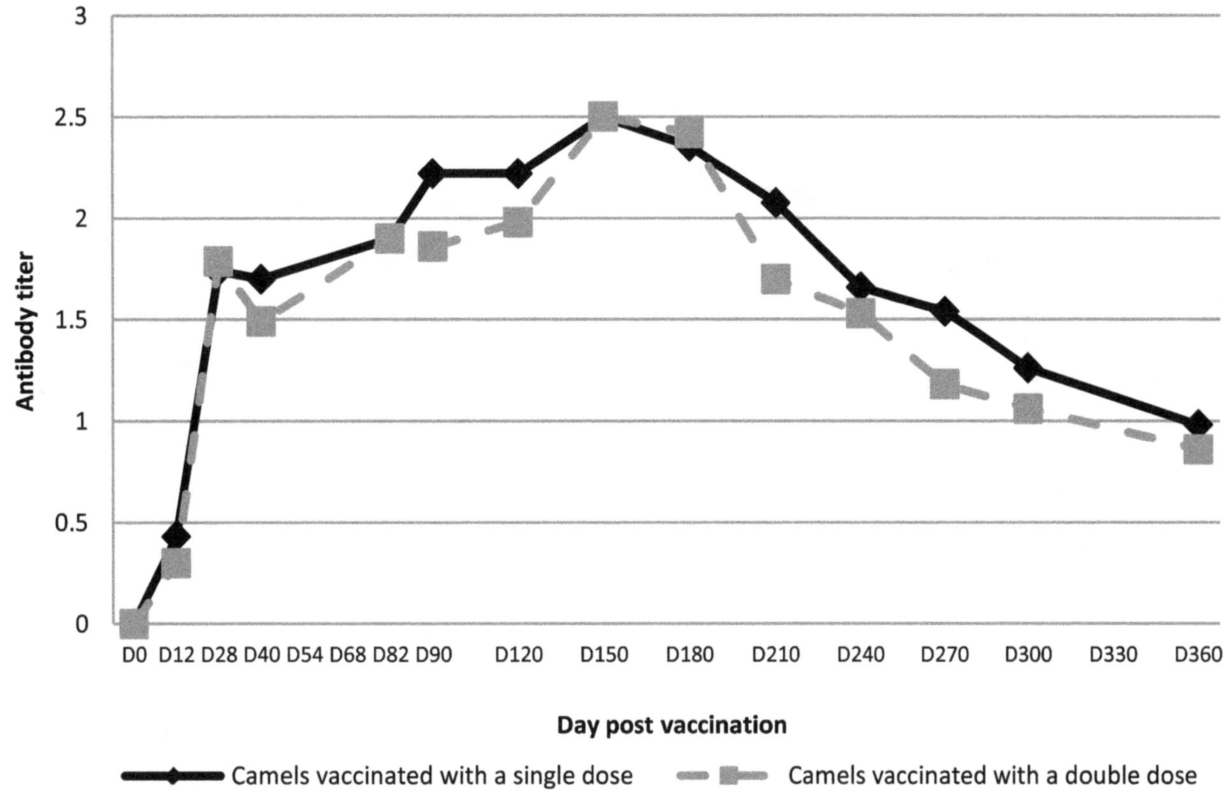

Fig. 1 Neutralizing antibody titres in camels vaccinated with a single and a double dose of live CL13T RVF vaccine. All camels were vaccinated subcutaneously (SC) with a dose of $10^6 TCID_{50}$ of the CL13T vaccine. Camels in group 1 received a single dose and camels of group 2 received a booster at day 30 after vaccination

months post-vaccination (Fig. 1). Similar antibody titers were detected in camels vaccinated once (group 1) and twice (group 2), showing that there was no significant increase in neutralizing antibody titers through the administration of a booster dose of the vaccine.

Significant differences ($p < 0.05$) in antibody titers were observed in the sera samples from camels tested by VN as compared to those tested by cELISA. Antibody titers measured by the two tests (VN and cELISA) remained similar for the first 3 months post-vaccination and then diverged to attain titers that were significantly different (Fig. 2). Results revealed a reduced sensitivity of the cELISA compared to the VN test for the detection of RVFV antibody (Fig. 2). It is important to note however that the cELISA kit used in this study has only been validated for use in ruminants. Thus, results indicate that this cELISA may not be optimized for use in camels and that the sensitivity of the assay may need to be improved before it can be recommended for routine diagnosis or for vaccination monitoring in camels.

Discussion

This study reveals that camels mounted a strong and long-lasting neutralizing antibody response when vaccinated with a single dose of the live CL13T RVF vaccine and that the vaccine is safe to use, producing no significant side-effects in the vaccinated animals. The neutralizing antibody response was similar to that observed in small ruminants and cattle after vaccination with the live RVF clone 13 vaccine [17, 18].

This is the first report that evaluates the safety and efficacy of a live attenuated thermostabilized RVF vaccine in camels. To be sure that this vaccine protects camels against RVF, challenge studies would need to be carried out. However in the case of RVF, neutralizing antibodies are known to be reliable predictor of protection after vaccination [17, 19]. The high levels of neutralizing antibodies observed in the vaccinated camels may indicate therefore that the CL13T vaccine is likely to be protective in camels for up to 12 months.

It is highly recommended to vaccinate livestock to prevent the occurrence of disease in susceptible animals and if possible virus amplifying hosts, in order to break the epidemiological transmission cycle. With the high densities of dromedary camels in many areas where RVF is present, it is extremely important to be able to protect camels, as well as other susceptible species.

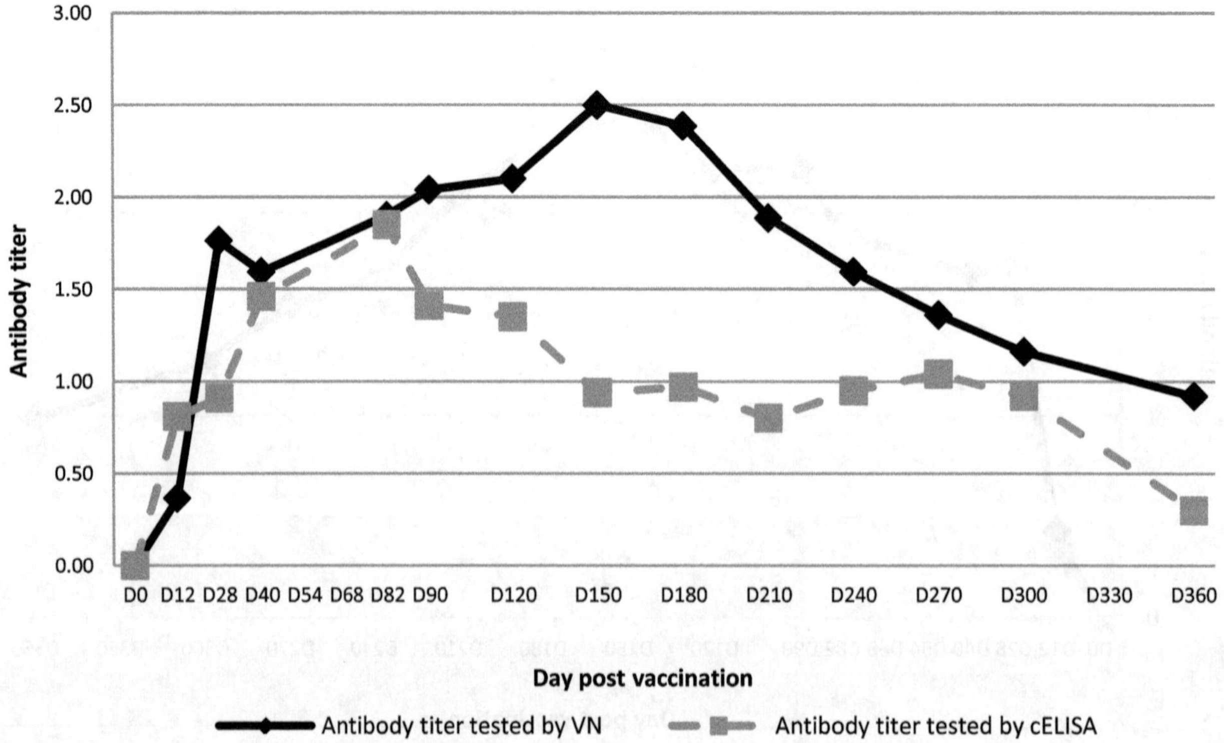

Fig. 2 Antibody titres of camels vaccinated with a live CL13T RVF vaccine tested by VN and cELISA. Neutralizing antibody were tested in all vaccinated camels by VN and cELISA test, a significant differences ($p < 0.05$) in antibody titers were observed

This is the first study that has evaluated the safety and immunogenicity of a live attenuated RVF vaccine in camels. A recent study, reported camel vaccination with a recombinant adenovirus encoding RVFV envelope glycoprotein. A lower antibody neutralizing titre was observed in camels comparatively to other species (sheep, goats and cattle) with a dose of 10^9 injected intramuscularly in the presence of an adjuvant [19]. No challenge was carried out for the protection testing.

Conclusions

In our study, the obtained antibody response in vaccinated camels was similar to that registered in sheep and better than cattle response with a dose of 10^6 only, injected by S/C route. Although this is a preliminary study, the presence of neutralization antibodies is likely to correlate with protection. To be noted that RVF protection of camels has never been tested by experimental infection and no challenge model has been developed for camels.

In summary, the study showed that the CL13T live attenuated vaccine is safe to use in camels and that a single dose of the vaccine stimulated strong and long-lasting neutralizing antibody response for up to 12 months. In the absence of any tested live vaccine for camels, the CL13T vaccine could be considered for camel protection against RVF after a field trial that include sufficient number of animals under the normal living conditions.

Abbreviation

CL13, clone 13; CL13T, clone 13 thermostable; PV, post-vaccination; RVF, Rift Valley fever; RVFV, Rift Valley fever virus; SC, subcutaneously; Vero, African Green monkey kidney cells; VN, virus-neutralization

Acknowledgements

All the authors have seen and approved the content and have contributed significantly to the work.

Funding

No funding was obtained for this study.

Authors' contributions

SD and ME planned and conceived the experiments; KT participated in the design and the follow up of the study; FG performed the safety and the potency testing, YN carried out the Elisa test; SD carried out other laboratory works; SD, ME, MME and CO analyzed the data and wrote the manuscript. All authors read and approved the final manuscript.

Competing interests

The authors declare that they have no competing interests.

Consent for publication

Not applicable.

Author details
[1]Research and Development Virology, Multi-Chemical Industry, Lot. 157, Z I, Sud-Ouest (ERAC) B.P: 278, Mohammedia 28810, Morocco. [2]Laboratory of Virology, Hygiene & Microbiology, Faculty of Sciences & Technics, University Hassan II Mohammedia-Casablanca, 20650 Mohammedia, Morocco. [3]School of Veterinary Medicine, University of the West Indies, St. Augustine, Trinidad and Tobago.

References

1. Meegan JM. The Rift Valley fever epizootic in Egypt 1977–78. 1. Description of the epizzotic and virological studies. Trans R Soc Trop Med Hyg. 1979; 73(6):618–23.
2. Balkhy HH, Memish ZA. Rift Valley fever: an uninvited zoonosis in the Arabian peninsula. Int J Antimicrob Agents. 2003;21(2):153–7.
3. Sissoko D, Giry C, Gabrie P, Tarantola A, Pettinelli F, Collet L, D'Ortenzio E, Renault P, Pierre V. Rift Valley Fever, Mayotte, 2007–2008. Emerg Infect Dis. 2009;15(4):568–70.
4. Easterday BC, Mc GM, Rooney JR, Murphy LC. The pathogenesis of Rift Valley fever in lambs. Am J Vet Res. 1962;23:470–9.
5. Coetzer JA. The pathology of Rift Valley fever. I. Lesions occurring in natural cases in new-born lambs. Onderstepoort J Vet Res. 1977;44(4):205–11.
6. Coetzer JA, Barnard BJ. Hydrops amnii in sheep associated with hydranencephaly and arthrogryposis with wesselsbron disease and rift valley fever viruses as aetiological agents. Onderstepoort J Vet Res. 1977; 44(2):119–26.
7. Flick R, Bouloy M. Rift Valley fever virus. Curr Mol Med. 2005;5(8):827–34.
8. Pepin M, Bouloy M, Bird BH, Kemp A, Paweska J. Rift Valley fever virus(Bunyaviridae: Phlebovirus): an update on pathogenesis, molecular epidemiology, vectors, diagnostics and prevention. Vet Res. 2010;41(6):61.
9. Daouam S, Fakri FZ, Ennaji MM, El Arkam A, Tadlaoui KO, Oura C, Elharrak M. Heat stability of the Rift Valley Fever Virus Clone 13 live vaccines. Trials Vaccinol. 2014;3:61–4.
10. Khafagy HA, Ebied MH, Abdelwahab MG, Saad MA. Clinical and immunological studies on live attenuated Rift Valley Fever vaccine. N Y Sci J. 2013;6:12–7.
11. Kaschula VR. The propagation and modification of strains of Rift Valley fever viruses in embryonated eggs and their use as immunizing agents for domestic ruminants. South Africa: Thesis Doctor of Veterinary Science, University of Pretoria; 1953.
12. Daouam SGF, EL Arkam A, Naouli Y, Jazouli M, Ennaji MM, Tadlaoui KO, Oura C, Elharrak M. Evaluation of the safety and efficacy of a live attenuated thermostable Rift Valley fever vaccine in Sheep, Goats and Cattle. J Vaccines Vaccin. 2015;6:295. doi:2157-7560.1000295.
13. El Mamy AB, Baba MO, Barry Y, Isselmou K, Dia ML, El Kory MO, Diop M, Lo MM, Thiongane Y, Bengoumi M, et al. Unexpected Rift Valley fever outbreak, northern Mauritania. Emerg Infect Dis. 2011;17(10):1894–6.
14. El-Harrak M, Martín-Folgar R, Llorente F, Fernández-Pacheco P, Brun A, Figuerola J, Jiménez-Clavero MÁ. Rift Valley and West Nile Virus Antibodies in Camels. North Afr Emerg Infect Dis. 2011;17(12):2372–4.
15. Swai ES, Sindato C. Seroprevalence of Rift Valley fever virus infection in camels (dromedaries) in northern Tanzania. Trop Anim Health Prod. 2015; 47(2):347–52.
16. Anyangu AS, Gould LH, Sharif SK, Nguku PM, Omolo JO, Mutonga D, Rao CY, Lederman ER, Schnabel D, Paweska JT, et al. Risk factors for severe Rift Valley fever infection in Kenya, 2007. Am J Trop Med Hyg. 2010;83(2 Suppl):14–21.
17. Dungu B, Louw I, Lubisi A, Hunter P, von Teichman BF, Bouloy M. Evaluation of the efficacy and safety of the Rift Valley Fever Clone 13 vaccine in sheep. Vaccine. 2010;28(29):4581–7.
18. von Teichman B, Engelbrecht A, Zulu G, Dungu B, Pardini A, Bouloy M. Safety and efficacy of Rift Valley fever Smithburn and Clone 13 vaccines in calves. Vaccine. 2011;29(34):5771–7.
19. Warimwe GM, Gesharisha J, Carr BV, Otieno S, Otingah K, Wright D, Charleston B, Okoth E, Elena LG, Lorenzo G, et al. Chimpanzee Adenovirus vaccine provides multispecies protection against Rift Valley fever. Sci Rep. 2016;6:20617.

Safety studies with the oral rabies virus vaccine strain SPBN GASGAS in the small Indian mongoose (*Herpestes auropunctatus*)

Steffen Ortmann[1], Ad Vos[1*], Antje Kretzschmar[1], Nomusa Walther[1], Christiane Kaiser[1], Conrad Freuling[2], Ivana Lojkic[3] and Thomas Müller[2]

Abstract

Background: Oral vaccination of the small Indian mongoose against rabies has been suggested as a potential tool to eliminate mongoose-mediated rabies on several Caribbean islands. A recently developed oral rabies virus vaccine strain, SPBN GASGAS, has already been shown to be efficacious in this reservoir species. Since, all available oral rabies vaccines are based on replication-competent viruses and vaccine baits are distributed unsupervised in the environment, enhanced safety standards for such vaccine types are required.

Results: The results of safety studies, including overdose, repeated doses, dissemination and different routes of administration, in the target species are presented. It was shown that the construct was apathogenic, irrespective of dose and route of administration. Even when it was inoculated directly in the brain, it did not induce rabies infection. Furthermore, the vaccine strain did not spread within the target species after direct oral instillation beyond the site of entry.

Conclusion: The vaccine strain SPBN GASGAS meets the safety requirements for live rabies virus vaccines in this target species, the small Indian mongoose.

Keywords: Rabies, Mongoose, Oral vaccination, Safety, SPBN GASGAS

Background

The small Indian mongoose (*Herpestes auropunctatus*), native to southern Asia, has been introduced to many islands worldwide for control of pest animals [1]. Since the mid-twentieth century, the species has been identified as a rabies reservoir on some of the Caribbean islands it has been introduced to, i.e. Cuba, Dominican Republic, Grenada and Puerto Rico [2]. As with other wildlife rabies reservoirs, attempts to control mongoose rabies in the Caribbean through culling have so far failed [1, 2]. Hence, oral vaccination of mongoose against rabies has been suggested as a more promising alternative [3, 4] and is presently under investigation in Puerto Rico [5]. Oral vaccination campaigns against rabies of different wildlife reservoir species has been successfully implemented in Europe and North America [6, 7]. Several experimental studies have shown that mongoose can be vaccinated against rabies by the oral route using the vaccine strain SPBN GASGAS [4, 8]. Also, field studies showed that baits were readily accepted by mongooses and can reach a high proportion of the target species [9–11]. Thus oral vaccination of small Indian mongooses against rabies seems a feasible approach as all three components of this concept (vaccine, bait and distribution system) are available.

However, besides being efficacious after a single dose, the vaccine should also meet certain safety standards; especially considering that all available oral rabies vaccines are based on replication-competent viruses. Furthermore, in contrast to parenteral administered vaccines, oral rabies vaccine baits are distributed in the environment without direct supervision. Therefore, an important prerequisite for the deliberate distribution of vaccine baits in the environment containing live replication competent viruses is a stringent safety assessment.

* Correspondence: Ad.Vos@idt-biologika.de
[1]IDT Biologika GmbH, Am Pharmapark, 06861 Dessau Rosslau, Germany
Full list of author information is available at the end of the article

In this paper, the safety studies in the potential target species, the small Indian mongoose, with the oral rabies virus vaccine strain SPBN GASGAS are presented. For the licensing of such vaccines in Puerto Rico, the Center of Veterinary Biologics of the Animal and Plant Health Inspection Service, United States Department of Agriculture (USDA/APHIS/CVB), is responsible. Detailed descriptions of the safety studies required can be found in the Code of Federal Regulation (Title 9 – Animals and Animal Products) [12] and Veterinary Services Memoranda [13]. However, unlike in the European Pharmacopoeia there is no dedicated chapter on oral rabies vaccines in these documents; the listed study protocols for live rabies virus vaccines are intended for parenteral administered vaccines. Thus, it became necessary to adapt the protocols in such a way that the recommended oral route of administration was investigated instead of intramuscularly injection. Besides the required dissemination study of the vaccine virus using the recommended route of administration (oral), animals also received the vaccine virus by the i.c. and i.m route. Repeated dose studies are required only for vaccines that need to be administered on multiple occasions in order to induce a protective immune response. For oral vaccination of mongoose against rabies a single dose SPBN GASGAS is sufficient [4, 8]. Hence, a repeated dose study is not compulsory. However, in the context of oral vaccination where any animal can locate and consume multiple vaccine baits distributed in the environment repeated dose studies are relevant for safety assessment; thus, a single high-titred overdose was administered. Furthermore, mongooses can come in contact with the vaccine virus on multiple occasions after bait distribution. To imitate such a situation, the animals were offered a vaccine dose on three occasions within 1 week. The selection of 7 days is based on the observation that most baits distributed in the environment are generally taken up within this time frame [14–17]. Also, stability of SPBN GASGAS over periods longer than 7 days in the environment is not guaranteed, especially considering the prevailing climatic conditions in Puerto Rico. Rabies lyssavirus is considered relatively thermo-instable and will rapidly lose its infectivity when exposed to elevated temperatures [18]. Shedding of vaccine virus in saliva and feces has been investigated during the dissemination and overdose studies; these results have been published previously and will not be presented here [19]. It was shown that the vaccine strain SPBN GASGAS was completely innocuous for the small Indian mongoose, irrespective of the route of administration and dose.

Methods

Animals

Male juvenile and adult mongooses were caught using baited box traps on the rabies-free island Korčula, Croatia, and transported to IDT Biologika GmbH (IDT), Germany. Each mongoose was housed in a cage individually (0.44 m^2 - including sleeping box) and identified by cage number. The cages were placed within the two rooms of an isolation unit. Temperature in the isolation unit was between 20 °C and 25 °C, humidity between 20% and 70%, the light regimen was 12 h light and 12 h darkness and the air exchange rate was 15 times per hour. The mongooses were fed with a standardised feed of the following composition throughout the study: 26% poultry, 22% fish scraps, 12% beef heart, 5% beef liver/ beef kidney, 12% green tripe, 16% grain premix for fur animals with vitamins, minerals and water (Schirmer und Partner, 09306 Döhlen, Germany). Every animal received 35 – 50 g feed per day according to individual consumption behaviour and need. Additionally, twice a week, the mongooses received some fruit or vegetables and a boiled egg. Water was offered ad libitum. Animals were checked at least once per day and the individual general health status, food intake and defecation was recorded. In case the mongoose needed to be sedated or euthanized the following capture procedure was followed; a small cage-trap with a fixation mechanism was placed in front of the sleeping box. Once the animals were trapped, they received an intramuscular injection into the thigh muscles of a hind leg with a solution of Ketamin (26.5 mg/kg; Ketamin 10%, MEDISTAR Arzneimittelvertrieb GmbH, Germany) and Xylazin (0.9 mg/kg; Sedaxylan®, Eurovet Animal Health B.V.; Netherland). The euthanasia at the end of the studies was done under deep sedation by an intracardial injection with Pentorbital-Natrium (450 mg/kg; Release® 500 mg/ml; Wirtschaftsgenossenschaft deutscher Tierärzte eG; Germany).

Vaccine

The vaccine strain SPBN GASGAS is derived from SAD L16, a cDNA clone of the oral rabies virus vaccine strain SAD B19 [19, 20]. SPBN GASGAS lacks the pseudogene (Ψ) and has been genetically modified by site-directed mutagenesis at the amino acid positions 194 and 333 of the glycoprotein [21]. Furthermore, the construct contains a second identical glycoprotein gene with the described modifications [22, 23]. Two different doses, $10^{7.7}$ and $10^{9.1}$ FFU/ml SPBN GASGAS, were used in the studies. The virus material was produced according to the protocol given by Vos et al. [24]. Material for the overdose study was concentrated via tangential flow filtration using ultrafiltration flat sheet cassettes with a Molecular Weight Cut Off (MWCO) of 300 kDa.

Study protocol

As mentioned, there is no dedicated monograph from the regulatory authorities for oral rabies vaccines available in the US. Therefore, small adaptations have been made to the existing guidelines that are intended for live rabies virus vaccines delivered parenterally; 9 CFR 113.312 "Rabies Vaccine, Live Virus" (Table 1). The number of animals per study was based on the minimum numbers required by the regulatory authorities; to compensate for potential losses for the long observation period in the overdose study several surplus animals were included.

Overdose

According to 9 CFR 113.312, it is required to administer 10 doses of high virus titer material i.m. and by infiltrating a major nerve of at least 10 animals each and observe them for 90 days. As the intended route of administration is by offering the animals a vaccine bait the protocol has been adapted and 14 animals received a single dose (0.7 ml) of high-titred SPBN GASGAS ($10^{9.1}$ FFU/ml) by direct oral application onto the mucosae of the *palatum durum*, cheeks and under the tongue. Subsequently, the animals were observed for 182 days post administration. Blood samples were collected on day 0, 28 and 182 post vaccine administration and examined for the presence of virus neutralizing antibodies (VNA). Finally, the brain of the animals was examined for the presence of rabies virus antigen at the end of the observation period.

Repeated dose

5 mongooses received a dose of 0.7 ml of the vaccine strain ($10^{7.7}$ FFU/ml) by direct oral application on study days 0, 3 and 7. The observation period ended 56 days after the first administration of the vaccine strain and all animals were euthanized. Subsequently, the brain was examined for the presence of virus antigen. Blood samples were collected from all animals on study days 0, 28 and 56 for determination of the antibody titre.

Dissemination

For this purpose 12 mongooses received one dose (0.7 ml) SPBN GASGAS with a titre of $10^{7.7}$ FFU/ml. On study days 1, 2, 3, 5, 7 and 10 post administration two treated animals were euthanized and subsequently organs and tissues were collected to test for the presence of the vaccine strain. The following tissue samples were collected of all animals from the oral cavity; regional lymphnodes (*lnn. Mandibularis, lnn. reteropharyngeales*), upper and lower mucosa, tongue, soft palate, tonsils (*tonsilla sublingualis, tonsilla lingualis, tonsilla palatine, tonsilla pharyngica*). Additionally, samples from the brain (*hippocampus, medulla oblongata, cerebrum* and *cerebellum*) and additional tissues from the lungs, kidneys, bladder, heart, colon, jejunum and ileum were collected. Blood samples were collected prior to vaccination and at the time point of euthanasia for determination of seroconversion.

Different routes of administration

According to 9 CFR 113.312, 5 animals each should receive the vaccine intramuscularly (i.m.) or by infiltrating a major nerve and its surrounding tissue. The selected routes of administration have been slightly adapted for the intended oral use. Besides injecting the vaccine strain i.m., it was also administered by direct oral administration (d.o.a.). The d.o.a.-treated animals received 1.0 ml ($10^{7.7}$ FFU/ml) of the vaccine strain by direct application onto the mucosae of the pharynx and oral cavity after sedation. The other group received 1.0 ml SPBN GASGAS ($10^{7.7}$ FFU/ml) divided over 4 injection sites; the thigh muscles of both hind limbs and in the muscles of both shoulder blades. One animal of each group ($n = 5$) was sacrificed on day 15, 20, 25, 30 and 35 post vaccine administration. Instead of infiltrating a major nerve, the vaccine strain was directly inoculated intracerebrally (i.c.) in 5 animals. These animals were put under anaesthesia and shaved along a line between the outer canthus and area of the medial cranial line. This point was disinfected with iodine solution. An incision of about 1 cm in length was performed in the cranial-caudal direction up to the cranial bone. Small blood losses were stopped by tamponade. The skin along the wound was displaced to the side, and the superimposed muscle layers freed from the cranium. A hole measuring about 0.2 cm in diameter was drilled through the skull (trepanation) using a drill (DREMEL® 8200, DREMEL Europe, Netherlands). Using a 23G cannula, an inoculum of 0.1 ml ($10^{7.7}$ FFU/ml) was applied 1.0 cm deep into the left half of the cerebrum. The wound was closed with two individual staples and freed

Table 1 Overview of safety studies conducted in the small Indian mongoose

Purpose	Number of animals	Observation period (days)	Dose (titre; volume)
Repeated dose (day 0, 3 & 7)	5	56	$10^{7.7}$ FFU/ml; 0.7 ml
Dissemination	12	1, 2, 3, 5, 7 & 10	$10^{7.7}$ FFU/ml; 0.7 ml
Overdose	14	182	$10^{9.1}$ FFU/ml; 0.7 ml
Different routes of administration	5 (i.m.)	15, 20, 25, 30 & 35	$10^{7.7}$ FFU/ml; 1.0 ml
	5 (d.o.a)	15, 20, 25, 30 & 35	$10^{7.7}$ FFU/ml; 1.0 ml
	5 (i.c.)	3, 6, 9, 15 & 30	$10^{7.7}$ FFU/ml; 0.1 ml

from clotted blood. On day 3, 6, 9, 15 and 30 post administration one animal was sacrificed. For all animals, the brain, salivary glands, and kidneys were collected and tested for the presence of the vaccine strain. In addition, the *Lnn. mandibularis* and *Lnn. retropharyngeales* were taken from the d.o.a group and in the i.m. group regional lymph nodes were additionally taken near the application site.

Diagnostic assays

Rabies viral antigen in the brain (Ammons' horn, cerebellum and Medulla oblongata) of animals was detected by the fluorescent antibody test (FAT) using commercial monoclonal FITC- labelled anti-rabies antibodies (SIFIN, Berlin, Germany) and defined positive - and negative controls [25]. Tissues samples (10 mg – 100 mg) other than brain were homogenized in a volume of 1000 µl sterile minimum essential medium (MEM-10, with 2% Streptomycin). Subsequently, RNA was extracted from 200 µl organ suspension using the commercial RNeasy kit (Qiagen, Germany) and screened for vaccine viral RNA using a rabies virus specific RT-qPCR essentially as described [26]. RT-qPCR positive tissue samples were subject to investigation for presence of replication competent vaccine strain in the Rabies Tissue Culture Infection Test (RTCIT) on murine neuroblastoma (Na42/13) cells [27]. Three consecutive passages were conducted to confirm a negative result. Also, in case brain samples were FAT-inconclusive, the samples were subsequently examined by RTCIT.

Sera were tested for the presence of VNA in a modified rapid fluorescence focus inhibition test (RFFIT) and the Fluorescent Antibody Viral Neutralization (FAVN) essentially as described by Moore et al [28] and Cliquet et al [29], respectively, using rabies lyssavirus CVS-11 as test virus and BHK21-BSR/5 (CCLV-RIE 0194/260) cells. While the FAVN was used in the overdose study, RFFIT was applied in the other three studies. In each assay, the calibrated WHO international standard immunoglobulin (2nd human rabies immunoglobulin preparation, National Institute for Standards and Control, Potters Bar, UK) or the calibrated OIE serum of dog origin adjusted to 0.5 international units (IU) and a naive bovine serum served as positive – and negative control, respectively. VNA titres were calculated using inverse interpolation as described and subsequently converted into concentrations expressed in international units (IU/mL) [30]. VNA titres equal or greater than 0.5 IU/ml were considered positive.

Results

Overdose

2 of the 14 animals were euthanized before the end of the observation period: on day 38 and 56 post vaccine administration. The clinical signs observed did not indicate rabies and no rabies virus antigen was detected by FAT in the brains of these animals. Upon necropsy, both animals showed a hepatitis of unknown origin. All other animals showed no impairment of general health throughout the study, including body weight loss, and tested negative for the presence of rabies virus antigen in the brain. All animals tested seronegative before vaccination and subsequently seroconverted, except for one animal, post vaccine administration (FAVN). The geometric mean titre (GMT) was 8.32 IU/ml [range: 0.06–30.81] and 8.36 IU/ml [range: 1.98–30.81] on day 28 and 182 post vaccine administration, respectively (Table 2).

Repeated dose

All animals remained healthy and no critical clinical findings were observed during the entire observation period of 56 days. The brains of all study animals tested negative for the presence of rabies virus antigen (FAT). All five animals tested seronegative prior to vaccine administration and all animals developed a detectable immune response after vaccine administration. The GMT was 4.39 IU/ml [range: 1.61–11.56) and 3.51 IU/ml [range: 2.33–5.66] on day 28 and 56 after the first dose was administered, respectively (Table 3).

Dissemination

All but two of the selected tissues samples collected after d.o.a tested PCR-negative. While rabies virus could be

Table 2 Serological results of the overdose study

Animal	B0 day 0	B1 day 28	B2 day 182
1	0.04	7.81	2.60
2	0.04	13.52	23.42
3	0.04	30.81	n.d.
4	0.04	30.81	30.81
5	0.04	0.06	n.d.
6	0.04	17.79	23.42
7	0.04	3.43	3.43
8	0.04	1.14	3.43
9	0.04	30.81	23.42
10	0.04	13.52	1.98
11	0.04	30.81	5.93
12	0.04	23.42	23.42
13	0.04	10.27	4.51
14	0.04	5.93	7.81
GMT	0.04	8.32	8.36
s.d.	–	11.70	10.93

n.d. not determined since no sample available since animal was removed from study prior to the end of the observation period, *GMT* geometric mean titre (IU/ml - FAVN), *s.d.* standard deviation

Table 3 Level of virus neutralizing antibodies in sera after repeated administration of SPBN GASGAS

Animal	B0 (day 0)	B1 (day 28)	B2 (day 56)
1	0.06	4.77	3.02
2	0.04	1.61	5.66
3	0.08	11.56	4.56
4	0.07	3.75	2.97
5	0.04	4.78	2.33
GMT	0.06	4.37	3.52
s.d.	0.02	3.73	1.37

day number of days after first dose administered, *GMT* geometric mean titre (IU/ml – RFFIT), *s.d.* standard deviation

isolated in RTCIT from a PCR-positive lung sample taken from an animal 1 day after oral administration, virus isolation of a PCR-positive *Tonsilla sublingualis* of another animal sampled on day 7 after application of the test material failed. Furthermore, all brain samples tested negative for the presence of rabies virus antigen. Seroconversion (> 0.5 IU/ml) was observed only in animals sacrificed 10 days after vaccine administration (Table 4).

Different routes of administration

All animals tested seronegative (< 0.5 IU/ml) prior to vaccine administration; GMT = 0.07 IU/ml, [range: 0.02–0.36 IU/ml]. During the observation period, none of the animals showed any signs of illness or died during this period, including the animals that received the vaccine strain i.c. With the exception of one lymph node sample from the hind leg collected on day 15 post vaccine administration (i.m.), all tissue samples tested negative by PCR. The positive lymph node sample was found negative for the presence of viable virus by RTCIT. No virus antigen was detected in the brain of all 5 animals; already 3 days post vaccine administration i.c. As the vaccine strain was directly inoculated in the brain, it can be concluded that it must have been rapidly cleared from the brain.

Discussion

The native range of the small Indian mongoose stretches from the Middle East to Myanmar [31]. It has also been introduced to many islands in the Pacific and Indian Oceans, the Caribbean and Adriatic seas and to continental South America and Europe; predominantly in the late 19th and early twentieth century [1, 31]. In the Caribbean, the small Indian mongoose is present on 33 islands [1], but only on 4 islands rabies in mongoose has been reported; Grenada, Dominican Republic, Cuba and Puerto Rico [2]. The first major outbreak attributed to the small Indian mongoose started in 1950 in Puerto Rico [32]. In its natural distribution area it has not been identified as an important vector of rabies. Also elsewhere, only sporadic cases of rabies in other mongoose species are reported; for example India, Sri Lanka, Israel, and Nigeria [33–36]. The only other region where rabies in mongooses has been well described and is regularly reported is southern Africa [37–39]. In order to eliminate mongoose rabies in the Caribbean population control measures have not been successful [1, 2] and hence alternative methods have been suggested [4, 10, 40, 41]. Since several years, Wildlife Services of the Animal and Plant Health Inspection Service, United States Department of Agriculture (USDA/APHIS/WS) is investigating the possibility of oral vaccination of mongoose against rabies in Puerto Rico [5]. One of the prerequisites for oral vaccination is a highly efficacious and safe vaccine for the target species. The results of the safety studies presented here showed that this vaccine strain SPBN GASGAS is innocuous for the target species, the small Indian mongoose, irrespective of dose and route administered. Even direct inoculation in the brain did not result in rabies infection. Also, repeated application of the construct did not induce any adverse reaction in the animals. After oral administration, the vaccine did not disseminate to any of the organs or tissues examined. Only in one lung sample taken 24 h after oral administration, the vaccine virus was re-isolated. The position of the lungs and the time of sampling in relation to time of application lead to the assumption that the vaccine was most likely aspirated into the lungs during

Table 4 Serological results of the dissemination study: RFFIT – IU/ml

sample day (post vacc.)	Animal											
	1	2	3	4	5	6	7	8	9	10	11	12
0	0.02	0.05	0.11	0.02	0.02	0.11	0.07	0.02	0.03	0.10	0.02	0.12
1	0.08	0.09										
2			0.08	0.08								
3					0.06	0.07						
5							0.04	0.19				
7									0.42	0.16		
10											5.43	10.03

forced administration under sedation. It is highly unlikely that the vaccine would enter the respiratory tract under natural condition when an animal consumes a bait. Interestingly, no virus was found in the palatine tonsils as this was determined as the primary site of uptake after oral administration [42]. Finally, no infectious vaccine virus was detected in fecal samples and saliva swabs collected during the overdose and dissemination study, although viral RNA was detected in several of these samples [19]. All mongooses of which blood samples were collected seroconverted with the exception of one animal (overdose study), indicating successful vaccine uptake (Tables 2-4). Outside the scope of the studies presented here, additional safety studies have to be performed in non-target species, since all species inhabiting an area where baits are distributed can locate and come in contact with the vaccine virus. Hence, a risk assessment has to be carried out identifying possible non-target species for which additional safety studies need to be conducted.

Conclusion

It can be concluded that the vaccine strain SPBN GASGAS fulfils the safety requirements for live rabies virus vaccines. Hence, this efficacious vaccine construct is a suitable candidate for oral vaccination of the small Indian mongoose against rabies.

Acknowledgements
We would like to acknowledge Ivan Budinski for capturing the animals and Jeannette Kliemt for her excellent diagnostic skills.

Funding
No external funding has been received.

Authors' contributions
SO, AK and AV were responsible for the study design. IL, CK, AK, WN and SO coordinated and supervised the animal studies and collection of samples. TM and CF were responsible for diagnostics. SO, TM and AV contributed writing the manuscript. All authors read and approved the final manuscript.

Competing interest
AK, SO, NW, CK and AV are full-time employee of IDT Biologika GmbH, a manufacturer of oral rabies vaccine baits. TM and CMF from the Friedrich-Loeffler-Institute received funding from IDT Biologika GmbH for research into mechanisms of oral rabies vaccination and serological response. IL – not applicable.

Ethics approval
All animals were kept in accordance with the prevailing guidelines and the in vivo studies were performed according to European guidelines on animal welfare, clinical endpoints, and care of the Federation of European Laboratory Animal Science Associations (FELASA). The required permits, including ethical approval, for the animal studies were obtained from the appropriate veterinary authorities in the federal state of Saxony Anhalt, Germany (Landesverwaltungsamt Sachsen – Anhalt, Referat Verbraucherschutz, Veterinärangelegenheiten, approval number AZ 42502-3-762). Approval and subsequent release of the captured animals was obtained by the custom veterinary officials in Croatia; TRACES documents for intra-community trade intra.hr.2016.0004862-V1 and intra.hr.2016.0005574-V1.

Consent for publication
not applicable.

Author details
[1]IDT Biologika GmbH, Am Pharmapark, 06861 Dessau Rosslau, Germany. [2]Institute of Molecular Virology and Cell Biology, Friedrich-Loeffler-Institute, Südufer 10, 17493 Greifswald, Insel Riems, Germany. [3]Department of Virology, Croatian Veterinary Institute, Svaská cesta 143, 10000 Zagreb, Croatia.

References

1. Barun A, Hanson CC, Campbell KJ, DI S. A review of the small Indian mongoose management and eradications on islands. In: Veitch CR, Clout MN, Towns DR, editors. Islands invasives: eradication and management. Gland: IUCN; 2011. p. 17–25.
2. Everard COR, Everard JD. Mongoose rabies in the Caribbean. Ann N Y Acad Sci. 1992;16:356–66.
3. Everard COR, Baer GM, Alls ME, Moore SA. Rabies serum neutralizing antibody in mongooses from Grenada. Trans R Soc Trop Med Hyg. 1981;75: 654–6.
4. Blanton JD, Meadows A, Murphy SM, Manangan J, Hanlon CA, Faber ML, Dietzschold B, Rupprecht CE. Vaccination of small Asian mongoose (Herpestes javanicus) against rabies. J Wildl Dis. 2006;42:663–6.
5. Berentsen AR, Johnson SR, VerCauteren KC, Gruver K, Boyd F, Gilbert AT, Chipman RB. Mongoose research by USDA wildlife Services in Puerto Rico, 2011 – 2015: implications for oral rabies vaccination. In: Abstracts RITA 2015, rabies in the Americas, Fort Collins, Colorado. p. 2015.
6. Müller T, Freuling CM, Wysocki P, Roumiantzeff M, Freney J, Mettenleiter TC, Vos A. Terrestrial rabies control in the European Union: historical achievements and challenges ahead. Vet J. 2015;203:10–7.
7. Rosatte R. Evolution of wildlife rabies control tactics. Adv Virus Res. 2011;79: 397–419.
8. Vos A, Kretzschmar A, Ortmann S, Lojkic I, Habla C, Müller T, Kaiser C, Hundt B, Schuster P. Oral vaccination of captive small Indian mongoose against rabies. J Wildl Dis. 2013;49:1033–6.
9. Linhart SB, Creekmore TE, Corn JL, Whitney MD, Snyder BD, Nettles VF. Evaluation of baits for oral rabies vaccination of mongooses: pilot field trials in Antigua, West Indies. J Wildl Dis. 1993;29:290–4.
10. Creekmore TE, Linhart SB, Corn JL, Whitney MD, Snyder BD, Nettles VF. Field evaluation of baits and baiting strategies for delivering oral vaccine to mongooses in Antigua, West Indies. J Wildl Dis. 1994;30:497–505.
11. Berentsen A, Johnson SR, VerCauteren KC. Bait matrix flavor preference by mongoose (Herpestes auropunctatus) in Puerto Rico: implications for oral rabies vaccination. Caribb J Sci. 2014;48:52–8.
12. 9 CFR 113.312 "Rabies Vaccine, Live Virus". https://www.gpo.gov/fdsys/pkg/CFR-2012-title9-vol1/pdf/CFR-2012-title9-vol1-sec113-312.pdf. Accessed 15 March 2016
13. United States Department of Agriculture, Animal and Plant Health Inspection Service. Veterinary Services Memoranda. https://www.aphis.usda.gov/aphis/ourfocus/animalhealth/veterinary-biologics/biologics-regulations-and-guidance/ct_vb_vs_memos. Accessed 15 March 2016.
14. Hadidian J, Jenkins SR, Johnston DH, Savarie PJ, Nettles VF, Manski D, Baer GM. Acceptance of simulated oral rabies vaccine baits by urban raccoons. J Wildl Dis. 1989;25:1–9.
15. Hable CP, Hamir AN, Snyder DE, Joyner R, French J, Nettles V, Hanlon C, Rupprecht CE. Prerequisites for oral immunization of free-ranging raccoons (Procyon lotor) with a recombinant rabies virus vaccine: study site ecology and bait system development. J Wildl Dis. 1992;28:64–79.
16. Blackwell BF, Seamans TW, White RJ, Patton ZJ, Bush RM, Cepek JD. Exposure time of oral rabies vaccine baits relative to baiting density and raccoon population density. J Wildl Dis. 2004;40:222–9.
17. Vos A, Sutor A, Selhorst T, Schwarz S, Pötzsch C, Staubach C, Müller T. The spatial and temporal disappearance of different oral rabies vaccine baits. Berl Munch Tierarztl Wochenschr. 2004;117:360–6.
18. Vos A, Neubert A. Thermo-stability of the oral rabies virus vaccines SAD B19 and SAD P5/88. Dtsch Tierarztl Wochenschr. 2002;109:428–32.

19. Vos A, Freuling C, Ortmann S, Kretzschmar A, Mayer D, Schliephake A, Müller T. An assessment of shedding with the oral rabies virus vaccine strain SPBN GASGAS in target and non-target species. Vaccine. 2018;36:811–7.
20. Schnell MJ, Mebatsion T, Conzelmann KK. Infectious rabies viruses from cloned cDNA. EMBO J. 1994;13:4195–203.
21. Faber M, Faber ML, Papaneri A, Bette M, Weihe E, Dietzschold B, Schnell MJ. A single amino acid change in rabies virus glycoprotein increases virus spread and enhances virus pathogenicity. J Virol. 2005;79:14141–8.
22. Faber M, Pulmanausahakul R, Hodawadekar SS, Spitsin S, McGettigan JP, Schnell MJ. Overexpression of the rabies virus glycoprotein results in enhancement of apoptosis and antiviral immune response. J Virol. 2002;76: 3374–81.
23. Faber M, Faber ML, Li J, Preuss MA, Schnell MJ, Dietzschold B. Dominance of a nonpathogenic glycoprotein gene over a pathogenic glycoprotein gene in rabies virus. J Virol. 2007;81:7041–7.
24. Vos A, Neumann G, Hundt B, Neubert A. Attenuated vaccines for veterinary use. In: Rupprecht C, Nagarajan T, editors. Current laboratory techniques in rabies diagnosis, research and prevention, volume 1. San Diego: Elsevier Academic Press; 2015. p. 237–44.
25. Dean DJ, Abelseth MK, Atanasiu P. The fluorescent antibody test. In: Meslin F-X, Kaplan MM, Koprowski H, editors. Laboratory techniques in rabies. 4th ed. Geneva: World Health Organization; 1996. p. 88–95.
26. Hoffmann B, Freuling CM, Wakeley PR, Rasmussen TB, Leech S, Fooks AR, Beer M, Müller T. Improved safety for molecular diagnosis of classical rabies viruses by use of a TaqMan real-time reverse transcription-PCR "double check" strategy. J Clin Microbiol. 2010;48:3970–8.
27. Webster WA, Casey GA. Virus isolation in neuroblastoma cell culture. In: Meslin FX, Kaplan MM, Kaprowski H, editors. Laboratory techniques in rabies. 4th ed. Geneva, World Health Organization; 1996. p. 96–104.
28. Moore S, Gilbert A, Vos A, Freuling C, Ellis C, Kliemt J, Müller T. Review of rabies virus antibodies from oral vaccination as a correlate of protection against lethal infection in animals. Trop Med Infect Dis. 2017;2:31.
29. Cliquet F, Aubert M, Sagné L. Development of a fluorescent antibody virus neutralisation test (FAVN test) for the quantitation of rabies-neutralising antibody. J Immunol Methods. 1998;212:79–87.
30. Müller T, Selhorst T, Burow J, Schameitat A, Vos A. Cross-reactive antigenicity in orally vaccinated foxes and raccoon dogs against European bat lyssavirus type 1 and 2. Dev Biol. 2006;125:195–204.
31. Barun A, Simberloff D, Tcrtkovic N, Pascal M. Impact of the introduced small Indian mongoose (Herpestes auropunctatus) on abundance and activity time of the introduced ship rat (Rattus rattus) and the small mammal community on Adriatic islands, Croatia. NeoBiota. 2011;11:51–61.
32. Tierkel ES, Arbona G, Rivera A, De Juan A. Mongoose rabies in Puerto Rico. Public Health Rep. 1952;67:274–8.
33. Mani RS, Moorkoth AP, Balasubramanian P, Devi K, Madhusudana SN. Rabies following mongoose bite. Indian J Med Microbiol. 2016;34:256–7.
34. Patabendige CGUA, Wimalaratne O. Rabies in mongooses and domestic rats in the Southern Province of Sri Lanka. Ceylon Med J. 2003;48:48–50.
35. Shimshony A. Epidemiology of emerging zoonoses in Israel. Emerg Infect Dis. 1997;3:229–38.
36. Atuman YJ, Adawa DAY, Okewole PA, Shamaki D, Audu SW, Mshelbwala PP, Ogunkoya AB. Detection of rabies antigens in the brain tissues of jackals and mongooses and its implications on public health and conservation goals in Bauchi state Nigeria. Scientific J Vet Adv. 2014;3:42–7.
37. Nel LH, Sabeta CT, von Teichman B, Jaftha JB, Rupprecht CE, Bingham J. Mongoose rabies in southern Africa: a re-evaluation based on molecular epidemiology. Virus Res. 2005;109:165–73.
38. Davis PL, Rambaut A, Bourhy H, Holmes EC. The evolutionary dynamics of canid and mongoose rabies virus in southern Africa. Arch Virol. 2007;152: 1251–8.
39. Van Zyl N, Markotter W, Nel LH. Evolutionary history of African mongoose rabies. Virus Res. 2010;150:93–102.
40. Everard CO, Everard JD. Mongoose rabies. Rev Infect Dis. 1988;10:S610-4.
41. Zieger U, Marston DA, Sharma R, Chikweto A, Tiwari K, Sayyid M, Louison B, Goharriz H, Voller K, Breed AC, Werling D, Fooks AR, Horton DL. The Phylogeography of rabies in Grenada, West Indies, and implications for control. PLoS Negl Trop Dis. 2014;8:e3251.
42. Vos A, Freuling CM, Hundt B, Kaiser C, Nemitz S, Neubert A, Nolden T, Teifke JP, Te Kamp V, Ulrich R, Finke S, Müller T. Oral vaccination of wildlife against rabies: differences among host species in vaccine uptake efficiency. Vaccine. 2017;35:3938–44.

18

Nutrient digestibility, organ morphometry and performance in vaccinated or non-vaccinated *Lawsonia intracellularis* infected piglets

Christian Visscher[1*], Jasmin Mischok[1], Saara Sander[1], Marion Schmicke[2], Eva-Ursula Peitzmeier[3], Isabel von dem Busche[3], Karl Rohn[4] and Josef Kamphues[1]

Abstract

Background: *Lawsonia intracellularis* is one of the world's most important infectious diseases in pork production with regard to economic losses. So far, studies are missing that describe the effects of a natural infection of piglets on the digestibility of nutrients, possible effects on performance and the morphometrics of the intestine depending on whether piglets are vaccinated, clinically healthy or clinically affected with regard to *Lawsonia intracellularis* induced diarrhoea.

Results: Digestibility studies were performed on a total of 27 eight-week-old piglets with naturally occurring *Lawsonia intracellularis* infection in a trial with three repetitions. Nine out of 27 animals were vaccinated as suckling pigs with a commercial *Lawsonia intracellularis* vaccine (vac; Enterisol®Ileitis). Half of the remaining 18 animals were without clinical signs of infection (non-vac/cs-), half showed moderate clinical signs of *Lawsonia intracellularis* induced diarrhoea (non-vac/cs+). All three groups were fed one identical complete diet *ad libitum*. Faecal shedding of *Lawsonia intracellularis* was found in all groups (25 out of 27 animals). Numerically, the mean excretion in the group non-vac/cs + (7.69 ± 1.65 $\log_{10}$ copies/ g faeces) was higher in comparison to the group non-vac/cs- (5.83 ± 2.35 $\log_{10}$ copies/ g faeces) and vaccinated animals (vac: 6.00 ± 2.89$\log_{10}$ copies/ g faeces). The average daily weight gain (ADG; Ø 8.66 day period) differed significantly (vac: 894^{a} ± 73.3, non-vac/cs-: 857^{ab} ± 86.3, non-vac/cs+: 785^{b} ± 137 g/day). The apparent total tract digestibility (ATTD) of nitrogen was significantly lower in clinically affected animals (vac: 83.0^{a} ± 1.72, non-vac/cs-: 83.9^{a} ± 2.03, non-vac/cs+: 80.7^{b} ± 2.57).The total length of the small intestine in clinically affected animals increased significantly (vac: 15.9^{ab} ± 1.57, non-vac/cs-: 14.6^{b} ± 1.12, non-vac/cs+: 16.2^{a} ± 1.37 m). The relative body weight depending on the length of the small intestine was lower for clinically affected animals (vac: 1.72^{a} ± 0.21, non-vac/cs-: 1.83^{a} ± 0.17, non-vac/cs+: 1.56^{b} ± 0.12 kg/m).

Conclusion: These studies show that clinically moderate *L. intracellularis* infections lead to significantly lower ADGs in comparison to vaccinated animals. The disease is also found in altered intestinal morphometry and reduced total N digestibility if clinical signs occur.

Keywords: *Lawsonia intracellularis* infection, Vaccination, Digestibility, Performance, IGF-1, Organ morphometrics

* Correspondence: Christian.Visscher@tiho-hannover.de
[1]Institute for Animal Nutrition, University of Veterinary Medicine Hannover, Foundation, Bischofsholer Damm 15, D-30173 Hannover, Germany
Full list of author information is available at the end of the article

Background

Infections with *Lawsonia intracellularis* (*L. intracellularis*) in pigs lead to economic losses both in the case of clinical manifestations and subclinical infections [1–4]. Lower performance results from reduced growth and an impaired feed efficacy [5–8]. The overall prolonged rearing and fattening period is a typical finding of subclinical infections [1, 9–11]. This is a common sign of an *L. intracellularis* infection in practice [2]. Clinically apparent infections are traditionally associated with diarrhoea and can be related to animal losses due to the haemorrhagic course named porcine haemorrhagic enteropathy [4, 12]. These may occur more frequently in individual stocks, but play a less important role overall [13].

In order to convert the absorbed nutrients at their highest rate into weight gain, a good state of health of the growing animals is essential. This excludes any avoidable activation of an inflammatory immune response, which might also be common for gastrointestinal infections [14]. High concentrations of proinflammatory cytokines often lead to a condition known as the systemic inflammatory response syndrome (SIRS) [15] which is often related to sickness symptoms like decreased feed and water intake [15, 16]. The reduced appetite is mediated by these aforementioned cytokines acting in the central nervous system [15–17]. There are findings indicating that Insulin-like growth factor 1 (IGF-1) is potent in attenuating sickness behaviour induced by tumour necrosis factor-alpha [17]. On the other hand there are indications that the immune response is hardly activated in the initial course of an infection with *L. intracellularis* [18].

In general, an immediate reduction in average daily feed intake (ADFI) for pigs affected by digestive bacterial infections can be estimated at 15% [19]. Nonetheless, also an impaired digestibility of the nutrients has to be considered in cases of an *L. intracellularis* infection. With regard to the pathomorphological changes in the intestines of infected pigs, it has to be assumed that due to the reduced permeability of the intestinal wall there is a reduced absorption of certain nutrients in cases of an *L. intracellularis* infection [20, 21]. For infections with porcine epidemic diarrhoea virus apparent total tract digestibility (ATTD) of dry matter (DM) and energy are decreased by 8 and 12%, respectively [22]. However, the digestibility of nutrients and the concentrations of nutrients in the digesta of the terminal ileum influence the length of the gastrointestinal tract [23]. This is particularly noticeable after weaning because here very fast adaptation can be seen in the form of elongation [23]. In general, the response of the gastrointestinal tract to ingestion of nutrients is a complex and closely controlled process [24]. Mechanical and chemical control mechanisms are involved in the short and long term. Due to the feed consumption there is a distension of hollow viscera along with activation of both elongation and tension mechanoreceptors [24]. There are simultaneously nutrient-sensing chemoreceptors in the upper gastrointestinal tract [24]. These are involved in detecting the presence of all main categories of nutrients in the lumen [24]. A leading mechanism of intestinal adaption to enteral nutrients is driven by humural factors like the intestinotrophic peptide glucagon-like peptide-2 (GLP-2) [25, 26]. Enteroendocrine L-cells secrete GLP-2 after direct stimulation by nutrients distally in the small intestine [25].

To date, no investigation has been carried out on how an infection with *L. intracellularis* might affect the digestibility of nutrients, performance, IGF-1 status and gastrointestinal tract morphometry as a result of natural exposure when non-vaccinated and vaccinated animals are compared.

Methods

Animal experiments were carried out according to German regulations. It was not an animal experiment requiring a notification or an approval according to the Animal Protection Act (§ 7, paragraph 2, sentence 3). Interventions before dissection were not carried out. The animals were killed according to § 4, paragraph 3 of the Animal Protection Act, exclusively to use their organs or tissues for scientific purposes.

Origin of animals, preparation and selection

All animals used in these trials came from one farm with 420 sows of Danish genetics (DK: Danish Landrace 50% x Yorkshire 50%). In total, 27 piglets (DK x Pietrain) were used in a trial with three repetitions. The sows in the herd were regularly vaccinated (Porcine Reproductive and Respiratory Syndrome Virus, Swine Influenza Virus, Porcine Parvovirus, *Erysipelothrix rhusiopathiae*, *Escherichia coli* + *Clostridium perfringens* dam vaccine) as were the piglets (Porcine Circovirus 2, *Mycoplasma hyopneumoniae* and *Haemophilus parasuis*). In the context of regular and long-term screening programmes, the herd showed no signs of *Salmonella* and *Brachyspira* infections. Clinical symptoms of an *L. intracellularis* infection (confirmed by pathogen detection in faeces) were, on the other hand, a common finding in piglets at an age of seven to nine weeks. Before the starting the experimental trials, additional results of serological analyses of piglets were obtained from the veterinarian of the herd. From these random tests in the rearing phase of piglets, it was found that there were no serological positive animals in the middle of this phase whereas at the end of the rearing phase, only 10% were still serological negative (data not shown).

The production system on the farm was organised in a two-week rhythm. During the trial period every two weeks approximately 50 piglets from a total of four to five complete litters were vaccinated with a commercial *L. intracellularis* vaccine (Enterisol® Ileitis, Boehringer Ingelheim Vetmedica GmbH, Ingelheim / Rhine, Germany) on the 21st day of life. The vaccination was done via oral drenching. Subsequently, the piglets were marked individually.

At weaning all 450 to 500 piglets in a group were placed in a piglet rearing compartment in groups of 12 to about 30 animals on fully slatted floors (Fig. 1). Non-vaccinated and vaccinated animals were mixed. From weaning to the presumed initial *L. intracellularis* infection time point, samples from the individual stables were tested for their *L. intracellularis* status by real-time PCR using established methods [27]. With the positive proof a change to a single-animal examination procedure took place. All piglets in a weaning group were clinically examined. Individual samples were collected from conspicuous animals with regard to faecal quality (healthy pigs with moderate to soft feaces consistency) and analysed by means of real-time PCR [27]. After obtaining the results, three conspicuous animals (no siblings) were taken from the appropriate weaning group (non-vac/cs+). At the same time three clinically healthy ones (non-vac/cs-) and three vaccinated animals (vac+) of the same age and identical weight were chosen from the group, if possible in a balanced gender relationship. All selected animals were transported to the Institute for Animal Nutrition, University of Veterinary Medicine Hannover, Foundation, Hannover, Germany.

Animal husbandry and experimental conditions

The pigs were housed individually in 3 × 1 m boxes during the entire trial period. The boxes were equipped with a nipple drinker, a 1 m long earthenware trough at one of the narrow sides of the box, an infrared warming lamp and (manipulable material). Visual contact to other animals was possible at all times. The boxes had a concrete floor. All three repetitions of the trial were performed identically.

Diet and digestibility trials

The pigs continued to receive the diet they were accustomed to on the farm. The diet contained 41.0% wheat, 35.0% barley, 18.0% soybean meal, 2.00% soybean oil and 4.00% of a mineral and vitamin supplement (MOVIKALIN Speed 10®, HS-Kraftfutterwerk, Ochtrup, Germany; Table 1).

The nutrient composition was in accordance with the official recommendation for piglets in Germany. The complete diet for all trial repetitions derived from one batch. The digestibility trial consisted of two phases starting with a 3-day adaptation period followed by a five-day collection period. The adaptation period was shortened to only three days due to the use of the identical diet already on the farm. In this way, the experiment still focused on the clinically conspicuous phase of the natural *L. intracellularis* infection. Chromium oxide (0.5%) was added to the diet as a marker for calculating the precaecal digestibility. The diet was offered *ad libitum*. The feed was changed once a day. Feed refusals were removed and the amount determined after drying at 103 °C. The collected faeces were weighed by means of electronic scales (Acculab, Sartorius AG, Göttingen, Germany) and then frozen. At the end of the collection period, an aliquot of the total amount of faeces was collected after thawing and homogenisation for further analysis.

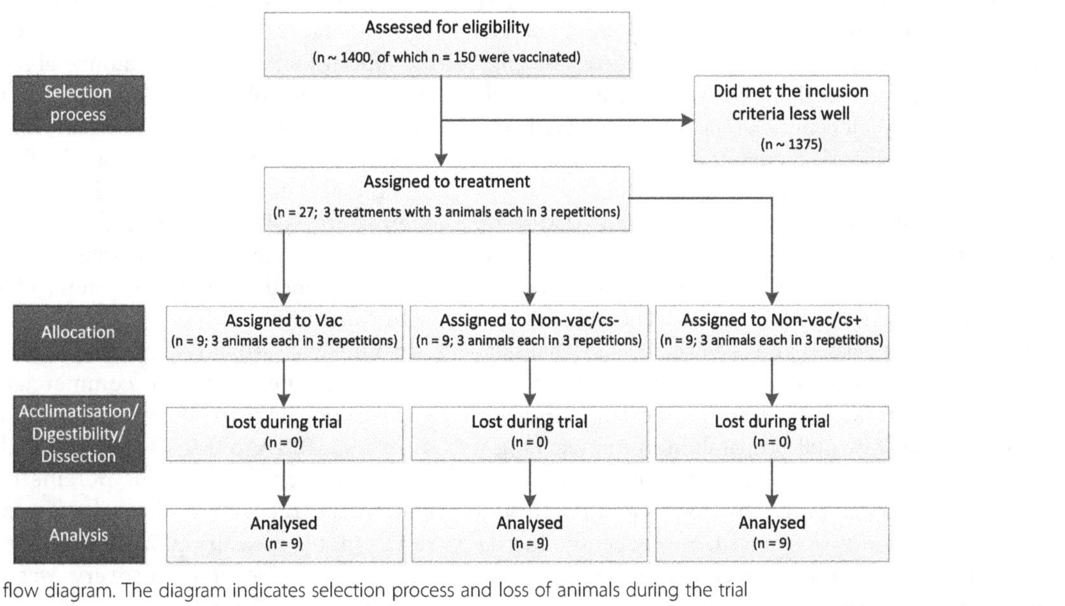

Fig. 1 Clinical trial flow diagram. The diagram indicates selection process and loss of animals during the trial

Table 1 Energy content and concentrations of ingredients in the diet for rearing piglets

Item		Content
Metabolisable Energy (ME, MJ)	per kg diet	13.8
Crude ash	g/kg DM	56.7
Crude fat		38.4
Crude fibre		26.9
Crude protein		201
Starch		480
Sugar		21.6
Lysin		16.5
Ca		9.88
P		6.38
Na		2.14
Cu	mg/kg DM	156
Zn		150
Se		0.44

Mineral and Vitamin supplement (4% of complete diet) contained 500,000 I.E Vit A, 50000 I.E. Vit. D3, 3000 mg Vit. E, 30 mg Jodine

Dissection

At day of the dissection the pigs were fed in a timely manner. There was an interval of nine hours between offering the fresh diet and death of each animal. In each repetition 3 out of 9 animals were dissected on the day of finishing the digestibility trial, the remaining animals on the following day. Prior to the dissection the animals were anaesthetised with neuroleptanalgesia by means of a combination of ketamine (Ursotamin® 10%, Serumwerke Bernburg, Bernburg, Germany; active ingredient: ketamine hydrochloride, dosage: 15 mg/kg body weight intramuscularly) and azaperone (Stresnil® 4% Janssen Animal Health, Neuss, Germany; active ingredient: azaperone, dosage: 2 mg/kg body weight intramuscularly). In the course of the dissection a blood sample was taken intracardially from the pigs. After that, pigs were euthanised with T61®intracardially (Intervet, Unterschleißheim, Germany; active ingredients: tetracaine hydrochloride, embutramide, mebenzonium iodide, dosage: 0.6 mL/10 kg body weight).

Before opening the abdominal cavity the naso-rump length of the animals was measured. The abdominal cavity was opened along the linea alba as well as a relief cut being performed in the flank region. The caecum was pre-placed, double-ligated and then removed. Other ligatures were placed directly between the pylorus and the jejunum and in front of the rectum. The removal of the stomach was done by dull preparation of the diaphragm and connective tissue. After placing an intestinal clamp on the cardia and severing the connection to the jejunum, the stomach was removed. Subsequently, the removal of the whole intestinal tract and the application of a ligature between the colon and the jejunum took place. Both the colon and the jejunum were freed from the mesenterium and their total length was measured in the filled state, also the length of the blind arm was measured. Digesta from the terminal small intestine for precaecal digestibility determination was taken in accordance with common procedures [22]. The contents of the different segments (stomach, small intestine, caecum, colon) were collected separately in plastic containers and used for further analysis.

Analytical methods

Diets were analysed by standard procedures in accordance with the official methods of the VDLUFA [28].The analyses were always performed in duplicate. The dry matter content was determined by drying to the weight constancy at 103 °C. The crude ash was analysed by means of incineration in the muffle furnace at 600 °C for 6 h. The total nitrogen content was determined by means of the analyser Vario Max® (Elementar, Hanau, Germany), which operates according to the principle of a catalytic tube combustion (DUMAS combustion method). The molecular nitrogen formed by reduction from nitric oxide was detected by a thermal conductivity detector and the nitrogen content was calculated by the device software. The crude protein content of the sample was calculated by multiplication with a constant factor of 6.25. The crude fat content was determined after acid hydrolysis in the Soxhlet apparatus. The content of crude fibre was determined after washing in diluted acids and alkalis by established methods. The determination of starch contents was carried out polarimetrically (Polatronic E, Schmidt und Haensch GmbH & Co., Berlin, Germany). The sugar content was analysed according to Luff-Schoorl by titration with sodium thiosulphate. The mineral content was determined in accordance with the official methods [28] by atomic absorption spectrometry (Unicam Solaar 116, Thermo, Dreieich, Germany). The analyses of the chyme were performed in principle by the identical methods as described for feeds.

The determination of mean *L. intracellularis* genome equivalents (GE) was done from the aliquot of the homogenised faeces via quantitative PCR according to established methods [29]. The numbers are shown in the logarithm of 10.

Insulin-like growth factor I (IGF-1) concentration was determined using a commercial radioimmunoassay acoording to the standard operation manual (A15729, IRMA IGF-I; Beckman Coulter, CA, USA). The assay was validated for porcine plasma by determining the recovery and an intra-assay coefficient of variation by measuring 20 times one sample within one test routine. The recovery was 94,5% and the intra-assay was 6,3%.

Statistical analyses

Normal distribution of the model residuals was confirmed by Kolmogorov-Smirnov-Test and visual assessment of q-q - plots. All data were included into a descriptive analysis with calculation of the arithmetic mean, standard deviation, minimum and maximum.

The influence of the factor group (vac, non-vac/cs-, non-vac/cs+) on the quantitative variables (Log10 genome equivalents; DM faeces, performance parameters, digestibility nutrients, organ morphometry parameters) was carried out by a one way variance analysis of variance (ANOVA) with REGWQ (Ryan-Einot-Gabriel-Welsch multiple Range-Test) post hoc test for multiple pairwise comparisons, concerning the experimentwise errorrate.

Analyses were carried out with the statistical software SAS, version 9.3 (SAS Institute, Cary, NC, USA), using SAS® Enterprise Guide 5.1. Differences were taken to be statistically significant when $P < 0.05$.

Results

The investigations were carried out on a total of 27 piglets. In all three repetitions of the trial, the general health status of each animal was checked at least twice a day. The 27 animals showed an undisturbed general state. Moderate clinical diarrhoea in all animals of the non-vaccinated, clinically affected group (non-vac/cs+) previously found on the farm was included in the study as a selection criteria (moderate diarrhoea induced by *L. intracellularis*).

Lawsonia intracellularis excretion and performance

Faecal shedding of *L. intracellularis* was found in all groups (25 out of 27 animals). There were no statistically significant differences in the absolute level of pathogen excretion (Table 2). Numerically, the mean excretion in the groups non-vac/cs- and vac was lower (– 1.87 or rather – 1.70 log units/g faeces). The clinically affected animals showed at the same time significantly lower faecal dry matter compared to the other two groups (– 10.6% compared to vac and – 13.9% compared to the group non-vac/cs-). Neither at the trial's start nor at the time of the dissection did the body masses differ between the three groups. The daily feed intake did not differ significantly between groups. Numerically, differences between the groups could be seen. The feed intake in the group non-vac/cs + was reduced by 10.2% and in group non-vac/cs- by 6.94% compared to the feed intake of vaccinated animals. However, the sample size included only 2 out of 3 trials. The average daily body weight gains (ADG) were significantly different between the clinically affected (non-vac/cs+) and the vaccinated group (vac). In the former, the growth was reduced by 12.2%. The non-vaccinated, clinically healthy animals showed no significant differences in average daily gains compared to one of the other groups. These were only 4.14% lower than for the group vac. The FCR did not differ between the groups.

In the animals' blood at the time of dissection the concentrations of IGF-1 were measured (Fig. 2). There were no significant differences in the IGF-1 levels between the three groups (Mean ± SD in ng/mL; vac: 285 ± 68.3; non-vac/cs-: 272 ± 57.1; non-vac/cs+: 226 ± 74.4).

Table 2 Overview on Lawsonia intracellularis excretion, dry matter content of faeces and growth performance

Item	Vac		Non-vac/cs-		Non-vac/cs+	
	Mean	SD	Mean	SD	Mean	SD
Log_{10} genome equivalents	6.00	2.89	5.83	2.35	7.69	1.65
DM faeces (g/kg DM)	23.6[a]	1.84	24.5[a]	1.68	21.1[b]	1.98
BW start (kg)	19.2	1.64	19.2	1.36	18.4	1.53
BW Dissection (kg)[c]	27.0	1.71	26.7	2.19	25.3	2.43
ADFI (kg DM/day)[d]	1.297	0.116	1.207	0.119	1.165	0.148
ADG (kg/day)	0.894[a]	0.073	0.857[ab]	0.086	0.785[b]	0.137
FCR (kg diet/kg ADG)	1.410	0.075	1.422	0.078	1.470	0.061

Vac vaccinated with Enterisol®Ileitis, *Non-vac/cs-* not vaccinated, clinically no signs, *Non-vac/cs +* not vaccinated, clinical signs

[a,b]Values within a row with different superscripts differ significantly at $P < 0.05$

[c]Dissection was done in 3 out of 9 animals 8 days after starting experiment, in 6 out of 9 piglets 9 days after start of experiment

[d]Due to technical detection problems, three values are missing from one of three repetitions

Digestibility of nutrients

There were no differences between the groups in regard to the precaecal digestibility of nutrients (Table 3).

The ATTD of the nutrients differed significantly only with respect to the crude protein (Table 4). The group with clinically affected animals showed a significantly lower N-digestibility (– 2.77% compared to group vac; – 3.81% compared to non-vac/cs-). The digestibility of organic matter, raw fat, crude fibre and starch did not differ significantly.

Morphometry of organs

The total length of the small intestine in clinically conspicuous animals was significantly longer (+ 1.60 m against group non-vac/cs-; Table 5). In relation to the nose-rump length, the body mass was significantly higher in vaccinated animals (+ 7.8% per m). That means, it is concentrated more mass per unit of length. Also, the clinically inconspicuous animals had a significantly higher body mass per m length of the small intestine (+ 17.3% per m) in relation to clinically conspicuous animals.

The vaccinated animals had the highest ADG (+ 15.4% per m) in proportion to the nose-rump length. Therefore, per unit body length more gain in body mass is concentrated. The vaccinated and also the clinically inconspicuous animals each had the highest ADG in

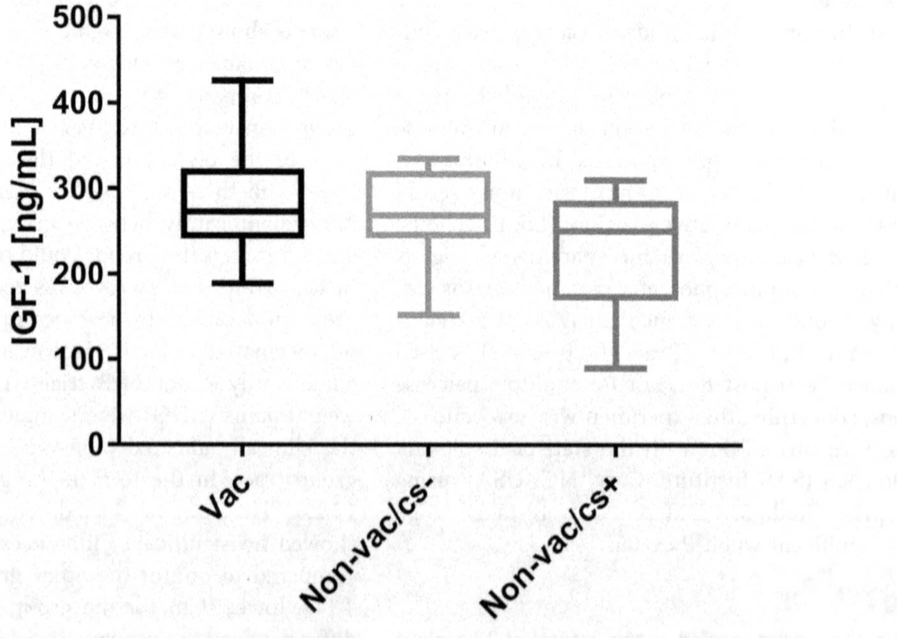

Fig. 2 Concentrations of IGF-1 levels in blood at dissection

relation to the length of the small intestine (+ 18.2% per m and + 21.5% per m).

Total mass of the caecum tissue (– 19.5% against group vac; – 17.3% against non-vac/cs-; Table 6) was significantly lower in clinically affected animals. Consequently, the relative body mass per mass of caecum was significantly increased in the presence of clinical signs of an *L. intracellularis* infection (+ 18.2%) relative to vaccinated animals. Vaccinated animals had the highest ADG (+ 13.0%) in relation to the mass of the stomach. There was a significantly reduced amount of stomach content (– 32.0% compared to group vac; – 31.4% compared to non-vac/cs-) in clinically conspicuous animals.

There were no significant differences between the groups regarding the ratio of the mass of the small intestine and the length of the small intestine. Numerically, the relation was highest for the non-vaccinated, clinically non-affected animals (in g/m; non-vac/cs-: 78.1 ± 6.39, vac: 74.6 ± 9.39, non-vac/cs+: 71.6 ± 6.98). There were also no significant differences between the mass of the small intestine and the mass of the stomach. Numerically, the mass of the small intestine was lowest in relation to the mass of the stomach in the clinically healthy animals (non-vac /cs-:4.72 ± 0.61; vac: 5.03 ± 0.55; non-vac/cs: 5.07 ± 0.68).

Table 3 Apparent precaecal digestibility values of organic matter, crude protein and starch in piglets

Diet component	Apparent precaecal digestibility rates (%)					
	Vac		Non-vac/cs-		Non-vac/cs+	
	Mean	SD	Mean	SD	Mean	SD
Organic matter	62.2	7.94	66.7	2.03	64.7	5.09
Crude protein	71.6	5.18	72.5	3.93	70.2	4.25
Starch	91.3	2.32	93.2	1.97	93.3	2.31

Vac vaccinated with Enterisol®Ileitis, *Non-vac/cs-* not vaccinated, clinically no signs, *Non-vac/cs +* not vaccinated, clinical signs
Values within a row with different superscripts differ significantly at $P < 0.05$ (significances are missing)

Discussion

Performance losses in the course of an *L. intracellularis* infection result from lower average daily gains and a feed conversion ratio which is worse [5–8]. The economic losses due to this infection with *L. intracellularis* in pigs are the main issue for the pig industry [1–4].

Table 4 Apparent total tract digestibility of organic matter and nutrients in piglets

Diet component	Apparent total tract digestibility (%)					
	Vac		Non-vac/cs-		Non-vac/cs+	
	Mean	SD	Mean	SD	Mean	SD
Organic matter	86.4	1.46	86.9	1.81	84.8	2.19
Crude fat	72.1	4.08	73.1	6.15	71.5	4.31
Crude fibre	18.8	7.64	22.9	10.2	14.4	15.3
Crude protein	83.0^{a}	1.72	83.9^{a}	2.03	80.7^{b}	2.57
Starch	98.9	0.27	99.0	0.15	98.8	0.26

Vac vaccinated with Enterisol®Ileitis, *Non-vac/cs-* not vaccinated, clinically no signs, *Non-vac/cs +* not vaccinated, clinical signs
^{a,b}Values within a row with different superscripts differ significantly at $P < 0.05$

Table 5 Morphometric parameters and relations between morphometric parameters as well as relations to performance in piglets

Parameter /Organ	Total value and relations of parameters					
	Vac		Non-vac/cs-		Non-vac/cs+	
	Mean	SD	Mean	SD	Mean	SD
Length (m)						
Nose-rump	0.89	0.03	0.90	0.03	0.90	0.05
Small intestine	15.9[ab]	1.57	14.6[b]	1.12	16.2[a]	1.37
Caecum	0.22	0.02	0.21	0.02	0.21	0.01
Colon	3.03	0.39	2.98	0.28	2.96	0.31
Relation body weight to nose rump and organ length (kg/m)						
Nose-rump	30.4[a]	1.44	29.7[ab]	1.59	28.2[b]	2.02
Small intestine	1.72[ab]	0.21	1.83[a]	0.17	1.56[b]	0.12
Caecum	123	7.83	126	18.9	123	11.3
Colon	8.98	0.95	9.03	1.11	8.60	1.03
Relation ADG to nose rump and organ length (g/m)						
Nose-rump	1010[a]	78.6	953[ab]	71.7	875[b]	128
Small intestine	57.1[a]	9.44	58.7[a]	6.57	48.3[b]	6.85
Caecum	4070	300	4056	635	3808	622
Colon	299	45.9	289	35.1	267	48.7

Vac vaccinated with Enterisol® Ileitis, *Non-vac/cs-* not vaccinated, clinically no signs, *Non-vac/cs +* not vaccinated, clinical signs
[a,b]Values within a row with different superscripts differ significantly at $P < 0.05$

Table 6 Organ mass and relation of body weight and average daily gains to mass of organs

Parameter / Organ	Total value and relations of parameters					
	Vac		Non-vac/cs-		Non-vac/cs+	
	Mean	SD	Mean	SD	Mean	SD
Mass (g)						
Stomach	236	31.2	243	22.6	230	22.1
Small intestine	1173	82.7	1142	124	1165	173
Caecum	74.8[a]	8.94	72.8[a]	14.6	60.2[b]	9.41
Colon	418	78.9	439	57.8	400	58.0
Relation body weight to organ mass (g/g)						
Stomach	115	10.6	110	7.40	110	7.46
Small intestine	23.1	1.95	23.5	2.60	22.0	2.72
Caecum	363[b]	32.2	376[ab]	54.0	429[a]	71.6
Colon	66.3	11.6	61.3	4.65	64.2	9.48
Relation ADG to organ mass (g/g)						
Stomach	3.83[a]	0.48	3.53[ab]	0.31	3.39[b]	0.34
Small intestine	0.76	0.06	0.75	0.09	0.68	0.12
Caecum	12.0	1.00	12.0	1.67	13.3	3.15
Colon	2.22	0.50	1.96	0.17	1.99	0.43

Vac vaccinated with Enterisol®Ileitis, *Non-vac/cs-* not vaccinated, clinically no signs, *Non-vac/cs +* not vaccinated, clinical signs
[a,b]Values within a row with different superscripts differ significantly at $P < 0.05$

Effects on performance

A high feed intake is the basic prerequisite for exploiting the performance potential of pigs [30, 31]. The first consequence of an infection is the reduced appetite and therefore lower feed intake [32]. In the present study, feed intake in the group non-vac/cs+ was only numerically reduced by 10.2% and in group non-vac/cs- by 6.94% compared to the feed intake of vaccinated animals. In the literature, there is up to now no direct comparison between these three types of groups. In a study with an experimental *L. intracellularis* infection, a reduced feed intake was observed in animals aged 28 to 49 days. When groups with different inoculation doses (counts per pig) were compared (7.2×10^7 to 3.8×10^5 and 7.2×10^7 to 2.2×10^6), the reduction in feed intake was 1.27% and 7.85%, respectively [33]. In another study the reduction in feed intake was 3.79% in pigs at 38 to 58 days of age after experimental infection (1.26×10^{10} *L. intracellularis* organisms in the inoculum) in comparison with animals treated with 50 ppm tylvalosin for 14 further days after experimental infection [34]. For viral intestinal infections (porcine epidemic diarrhoea = PED), there are also significant effects on performance. After a 4-day acclimatisation period, the infection with PED resulted in a reduced feed intake of 11.5% over a period of 21 days [22]. In a recent meta-analysis on the effects of infections on feed intake due to bacterial infections of the digestive system (mainly *E. coli* in piglets) the reduction was 15% [19]. In conclusion, an infection with *L. intracellularis* in the acute phase seems to have a somewhat lower effect on the feed intake than viral or classical bacterial intestinal infection in piglet rearing. In the present study, the effects of an *L. intracellularis* infection on the feed intake were higher in percentage terms than in the literature [8, 34]. This can be interpreted as the effect of strict division of animals into three groups according to clinical appearance and vaccination status. At the same time, it should be borne in mind that the experimental approach here per se may reflect the natural conditions in the field best because naturally - infected, conspicuous animals have been selected. Experiments with an artificial infection are not possible in the classical sense due to the lack of possibility of cultural cultivation. For that reason usually strains of *L. intracellularis* are freshly harvested from McCoy cells [35–37]. On the other hand, digestibility studies in animals with a natural microbiome for an *L. intracellularis* infection may simulate the conditions in the field better. This is because interactions between the natural composition of the microbiome in pigs and nutrient digestibility are proven [38]. This is the reason why in the present study unlike in conventional studies with experimental infection, animals from a farm with an early field infection were used.

Growth factor and inflammation

The Insulin-like growth factor I is an important anabolic hormone that mediates growth and development of individuals [39]. IGF-1 is probably also a useful biomarker of growth performance for comparing pigs from the same herd [40]. In the present study no significant differences in the serum levels of IGF-1 were found. In general, it is stated that the variation in hepatic IGF-1 expression is probably due to the natural variability observed in the young growing pigs. Therefore, this might have an influence on the statistically significant gained results [40].

Numerically, the vaccinated animals had the highest mean values (285 ng / mL). Non-vaccinated, clinically healthy animals (– 4.72%) and pigs with clinical signs of infection (– 20.9%) had lower IGF-1 concentrations in the serum at the time of dissection.

From literature it is known that pigs with higher post-weaning average daily gains have significantly increased odds of elevated IGF-1 expression in the liver [39]. For example in the named study, the pig with the highest average daily gain (556 g/day) was 1073 (95% CI: 16.02–71,892) times more likely to have higher IGF-1 expression than the pig with the lowest gain (140 g/day; $P < 0.01$) [39].

In a five-week feeding experiment with piglets on the effects of antibiotics (22.7 ppm of chlortetracycline, 22.7 ppm of sulfamethazine, and 11.4 ppm of penicillin) the levels of IGF-1 in untreated animals were significant lower (– 19.2%; 105 vs. 131 ng/mL $p < 0.001$; [41]). This observation was accompanied by a decrease in average daily gains of 20.6% ($p < 0.01$; [41]). From studies on growing pigs, it has been known for a long time that restrictive feeding is associated with lower IGF-1 levels in the serum [42]. In general, this is in accordance with the results found here with a lower feed intake in clinically conspicuous animals. Therefore, higher IGF-1 concentrations may be the explanation for the numerically higher feed consumption and the increased average daily gains in the vaccinated group.

Nutrient digestibility and morphometry of organs

One of the characteristics of an infection with the pathogen *L. intracellularis* in pigs is a downregulation of various genes in the enterocytes. These play an important role in the mechanisms of nutrient absorption [21]. Therefore, it can be assumed that an infection with *L. intracellularis* can have an influence on the digestibility of nutrients. No significant differences were found in the study with regard to the precaecal digestibility of the nutrients, although numerically the digestibility rate of nitrogen decreased by 2.3% percentage points in the presence of clinical manifestations of the disease (non-vac/cs + vs. non-vac/cs-). Until now, there is no comparative study dealing with the influence of this relevant infectious agent of the pig on digestibility of nutrients [22]. For porcine reproductive and respiratory syndrome virus, porcine epidemic diarrhoea virus and a co-infection from both illnesses no significant influence on the ileal digestibility was seen [22]. This is consistent with results found here.

The response of the gastrointestinal tract to ingested nutrients is a complex and closely controlled process [24]. A leading mechanism of intestinal adaptation to enteral availability nutrients is driven by humoral factors like the intestinotrophic peptide glucagon-like peptide-2 (GLP-2) [25]. Enteroendocrine L-cells secrete GLP-2 after direct stimulation by nutrients present in the ileal digesta [25]. GLP-2 is responsible for the adjustment control of the intestinal absorption area and nutrient availability [43]. Within a few days massive adjustments are possible [43]. For example, a reduction in the mass of the small intestine in rats within 6 days could be detected in 34% of cases with parenteral nutrition [43]. Therefore, low digestibility rates of nutrients in the small intestine cause the intestine to react with a morphometric adjustment in the form of growth. This could be the explanation for the fact that a disease might not directly influence the precaecal digestibility of nutrients. However, the result of this adaptation is a longer intestine or higher relative intestinal mass or both. Thus, the relative efficiency of the digestive organs per se might be reduced. Indications for such organ adaptations could also be found in this study. Relative to the length of the small intestine, the clinically conspicuous animals had the smallest body mass and relative to the organ mass of the small intestine, they had, numerically, the smallest body mass. In relation to the organ length, the group of clinically conspicuous animals had significantly lower average daily weight gains.

In the present study, it was seen that average total tract digestibility of nitrogen was significantly reduced in clinically affected animals. This was also demonstrated in the above-mentioned study for the combined infection of PRRSV and PED [22]. The total digestibility of the dry matter, nitrogen and the gross energy was also reduced [22]. While in the aforementioned study the reduction in nitrogen digestibility was 12.8% [22], it was only 3.81% for the clinically conspicuous animals in the present study.

It can be presumed that mucosal alterations might lead to increased presence of nitrogen compounds in the intestine as hypothesised for *Brachyspira* infection in swine [44]. This might be due to the increased amounts of endogenous nitrogen in the distal parts of the small intestine and parts of the large intestine. It is known that *L. intracellularis* is also a prevalent cause of naturally acquired colitis in pigs. About 25% of endogenous nitrogen originates from the large intestine while 59.9% originates from the small intestine [45]. The reabsorption of endogenous nitrogen (total 10.7 g) amounted to 79% towards the end of the small intestine and 88% for the whole digestive tract [46] for an nitrogen-intake of 23.6 g/day. Other authors calculated for higher endogenous secretion (18.1 g for 40 g nitrogen-intake a day [47] and 16.1 g for 35 g nitrogen-intake [48] with reabsorption up to the end of the digestive tract from 90% or rather 78%). Therefore a lower reabsorption of endogenous nitrogen could be a reason for a lower digestibility of nitrogen in clinically apparent piglets.

Conclusion

This study clearly shows that the performance of pigs is adversely affected by an *L. intracellularis* infection. The lower average weight gain is primarily caused by a lower feed intake. The precaecal digestibility of the nutrients was not reduced significantly. Adaptation mechanisms lead to increased length and relative mass of the small intestine in diseased animals. Therefore, the relative efficiency of nutrient utilisation might be adversely affected. In the case of vaccinated animals, the lowest effects of an *L. intracellularis* infection were observed concerning the performance of the animals.

Abbreviations

ADFI: Average daily feed intake; ADG: Average daily gains; ATTD: Apparent total tract digestibility; DK: Danish Landrace 50% x Yorkshire 50%; DM: Dry matter; FCR: Feed conversion ratio; GLP-2: Glucagon-like peptide-2; IGF-1: Insulin-like growth factor 1; ME: Metabolizable Energy; Non-vac/cs-: Not vaccinated, clinically no signs; Non-vac/cs +: Not vaccinated, clinical signs; PRRSV: Porcine Reproductive and Respiratory Syndrome Virus; PED: Porcine epidemic diarrhoea; ST: *Salmonella typhimurium*; Vac : vaccinated with Enterisol®Ileitis

Acknowledgements

We would like to thank the farmer who provided the animals from his stock for these studies and Frances Sherwood-Brock for editing the manuscript to ensure correct English.

Funding

The study was financially supported by Boehringer Ingelheim Vetmedica GmbH, D-55216 Ingelheim am Rhein, Germany. The role of the funding body was merely financial for purchasing the materials and the analysis of the data for the trials at the Institute for Animal Nutrition, University of Veterinary Medicine Hanover, Foundation. They did not have any role in the collection, interpretation, analysis and writing of the data.

Authors' contributions

CV and JK were the initiators of the idea. CV and JK designed the study. KR was responsible for designing the study in statistical terms. E-UP, IvdB, CV and JM visited the farm, selected the animals and were responsible for clinical investigations as well as for taking the samples. Investigations and analyses at the university were made by JM, CV and SS. MS performed the analysis of IGF-1. JM, CV and KR did the statistics. CV wrote the paper. All authors critically revised the manuscript and approved the final version of the manuscript. All authors agreed to be accountable for all aspects of the work.

Ethics approval and consent to participate

The animals were killed according to § 4, paragraph 3 of the Animal Protection Act, exclusively to use their organs or tissues for scientific purposes ("Tötungsanzeige beim Tierschutzbeauftragten der Stiftung Tierärztliche Hochschule Hannover vom 16.07.2012"). The animals had to be brought to the university, since the killing of the animals for organ removal may not take place on the farm legally. The animals came from a farm where animals excreted *Lawsonia intracellularis* with their faeces in consequence of a natural infection. Some of the animals had already been immunized against *Lawsonia intracellularis* with a commercially available vaccine at the time of removal according to the farmer's decision. All animals were healthy at the time of removal, differing only in faecal consistency. The animals showed no diarrhea. The animals came from different boxes. The removal of organs for scientific purposes can only be justified if the collection of samples also reflects natural conditions of digestive physiology, i.e. the feed intake must be undisturbed for several days. Experience has shown that stabling at least two previously unknown animals together to form a group would have meant an additional adaptation phase lasting several days in which the animals would have to get used to each other and form a hierarchy and, therefore, an undisturbed feed intake would have been achieved. This would have been associated with considerable and prolonged stress for the animals. Also, in Germany, the legal requirements (§ 28 Paragraph 1 Sentence 2 of the Animal Welfare Animal Husbandry Ordinance "Tierschutz-Nutztierhaltungsverordnung") make it mandatory to avoid regrouping as far as possible. Economic efficiency, labour and cost savings are no justification for this. Should a regrouping nevertheless become necessary, sufficient alternative, retreat and covering possibilities for inferior animals must be created (Annex I Chap. 2 D Nr. 2 S. 3 RL 2008/120/EG). The legal requirements show that legislation at national and EU level assumes or has recognised that the stress associated with regrouping the pig is a significant impairment of welfare, which can only be justified on reasonable grounds. Against the background of the short keeping period of only a few days until killing, the considerable strain on the animals due to regrouping would not have been justifiable from the point of view of animal welfare. The boxes were designed in such a way that there was no social isolation, as the pigs had visual, auditory and olfactory contact with each other and the possibility of physical contact existed at any time. Therefore, animal experiments were carried out according to German regulations. It was not an animal experiment requiring a notification or an approval according to the Animal Protection Act (§ 7, paragraph 2, sentence 3).

Consent for publication

Not applicable.

Competing interests

The authors declare that they have no competing interests.

Author details

[1]Institute for Animal Nutrition, University of Veterinary Medicine Hannover, Foundation, Bischofsholer Damm 15, D-30173 Hannover, Germany. [2]Clinic for Cattle, University of Veterinary Medicine Hannover, Foundation, Bischofsholer Damm 15, D-30173 Hannover, Germany. [3]Tierarztpraxis Dr. Peitzmeier, Meente 24, D-32479 Hille, Germany. [4]Institute for Biometry, Epidemiology and Information Processing, University of Veterinary Medicine Hannover, Foundation, Bünteweg 2, D-30559 Hannover, Germany.

References

1. McOrist S, Smith SH, Green LE. Estimate of direct financial losses due to porcine proliferative enteropathy. Vet Rec. 1997;140(22):579–81.
2. Lawson GHK, Gebhart CJ. Proliferative enteropathy. J Comp Pathol. 2000; 122(2–3):77–100.
3. McOrist S. Defining the full costs of endemic porcine proliferative enteropathy. Vet J. 2005;170(1):8–9.

4. Jacobson M, Fellstrom C, Jensen-Waern M. Porcine proliferative enteropathy: an important disease with questions remaining to be solved. Vet J. 2010; 184(3):264–8.
5. Brandt D, Kaim U, Baumgartner W, Wendt M. Evaluation of Lawsonia intracellularis infection in a group of pigs in a subclinically affected herd from weaning to slaughter. Vet Microbiol. 2010;146(3–4):361–5.
6. Pedersen KS, Skrubel R, Stege H, Angen O, Stahl M, Hjulsager C, Larsen LE, Nielsen JP. Association between average daily gain, faecal dry matter content and concentration of Lawsonia intracellularis in faeces. Acta Vet Scand. 2012;54:58.
7. Johansen M, Nielsen M, Dahl J, Svensmark B, Baekbo P, Kristensen CS, Hjulsager CK, Jensen TK, Stahl M, Larsen LE, et al. Investigation of the association of growth rate in grower-finishing pigs with the quantification of Lawsonia intracellularis and porcine circovirus type 2. Prev Vet Med. 2013; 108(1):63–72.
8. Collins AM, Barchia IM. The critical threshold of Lawsonia intracellularis in pig faeces that causes reduced average daily weight gains in experimentally challenged pigs. Vet Microbiol. 2014;168(2–4):455–8.
9. Veenhuizen M, Elan T, Soensken N: The potential economic impact of porcine proliferative enteropathy on the US swine industry. In: 15° Congress IPVS: 1998; 1998: 64.
10. Hardge T, Nickoll E, Grunert H, Elbers K, Langbein U, Keller C, Bleier T, Pohlenz J, Ohlinger V, Schroeder B. Prevention of porcine proliferative enteropathy (PPE) by vaccination–efficacy and economics in European farms. Pig J. 2004;54:17–34.
11. Kroll JJ, Roof MB, Hoffman LJ, Dickson JS, Harris DL. Proliferative enteropathy: a global enteric disease of pigs caused by Lawsonia intracellularis. Anim Health Res Rev. 2005;6(2):173–97.
12. Holyoake P, Cutler R. Outbreaks of proliferative haemorrhagic enteropathy on two pig farms. Aust Vet J. 1995;72(7):253–6.
13. McOrist S, Gebhart C. Proliferative enteropathy. Diseases of Swine 10th ed Ames. Iowa: Blackwell Publishing; 2012. p. 811–20.
14. Elsasser TH, Caperna TJ, Li C-J, Kahl S, Sartin JL. Critical control points in the impact of proinflammatory immune response on growth and metabolism. J Anim Sci. 2008;86:E105–25.
15. Kelley KW, Bluthe RM, Dantzer R, Zhou JH, Shen WH, Johnson RW, Broussard SR. Cytokine-induced sickness behavior. Brain Behav Immun. 2003;17:S112–8.
16. Johnson RW. Immune and endocrine regulation of food intake in sick animals. Domest Anim Endocrinol. 1998;15(5):309–19.
17. Bluthe RM, Kelley KW, Dantzer R. Effects of insulin-like growth factor-I on cytokine-induced sickness behavior in mice. Brain Behav Immun. 2006;20(1): 57–63.
18. Jacobson M, Andersson M, Lindberg R, Fossum C, Jensen-Waern M. Microarray and cytokine analyses of field cases of pigs with diarrhoea. Vet Microbiol. 2011;153(3–4):307–14.
19. Pastorelli H, van Milgen J, Lovatto P, Montagne L. Meta-analysis of feed intake and growth responses of growing pigs after a sanitary challenge. Animal. 2012;6(6):952–61.
20. Vannucci FA, Gebhart CJ. Recent advances in understanding the pathogenesis of Lawsonia intracellularis infections. Vet Pathol. 2014;51(2): 465–77.
21. Vannucci FA, Foster DN, Gebhart CJ. Laser microdissection coupled with RNA-seq analysis of porcine enterocytes infected with an obligate intracellular pathogen (Lawsonia intracellularis). BMC Genomics. 2013;14:421.
22. Schweer WP, Schwartz K, Burrough ER, Yoon KJ, Sparks JC, Gabler NK. The effect of porcine reproductive and respiratory syndrome virus and porcine epidemic diarrhea virus challenge on growing pigs I: growth performance and digestibility. J Anim Sci. 2016;94(2):514–22.
23. Cera KR, Mahan DC, Cross RF, Reinhart GA, Whitmoyer RE. Effect of age, weaning and Postweaning diet on small intestinal growth and Jejunal morphology in young swine. J Anim Sci. 1988;66(2):574–84.
24. Farre R, Tack J. Food and symptom generation in functional gastrointestinal disorders: physiological aspects. Am J Gastroenterol. 2013;108(5):698–706.
25. Tappenden KA. Mechanisms of enteral nutrient-enhanced intestinal adaptation. Gastroenterology. 2006;130(2):S93–9.
26. Ahlfänger B. Investigations on influences of an exocrine pancreatic insufficiency on the length and the histological morphology of the small intestine in young pigs. Hannover: University of Veterinary Medicine Hannover, Foundation; 2016.
27. Nathues H, Holthaus K, Beilage EG. Quantification of Lawsonia intracellularis in porcine faeces by real-time PCR. J Appl Microbiol. 2009;107(6):2009–16.
28. Naumann C, Bassler R. Methoden der landwirtschaftlichen Forschungs-und Untersuchungsanstalt, Biochemische Untersuchung von Futtermitteln. In: Methodenbuch III (einschließlich der achten Ergänzungen). Darmstadt: VDLUFA; 2012.
29. Holthaus K. Quantitativer Nachweis von Lawsonia intracellularis mittels real-time PCR in Kotproben von Schweinen. Hannover: University of Veterinary medicine Hannover, Foundation; 2008.
30. Rauw WM, Soler J, Tibau J, Reixach J, Raya LG. Feeding time and feeding rate and its relationship with feed intake, feed efficiency, growth rate, and rate of fat deposition in growing Duroc barrows. J Anim Sci. 2006;84(12): 3404–9.
31. Hermesch S, Kanis E, Eissen JJ. Economic weights for feed intake in the growing pig derived from a growth model and an economic model. J Anim Sci. 2003;81(4):895–903.
32. Klasing KC. Negative consequences of immune response: what can be done by nutritionists? Proc Soc Nutr Physiol. 2006;15:17–23.
33. Paradis M, McKay R, Wilson J, Vessie G, Winkelman N, Gebhart C, Dick C. Subclinical ileitis produced by sequential dilutions of *Lawsonia intracellularis* in a mucosal homogenate challenge model. In: Proceedings of the American Association of Swine Veterinarians Annual Meeting. 2005:189–191.
34. Guedes RMC, Franca SA, Machado GS, Blumer MA, Cruz ECD. Use of tylvalosin-medicated feed to control porcine proliferative enteropathy. Vet Rec. 2009;165(12):342–6.
35. Collins A, Love RJ, Pozo J, Smith SH, McOrist S. Studies on the ex vivo survival of Lawsonia intracellularis. Swine Health Prod. 2000;8(5):211–5.
36. Wattanaphansak S, Gebhart C, Olin M, Deen J. Measurement of the viability of Lawsonia intracellularis. Can J Vet Res. 2005;69(4):265–71.
37. Borewicz KA, Kim HB, Singer RS, Gebhart CJ, Sreevatsan S, Johnson T, Isaacson RE. Changes in the porcine intestinal microbiome in response to infection with Salmonella enterica and Lawsonia intracellularis. PLoS One. 2015;10(10):e0139106.
38. Vigors S, Sweeney T, O'Shea CJ, Kelly AK, O'Doherty JV. Pigs that are divergent in feed efficiency, differ in intestinal enzyme and nutrient transporter gene expression, nutrient digestibility and microbial activity. Animal. 2016;10(11):1848–55.
39. Slifierz MJ, Friendship R, de Lange CFM, Slavic D, Grgic H, Farzan A. Immunomodulatory factors and infectious agents associated with the hepatic gene expression of the IGF system in nursery pigs. Animal. 2014; 8(5):844–51.
40. Slifierz MJ, Friendship R, de Lange CFM, Rudar M, Farzan A. An epidemiological investigation into the association between biomarkers and growth performance in nursery pigs. BMC Vet Res. 2013;9:247.
41. Hathaway MR, Dayton WR, White ME, Henderson TL, Henningson TB. Serum insulin-like growth factor I (IGF-I) concentrations are increased in pigs fed antimicrobials. J Anim Sci. 1996;74(7):1541–7.
42. Therkildsen M, Vestergaard M, Busk H, Jensen MT, Riis B, Karlsson AH, Kristensen L, Ertbjerg P, Oksbjerg N. Compensatory growth in slaughter pigs-in vitro muscle protein turnover at slaughter, circulating IGF-I, performance and carcass quality. Livest Prod Sci. 2004;88(1–2):63–75.
43. Chance W, Foley-Nelson T, Thomas I, Balasubramaniam A. Prevention of parenteral nutrition-induced gut hypoplasia by coinfusion of glucagon-like peptide-2. Am J Physiol-Gastr L. 1997;273(2):G559–63.
44. Skrlep M, Batorek N, Bonneau M, Fazarinc G, Segula B, Candek-Potokar M. Elevated fat skatole levels in immunocastrated, surgically castrated and entire male pigs with acute dysentery. Vet J. 2012;194(3):417–9.
45. Nyachoti CM, deLange CFM, McBride BW, Schulze H. Significance of endogenous gut nitrogen losses in the nutrition of growing pigs: a review. Can J Anim Sci. 1997;77(1):149–63.
46. Souffrant W, Rerat A, Laplace J, Darcy-Vrillon B, Köhler R, Corring T, Gebhardt G, Bernard F, Jähnichen M, Schneider B. Exogenous and endogenous contributions to nitrogen fluxes in the digestive tract of pigs fed a casein diet. III Recycling of endogenous nitrogen. Reprod Nutr Dev. 1993;33(4): 373–82.
47. Low A. Endogenous nitrogen evaluation from absorption studies [digestive absorption of endogenous nitrogen, pigs]. Colloques de l'INRA (France) 1982.
48. Krawielitzki K, Zebrowska T, Schadereit R, Kowalczyk J, Hennig U, Wünsche J, Herrmann U. Determining of nitrogen absorption and nitrogen secretion in different sections of the pig's intestine by digesta exchange between 15N labelled and unlabelled animals. Arch Anim Nutr. 1990;40(1–2):25–37.

19

Exploratory field study on the effect of Porcine circovirus 2 (PCV2) sow vaccination on serological, virological and reproductive parameters in a PCV2 subclinically infected sow herd

Salvador Oliver-Ferrando[1], Joaquim Segalés[2,3], Sergio López-Soria[1], Antonio Callén[4], Olivier Merdy[5], François Joisel[6] and Marina Sibila[1*]

Abstract

Background: This study sought to evaluate the effect of sow vaccination against *Porcine circovirus 2* (PCV2) on reproductive parameters during two consecutive reproductive cycles. The study was performed in a PCV2 subclinical infected breeding herd (PCV2 circulation but absence of major reproductive problems). Ninety-four pregnant sows were primo-immunized with a commercial PCV2 vaccine and ninety-seven were injected with phosphate-buffered saline at 6 and 3 weeks before the first studied farrowing, and then boosted at 2 weeks before the second one. Blood samples were taken throughout the study to assess PCV2 DNA load and antibodies. At farrowing, main reproductive parameters and piglet vitality index were registered. In addition, in those litters with more than three mummified or stillborn piglets, microscopic examination and PCV2 antigen detection in foetal myocardium was done.

Results: Vaccinated sows showed significantly higher antibody levels compared to the non-vaccinated counterparts. PCV2 DNA was only detected at farrowing in 2 (4.2%) non-vaccinated sows. Vaccinated sows had 1.3 more live-born piglets per litter at the second cycle than non-vaccinated counterparts. Piglets from vaccinated sows had significantly higher (+ 12.7%) vitality score than the ones born from non-vaccinated sows. No PCV2 compatible lesions neither PCV2 antigen were detected in the tested foetal hearts.

Conclusions: The present study represents a first attempt to demonstrate that PCV2 sow vaccination may have a positive influence on prolificacy and vitality of the offspring in a subclinical infected breeding herd. However, since reproductive outcomes at farm level may be affected by a number of factors, further studies would be needed to confirm this association.

Keywords: *Porcine circovirus 2* (PCV2), PCV2 subclinical infection (PCV2-SI), Vaccine efficacy, Sow, Reproduction

* Correspondence: marina.sibila@irta.cat
[1]IRTA, Centre de Recerca en Sanitat Animal (CReSA, IRTA-UAB), Campus de la Universitat Autònoma de Barcelona, 08193 Bellaterra, Spain
Full list of author information is available at the end of the article

Background

Porcine circovirus 2 (PCV2) is a small and ubiquitous single-stranded DNA virus with a great economic importance for the swine industry [1]. This virus is linked to a number of diseases collectively named Porcine circovirus diseases (PCVD) [2]. Among these, PCV2 has been shown to be involved in reproductive disorders in sows such as return-to-oestrus, late term abortions and increased number of mummified, stillborn and non-viable piglets at birth [3–8], as well as early embryo mortality [7, 9]. In this context, PCV2 can be transmitted to the embryos as soon as they get rid of the zona pellucida [10], to the foetus through the placenta [11] and to the new-born piglets by colostrum [12]. Under experimental conditions, some studies have demonstrated that infection of sows by both artificial insemination (AI) with PCV2-spiked semen or PCV2 inoculation can cause foetal infection and reproductive disorders [5, 13]. Moreover, foetal infections and reproductive abnormalities have been reproduced by intrauterine inoculation of foetuses or foetal liquids [14–16]. However, at farm level, it is feasible that a proportion of PCV2 effects on reproduction are linked to embryonic death [7, 10], which nowadays is still beyond the diagnostic capacity. This overall situation leads to the fact that clinical and noticeable reproductive disease (PCV2-RD) attributed to PCV2, at field level, is infrequent [6, 11, 17].

PCV2 vaccination in sows prior to farrowing is focused on the protection of the offspring by antibody transfer through the colostrum. This strategy has resulted in prevention of PCV2-systemic disease (PCV2-SD) [18], decrease of viremia [19–21] and PCV2 tissue load [22] in their progeny, and improvement of the average daily weight gain (ADWG) in subclinically infected finisher pigs [23]. Despite these facts, it has been demonstrated that sow vaccination does not fully prevent PCV2 vertical transmission [24–27].

In contrast, influence of PCV2 sow vaccination on reproductive parameters has been poorly investigated. As for example, this type of problems has been tackled as a secondary goal and in a very limited number of sows (1-3 sows per group) in some experimental studies [24, 25, 27]. At farm level, this issue has only been assessed in two peer-reviewed studies: firstly in one farm suffering from PCV2-SD in growing pigs but without evident reproductive problems (PCV2-SI scenario in the sow herd) [23] and, secondly, in one farm with PCV2-SD among weaners and serious reproductive problems in sows [28]. Whereas in the first study no significant differences on the main reproductive parameters between treatments were detected, in the second one an improvement of all measured reproductive parameters were recorded. However, information about the effect of this vaccination strategy on reproductive parameters in a farm with neither reproductive nor PCV2-SD problems (scenario resembling a situation of most breeding herds) is missing in the peer-reviewed literature. Thus, the current work was aimed to evaluate the potential effects of sow vaccination against PCV2 on serological (ELISA), virological (quantitative PCR (qPCR)) and reproductive parameters during two consecutive reproductive cycles in a PCV2 subclinical infection (PCV2-SI) scenario (PCV2 circulation in the breeding herd but absence of clinical reproductive problems).

Methods

Farm selection

The study was conducted in a 1900-sow farm located in Catalonia (Spain). This farm worked with weekly farrowing batches in all-in/all-out management system. The vaccination program applied by routine included sow immunization against *Porcine reproductive and respiratory syndrome virus* (PRRSV), *Aujeszky's disease virus*, *Swine influenza virus*, *Porcine parvovirus*, *Erysipelothrix rhusiopathiae*, *Escherichia coli* and *Clostridium perfringens*. Piglets were vaccinated against *Mycoplasma hyopneumoniae* and PCV2 at 5 days pre-weaning and at weaning, respectively. Weaning was performed at 3 weeks of age. Moreover, no signs of any major pig diseases were present and herd immunity status against PRRSV was deemed as "positive-stable" (II-A) [29].

This farm had average reproductive parameter performance in line with the average Spanish national records (www.bdporc.irta.es) and did not suffer from PCVD clinical signs. Prior to the start of the study, PCV2 antibody detection was confirmed (Ingezim Circo IgG 11.PCV.K1®, Ingenasa, Madrid, Spain) in 7 out of 7 (100%) gilts and in 33 out of 38 (87%) sows of different parity that have never been vaccinated before against PCV2 (Fig. 1). In addition, antibody levels were heterogeneous (ranging from 0.20 to 1.49 ELISA *S*/*P* values), with a decreasing value trend in older sows.

Study design

One hundred and ninety-one healthy sows were selected in three consecutive farrowing batches at 6 weeks pre-farrowing. These animals were individually ear-tagged and distributed in two treatment groups (Table 1). Randomization was performed according to parity (from 1 to 8) and the number of total-born and live-born piglets at the former farrowing. The comparability of the obtained groups was also checked for number of piglets weaned in the previous farrowing. Sample size was calculated using the expected differences between treatment groups in terms of magnitude of the parameters used for randomization. For this purpose, a statistical and qualitative data analysis software (GPower, University of Düsseldorf) was used. The study was conducted in two

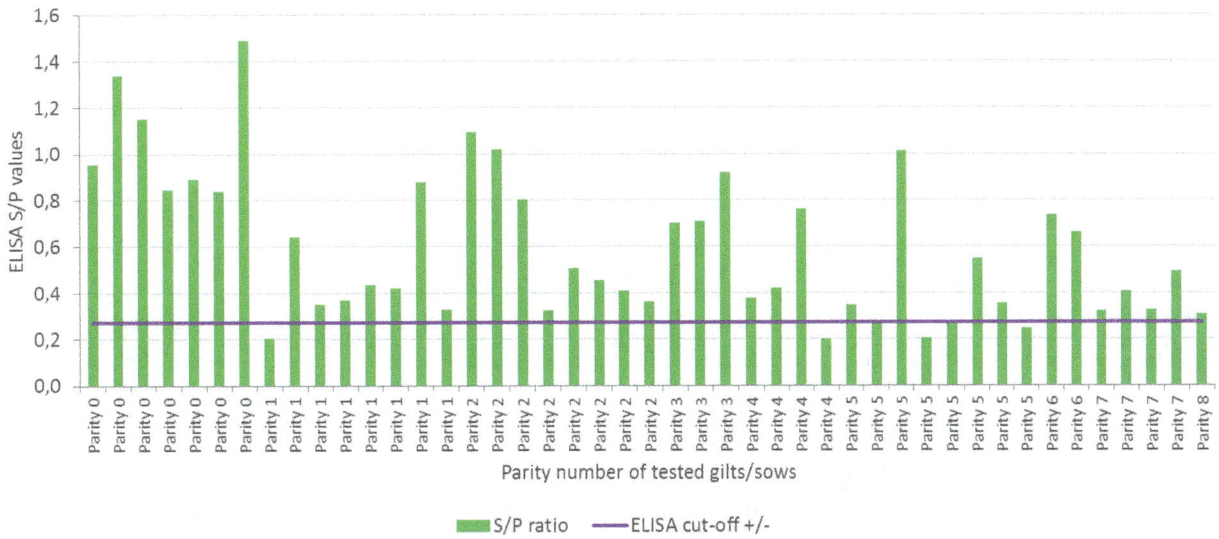

Fig. 1 Individual PCV2 ELISA S/P results in serum samples from gilts and sows with different parity number prior to the start of the study (farm screening)

consecutive reproductive cycles. Sows were vaccinated by intramuscular injection with 2 mL of a commercial inactivated PCV2 vaccine (CIRCOVAC®, Batch number: L414725) at time points indicated in Table 1. Non-vaccinated sows received 2 ml of phosphate buffer saline (PBS) at the same time points and by the same route. Animals with different treatments were located comingled in the same gestation pens as well as in the same farrowing unit rooms.

Study design is represented in Table 2. Any abnormality related to general state, condition of the skin, hair and mucosa, respiratory, digestive and nervous signs, and locomotive problems was registered at different time points. At the end of the first experimental reproductive cycle, as part of routine breeder management, sows with major pathologies (lameness, injuries, etc.) and high parity (older sows) were excluded from the study. In addition, those sows showing return-to-oestrus (non-pregnant ones) in regards their counterparts, were registered and removed from the second cycle. Furthermore, sow mortality was also recorded.

Blood samples from a randomly selected subpopulation of sows ($n = 48$ per treatment group) were taken at different time points throughout the first (at vaccination, farrowing and weaning) and second (at farrowing) gestational cycle (Table 2). Once in the laboratory, these samples were allowed clotting, and were centrifuged at 3200 rpm during 20 min at 4 °C. All sera were aliquoted and stored at − 20 °C until testing.

In each reproductive cycle, the following reproductive parameters were registered: return-to-oestrus, abortion rate, interval between expected and real farrowing date, weaning-to-fertile mating interval and number of live-born, mummified, stillborn, crushed and weaned piglets per litter.

All piglets issued from the studied sows (first and second gestational cycle) were ear-tagged, gender recorded and assigned a vitality index (VI) (see section Vitality index scoring method). Cross-fostering was only allowed within sows of the same treatment group and, when possible, within the same parity group (1st parity; 2nd-4th parity; 5th-8th parity). Moreover, from those litters with more than three mummified or stillborn foetuses, heart samples were taken and fixed in 10% neutral-buffered formalin for further histopathological analysis and PCV2 antigen detection by

Table 1 Treatment distribution of sows and vaccination schedule in both gestational cycles

Population	N[b]	Group	Treatment	Volume and doses		Number of sows bled
				First gestational cycle	Second gestational cycle	
Sows	94 (75)	V	PCV2 vaccine[a]	2 ml at 6 and 3 weeks pre-farrowing	2 ml at 2 weeks pre-farrowing	48
	97 (75)	NV	PBS			48

V vaccinated, *NV* non-vaccinated
[a]Animals were vaccinated with CIRCOVAC®
[b]In parentheses, number of sows remaining for the second gestational cycle in each group

Table 2 Study design schedule

Population	First gestational cycle				Second gestational cycle			
	6 weeks pre-farrowing	3 weeks pre-farrowing	Farrowing	Weaning	AI	2 weeks pre-farrowing	Farrowing	Weaning
Sows	CS	CS	CS	CS		CS	CS	CS
	T	T				T		
	BL		BL	BL			BL	
			RP				RP	
Piglets			S	CS			S	CS
			CS				CS	
			VI				VI	

AI artificial insemination, *CS* clinical signs, *T* treatment application, *BL* blood sampling, *RP* reproductive parameters assessment, *S* sex recording, *VI* vitality index

immunohistochemistry (IHC) (see section Histopathology and IHC in heart of foetuses). All piglets included in the study were monitored for clinical signs and mortality during lactation.

Housing conditions, feeding system, feed characteristics and health management remained consistent along the course of the trial, and were the same for both experimental groups. The present study was approved by the Ethics Committee for Animal Experimentation from the *Universitat Autònoma de Barcelona* and the Animal Experimentation Commission from the local government (*Dpt. de Medi Ambient i Habitatge from the Generalitat de Catalunya*; Reference 5796).

Vitality index scoring method

The vitality of the piglets (within the first 3 h of life, approximately) was assessed according to a previously published index [30]. The behavioral variables evaluated were the following:

- Udder stimulation (U): 0 = no head movements, no emulating udder stimulation movements or no searching behavior within 30 s; 1 = head movements, emulating udder stimulation movements or searching behavior within 30 s.
- Number of completed circles around the enclosure (NCC): 0 = Not able to turn piglet body axis 360° from its initial orientation nor able to walk along the limits of the bucket; 1 = Able to turn piglet body axis 360° from its initial orientation or walk along the limits of the bucket once within 30 s; 2 = Able to turn piglet body axis 360° from its initial orientation or walk along the limits of the bucket at least twice within 30 s.

Histopathology and IHC in heart of foetuses

After fixation by immersion in 10% neutral-buffered formalin and embedding in paraffin, tissue sections were processed routinely for haematoxylin/eosin (HE) staining. These samples were examined under a light microscope for the evaluation of potential microscopic lesions.

For IHC technique, serial sections (3 μm) were dewaxed in xylene and rehydrated through graded alcohols. Endogenous peroxidase was blocked with 3% of H_2O_2 (30%) in methanol during 30 min, followed by a 5-min wash in distilled water. Sections were then subjected to proteolytic enzyme digestion with protease type XIV (Sigma, Madrid, Spain) at a concentration of 0.1% in PBS for 8 min at 37 °C. After digestion, the sections were washed three times during 5 min in PBS. Then, these sections were incubated for 1 h at room temperature with 2% of bovine serum albumin (Sigma, Madrid, Spain) in PBS. A specific monoclonal antibody (isotype IgG2a) (Ingenasa, Madrid, Spain) against PCV2 Cap protein was applied at a 1 in 1000 dilution in 2% of bovine serum albumin in PBS (pH 7.4) to tissue sections and incubated overnight at 4 °C. Sections were then washed three times in PBS for 5 min. After washing, sections were incubated for 45 min with peroxidase-labelled polymer-horseradish peroxidase conjugated to goat anti-mouse immunoglobulins (Envision 1 System-HRP-DAB; Dako, Barcelona, Spain). Staining was completed by incubation with 3,3′diaminobenzidine chromogen solution (Envision 1 System-HRP-DAB; Dako, Barcelona, Spain). Sections were counterstained with Mayer's haematoxylin, dehydrated, and mounted. Samples were examined under a light microscope for the analysis of immunostaining.

DNA extraction and real-time quantitative PCR

DNA was extracted from 200 μl of serum by using the MagMAX™ Pathogen RNA/DNA Kit (Applied Biosystems) following the manufacturer's instructions. DNA obtained was suspended in 90 μl of elution solution. To quantify PCV2 DNA in serum samples, a real-time qPCR assay (LSI VetMAX™ Porcine Circovirus Type 2-Quantification, Life Technologies) was performed. Each extraction and qPCR plate included negative controls where DNA was substituted for diethylpyrocarbonate

(DEPC)-treated water. In addition, each sample reaction had an internal positive control (IPC) to monitor DNA extraction and amplification procedures. Viral concentrations were expressed as the mean $\log_{10}$ PCV2 genome copies/mL ± standard deviation (SD).

Indirect ELISA for detecting anti-PCV2 IgG antibodies

All serum samples were tested by Ingezim Circo IgG 11.PCV.K1® assay (Ingenasa, Madrid, Spain). Optical density (OD) was measured at 450 nm by PowerWave XS reader (BioTek). Mean positive cut-off was established at 0.3 OD (± SD) following kit's instructions (positive cut-off = OD of negative control + 0.25). ELISA results were expressed as mean S/P ratio (OD of sample/OD of positive control for each ELISA plate) ± SD.

Statistical analyses

Statistical analyses were carried out using SAS v9.4, SAS Institute Inc., Cary, NC, USA. Significance level was set at $p < 0.05$. Proportion of animal mortality and exclusion rates between vaccinated and non-vaccinated sows was compared using Fisher exact test and Chi-square test, respectively. Reproductive parameters from all sows included in the study were analyzed and compared between experimental groups within each reproductive cycle (intra-cycle comparison) using the non-parametric Wilcoxon test. In addition, reproductive parameters from those sows farrowing in both reproductive cycles were compared between cycles (inter-cycle comparison) using generalized linear mixed models. Treatment, cycle and their interaction were considered as a fixed effects and sow as a random effect. Percentage of positive qPCR serum samples and mean $\log_{10}$ PCV2 copies/mL among those qPCR positive samples were compared at each sampling point using Fisher exact tests and Wilcoxon tests, respectively. ELISA S/*P* values were analyzed using a linear mixed model. For the analysis of VI (U and NCC), clinical signs in piglets and piglet mortality during lactation generalized linear mixed models were used. Treatment was considered as a fixed effect and sow as a random effect.

Results

Clinical signs in sows

No evident clinical signs were observed in any of the sows, but one, throughout the study. The particular affected sow was from the vaccinated group and developed severe lameness at the end of the first reproductive cycle, when it was excluded from the study.

Mortality and exclusion in sows

Mortality and exclusion rates and reason of exclusion are detailed in Table 3. In both reproductive cycles, non-vaccinated sows showed numerically higher (but not significant) mortality than the vaccinated ones. Moreover, no statistically significant differences among treatment groups were observed between the two reproductive cycles with regards to the number of excluded females and the exclusion reason.

Reproductive parameters

Comparison between experimental groups within each reproductive cycle (intra-cycle comparison)

Main reproductive parameters for each treatment group at first and second reproductive cycles are listed in Table 4. Number of live-born piglets at the second cycle was significantly ($p < 0.05$) higher (+ 1.3 piglets/sow) in the vaccinated group. In addition, a tendency of higher number of weaned piglets (+ 0.8) in vaccinated sows was observed ($p < 0.1$). Moreover, most reproductive parameters (return-to-oestrus [− 0.6%], interval between expected and real farrowing date [− 0.3 days] and number of mummified [− 0.1] piglets per litter) were numerically better for the vaccinated group in the second cycle. Whereas at first reproductive cycle number of stillborn piglets per litter was significantly higher in the vaccinated group, at the second period this parameter was numerically higher in the non-vaccinated one. Besides, number of crushed piglets at birth was numerically higher in the vaccinated group at first and second cycles. Regarding the abortions, there was only one abortion in each cycle for each treatment group. In addition, piglets from vaccinated sows had significantly higher vitality

Table 3 Number and percentage (in brackets) of dead and excluded sows and reason of exclusion

	Treatment	V ($n = 94$)	NV ($n = 97$)
Mortality in first reproductive cycle		2 (2.13%)	5 (5.15%)
Exclusion at the end of the first reproductive cycle	Return to oestrus	13 (13.83%)	14 (14.43%)
	Culling. Old sow	2 (2.13%)	1 (1.03%)
	Culling. Lameness	1 (1.06%)	0 (0%)
	Human mistakes (vaccination, misplaced sows…)	1 (1.06%)	2 (2.06%)
	TOTAL excluded animals	17 (18.09%)	17 (17.53%)
Mortality in second reproductive cycle		0 (0%)	2 (2.67%)

No statistically significant differences ($p < 0.05$) among experimental groups were observed
V vaccinated, *NV* non-vaccinated

Table 4 Reproductive parameters (mean ± SD) in PCV2 vaccinated (V) and non-vaccinated (NV) sows during both cycles

	First gestational cycle		Second gestational cycle	
	V (n = 94)	NV (n = 97)	V (n = 75)	NV (n = 75)
Interval between expected and real farrowing date (days)	0.45 ± 2.07[a]	0.73 ± 1.36[a]	0.72 ± 1.57[a]	1.00 ± 1.33[a]
Live-born*/litter	14.34 ± 3.24[a]	13.61 ± 3.12[a]	15.42 ± 3.43[a]	14.16 ± 3.45[b]
Crushed/litter	0.53 ± 0.84[a]	0.43 ± 0.66[a]	0.95 ± 1.16[a]	0.73 ± 1.13[a]
Mummified/litter	0.35 ± 0.62[a]	0.44 ± 0.87[a]	0.38 ± 0.70[a]	0.47 ± 0.74[a]
Stillborn/litter	1.45 ± 1.72[a]	0.88 ± 1.36[b]	0.88 ± 1.05[a]	1.24 ± 1.35[a]
Weaned/litter	12.35 ± 2.89[a]	12.06 ± 2.71[a]	12.82 ± 2.75[a]	12.01 ± 3.31[a]
Vitality index (%)**-U				
○ 1 (positive score)	91.91[a]	79.87[b]	97.14[a]	89.35[a]
Vitality index (%)**-NCC				
○ ≥ 1 (positive score)	23.40[a]	10.69[b]	22.86[a]	10.19[b]
Weaning to fertile mating interval (days)	4.51 ± 2.53[a]	4.49 ± 2.67[a]	NA	NA
Abortion (%)	0[a]	1.0[a]	1.3[a]	0[a]

Different letters in superscript mean statistically significant differences ($p < 0.05$) among experimental groups within each reproductive cycle
NA: not available
*including crushed piglets at birth
**This index was calculated only from piglets of three or less hours of life

than the ones derived from non-vaccinated sows in both reproductive cycles. Specifically, piglets from vaccinated group showed higher percentage of head movements emulating the udder searching (statistically significant at first cycle) and greater mobility (statistically significant in both cycles) during the 30 tested seconds than the ones from non-vaccinated group.

Comparison of each experimental group between reproductive cycles (inter-cycle comparison)

In the second cycle, vaccinated sows had significantly different number of live-born (+ 1.17), crushed (+ 0.34) and stillborn (– 0.55) piglets per litter in comparison to the same sows (n = 75) in the first reproductive cycle. Moreover, non-vaccinated sows (n = 75) showed at their second cycle significantly higher number of crushed (+ 0.32) and stillborn (+ 0.36) piglets per litter than in their previous cycle. No statistically significant differences between cycles were observed for the rest of the parameters.

Clinical signs and mortality in suckling piglets

In the first cycle, although the number of sows included in the study was 94 and 97 for the vaccinated and non-vaccinated groups, respectively, the number of litters monitored during the first lactation period was 93 and 96, since there was one premature farrowing and one abortion in the vaccinated and non-vaccinated groups, respectively. In this context, 9 out of 93 (9.7%) and 10 out of 96 (10.4%) litters from vaccinated and non-vaccinated sows, respectively, evidenced diarrhoea. Besides, 65 out of 1333 (4.9%) and 53 out of 1307 (4.1%) piglets from vaccinated and non-vaccinated sows, respectively, showed neurological signs clinically attributed to *Streptococcus suis (S. suis)* infection. In the second suckling period, 8 out of 74 (10.8%) and 9 out of 75 (12%) litters from vaccinated and non-vaccinated sows, respectively, suffered from diarrhoea. In addition, prevalence of *S.suis*-like infections was reduced, recording only 3 out of 1141 (0.3%) and 2 out of 1062 (0.2%) clinical cases in piglets from vaccinated and non-vaccinated sows, respectively. No statistically significant differences between treatments in terms of diarrhoea and neurological signs were observed for any of the two lactation periods.

Piglet mortality rate (including crushed piglets around birth) in lactation was 13.9% and 16.8% for piglets from vaccinated sows at first and second cycles, respectively. Similarly, pre-weaning mortality rate in piglets from non-vaccinated sows was 11.4% and 15.2% at first and second suckling periods, respectively. However, no statistically significant differences among treatment groups were observed in any of the two lactation periods.

Microscopic evaluation and PCV2 antigen detection in foetal heart tissues

Although, 14 litters (7.33%) from the first farrowing cycle had more than three mummified or stillborn piglets, only 2 of them were sampled. On the contrary, at second farrowing cycle, foetal heart samples from all the litters (n = 11, 7.33%) presenting high number of mummified or stillborn piglets were taken and evaluated. No microscopic lesions associated to PCV2 infection or PCV2 antigen were observed in myocardium of mummified or stillborn piglets from all the tested litters.

Quantification of PCV2 DNA in sow serum samples

All vaccinated sows were qPCR negative (48 out of 48) throughout the study, whilst 2 out of 48 (4.17%) non-vaccinated sows were qPCR positive (mean viral load: 4.15 $\log_{10}$ PCV2 copies/mL) at farrowing sampling of the first reproductive cycle. No statistically significant differences between treatment groups were observed.

Anti-PCV2 IgG antibody levels in sow serum samples

The course of antibodies against PCV2 for sows of the two treatment groups is shown in Fig. 2. From 6 weeks before farrowing to sampling at delivering of first gestational cycle, vaccinated group showed an increase of ELISA S/*P* values, resulting in significantly higher ($p < 0.05$) antibody levels compared to the ones from the non-vaccinated group at farrowing and weaning. In the second gestational cycle, ELISA S/P values from vaccinated sows increased again, reaching the maximum difference with the antibody levels from the non-vaccinated counterparts.

Discussion

The objective of the present study was to evaluate the potential effect of sow PCV2 vaccination in a PCV2 subclinically infected breeding herd (PCV2 circulation but absence of overt reproductive problems). The supporting evidence of a subclinical infection was the presence of seropositive gilts and sows before starting the trial together with the low percentage of viremic animals (less than 5%) detected within the studied sow population. This low prevalence would resemble the situation of other PCV2-SI farms [31–33]. In parallel, in order to have additional information about the PCV2 infection status at the time when the study was carried out, blood samples from 12 gilts at acclimatization were taken and tested by qPCR. Indeed, PCV2 DNA was detected in 2 out of those 12 gilts (16.7%, data not shown), corroborating the PCV2-SI in the studied scenario.

Three criteria have to be fulfilled to diagnose a clinical case of PCV2-RD during late gestation [6]: 1) presence of clinical signs associated to late reproductive disorders (abortions, increased number of mummified, stillborn piglets at birth, etc.), 2) microscopic lesions in foetal heart or lymphoid tissues, and 3) detection of PCV2 antigen or DNA in those foetal tissues. In addition, return-to-oestrus problems have also been associated to PCV2-RD at early gestation [34]. The negative results of histopathology and IHC in all tested foetuses from litters with high number of mummies and stillbirths indicated that these findings were not apparently related to PCV2. Therefore, as expected, the present farm was not suffering from PCV2-RD (late reproductive failures or return-to-oestrus), since the average of all reproductive parameters were within normal ranges according to the Spanish national records.

In the present farm conditions, the PCV2 vaccination strategy applied (primo-immunization at 6 and 3 weeks pre-partum and a booster at 2 weeks before the subsequent farrowing) led to a significantly higher antibody response throughout the study period with regard to their non-vaccinated counterparts. This fact tallies with other studies where sow vaccination before mating or farrowing elicited a high antibody response [31], including neutralizing antibodies [35], in serum. In fact, the increase of antibody levels measured by the used ELISA kit is

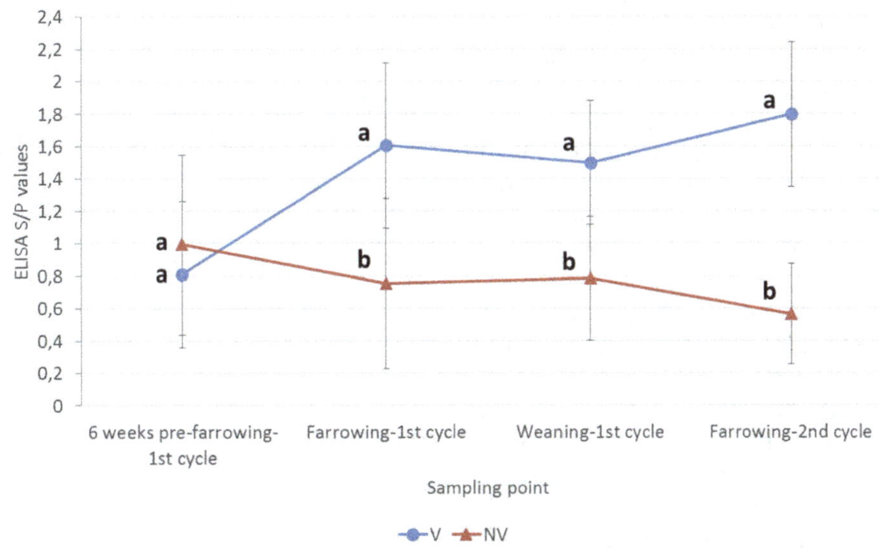

Fig. 2 PCV2 ELISA S/P results (mean ± SD) in serum samples taken from the sows included in the study during the first (6 weeks pre-farrowing, farrowing, weaning) and second (farrowing) reproductive cycle. Different letters in superscript mean statistically significant differences ($p < 0.05$) among experimental groups at each sampling point

apparently correlated with PCV2 neutralizing antibody values [36], although these were not specifically measured in this study. Besides, the booster vaccination at the second cycle resulted in higher antibody levels than the ones observed after first cycle vaccination, suggesting a potential greater protection for both sows and piglets. At reproductive level, sows immunized with the PCV2 vaccine showed a significantly ($p < 0.05$) higher number of live-born piglets and tend ($p < 0.1$) to have higher number of weaned piglets per litter at the second gestational cycle. In this study, sow vaccination at first cycle was applied at a relatively late time during pregnancy when the litter size is already established; therefore, the potential impact of PCV2 vaccination on litter size was only expected after second cycle vaccination. This effect on reproductive parameters is in line with those observed by Pejsak et al. [28], but in disagreement with the ones reported by Kurmann et al. [23]. The first trial [28] was conducted in a farm with important reproductive problems (most likely related to PCV2-RD) and sporadic PCV2-SD cases. In that study, the application of a 3-year PCV2 vaccination in boars, gilts (at acclimatization) and sows (before farrowing) resulted in the improvement of all measured reproductive parameters (insemination rate, number of live-born and weaned piglets per litter and birth weight). These positive effects were more evident after several months of vaccine application, resembling the findings of the present study. On the contrary, in the other study [23], the application of PCV2 vaccine at 4 and 2 weeks before AI and 4 weeks pre-partum during 14 months in two farms with a history of recurrent PCV2-SD in growing pigs but with no apparent reproductive problems in sows did not culminate in better reproductive parameters. Therefore, to the authors' knowledge, the current study represents the first approach in the peer-reviewed literature to show the potential benefits of PCV2 sow vaccination on reproductive parameters in a subclinically infected sow herd. It must be kept in mind, however, that reproductive performance may be influenced by other factors at farm level [37]; in consequence, although the number of studied sows is relatively high, the present study should be considered of exploratory nature and a higher number of sows and production cycles would be needed to validate obtained results.

Curiously enough, at the first farrowing post-vaccination, the number of stillborns per litter was significantly higher in the vaccinated group. The cause of this result is unknown, as there was no evidence of any factor that could adversely affect this parameter. Nevertheless, at the second gestational cycle this situation was reversed, since vaccinated and non-vaccinated groups significantly reduced and increased the number of stillborn piglets, respectively. Generally, 10 to 15% of piglets are born dead in pig farms [38]; therefore, the stillborn rate reported in the present study falls within regular values in both reproductive cycles. This parameter might be related to hypoxia during farrowing since the number of stillbirths increases in cases of high litter size, prolonged farrowing time and high birth weight [39, 40]. Besides, stillbirth can be associated with other factors such as environmental temperature, sow parity, farrowing induction, infectious diseases, mycotoxins and uterine capacity [41].

Moreover, piglets from vaccinated sows had higher vitality (in the first three hours of life) than the animals issued from non-vaccinated ones in both reproductive cycles. This finding was subjectively reported in a farm with major reproductive problems, most probably related to PCV2, using the same vaccine than the present study [28]. Besides, since VI was higher in piglets coming from vaccinated sows, one would expect to have less crushed piglets in that group. However, vaccinated sows showed higher (but non-significantly) number of crushed piglets. Most probably, this was a fortuitous event and not associated to piglet vitality, since crushing is related to other factors such as sow behaviour (depends of the sow genetics), design of farrowing crates and management practices [42].

Conclusions

After two reproductive cycles, sows vaccinated against PCV2 experienced significantly higher antibody levels, prolificacy and vitality of their offspring. However, as reproductive performance may be influenced by multiple factors, the present study represents a further investigation of the PCV2 sow vaccination effects on reproductive parameters under a PCV2 subclinical infection scenario.

Abbreviations

ADWG: Average daily weight gain; AI: Artificial insemination; BL: Blood sampling; CS: Clinical signs; DEPC: Diethylpyrocarbonate; DNA: Deoxyribonucleic acid; ELISA: Enzyme-linked immunosorbent assay; HE: Haematoxylin/eosin; Ig: Immunoglobulin; IHC: Immunohistochemistry; IPC: Internal positive control; NCC: Number of completed circles around the enclosure; NV: Non-vaccinated; OD: Optical density; PBS: Phosphate buffer saline; PCR: Polymerase chain reaction; PCV2: *Porcine circovirus 2*; PCV2-RD: PCV2 reproductive disease; PCV2-SD: PCV2 systemic disease; PCV2-SI: PCV2 subclinical infection; PCVD: Porcine circovirus disease; PRRSV: *Porcine reproductive and respiratory syndrome virus*; qPCR: Quantitative PCR; RP: Reproductive parameters; S: Sex recording; S. suis: *Streptoccocus suis*; S/P: Sample to positive; SD: Standard deviation; T: Treatment application; U: Udder stimulation; V: Vaccinated; VI: Vitality index

Acknowledgments

The authors would like to thank Eva Huerta, Anna Llorens, Patricia Pleguezuelos, Rosa López and Diego Pérez and to the farm animal caretakers and veterinarian for their willingness to collaborate in the study.

Funding

This work was funded by Merial S.A.S. and by *Secretaria d'Universitats i Recerca del Departament d'Economia i Coneixement de la Generalitat de Catalunya* (DI2013-0013) and CERCA Programme.

Authors' contributions
SOF participated in the design of the study, was involved in the field trial, performed the laboratory tests and drafted the manuscript. SLS contributed to the design, coordination and execution of the field trial. OM and FJ conceived the study and participated in its design. MS, JS and AC collaborated in the study design, were involved in the field trial, participated in the data analysis and results interpretation. All authors critically read and contributed to the manuscript, approving its final version.

Competing interests
AC, OM and FJ were employees of the vaccine manufacturer (Merial) at the time the experiment was designed and conducted.

Author details
[1]IRTA, Centre de Recerca en Sanitat Animal (CReSA, IRTA-UAB), Campus de la Universitat Autònoma de Barcelona, 08193 Bellaterra, Spain. [2]UAB, Centre de Recerca en Sanitat Animal (CReSA, IRTA-UAB), Campus de la Universitat Autònoma de Barcelona, 08193 Bellaterra, Spain. [3]Departament de Sanitat i Anatomia Animals, Facultat de Veterinària, UAB, 08193 Bellaterra, Spain. [4]Veterinarian, Zaragoza, Spain. [5]Agronomist, Lyon, France. [6]Private veterinary consultant, Lyon, France.

References
1. Segalés J, Kekarainen T, Cortey M. The natural history of porcine circovirus type 2: from an inoffensive virus to a devastating swine disease? Vet Microbiol. 2013;165:13–20.
2. Allan G, Krakowa S, Ellis J. PCV2; ticking time bomb?. Pig Prog. 2002;18:14–5.
3. Brunborg IM, Jonassen CM, Moldal T, Bratberg B, Lium B, Koenen F, Schonheit J. Association of myocarditis with high viral load of porcine circovirus type 2 in several tissues in cases of fetal death and high mortality in piglets. A case study. J Vet Diagn Investig. 2007;19:368–75.
4. West KH, Bystrom JM, Wojnarowicz C, Shantz N, Jacobson M, Allan GM, Haines DM, Clark EG, Krakowka S, McNeilly F, Konoby C, Martin K, Ellis JA. Myocarditis and abortion associated with intrauterine infection of sows with porcine circovirus 2. J Vet Diagn Investig. 1999;11:530–2.
5. Madson DM, Patterson AR, Ramamoorthy S, Pal N, Meng XJ, Opriessnig T. Reproductive failure experimentally induced in sows via artificial insemination with semen spiked with porcine circovirus type 2. Vet Pathol. 2009;46:707–16.
6. Madson DM, Opriessnig T. Effect of porcine circovirus type 2 (PCV2) infection on reproduction: disease, vertical transmission, diagnostics and vaccination. Anim Health Res Rev. 2011;12:47–65.
7. Mateusen B, Maes DG, Van Soom A, Lefebvre D, Nauwynck HJ. Effect of a porcine circovirus type 2 infection on embryos during early pregnancy. Theriogenology. 2007;68:896–901.
8. Ladekjaer-Mikkelsen AS, Nielsen J, Storgaard T, Botner A, Allan G, McNeilly F. Transplacental infection with PCV-2 associated with reproductive failure in a gilt. Vet Rec. 2001;148:759–60.
9. Kim J, Jung K, Chae C. Prevalence of porcine circovirus type 2 in aborted fetuses and stillborn piglets. Vet Rec. 2004;155:489–92.
10. Mateusen B, Sanchez RE, Van Soom A, Meerts P, Maes DG, Nauwynck HJ. Susceptibility of pig embryos to porcine circovirus type 2 infection. Theriogenology. 2004;61:91–101.
11. Pensaert MB, Sanchez RE Jr, Ladekjaer-Mikkelsen AS, Allan GM, Nauwynck HJ. Viremia and effect of fetal infection with porcine viruses with special reference to porcine circovirus 2 infection. Vet Microbiol. 2004;98:175–83.
12. Shibata I, Okuda Y, Kitajima K, Asai T. Shedding of porcine circovirus into colostrum of sows. J Vet Med B Infect Dis Vet Public Health. 2006;53:278–80.
13. Park JS, Kim J, Ha Y, Jung K, Choi C, Lim JK, Kim SH, Chae C. Birth abnormalities in pregnant sows infected intranasally with porcine circovirus 2. J Comp Pathol. 2005;132:139–44.
14. Johnson CS, Joo HS, Direksin K, Yoon KJ, Choi YK. Experimental in utero inoculation of late-term swine fetuses with porcine circovirus type 2. J Vet Diagn Investig. 2002;14:507–12.
15. Yoon KJ, Jepsen RJ, Pogranichniy RM, Sorden S, Stammer R, Evans LE. A novel approach to intrauterine viral inoculation of swine using PCV type 2 as a model. Theriogenology. 2004;61:1025–37.
16. Sanchez RE Jr, Nauwynck HJ, McNeilly F, Allan GM, Pensaert MB. Porcine circovirus 2 infection in swine foetuses inoculated at different stages of gestation. Vet Microbiol. 2001;83:169–76.
17. Karuppannan AK, Ramesh A, Reddy YK, Ramesh S, Mahaprabhu R, Jaisree S, Roy P, Sridhar R, Pazhanivel N, Sakthivelan SM, Sreekumar C, Murugan M, Jaishankar S, Gopi H, Purushothaman V, Kumanan K, Babu M. Emergence of porcine circovirus 2 associated reproductive failure in southern India. Transbound Emerg Dis. 2016;63:314–20.
18. Pejsak Z, Podgorska K, Truszczynski M, Karbowiak P, Stadejek T. Efficacy of different protocols of vaccination against porcine circovirus type 2 (PCV2) in a farm affected by postweaning multisystemic wasting syndrome (PMWS). Comp Immunol Microbiol Infect Dis. 2010;33:e1–5.
19. O'Neill KC, Hemann M, Gimenez-Lirola LG, Halbur PG, Opriessnig T. Vaccination of sows reduces the prevalence of PCV-2 viraemia in their piglets under field conditions. Vet Rec. 2012;171:425.
20. Fraile L, Sibila M, Nofrarías M, López-Jimenez R, Huerta E, Llorens A, López-Soria S, Pérez D, Segalés J. Effect of sow and piglet porcine circovirus type 2 (PCV2) vaccination on piglet mortality, viraemia, antibody titre and production parameters. Vet Microbiol. 2012;161:229–34.
21. Dvorak CMT, Payne BJ, Seate JL, Murtaugh MP. Effect of maternal antibody transfer on antibody dynamics and control of porcine circovirus type 2 infection in offspring. Viral Immunol. 2018;31:40–6.
22. Opriessnig T, Patterson AR, Madson DM, Pal N, Ramamoorthy S, Meng XJ, Halbur PG. Comparison of the effectiveness of passive (dam) versus active (piglet) immunization against porcine circovirus type 2 (PCV2) and impact of passively derived PCV2 vaccine-induced immunity on vaccination. Vet Microbiol. 2010;142:177–83.
23. Kurmann J, Sydler T, Brugnera E, Buergi E, Haessig M, Suter M, Sidler X. Vaccination of dams increases antibody titer and improves growth parameters in finisher pigs subclinically infected with porcine circovirus type 2. Clin Vaccine Immunol. 2011;18:1644–9.
24. Madson DM, Patterson AR, Ramamoorthy S, Pal N, Meng XJ, Opriessnig T. Effect of porcine circovirus type 2 (PCV2) vaccination of the dam on PCV2 replication in utero. Clin Vaccine Immunol. 2009;16:830–4.
25. Madson DM, Patterson AR, Ramamoorthy S, Pal N, Meng XJ, Opriessnig T. Effect of natural or vaccine-induced porcine circovirus type 2 (PCV2) immunity on fetal infection after artificial insemination with PCV2 spiked semen. Theriogenology. 2009;72:747–54.
26. Gerber PF, Garrocho FM, Lana AM, Lobato ZI. Fetal infections and antibody profiles in pigs naturally infected with porcine circovirus type 2 (PCV2). Can J Vet Res. 2012;76:38–44.
27. Hemann M, Beach NM, Meng XJ, Wang C, Halbur PG, Opriessnig T. A live-attenuated and an inactivated chimeric porcine circovirus (PCV)1-2 vaccine are both effective at inducing a humoral immune response and reducing PCV2 viremia and intrauterine infection in female swine of breeding age. Can J Vet Res. 2014;78:8–16.
28. Pejsak Z, Kusior G, Pomorska-Mol M, Podgorska K. Influence of long-term vaccination of a breeding herd of pigs against PCV2 on reproductive parameters. Pol J Vet Sci. 2012;15:37–42.
29. Holtkamp DJ, Polson DD, Torremorell M, Morrison B, Classen DM, Becton L, Henry S, Rodibaugh MT, Rowland RR, Snelson H, Straw B, Yeske P, Zimmerman J. Terminology for classifying the porcine reproductive and respiratory syndrome virus (PRRSV) status of swine herds. Tierarztl Prax Ausg G Grosstiere Nutztiere. 2011;39:101–12.
30. Muns R, Manzanilla EG, Sol C, Manteca X, Gasa J. Piglet behavior as a measure of vitality and its influence on piglet survival and growth during lactation. J Anim Sci. 2013;91:1838–43.
31. Sibila M, Fraile L, Ticó G, López-Soria S, Nofrarías M, Huerta E, Llorens A, López-Jimenez R, Pérez D, Segalés J. Humoral response and colostral antibody transfer following 'one-dose' pre-mating vaccination of sows against porcine circovirus type-2. Vet J. 2013;197:881–3.
32. Feng H, Blanco G, Segalés J, Sibila M. Can porcine circovirus type 2 (PCV2) infection be eradicated by mass vaccination? Vet Microbiol. 2014;172:92–9.
33. Eddicks M, Koeppen M, Willi S, Fux R, Reese S, Sutter G, Stadler J, Ritzmann M. Low prevalence of porcine circovirus type 2 infections in farrowing sows and corresponding pre-suckling piglets in southern German pig farms. Vet Microbiol. 2016;187:70–4.
34. Segalés J. Porcine circovirus type 2 (PCV2) infections: clinical signs, pathology and laboratory diagnosis. Virus Res. 2012;164:10–9.
35. Gerber PF, Garrocho FM, Lana AM, Lobato ZI. Serum antibodies and shedding of infectious porcine circovirus 2 into colostrum and milk of vaccinated and unvaccinated naturally infected sows. Vet J. 2011;188:240–2.
36. Oliver-Ferrando S, Segalés J, López-Soria S, Callén A, Merdy O, Joisel F, Sibila M. Evaluation of natural porcine circovirus type 2 (PCV2) subclinical

infection and seroconversion dynamics in piglets vaccinated at different ages. Vet Res. 2016;47:121.
37. Koketsu Y, Tani S, Iida R. Factors for improving reproductive performance of sows and herd productivity in commercial breeding herds. Porcine health management. 2017;3:1.
38. Baxter EM, Jarvis S, D'Eath RB, Ross DW, Robson SK, Farish M, Nevison IM, Lawrence AB, Edwards SA. Investigating the behavioural and physiological indicators of neonatal survival in pigs. Theriogenology. 2008;69:773–83.
39. Canario L, Cantoni E, Le Bihan E, Caritez JC, Billon Y, Bidanel JP, Foulley JL. Between-breed variability of stillbirth and its relationship with sow and piglet characteristics. J Anim Sci. 2006;84:3185–96.
40. Wittenburg D, Guiard V, Teuscher F, Reinsch N. Analysis of birth weight variability in pigs with respect to liveborn and total born offspring. J Anim Breed Genet. 2011;128:35–43.
41. Vanderhaeghe C, Dewulf J, de Kruif A, Maes D. Non-infectious factors associated with stillbirth in pigs: a review. Anim Reprod Sci. 2013;139:76–88.
42. Kirkden RD, Broom DM, Andersen IL. Invited review: piglet mortality: management solutions. J Anim Sci. 2013;91:3361–89.

20

Responses to dietary levels of methionine in broilers medicated or vaccinated against coccidia under *Eimeria tenella*-challenged condition

Anqiang Lai[1], Guozhong Dong[1*], Daijun Song[1], Tan Yang[2] and Xiaolong Zhang[2]

Abstract

Background: Coccidiosis is a prevalent problem in chicken production. Dietary addition of coccidiostats and vaccination are two approaches used to suppress coccidia in the practical production. Methionine (Met) is usually the first limiting amino acid that plays important roles in protein metabolism and immune functions in chickens. The present study is aimed to investigate whether increasing dietary Met levels will improve the anticoccidial effects in broilers medicated or vaccinated against coccidia under *Eimeria (E.) tenella*-challenged condition. Two thousand male Partridge Shank broiler chicks were obtained from a hatchery. After hatch, birds were weighed, color-marked and allocated equally into two anticoccidial treatments, namely medicated and vaccinated groups. Chicks were either fed, from 1 d of age, diets containing coccidiostat (narasin) or diets without the coccidiostat but were inoculated with an anticoccidial vaccine at 3 d of age. At 22 d of age, 1080 chicks among them were randomly allocated evenly into 6 groups under a 2×3 treatment with 2 anticoccidial programs and 3 dietary methionine (Met) levels. Chicks medicated or vaccinated against coccidia were fed diets containing 0.45%, 0.56% or 0.68% of Met from 22 to 42 d of age. All chicks were orally introduced with an amount of 5×10^4 sporulated oocysts of *E. tenella* at 24 d of age. The growth performance, serum anti-oxidative indexes, intestinal morphology, cecal lesion scores, fecal oocyst counts and immune parameters were measured.

Results: The results showed increasing dietary Met level from 0.45% to 0.56% and 0.68% improved weight gain and feed conversion of broilers medicated against coccidia. In contrast, higher dietary levels of Met did not improve growth performance of the vaccinated chickens. Higher Met levels helped the medicated chickens resist *E. tenella* infection, as indicated by improved intestinal morphology and immune functions as well as decreased cecal lesion and fecal oocyst counts.

Conclusions: Anticoccidial vaccination is a better strategy for controlling coccidiosis than feeding narasin, due to not only greater growth performance, but also the lower Met supplementation. Furthermore, higher dietary Met levels improved growth performance of chickens medicated rather than vaccinated against coccidia under *E. tenella*-challenged condition.

Keywords: Methionine, Anticoccidial drug, Vaccination, *E. tenella*, Broilers

* Correspondence: gzdong@swu.edu.cn
[1]College of Animal Science and Technology, Southwest University, Beibei, Chongqing 400716, People's Republic of China
Full list of author information is available at the end of the article

Background

Methionine (Met) is the first limiting amino acid in broiler chickens fed maize-soybean diets [1]. Supplementation with Met in the diets is usually necessary to ensure the proper functions in protein metabolism and immune function. Met, like other amino acids, is the component of tissue proteins, thus serves as substrates for protein synthesis. In addition, Met participates in the methyl group metabolism, which includes both transmethylation and remethylation pathways and the transsulfuration pathway [2, 3]. Biological methylation of DNA, RNA, and protein is a critical approach for both pre-transcriptional and post-transcriptional regulations [4–6]. Through the transsulfuration, Met serves as a precursor for the synthesis of other sulfur amino acids, notably cystine, and several other metabolites, including glutathione (GSH), coenzyme A, taurine and inorganic sulfur [3]. GSH and taurine are essential compounds for host defense against oxidative stress. Met is also known to play critical roles in both cellular and humoral immunities of chickens. Dietary Met is involved in antibody production and cell-mediated immune responses in broilers [7]. Met deficiency can cause pathological and ultrastructural changes of thymus, reduce serum interlukin-2 (IL-2) contents and the T-cell population, and induce impaired proliferative function of T-cells and increased percentage of apoptotic cells in spleen [1]. There is evidence that Met metabolite, GSH, regulates nuclear transcription factor κB pathway, T-helper cell function and antibody and interferon-γ (IFN-γ) production in response to immunological challenges [7]. Therefore, the involvement of Met in immune function is probably related to the synthesis of antibodies, cytokines and other cytotoxic substances as well as the regulation of gene expression, signaling pathways and cellular redox state [7].

Coccidiosis, caused by several species of *Eimeria*, is prevalent in the poultry industry and continues to cause the most severe health and welfare problems. Malabsorption and diarrhea are typical symptoms of coccidiosis. Chickens with coccidiosis thus have depressed growth rate, impaired feed conversion rate, and, in worst cases, increased mortality [8]. Dietary addition of coccidiostats and vaccination against coccidia are two primary strategies for coccidiosis control, which effectively decrease the incidences and severity of coccidiosis [9]. Their protective effects against coccidial infection are supposed to ensure a normal gut function for the absorption of amino acids in diets.

However, both strategies have their shortcomings. The use of coccidiostats over the past 50 years has caused some degree of resistance of *Eimeria* strains, which conversely decreases anticoccidial effectiveness of drugs [9]. But to what extent drug-tolerant *Eimeria* strains influence the nutrient absorption of chicks remains unclear. Coccidial vaccination is generally associated with secondary enteritis, or even sporadically, necrotic enteritis incidence [9]. In addition, the immune regulatory actions of vaccines pose significant impact on the metabolism of certain amino acids, like Met. Amino acid metabolism is markedly altered to support the enhanced metabolic flows and cellular synthesis during the inflammatory and immune responses [10]. It has been found that the loss of urinary N is increased with the immune responses, which suggests an increased expenditure of endogenous amino acid sources [10]. The availability of amino acids influences aspects of the immune responses, which depend upon increased DNA and protein synthesis during lymphocyte replication and antibody synthesis. Previous research has suggested that Met supplemental level should be above the NRC (1994) recommendations under various catabolic conditions [11]. Maroufyan et al. [11] found that feeding Met at the level of twice NRC (1994) recommendation enhanced immune response in broiler chickens challenged by infectious bursal disease. Mirzaaghatabar et al. [2] discovered that feeding a diet containing 1.2% Met has improved humoral immunity and production performance of chickens compared to 0.45% Met. A study performed in various genotypes of broilers shows that antibody titers against antigens derived from sheep red blood cells were increased with the concentrations of Met from 3.91 to 5. 54 g/kg in the diets [12].

However, the effects of dietary Met levels on the resistance to coccidia in broilers under different anticoccidial programs remain unclear. Therefore, this study is aimed to investigate whether increasing dietary Met levels will improve the anticoccidial effects and growth performance in broilers medicated or vaccinated against coccidia under *Eimeria (E.) tenella*-challenged condition.

Methods

Experimental design and procedures

Two thousand male Partridge Shank broiler chicks were obtained from a hatchery in which eggs were set and hatched in a common incubator. After hatch, birds were weighed, color-marked and allocated equally into two anticoccidial treatments, namely medicated and vaccinated groups. In the medicated group, chicks were fed diets always containing 60 mg/kg narasin (an anticoccidial drug) in the starter diet and the grower diet, whereas chicks in the vaccinated group were inoculated with an anticoccidial live vaccine (1 dose per bird, 7-valent anticoccidial live vaccine, Schering-Plough, Shanghai, China) at 3 d of age without dietary addition of anticoccidial drugs. All chicks received a complete starter diet (Table 1) that meets the Feeding Standard of Chickens [13]. Feed and water were available to the birds ad libitum. For the first 7 days, the chicks were housed in stainless

Table 1 Composition and nutrient levels (air-dry basis, %) of the starter diet (1–21 d of age)

Ingredient	Content
Corn	55.04
Wheat	5.00
Dehulled soybean meal	35.00
Soybean oil	1.30
Dicalcium phosphate	1.85
Limestone	1.16
Choline chloride	0.10
Salt	0.32
L-lysine·HCl	0.03
Vitamin Premix[a]	0.10
Trace-element premix[b]	0.10
Total	100
Nutrient level[c]	Content
ME (Mcal/kg)	2.90
Crude protein	21.00
Lysine	1.07
Methionine	0.31
Methionine+cystine	0.68
Threonine	0.76
Calcium	1.00
Available phosphorus	0.45

[a]Provided per kg of diet: vitamain A, 8000 IU; vitamain D_3,2000 IU; vitamain E,15 IU; vitamain K_3, 1.5 mg; thiamine, 2 mg; riboflavin, 5 mg; pyridoxine, 5 mg; vitamain B_{12}, 0.02 mg; folic acid, 0.7 mg; nicotinic acid, 40 mg; pantothenic acid, 12 mg; biotin, 0.2 mg
[b]Provided per kg of diet: copper, 10 mg (as copper sulfate); iron, 90 mg (as ferrous sulfate); manganese, 100 mg (as manganese sulfate); zinc, 100 mg (as zinc sulfate); selenium, 0.3 mg (as sodium selenite); iodine, 0.5 mg (as calcium iodate)
[c]ME is metabolizable energy and is a calculated value. Other nutrient levels are measured values

steel battery cages (68 cm × 70 cm, five birds/cage) in a temperature-controlled house with continuous lighting. The temperature of the room was maintained at 32 to 34 °C for the first 3 d and then reduced by 2 to 3 °C per week to a final temperature of 20 °C. Birds were protected against Newcastle disease, infectious bursal disease, avian influenza and fowl pox according to the routine vaccination schedule. Chicks were transferred at 7 d of age into floor pens with free water and feed access as well as constant illumination. The floor of each pen was bedded with rice hull. From 22 to 42 d of age, 1080 chicks among them were randomly allocated evenly into 6 groups under a 2 × 3 treatment with 2 anticoccidial programs and 3 dietary Met levels. Chicks medicated or vaccinated against coccidia were fed diets containing 0.45%, 0.56 or 0.68% of Met from 22 to 42 d (Table 2). These dietary Met levels are equivalent to 100%, 125% and 150% of the growing broiler requirement, respectively [13]. Each experimental treatment was replicated in six separate pens with 30 chicks per pen. All chicks were orally introduced with an amount of 5×10^4 sporulated oocysts of *E. tenella* at 24 d of age.

Performance measurements and fecal oocyst counts

Average daily gain (ADG), average daily feed intake (ADFI) and feed to gain ratio (F/G) were measured through d 22 to d 42. Mortality data were collected and recorded on a daily basis, and the mortality was low in all treatment groups. Excreta was observed daily after oocyst challenge and oocyst counts were determined in excreta samples taken from each pen on d 6 and d 7 after challenge. Oocysts population was enumerated by microscopy according to the procedure of Long and Joyner [14]. The final oocyst counts were the average of those on d 6 and d 7 after challenge.

Blood and intestinal sample collection and processing

At 42 d of age, 30 birds per treatment were randomly selected (6 pens per treatment and 5 birds from each pen) after feed deprivation for 12 h. Blood samples (about 5 mL each) were taken from the wing vein and centrifuged at 3000×g for 15 min at 4 °C to separate serum, which was frozen at − 20 °C for further analysis. Blood samples for testing $CD4^+$ and $CD8^+$ lymphocyte populations (about 5 ml each), which were taken from wing vein, were stored in EDTA anticoagulation tubes. After blood collection, birds were killed by cervical dislocation. The ileum and cecum were separated and excised for histological examination. Intestinal contents from the cecum were dissolved into 0.9% NaCl solution (1:1, *v*/v) and then centrifuged at 10000×g for 1 min. The supernatant was used to detect the concentration of secreted immunoglobulin A (sIgA) in the lumen. The cecal tonsils were separated and stored in liquid nitrogen until Reverse transcription-PCR (RT-PCR) analysis.

Histological examination

The lesion scores of the cecum were determined and recorded according to the method of Johnson et al. [15]. The lesion scores range from 0 (no gross lesion) to 4 (most severe gross lesion). One-cm section of ileum was fixed in 4% paraformaldehyde solution, dehydrated and embedded in paraffin. The section was cut 4 μm long and stained with hematoxylin-eosin. The villus length (VH), crypt depth (CD), and VH to CD ratio (V/C) were measured by a Nikon phase contrast microscope coupled with a Micro Comp integrated digital imaging analysis system (Nikon Eclipse 80i, Nikon Corp., Tokyo, Japan).

Table 2 Composition and nutrient levels (air-dry basis, %) of grower diets (22–42 d of age)

	Medicated groups[d]			Vaccinated groups		
Met concentrations:	0.45%	0.56%	0.68%	0.45%	0.56%	0.68%
Ingredients						
Corn	60.41	60.29	60.05	60.41	60.29	60.05
Wheat	5.00	5.00	5.00	5.00	5.00	5.00
Dehulled soybean meal	28.50	28.50	28.50	28.50	28.50	28.50
Soybean oil	2.50	2.60	2.70	2.50	2.60	2.70
Dicalcium phosphate	1.60	1.60	1.60	1.60	1.60	1.60
Limestone	1.20	1.20	1.20	1.20	1.20	1.20
L-Lysine·HCl	0.03	0.03	0.03	0.03	0.03	0.03
Choline chloride	0.10	0.10	0.10	0.10	0.10	0.10
Salt	0.31	0.31	0.31	0.31	0.31	0.31
Vitamin Premix[a]	0.10	0.10	0.10	0.10	0.10	0.10-
Trace-element premix[b]	0.10	0.10	0.10	0.10	0.10	0.10
DL-methionine	0.15	0.27	0.39	0.15	0.27	0.39
Total	100	100	100	100	100	100
Nutrient levels[c]						
ME (Mcal/kg)	3.00	3.00	3.00	3.00	3.00	3.00
Crude protein	18.50	18.50	18.50	18.50	18.50	18.50
Methionine	0.45	0.56	0.68	0.45	0.56	0.68
Lysine	1.00	1.00	1.00	1.00	1.00	1.00
Threonine	0.65	0.65	0.65	0.65	0.65	0.65
Calcium	0.95	0.95	0.95	0.95	0.95	0.95
Available phosphorus	0.40	0.40	0.40	0.40	0.40	0.40

[a]Provided per kg of diet: vitamin A, 8000 IU; vitamin D_3,2000 IU; vitamin E,15 IU; vitamin K_3, 1.5 mg; thiamine, 2 mg; riboflavin, 5 mg; pyridoxine, 5 mg; vitamin B_{12}, 0.02 mg; folic acid, 0.7 mg; nicotinic acid, 40 mg; pantothenic acid, 12 mg; biotin, 0.2 mg

[b]Provided per kg of diet: copper, 10 mg (as copper sulfate); iron, 90 mg (as ferrous sulfate); manganese, 100 mg (as manganese sulfate); zinc, 100 mg (as zinc sulfate); selenium, 0.3 mg (as sodium selenite); iodine, 0.5 mg (as calcium iodate)

[c]ME is metabolizable energy and is a calculated value. Other nutrient levels are measured values

[d]Anticoccidial drug (narasin, 60 mg/kg diet) was added to diets in medicated groups, and an anticoccidial 7-valent live vaccine was inoculated in vaccinated groups

Enzyme-linked immunosorbent assay (ELISA)

sIgA levels in cecal lumina were examined using the commercially available ELISA kit (Sigma, St. Louis, MO, USA) following the manufacture protocols. Briefly, a 96 well coated with one specific antibody at the bottom was incubated at the room temperature. After washing, suitably diluted samples were added to designated wells with subsequent addition of secondary antibodies and ortho-phenylenediamine. Following an incubation period, the reaction was stopped with H_2SO_4 and the absorbance was determined at 492 nm in Multiskan ELISA plate reader (Thermolabsystems, Finland).

RT-PCR assays

Total RNA was isolated from the cecal tonsil tissues using TRIzol Reagent (TaKaRa, Dalian, Liaoning, China). Reverse transcription of total RNA was completed using Prime Script RT Reagent Kit (TaKaRa). Primers for RT-PCR were presented in Table 3. PCR was performed with a 7500 Fast Real-Time PCR System (Applied Biosystems,

Table 3 Sequences of primers for the PCR assay

Gene[a]	Forward(5'-3')	Reverse(5'-3')
IL-2	TCTTTGGCTGTATTTCGGTAG	CTTTATTAATGTTTGAAGAGGTTTC
IFN-γ	AGCCGCACATCAAACACAT	TCACCTTCTTCACGCCATC
TNF-α	CTTGGCTGTCGTGTGGTGG	CGTGGGCATTGCAATTTGG
β-tubulin	GCGTTATTTGACTGTGGCG	GGAGCTGTTCTTGGTCTGGA

[a]*IL-2*: interleukin-2; *IFN-γ*: interferon-γ; *TNF-α*: tumor necrosis factor-α

MA, USA), and data were analyzed with the $2^{-\Delta\Delta CT}$ method. β-tubulin expression was used as an internal control to calculate the relative expression levels of targeted genes (Table 3). The mRNA level of each targeted gene for the control birds was assigned a value of one.

Flow cytometry

Flow cytometry was used to assay $CD4^+$ and $CD8^+$ lymphocyte populations in peripheral blood. The fluorescein isothiocyanate (FITC)-$CD4^+$ and phycoerythrin (PE)-$CD8^+$ mouse anti-chicken antibodies (SouthernBiotech, Birmingham, USA) and blood samples were added to each tube and mixed by gentle shaking at 4 °C for 30 min. Erythrocytes were then lysed with 2 mL of Lysing Solution (Becton Dickinson (BD), Franklin Lakes, NJ, USA) at room temperature for 20 min. The lysate was centrifuged at 1500×g for 5 min and the supernatant was removed. The pellet was resuspended in phosphate-buffered saline (PBS). The lysate was centrifuged again at 1500×g for 5 min, the supernatant was removed, and the pellet was resuspended in 500 mL of PBS for assay performed on a flow cytometer (Coulter XL FCM, Beckman Coulter, Brea, CA, USA).

Measurements of anti-oxidative indexes

GHS peroxidase (GPx) in the serum was tested using detection kits (Beyotime Biotechnology, Shanghai, China), according to the manufacturer's instructions. Total antioxidant capacity (T-AOC) of the serum was measured using the azino-diethyl-benzthiazoline sulfate (ABTS) method. Incubation of ABTS with H_2O_2 and a peroxidase (metmyoglobin) results in the production of the blue-green radical cation $ABTS^+$. Antioxidants in the serum suppress this color production proportionally to their concentration. The system was standardized using Trolox, a water-soluble vitamin E analogue. The results were expressed as mmol Trolox equivalent. In malondialdehyde (MDA) assay, 2 mL 0.6% thiobarbituric acid was added to 2 mL of the serum in a 10 mL tube. This tube was next kept in boiling water for 15 min and placed on ice to cool down, before the optical density was measured at 532 nm. The results were expressed as nmol MDA/mL.

Statistical analysis

Statistical analyses were performed using the general linear procedure of the SAS software (Version 9.1; SAS Institute Inc., Cary, NC, USA). A two (anticoccidial programs) by three (dietary Met levels) factorial arrangement of treatments in a randomized complete block design was employed in the analysis of variance. All data were analyzed using anticoccidial programs, dietary Met levels, and their interactions as main effects. Differences among treatment means were classified by Duncan's multiple range test and significant difference was defined at $P < 0.05$. Results are reported as mean ± standard deviation.

Results

Growth performance of chickens

Under *E. tenella*-challenged conditions, anticoccidial programs and dietary Met levels had significant effects on final weight, ADG and ADFI ($P < 0.05$ or 0.01; Table 4). F/G ratio was influenced only by dietary Met levels ($P < 0.05$). There were interactions between anticoccidial programs and dietary Met levels for final weight, ADG and F/G ratio ($P < 0.01$). With regard to the anticoccidial programs, the vaccinated chicks displayed better or identical performance than the medicated chicks except for the high diet Met level (0.68%). In regard to dietary Met levels, feeding 0.45% Met to medicated chicks and 0.68% Met to vaccinated chicks resulted in the lowest final weight, and medicated chickens showed increased ADG and decreased F/G ratio with increasing dietary Met concentrations from 0.45 through to 0.68% ($P < 0.05$). For medicated chickens, high supplemental levels of Met had no effects on ADFI ($P > 0.05$). In contrast, feeding 0.68% Met to vaccinated chickens decreased final weight, ADG and ADFI compared to 0.45% and 0.56% Met ($P < 0.05$). Increasing dietary levels of Met had no beneficial effects on F/G ratio in vaccinated chickens ($P > 0.05$).

Intestinal morphology and the number of excreted coccidial oocysts

The VH, V/C, cecal lesion scores and excreted oocyst numbers were influenced by anticoccidial programs ($P < 0.05$ or 0.01; Table 5). Dietary Met levels changed the VH, CD, V/C, cecal lesion scores and excreted oocyst numbers ($P < 0.05$). For all these indexes, anticoccidial programs and dietary Met levels had an interaction ($P < 0.05$ or 0.01). Medicated chickens showed increased VH and V/C after feeding 0.56% and 0.68% Met compared to 0.45% Met ($P < 0.05$). The CD was decreased after medicated chickens were fed 0.56% and 0.68% Met ($P < 0.05$). However, vaccinated chickens had decreased VH after increasing Met levels ($P < 0.05$). Feeding high levels of Met had no effect on CD of vaccinated chickens ($P > 0.05$). Feeding 0.68% Met decreased V/C in vaccinated chickens ($P < 0.05$).

Vaccinated chickens showed lower cecal lesion scores and excreted coccidial oocysts than medicated chickens, irrespective of Met levels in diet (Table 5). Medicated chickens fed 0.56 and 0.68% Met showed decreased cecal lesion scores ($P < 0.05$). But, vaccinated chickens fed 0.68% Met exhibited increased cecal lesion scores, compared with those fed 0.45% and 0.56% Met ($P < 0.05$). The number of excreted

Table 4 Growth performance of chickens after indicated treatments[1]

	Medicated groups			Vaccinated groups			P value		
Met[2] concentrations:	0.45%	0.56%	0.68%	0.45%	0.56%	0.68%	Anticoccidial program	Met levels	Anticoccidial program × Met levels
Initial BW (g)	466 ± 12	470 ± 14	460 ± 8	470 ± 10	463 ± 11	466 ± 7	0.754	0.499	0.303
Final BW (g)	1187 ± 10^d	1221 ± 19^{bc}	1212 ± 12^c	1244 ± 14^a	1230 ± 0.17^b	1196 ± 13^d	0.004	0.009	<.001
ADFI (g/d)	87.23 ± 0.93^b	87.53 ± 1.66^b	86.69 ± 1.11^b	89.42 ± 0.94^a	89.47 ± 2.56^a	86.47 ± 2.01^b	0.027	0.014	0.166
ADG (g/d)	36.06 ± 0.32^c	37.58 ± 0.94^b	37.61 ± 0.76^b	38.73 ± 0.93^a	38.36 ± 1.11^{ab}	36.50 ± 0.72^c	0.008	0.035	<.001
F/G	2.42 ± 0.02^a	2.33 ± 0.03^b	2.31 ± 0.04^b	2.31 ± 0.03^b	2.33 ± 0.03^b	2.37 ± 0.05^b	0.188	0.032	<.001

[1]An anticoccidial drug (narasin, 60 mg/kg diet) was added to diets in medicated groups, and an anticoccidial 7-valent live vaccine was inoculated in vaccinated groups

[2]*Met* methionine, *BW* body weight, *ADFI* average daily feed intake, *ADG* average daily gain, *F/G* feed to gain ratio

[a,b,c,d]The data of the same row not sharing a lowercase letter differ ($P < 0.05$; $n = 180$)

coccidial oocysts was decreased when medicated chickens were fed 0.56% and 0.68% Met ($P < 0.05$). High supplemental levels of Met in the diet did not affect the number of excreted coccidial oocysts in vaccinated chicks.

Immune responses of chickens

Anticoccidial programs had no effects on the percentages of $CD4^+$ cells in the blood and the mRNA expression of *IFN-γ* in the cecal tonsil tissue ($P > 0.05$), but influenced $CD8^+$ cell percentages, $CD4^+/CD8^+$, cecal luminal sIgA levels and the mRNA expression of *TNF-α* and *IL-2* ($P < 0.05$ or 0.01; Table 6). Dietary Met levels impacted on all these indexes, and had interactions with anticoccidial programs for them ($P < 0.05$ or 0.01). The data showed that increasing dietary Met concentrations to 0.56% and 0.68% elevated the percentages of blood $CD4^+$ cells in medicated chicks ($P < 0.05$). However, the increase in dietary Met concentrations decreased the $CD4^+$ cell percentages in vaccinated chickens ($P < 0.05$). $CD8^+$ cell percentages in medicated chickens were notably increased as well after feeding 0.56% and 0.68% Met ($P < 0.05$). In vaccinated chickens, $CD8^+$ cell percentages were reduced after feeding 0.68% Met ($P < 0.05$). The $CD4^+/CD8^+$ was not influenced by Met concentrations in the diet in medicated chickens ($P > 0.05$), but decreased by high diet Met concentrations in vaccinated chickens ($P < 0.05$).

Feeding 0.56% and 0.68% Met was associated with elevated sIgA level in medicated chickens ($P < 0.05$), but had no effect on sIgA level in vaccinated chickens ($P > 0.05$). When Met concentrations in the diet for medicated chickens were increased to 0.56 and 0.68%, *TNF-α* and *IL-2* mRNA expression levels were dramatically increased ($P < 0.05$). mRNA expression of *TNF-α* and *IL-2* in vaccinated chickens was not affected by dietary Met concentrations. *IFN-γ* mRNA expression was increased in medicated chickens, but decreased in

Table 5 Intestinal morphology and coccidian oocyst numbers after indicated treatments[1]

	Medicated groups			Vaccinated groups			P value		
Met[2] concentrations:	0.45%	0.56%	0.68%	0.45%	0.56%	0.68%	Anticoccidial program	Met levels	Anticoccidial program × Met levels
VH (um)	845.73 ± 90.97^d	907.96 ± 100.88^{bc}	912.49 ± 111.38^b	923.37 ± 102.59^a	905.36 ± 100.60^{bc}	899.85 ± 95.98^c	0.027	0.033	0.009
CD (um)	124.17 ± 15.52^a	112.64 ± 14.08^b	109.84 ± 13.23^b	113.91 ± 15.23^b	112.21 ± 11.34^b	113.15 ± 12.59^b	0.069	0.040	0.039
V/C	6.90 ± 0.60^d	8.09 ± 0.82b^c	8.38 ± 1.07^a	8.15 ± 0.78^b	8.12 ± 0.98^b	8.00 ± 0.90^c	0.031	0.038	0.006
Score	0.89 ± 0.11^a	0.75 ± 0.09^b	0.68 ± 0.06^c	0.46 ± 0.05^e	0.48 ± 0.05^e	0.59 ± 0.07^d	0.008	0.019	0.006
ON (× 10^5/g)	1.47 ± 0.18^a	1.05 ± 0.13^b	1.00 ± 0.09^b	0.39 ± 0.02^c	0.41 ± 0.04^c	0.42 ± 0.05^c	0.004	0.025	0.008

[1]An anticoccidial drug (narasin, 60 mg/kg diet) was added to diets in medicated groups, and an anticoccidial 7-valent live vaccine was inoculated in vaccinated groups

[2]*Met* methionine, *VH*, villus height, *CD*, crypt depth, *V/C* VH to CD ratio; Score: the lesion scores of the cecum; ON: oocyst output

[a,b,c,d,e]The data of the same row not sharing a lowercase letter differ ($P < 0.05$, $n = 30$)

Table 6 Blood immune cell percentages, cecal luminal sIgA contents and the mRNA expression of cytokines in cecal tonsils after indicated treatments[1]

	Medicated groups			Vaccinated groups			*P* value		
Met[2] concentrations:	0.45%	0.56%	0.68%	0.45%	0.56%	0.68%	Anticoccidial program	Met levels	Anticoccidial program × Met levels
CD4 (%)	9.72 ± 1.05[c]	12.27 ± 1.36[a]	12.12 ± 1.33[a]	12.95 ± 1.42[a]	10.85 ± 1.27[b]	10.61 ± 1.17b[c]	0.092	0.028	0.002
CD8 (%)	8.51 ± 0.92[d]	11.16 ± 1.23[a]	10.96 ± 1.08[ab]	10.24 ± 1.14[b]	9.51 ± 1.03[bc]	9.21 ± 0.99[c]	0.045	0.015	0.005
CD4/CD8	1.15 ± 0.11[b]	1.10 ± 0.11[b]	1.11 ± 0.13[b]	1.27 ± 0.12[a]	1.14 ± 0.12[b]	1.16 ± 0.13[b]	0.023	0.041	0.003
sIgA (mg/mL)	1.30 ± 0.19[b]	1.47 ± 0.22[a]	1.52 ± 0.27[a]	1.50 ± 0.24[a]	1.49 ± 0.21[a]	1.50 ± 0.28[a]	0.028	0.037	0.008
TNF-α	1.09 ± 0.11[b]	1.39 ± 0.20[a]	1.47 ± 0.26[a]	0.83 ± 0.09[c]	0.87 ± 0.10[c]	0.81 ± 0.07[c]	0.008	0.035	0.025
IL-2	1.04 ± 0.09[b]	1.27 ± 0.14[a]	1.23 ± 0.18[a]	0.97 ± 0.11[b]	0.95 ± 0.09[b]	0.98 ± 0.07[b]	0.013	0.039	0.031
IFN-γ	1.10 ± 0.14[e]	1.54 ± 0.25[c]	1.62 ± 0.29[b]	1.76 ± 0.33[a]	1.33 ± 0.22[d]	1.14 ± 0.13[e]	0.074	0.005	0.001

[1]An anticoccidial drug (narasin, 60 mg/kg diet) was added to diets in medicated groups, and an anticoccidial 7-valent live vaccine was inoculated in vaccinated groups
[2]*Met* methionine, *CD4* CD4+ cells, *CD8* CD8+ cells, *sIgA* secreted immunoglobulin A, *TNF-α* tumor necrosis factor-α, *IL-2* interleukin-2, *IFN-γ* interferon-γ
[a,b,c,d,e]The data of the same row not sharing a lowercase letter differ ($P < 0.05$, n = 30)

vaccinated chickens, with Met level increased to 0.56% and 0.68% ($P < 0.05$). Feeding 0.45% Met to vaccinated chickens had the highest *IFN-γ* mRNA expression among all treatments.

The serum anti-oxidative parameters of chickens

As indicated in Table 7, anticoccidial programs had no effect on serum MDA concentration ($P > 0.05$), but impacted on GPx activity and T-AOC ($P < 0.05$). Dietary Met levels affected all these indexes ($P < 0.05$). There were interactions between anticoccidial programs and dietary Met levels for GPx activity and T-AOC ($P < 0.05$). Serum GPx activity in medicated chickens was increased by feeding 0.56% Met ($P < 0.05$), compared to 0.45% Met. But the beneficial effect was not evident by feeding 0.68% Met ($P > 0.05$). High Met levels in diets did not affect serum GPx activity in vaccinated chickens ($P > 0.05$).

Compared to 0.45% Met, feeding 0.56 and 0.68% Met increased MDA in serum to 8.62 ($P < 0.05$) and 10.84 nmol/mL ($P < 0.01$) from 6.93 nmol/mL in medicated chickens, and to 8.66 ($P < 0.05$) and 9.40 nmol/mL ($P < 0.05$) from 7.74 nmol/mL in vaccinated chickens. Serum T-AOC in medicated chickens was enhanced by feeding 0.56% Met ($P < 0.05$), but not by feeding 0.68% Met ($P > 0.05$). High Met levels in diets did not affect T-AOC in serum in vaccinated chickens ($P > 0.05$).

Discussion

Coccidiosis is a major parasitic disease of poultry, associated with malabsorption, inefficient feed utilization, impaired growth rate and increased mortality in broilers. *E. tenella* is one of seven species of coccidia that infect chickens. After the oocysts are ingested by chickens, they experience the excystation to generate the invasive

Table 7 The serum anti-oxidative parameters after indicated treatments[1]

	Medicated groups			Vaccinated groups			*P* value		
Met[2] concentrations:	0.45%	0.56%	0.68%	0.45%	0.56%	0.68%	Anticoccidial program	Met levels	Anticoccidial program × Met levels
GPx (U/mL)	1285.26 ± 172.80[b]	1392.71 ± 194.74[a]	1321.81 ± 186.24[ab]	1240.43 ± 157.82[b]	1266.49 ± 160.72[b]	1265.93 ± 161.22[b]	0.042	0.038	0.021
MDA (nmol/mL)	6.93 ± 0.72[e]	8.62 ± 0.89[c]	10.64 ± 1.11[a]	7.74 ± 0.99[d]	8.66 ± 1.19[c]	9.40 ± 1.34[b]	0.102	0.015	0.207
T-AOC (mmol Trolox)	9.55 ± 1.07[b]	10.36 ± 1.96[a]	9.85 ± 1.53[ab]	8.46 ± 0.93[c]	8.77 ± 1.01[bc]	8.79 ± 1.17[bc]	0.023	0.032	0.035

[1]An anticoccidial drug (narasin, 60 mg/kg diet) was added to diets in medicated groups, and an anticoccidial 7-valent live vaccine was inoculated in vaccinated groups
[2]*Met* methionine, *GPx* glutathione peroxidase, *MDA* malondialdehyde, *T-AOC* total antioxidant capacity
[a,b,c,d,e]The data of the same row not sharing a lowercase letter differ ($P < 0.05$, *n* = 30)

sporozoites, which penetrate into epithelial cells of the intestinal mucosa, often causing serious damage to the physical integrity and normal functions of the gut particularly in domestic chickens [16]. Previous study demonstrated that coccidial challenge reduced the amounts of L-Met absorption of broilers by 52% compared to unchallenged controls [17]. Anticoccidial drugs are extensively adopted to combat coccidial infection in the poultry industry, but their influences on Met absorption and requirement of growing broilers challenged by *E. tenella* are seldom investigated. In the present study, chicks were challenged with *E. tenella* by oral gavage of the sporulated oocysts, and were also provided diets containing narasin to control coccidiosis. In this case, feeding increased Met (0.56% and 0.68%) to medicated chicks improved the growth performance compared to 0.45% Met. Previous reports showed that feeding increased Met either had no effects or decreased the growth performance of chicks that were not challenged by coccidia [18, 19]. In general, 1.2% Met is a tolerable excess level that would not depress voluntary food intake or growth rate of broilers [20]. Increasing dietary Met level beyond this value linearly decreased weight gain, feed intake, and feed efficiency of chickens, which is probably due to the toxicity of the sulfur amino acids [21, 22]. Narasin itself has no effect on production performance and nutrient utilization in broiler chickens [23]. Our data, thus, suggest an increased Met requirement of broiler chickens given narasin under *E. tenella* -challenged conditions.

There is increasing concern about rising levels of drug resistance of *Eimeria* species. Narasin is an ionophore coccidiostat, processing a potent, broad-spectrum anticoccidial activity against *Eimeria* species. The control mechanism of ionophore coccidiostats is altering the ion transport and disrupting osmotic balance, which can damage the coccidial sporozoites during their release into the lumen [24]. However, the extensive and long-term use in chemotherapy to control coccidiosis leads to the generation of drug resistance. Peek and Landman [25] found that one isolated *E. tenella* from Dutch broilers in 1996 was sensitive to narasin, however, two isolated *E. tenella* in 1999 showed resistance to narasin. Another study found that replacing a proportion of nicarbazin with narasin results in reduced sensitivity to most coccidial species [26]. Due to drug resistance, some *E. tenella* probably still survive after the exposure to narasin and cause malabsorption and inefficient feed utilization of chickens. This may partly explain the increased Met requirement of the medicated broiler chickens under *E. tenella*-challenged conditions. In addition, we found that feeding increased Met to medicated chickens improved small intestinal morphology, as indicated by the improved VH, CD and V/C as well as reduced cecal lesion and fecal oocyst output. Immunological assays further revealed that immune functions of chickens fed anticoccidial drug were enhanced with the increase of Met levels in diet. These data suggested that increasing Met levels in diet helped medicated chickens antagonize the challenge of *E. tenella* through the stimulation of immune functions. Met is known to play an important role in the immune functions by regulating antibody production and cell-mediated immune responses. We hypothesized that anticoccidial drug narasin may be incapable of most effectively controlling the number of *E. tenella* probably due to the drug resistance under a heavy load of *E. tenella* infection. Many survived *E. tenella* induced the host immune response that is conducive to eliminating these pathogenic microorganisms. Increased Met in diet just meets the increased requirement for the stimulated immune functions. Following exposure to *Eimeria* species either naturally or via vaccination, chicks gradually develop acquired immunity and become resistant to reinfection of coccidia [9, 16]. *Eimeria* infection can induce a significant increase of $CD8^+$ cells in the intraepithelial leucocytes, tonsil lymphocytes and peripheral blood [27–30]. $CD4^+$ cells were also increased in the intraepithelial leucocytes, but decreased in the peripheral blood and spleen [29, 31]. The decrease in CD4+ cells was observed after primary infection of *Eimeria*, but not the secondary infection [29, 31]. To understand the role of these T cells in the protection against coccidiosis, previous experiments studied the response of immunosuppressed chickens by elimination of specific T cells to coccidial challenge. The selective depletion of $CD4^+$ cells reduced *IFN-γ* mRNA expression in the cecal tonsil and intraepithelial lymphocytes and increased production of oocysts of *E. tenella* in chicks [28, 32], which suggests the important role of $CD4^+$ lymphocytes in controlling primary infection with *E. tenella*. The selective elimination of $CD8^+$ cells resulted in the exacerbation of disease as evidenced by increased oocyst shedding after secondary infection with *E. tenella* or *E. acervulina* [32]. It is known that $CD4^+$ cells play an important helper function in protective immune responses, and $CD8^+$ cells act as effector cells in these processes [33]. Both CD4+ and CD8+ cells are responsible for the IFN-γ production [33]. IFN-γ production is higher in chicks infected with *Eimeria* species compared with non-infected chicks, and higher levels of IFN-γ coincide with a protective immune response to the infection [27]. Previous study found that pretreatment with cultural supernatants containing IFN-γ inhibited the intracellular development of *E. tenella* [34, 35]. Apart from IFN-γ, factors like IL-2 and IgA are induced for the resistance to *E. tenella*, as reviewed by Lillehoj et al. [35]. Although coccidial vaccination confers the protection of the host from coccidial infection, the enhanced immune functions likely increase Met consumption for the synthesis of more immunity-related proteins. Thus, it is necessary theoretically to increase Met supply to meet this specific requirement. Unexpectedly, in the present study, feeding a diet containing 0.56% Met had no growth stimulating effect on vaccinated chickens, compared to 0.45% Met. The increment of Met to 0.68% conversely decreased the feed intake and weight gains. In addition, we found that supplementation with high Met levels decreased $CD4^+$ and $CD8^+$ cells in the blood and suppressed *IFN-γ* mRNA expression in cecal tonsils, suggesting an inhibited immune function against *E. tenella*. Maybe the reason is that coccidial vaccination confers the protection of the host from coccidial infection, so 0.45% Met is sufficient for chickens vaccinated. Excess Met could be detrimental to the antioxidative system and immune function. It was reported that feeding Met-sufficient diets (containing 0.50 and 0. 70% Met) decreased the growth, feed intake and efficiency of feed utilization of chickens that were injected with some components of microbial pathogens, like *Escherichia coli* lipopolysaccharide or heat-killed *Staphylococcus aureus* [36]. This study suggests that Met-sufficient diet contributes to the generation of immunologic stress upon the stimulation by the immunogens. In the status of immunologic stress, increased releases of cytokines, including IL-1 and TNF-α, are associated with increased production of adrenocorticotropin and thyroxin-stimulating hormones. These metabolism-related hormones may be implicated in the poor growth performance. There is evidence indicating that TNF-α plays biphasic roles following *E. tenella* infection. TNF-α leads to the development of a protective immunity on the one hand, but, on the other hand, it participates in the pathogenesis of coccidiosis, because treatment of chickens with antibodies against TNF-α results in a partial abrogation of *E. tenella*-induced body weight loss in chickens [35]. Although *TNF-α* mRNA expression in cecal tonsils of the vaccinated chickens was not affected by increased diet Met levels, it was unclear whether the influence on TNF-α occurs in other immune organs, such as the spleen and intraepithelial lymphocytes. Further studies are warranted to investigate TNF-α alterations in these locations.

Eimeria infection increases the activity of NADPH oxidase, an important enzyme for production of oxidative species in infected mucosa [37]. It is known that Met serves as a precursor for the synthesis of GSH and taurine and hence plays a role in the defense against oxidative stress. It has reported that feeding 0.5% Met promotes the synthesis of the GSH and GPx activity in the liver of growing chicks co-fed increased unsaturated fats [38]. Broilers given a diet containing 0.59% Met have a higher hepatic GSH: GSH disulphide ratio than those given a diet containing 0.49% Met at day 21. In addition, broilers given high dietary Met have enhanced serum superoxide dismutase activity and decreased MDA content at day 7 [39]. Wen et al. [40] found that feeding 0. 57% Met increases T-AOC in breast muscle of fast-growing broilers compared to 0.44% Met. These studies suggest that a higher dietary Met concentration improves antioxidant status in broilers. Under heat stress conditions, feeding high levels of Met to broilers contributes to increased expression levels of genes related to antioxidant activity, including cystathionine β-synthase, GSH synthetase and GPx [41]. In the present study, increasing dietary Met concentrations from 0.45% to 0.56% was associated with increased GPx activity and T-AOC in serum in medicated chickens. But, the increase in dietary Met concentrations had no such effect in vaccinated chickens. MDA is one of the final products of polyunsaturated fatty acids peroxidation. As polyunsaturated fatty acids are highly susceptible to oxidative species compared with other macromolecular substances, such as protein and DNA, MDA is considered as a sensitive biomarker of oxidative stress. We found that dietary Met increased serum MDA levels in both medicated and vaccinated chickens in a dose-dependent manner. It is likely that feeding high levels of Met increases production of oxidative species in chickens under specific conditions, although Met can contribute to the synthesis of antioxidant products and enzymes.

Conclusions

In the present study, vaccinated chickens that were given 0.45% Met showed greater growth performance than medicated chickens that were provided basal (0.45%) or even increased levels of Met. Therefore, inoculation with anticoccidial vaccine is a better strategy for controlling coccidiosis than feeding narasin, not only due to greater growth performance obtained by the vaccination, but also due to the lower Met supplementation to achieve optimized performance. Furthermore, the present study for the first time revealed that high dietary Met levels benefit the growth performance of mediated chickens under *E. tenella*-challenged condition, but has no beneficial effects on that of vaccinated chickens.

Abbreviations

ADFI: Average daily feed intake; ADG: Average daily gain; CD: Crypt depth; *E. acervulina*: *Emeria acervulina*; *E. tenella*: *Emeria tenella*; F/G: Feed to gain ratio; GPx: Glutathione peroxidase; GSH: Glutathione; IFN-γ: Interferon-γ; Ig: Immunoglobulin; IL-2: Interleukin-2; MDA: Malondialdehyde; Met: Methionine; ON: Oocyst output; PBS: Phosphate-buffered saline; T-AOC: Total antioxidant capacity; TNF-α: Tumor necrosis factor-α; V/C: VH to CD ratio; VH: Villus height

Acknowledgements

The authors gratefully acknowledge the participation, expertise, and dedication of the entire staff of the Sichuan Giant Star Company's Poultry Farm.

Funding
This work was supported by Fundamental Research Funds for the Central Universities (XDJK2017A003) and the Innovation Team Building Program in Chongqing universities (CXTDG201602004) as well as funds for poultry fundamental research from Sichuan Giant Star Company.

Authors' contributions
AL, GD, DS, and TY conceived the study, performed the statistical analysis and drafted the manuscript. AL and XZ participated in animal experiments. GD managed the entire experiments and revised the manuscript. All authors read and approved the final manuscript.

Competing interests
The authors declare that they have no competing interests.

Author details
[1]College of Animal Science and Technology, Southwest University, Beibei, Chongqing 400716, People's Republic of China. [2]Sichuan Giant Star Company's Experimental Station, Leshan, Sichuan 614800, People's Republic of China.

References
1. Wu BY, Cui HM, Xi P, Fang J, Cui W, Liu XD. Effect of methionine deficiency on the thymus and the subsets and proliferation of peripheral blood T-cell, and serum IL-2 contents in broilers. J Integr Agr. 2012;11:1009–19.
2. Mirzaaghatabar F, Saki AA, Zamani P, Aliarabi H, Hemati Matin HR. Effect of different levels of diet methionine and metabolisable energy on broiler performance and immune system. Food Agr Immunol. 2011;22:93–103.
3. Métayer S, Seiliez I, Collin A, Duchêne S, Mercier Y, Geraert PA, Tesseraud S. Mechanisms through which sulfur amino acids control protein metabolism and oxidative status. J Nutr Biochem. 2008;19:207–15.
4. Gao F, Das SK. Epigenetic regulations through DNA methylation and hydroxymethylation: clues for early pregnancy in decidualization. Biomol Concepts. 2014;5:95–107.
5. Brocard M, Ruggieri A, Locker N. m6A RNA methylation, a new hallmark in virus-host interactions. J Gen Virol. 2017;98:2207–14.
6. Jin W, Peng J, Jiang S. The epigenetic regulation of embryonic myogenesis and adult muscle regeneration by histone methylation modification. Biochem Biophys Rep. 2016;6:209–19.
7. Li P, Yin YL, Li D, Kim SW, Amino WG. Acids and immune function. Br J Nutr. 2007;98:237–52.
8. Amerah AM, Ravindran V. Effect of coccidia challenge and natural betaine supplementation on performance, nutrient utilization, and intestinal lesion scores of broiler chickens fed suboptimal level of dietary methionine. Poult Sci. 2015;94:673–80.
9. Kitandu A, Juranová R. Progress in control measures for chicken coccidiosis. Acta Vet Brno. 2006;75:265–76.
10. Grimble RF, Grimble GK. Immunonutrition: role of sulfur amino acids, related amino acids, and polyamines. Nutrition. 1998;14:605–10.
11. Maroufyan E, Kasim A, Yong Meng G, Ebrahimi M, Teck Chwen L, Mehrbod P, Kamalidehghan B, Soleimani Far jam A. Effect of dietary combination of methionine and fish oil on cellular immunity and plasma fatty acids in infectious bursal disease challenged chickens. Scientific World J. 2013;2013: 531397.
12. Rama Rao SV, Praharaj NK, Ramasubba Reddy V, Panda AK. Interaction between genotype and dietary concentrations of methionine for immune function in commercial broilers. Br Poult Sci. 2003;44:104–12.
13. Chinese Ministry of Agriculture. Feeding standard of chickens (NY/T 33–2004). Beijing: China Agriculture Press; 2004.
14. Long PL, Joyner LPA. Guide to laboratory techniques used in the study and diagnosis of avian coccidiosis. Folia Vet Lat. 1976;6:201–17.
15. Johnson J, Reid WM. Anticoccidial drugs: lesion scoring techniques in battery and floor-pen experiments with chickens. Exp Parasitol. 1970;28:30–6.
16. Yun CH, Lillehoj HS, Lillehoj EP. Intestinal immune responses to coccidiosis. Dev Comp Immunol. 2000;24:303–24.
17. Ruff MD, Edgar SA. Reduced intestinal absorption in broilers during Eimeria mitis infection. Am J Vet Res. 1982;43:507–9.
18. Takahashi K, Horiguchi M. Effects of excess and deficiency of dietary methionine on mixed-function oxidase system of hepatic microsomes in male broilers. Comp Biochem Physiol A Comp Physiol. 1991;100:1049–52.
19. Swain BK, Johri TS. Effect of supplemental methionine, choline and their combinations on the performance and immune response of broilers. Brit Poultry Sci. 2000;41:83–8.
20. Scherer CS, Baker DH. Excess dietary methionine markedly increases the vitamin B-6 requirement of young chicks. J Nutr. 2000;130:3055–8.
21. Han Y, Baker DH. Effects of excess methionine or lysine for broilers fed a corn-soybean meal diet. Poult Sci. 1993;72:1070–4.
22. Acar N, Barbato GF, Patterson PH. The effect of feeding excess methionine on live performance, carcass traits, and ascitic mortality. Poult Sci. 2001;80: 1585–9.
23. Kalmendal R, Tauson R. Effects of a xylanase and protease, individually or in combination, and an ionophore coccidiostat on performance, nutrient utilization, and intestinal morphology in broiler chickens fed a wheat-soybean meal-based diet. Poult Sci. 2012;91:1387–93.
24. Shaw AL, van Ginkel FW, Macklin KS, Blake JP. Effects of phytase supplementation in broiler diets on a natural Eimeria challenge in naive and vaccinated birds. Poult Sci. 2011;90:781–90.
25. Peek HW, Landman WJ. Resistance to anticoccidial drugs of Dutch avian Eimeria spp. field isolates originating from 1996, 1999 and 2001. Avian Pathol. 2003;32:391–401.
26. Bafundo KW, Cervantes HM, Mathis GF. Sensitivity of Eimeria field isolates in the United States: responses of nicarbazin-containing anticoccidials. Poult Sci. 2008;87:1760–7.
27. Breed DG, Dorrestein J, Schetters TP, Waart LV, Rijke E, Vermeulen AN. Peripheral blood lymphocytes from E. Tenella infected chickens produce gamma-interferon after stimulation in vitro. Parasite Immunol. 1997;19:127–35.
28. Yun CH, Lillehoj HS, Choi KD. Eimeria tenella infection induces local gamma interferon production and intestinal lymphocyte subpopulation changes. Infect Immun. 2000;68:1282–8.
29. Bessay M, Le Vern Y, Kerboeuf D, Yvoré P, Quéré P. Changes in intestinal intra-epithelial and systemic T-cell subpopulations after an Eimeria infection in chickens: comparative study between E acervulina and E tenella. Vet Res. 1996;27:503–14.
30. Hong YH, Lillehoj HS, Lillehoj EP, Lee SH. Changes in immune-related gene expression and intestinal lymphocyte subpopulations following Eimeria maxima infection of chickens. Vet Immunol Immunopathol. 2006;114: 259–72.
31. Breed DG, Dorrestein J, Vermeulen AN. Immunity to Eimeria tenella in chickens: phenotypical and functional changes in peripheral blood T-cell subsets. Avian Dis. 1996;40:37–48.
32. Trout JM, Lillehoj HS. T lymphocyte roles during Eimeria acervulina and Eimeria tenella infections. Vet Immunol Immunopathol. 1996;53:163–72.
33. Breed DG, Schetters TP, Verhoeven NA, Vermeulen AN. Characterization of phenotype related responsiveness of peripheral blood lymphocytes from Eimeria tenella infected chickens. Parasite Immunol. 1997;19:563–9.
34. Bumstead JM, Topham SJ, Tomley FM. Inhibition of the development of Eimeria tenella in cultured bovine kidney cells by a soluble factor produced by peripheral blood lymphocytes from immune chickens. Parasitology. 1998;117:39–47.
35. Lillehoj HS, Min W, Dalloul RA. Recent progress on the cytokine regulation of intestinal immune responses to Eimeria. Poult Sci. 2004;83:611–23.
36. Klasing KC, Barnes DM. Decreased amino acid requirements of growing chicks due to immunologic stress. J Nutr. 1988;118:1158–64.
37. Allen PC. Production of free radical species during Eimeria maxima infections in chickens. Poult Sci. 1997;76:814–21.
38. Németh K, Mézes M, Gaál T, Bartos A, Balogh K, Husvéth F. Effect of supplementation with methionine and different fat sources on the glutathione redox system of growing chickens. Acta Vet Hung. 2004;52: 369–78.

39. Chen YP, Chen X, Zhang H, Zhou YM. Effects of dietary concentrations of methionine on growth performance and oxidative status of broiler chickens with different hatching weight. Br Poult Sci. 2013;54:531–7.
40. Wen C, Jiang XY, Ding LR, Wang T, Zhou YM. Effects of dietary methionine on growth performance, meat quality and oxidative status of breast muscle in fast- and slow-growing broilers. Poult Sci. 2017;96:1707–14.
41. Del Vesco AP, Gasparino E, Grieser Dde O, Zancanela V, Soares MA, Neto AR. Effects of methionine supplementation on the expression of oxidative stress-related genes in acute heat stress-exposed broilers. Br J Nutr. 2015; 113:549–59.

21

Efficacy of an adenovirus-vectored foot-and-mouth disease virus serotype: a subunit vaccine in cattle using a direct contact transmission model

John G. Neilan[1*], Christopher Schutta[1], José Barrera[2,3], Melia Pisano[3,4], Laszlo Zsak[1], Ethan Hartwig[5], Max V. Rasmussen[1], Barbara J. Kamicker[3], Damodar Ettyreddy[6], Douglas E. Brough[6], Bryan T. Butman[6] and David A. Brake[7]

Abstract

Background: A direct contact transmission challenge model was used to simulate natural foot-and-mouth disease virus (FMDV) spread from FMDV A24/Cruzeiro/BRA/55 infected 'seeder' steers to naïve or vaccinated steers previously immunized with a replication-deficient human adenovirus-vectored FMDV A24/Cruzeiro/BRA/55 capsid-based subunit vaccine (AdtA24). In two independent vaccine efficacy trials, AdtA24 was administered once intramuscularly in the neck 7 days prior to contact with FMDV A24/Cruzeiro/BRA/55-infected seeder steers.

Results: In Efficacy Study 1, we evaluated three doses of AdtA24 to estimate the 50%/90% bovine protective dose ($BPD_{50/90}$) for prevention of clinical FMD. In vaccinated, contact-challenged steers, the $BPD_{50/90}$ was 3.1×10^{10} / 5.5×10^{10} AdtA24 particles formulated without adjuvant. In Efficacy Study 2, steers vaccinated with 5×10^{10} AdtA24 particles, exposed to FMDV A24/Cruzeiro/BRA/55-infected seeder steers, did not develop clinical FMD or transmit FMDV to other vaccinated or naïve, non-vaccinated steers. In contrast, naïve, non-vaccinated steers that were subsequently exposed to FMDV A24/Cruzeiro/BRA/55-infected seeder steers developed clinical FMD and transmitted FMDV by contact to additional naïve, non-vaccinated steers. The AdtA24 vaccine differentiated infected from vaccinated animals (DIVA) because no antibodies to FMDV nonstructural proteins were detected prior to FMDV exposure.

Conclusions: A single dose of the AdtA24 non-adjuvanted vaccine conferred protection against clinical FMD at 7 days post-vaccination following direct contact transmission from FMDV-infected, naïve, non-vaccinated steers. The AdtA24 vaccine was effective in preventing FMDV transmission from homologous challenged, contact-exposed, AdtA24-vaccinated, protected steers to co-mingled, susceptible steers, suggesting that the vaccine may be beneficial in reducing both the magnitude and duration of a FMDV outbreak in a commercial cattle production setting.

Keywords: Foot-and-mouth disease virus, FMDV A24/Cruzeiro/BRA/55, Replication-deficient human adenovirus vectored vaccine, DIVA, Vaccine efficacy

* Correspondence: John.Neilan@st.dhs.gov
[1]U.S. Department of Homeland Security Science and Technology Directorate, Plum Island Animal Disease Center, P.O. Box 848, Greenport, NY 11944, USA
Full list of author information is available at the end of the article

Background

Foot-and-mouth disease (FMD) afflicts cloven-hooved animals, including cattle, pigs, sheep, goats, and buffalo and is enzootic throughout most of Africa and Asia. In most susceptible animals, FMD is characterized by pedal and oronasal vesicular lesions. The causative agent, foot-and-mouth disease virus (FMDV), a *Picornaviridae* RNA virus, encodes capsid proteins, nonstructural proteins and proteases (reviewed [1]). There are seven FMDV serotypes, and numerous strains within each serotype that often fail to confer intra-serotype immunity following immunization. Many FMD endemic and epizootic countries currently control outbreaks through annual or semi-annual vaccination with conventional, inactivated vaccines. However, in FMD-free countries, next generation recombinant FMD vaccines produced without the use of virulent FMDV strains are more advantageous than inactivated vaccines, especially for a rapid response against newly emerging FMDV topotypes/viral lineages that are a poor antigenic match against current vaccines. For example, the FMDV capsid gene sequence from an outbreak strain can be obtained following virus isolation, rapidly synthesized, and inserted into a standardized viral-vector vaccine production platform. In the event of an outbreak in a FMD-free country, a 'vaccinate to retain' versus a 'vaccinate to remove' policy would benefit from a recombinant FMD subunit vaccine. The AdtA24 described below, based on the AdtFMD vaccine platform, is genetically deleted in antibody epitopes used in current FMD serological diagnostic tests and thus can differentiate infected from vaccinated animals (DIVA).

The FMDV main transmission route in nature is by aerosol or direct contact (reviewed [2, 3]). Numerous FMD inactivated vaccine studies demonstrating clinical FMD protection using indirect or direct challenge models in livestock have been reported (reviewed [4]). Cattle vaccinated with a conventional FMDV serotype O vaccine were assessed for clinical FMD and the ability to transmit FMDV following indirect co-housing with previously infected pigs for various times post-vaccination [5]. Results demonstrated that cattle vaccinated 21 days prior to challenge were protected against clinical FMD and failed to transmit FMDV to susceptible cattle. When the interval between vaccination and infected pig contact exposure was shortened, mixed results were observed, leading to the recommendation that in the event of an outbreak, FMD-vaccinated cattle should be sequestered from non-vaccinated cattle for a minimum of three weeks. Additional studies using FMD high potency vaccines and indirect aerosol challenge from infected pigs at 2–4 days post-vaccination (dpv) confirmed that vaccinated cattle and pigs were protected against clinical FMD [6, 7]. In a swine direct contact challenge model, when FMDV serotype O vaccinated pigs were directly exposed to infected pigs for only 2 h, the majority of vaccinated pigs developed clinical FMD [8]. Another study using vaccinated pigs followed by a 9 h direct challenge period reported similar findings [9]. Additional studies using vaccinated cattle directly exposed to FMDV-infected naïve cattle indicated that normal dose or high potency vaccinated cattle were fully protected 3 weeks post-vaccination following subsequent exposure to infected cattle for 5 days [10, 11]. However, protection was reduced to 70–75% when a shorter, 10 day vaccine-to-challenge interval was used [12].

A few studies have evaluated the effectiveness of next generation FMD vaccines in contact challenge models. Protection using adenovectored FMD-vaccinated pigs subsequently challenged by direct contact with infected pigs has been reported [13, 14]. We recently reported that a replication deficient, recombinant human adenovirus serotype 5 vectored (Ad5) adjuvant-free vaccine co-expressing the P1 capsid from FMDV A24/Cruzeiro/BRA/55 and 3C protease genes of FMDV A12/119/Kent/UK/32 (AdtA24) was efficacious at 7 dpv in cattle using a intradermolingual (IDL) direct challenge model [15] and enabled DIVA prior to challenge. This AdtA24 vaccine also passed five safety evaluations: no adverse effects on calves, no reversion to virulence, no shedding from vaccinees to naïve animals, no excretion in milk from lactating dairy cows, and < 4% transient injection site reactions in 500 beef and dairy cattle evaluated under field conditions [16]. In order to expand these initial studies, we assessed AdtA24 vaccine efficacy in cattle using two different direct contact FMDV challenge experimental designs.

Methods

Animals

Healthy Holstein cross-bred steers, three to six months of age and 130–230 kg were purchased from an Association for the Assessment and Accreditation of Laboratory Animal Care accredited livestock facility. Animal care and study conduct were in compliance with the guidelines of and approved by the Plum Island Animal Disease Center (PIADC) Institutional Biosafety Committee and the Institutional Animal Care and Use Committee. Steers were acclimated and housed in the PIADC BSL-3 Ag animal facility. Prior to vaccination, steers were randomly allocated to treatment groups.

Experimental FMD vaccine

The AdtA24 vaccine vector was produced by GenVec, Inc. (Gaithersburg, MD) as previously summarized [15, 17, 18]. AdtA24 contains the P1-2A coding regions from FMDV A24/Cruzeiro/BRA/55, and the partially deleted (missing the amino terminus six amino acids) 3B1, complete 3B2, 3B3, and 3C nonstructural protein coding regions from FMDV A12/119/Kent/UK/32. For each vaccine lot, total particle units (PU) were quantified by HPLC [17], and all vaccines were stored at -80 °C. On the day of vaccination, thawed vaccines were diluted in final formulation buffer (FFB; Lonza). No adjuvants were used in these studies and for each study, baseline serum samples were collected immediately prior to vaccination (Day 0). Steers were inoculated intramuscularly (IM) in the cleidooccipitalis muscle with a single 2 ml injection with placebo (FFB) for control animals or one of the AdtA24 vaccine doses listed below for each study.

Challenge virus preparation and administration

FMDV A24/Cruzeiro/BRA/55 challenge virus (1×10^4 bovine infectious dose 50% /0.4 mL) was prepared and administered by the intradermal lingual (IDL) route to naïve control or naïve 'seeder' steers. Each steer received four, 0.1 ml injections in the tongue, as described previously [15, 18].

Experimental study designs

Efficacy study 1

The objective was to determine the AdtA24 immunogenic properties of three different vaccine doses and to evaluate their efficacy to protect cattle against experimental FMDV contact challenge at 7-days post-vaccination. Six steers per group were allocated for T1, T2 and T3, four steers to T4, and eight 'seeder' steers to T5 (Fig. 1a). AdtA24 treatments groups were: T1, 5×10^{10} PU (High dose); T2, 1.25×10^{10} PU (Medium dose); T3, 3.1×10^9 PU (Low dose). Primary (1°) Naïve, contact-challenged steers (T4) received FFB. Following injections, T1-T4 steers were co-mingled in the same pen and room. On Day 6, T5 'seeder' steers were infected via the IDL route, housed for 24 h in a separate pen in the same room housing T1-T4 steers, and then all 30 steers were allowed to intermingle starting on Day 7 (0 dpcc). The ratio of vaccinated (T1-T3) to infected steers (T5) was 18:8 (2.25:1) during 0–2 dpcc, Once the naïve contact (T4) and infected steers (T5) developed full clinical disease (pedal lesions on all 4 hooves)(3–6 dpcc) T4-T5 steers were from the co-mingling pen to another pen located in the same room through study durations (21 dpcc). Serum samples were collected weekly for the virus neutralization test starting on the day of vaccination (prior to AdtA24 administration). Oral and nasal swabs (Dacron polyester) were collected on 0–5 dpcc to detect the presence of FMDV by rRT-PCR.

Efficacy study 2

The main objective was to determine if a single high (emergency) dose of AdtA24 could prevent primary vaccinated 'donor' cattle contact exposed to FMDV infected cattle, from subsequent FMDV transmission to non-vaccinated, naïve cattle. On Day − 7, twelve T2 1° steers were vaccinated with 5×10^{10} PU AdtA24 and six T3 1° naïve steers were injected with a placebo (FFB). Between Day − 7 and Day − 1, the T2 1° and T3 1° naïve steers were co-mingled with ten T1 'seeder' steers which were IDL challenged with A24/Cruzeiro/BRA/55 on Day 0. (Fig. 1b). After 2 days post contact challenge (2 dpcc) by the 10 T1 IDL-challenged seeder steers: (i) three T2 1° vaccinated and exposed steers were moved into Room 1 that housed T4 AdtA24 secondary (2°) vaccinated steers ($n = 4$) previously immunized on Day − 5, (ii) three T2 1° vaccinated and exposed steers were moved into Room 2 that housed four T5 non-vaccinated (2° naïve) steers, and (iii) three T3 placebo-injected (1° naïve and exposed) steers were moved into Room 3 that housed four T6 recipient non-vaccinated (2° naïve) steers. This same allocation method was repeated 24 h later (after 3 dpcc) with the remaining six T2 1° vaccinated and exposed steers and three T3 placebo-injected (1° naïve and exposed) steers. Steers were then co-mingled within each room (10 steers/room; Rooms 1–3) for an additional 36 days (study termination). For the initial study phase during 0–2 dpcc, the ratio of donor vaccinated to naïve steers was 0.75:1, and decreased to 0.46:1 on 2–3 dpcc. For the subsequent 4–43 dpcc study phase, the ratio of T2 donor vaccinates to T4 recipient vaccinates or T5 recipient naïve steers was 1:1. Serum samples were collected weekly for the virus neutralization test and to detect antibodies to the FMDV nonstructural proteins starting on the day of vaccination (prior to AdtA24 administration). Plasma samples were collected daily on 0–7 and 9 dpcc. Oral (mouth) and nasal samples were separately collected on 0, 2, and 4 dpcc, and probang samples on 29–30, 36–37, and 42–43 dpcc to detect the presence of FMDV by rRT-PCR.

Clinical observations and analytical assays

Trained scientists, through masked treatment allocation, performed clinical observations (lesions). Following IDL challenges, the presence or absence of clinical FMD in sedated steers was assessed twice per week through the study termination date. FMD clinical signs and lesions used the following criteria: negative, no pedal or oronasal (lip, mouth or nose) vesicular lesions; positive, one or more pedal or oronasal vesicular lesions.

Virus neutralization test (VNT)

Beginning on the day of vaccination, serum samples were collected weekly, prior to administration of any treatments, heat inactivated (56 °C, 30 min), and stored at -20 °C. FMDV A24/Cruzeiro/BRA/55 VNT titers were determined on BHK21 [C13] (ATCC® CCL10™) cells, measuring cytopathic effect, as previously described [15]. The VNT geometric mean titers (GMT) were calculated using a value of 0.6 $\log_{10}$ for samples that were below the limit of detection.

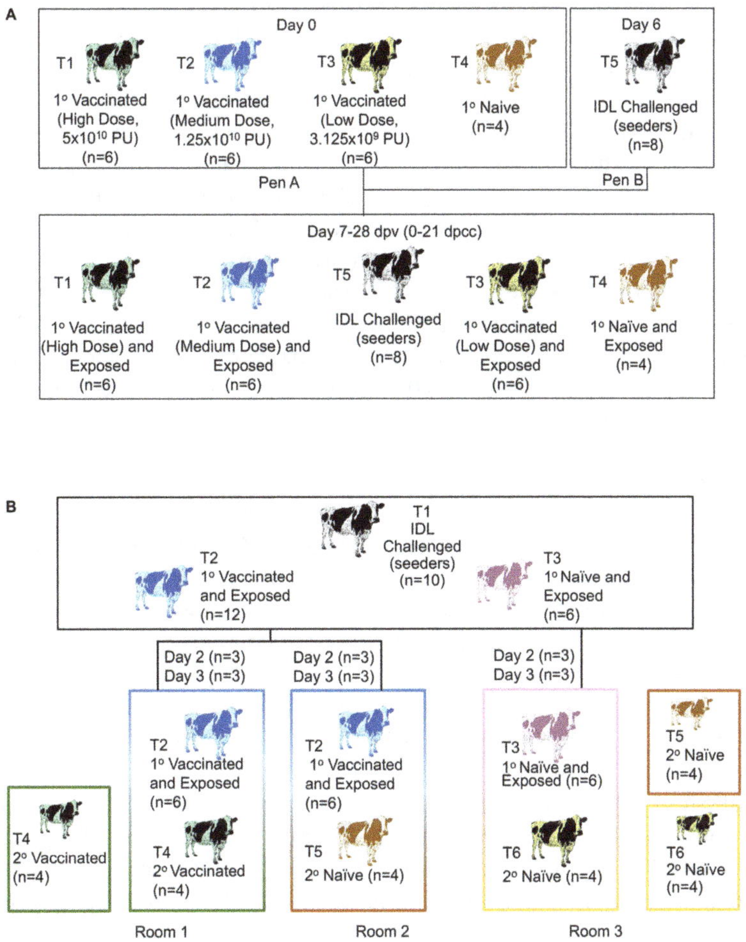

Fig. 1 a. Efficacy Study 1 Experimental Design: Evaluation of vaccinated and non-vaccinated steers following contact with FMDV-infected steers. Top row: A total of 18 steers vaccinated with either a high, medium or low dose of AdtA24 vaccine and 4 naïve steers were co-mingled beginning 7 dpv with 8 steers that were directly infected with FMDV 24 h earlier (6 dpv). **b**. Efficacy Study 2: Experimental Design: Evaluation of vaccinated and non-vaccinated steers in contact with FMDV-exposed steers. Top row: 12 "primary (1°) vaccinated and exposed" T2 steers were vaccinated with 5×10^{10} particle units of AdtA24 7 days prior to co-mingling with 10 T1 steers that were infected with FMDV via the intradermolingual (IDL) route on Day 0. The 10 T1 IDL-challenged 'seeder' steers were mingled with 12 T2 AdtA24 "1° vaccinated and exposed" steers for 2 ($n = 6$ steers) and 3 days ($n = 6$ steers) and with 6 T3 "1° naïve and exposed" steers for 2–3 days (3 steers for each day of duration). Bottom rows: for the next 41 days, 4 T4 2° vaccinated + 6 T2 1° vaccinated and exposed steers were in room 1; 4 T5 2° naïve + 6 T2 1° vaccinated and exposed steers were in room 2; 4 T6 2° naïve + 6 T3 1° naïve steers were in room 3

A test sample was scored positive if the VNT titer was ≥0.9 $\log_{10}$.

Detection of FMDV or FMDV nucleic acid

Clinical samples

LFBK$\alpha_v\beta_6$ cells (kindly provided by M. LaRocco, USDA Agricultural Research Service, PIADC [19, 20]) were used to detect FMDV from plasma, oral, nasal, and probang samples based on cytopathic effect [18]. Oral and nasal swabs were placed separately into chilled transport medium, mixed, removed, and samples frozen at -70 °C. Thawed, centrifuged, and clarified samples (Spin-X centrifuge tube filters) were tested. FMDV nucleic acid in plasma, oral, and nasal samples was detected by Real-Time Reverse Transcriptase-Polymerase Chain Reaction (rRT-PCR) [18, 21]. A sample C_t value < 40 was scored as positive. Oral and nasal results are reported together (i.e., oronasal fluids).

Air samples

In Efficacy Study 2, to detect circulating FMDV nucleic acid by rRT-PCR, two air filter samples were collected on opposite sides of each room for all three rooms daily for 18 days (2–20 dpcc) and then on alternate days until 43 dpcc. Air sampling was performed as previously described [22] and filters were replaced every 24 h. A sample was considered positive if the Ct value was < 40 in at least one air filter/room. Samples for each room were tested separately and results are shown for each room.

Detection of antibodies to FMDV non-structural proteins (NSP)
During both studies, weekly serum samples were collected to detect antibodies to FMDV 3ABC NSPs using the PrioCHECK® FMDV NS ELISA (ThermoFisher Scientific), according to manufacturer's instructions. A serum sample was considered positive if the percent inhibition was ≥50%.

Data analysis
Serum VNT geometric mean titers and standard deviations were calculated (Microsoft Excel). Comparisons between treatments within an experiment were done using unpaired one- or two-tailed T-tests (Excel). *p*-values ≤0.05 were considered significant. BPD_{50} and BPD_{90} values were calculated by the Spearman-Kärber method using lesion data obtained on 14 dpcc [23].

Results

Efficacy – Study 1
On the day of contact challenge (7 dpv/0 dpcc), 100%, 100%, and 67% of T1-T3 vaccinates, respectively had FMDV A24/Cruzeiro/BRA/55 VNT titers (Table 1). VNT responses were vaccine dose-dependent, and the T1 GMT (2.2 ± 0.2) was statistically higher compared to T2 (1.5 ± 0.5) ($p = 0.01$) and T3 (1.1 ± 0.5) ($p < 0.001$). On 3 days post-challenge, all eight IDL-infected seeder steers (T5) had pedal lesions on all four hooves except for one with three hooves with lesions, and all had oronasal lesions. Two of four 1° naïve contact controls (T4) developed pedal lesions by 3dpcc: one had two and the other had four hooves affected. On 7 dpcc, all four T4 steers were positive on all hooves. In T1-T3 vaccinates, protection against clinical FMD (e.g., any vesicular lesion) was vaccine dose-dependent, since 50% of T1 high dose vaccinates were completely protected compared to 33% and 0% of T2, medium dose, and T3, low dose, vaccinates. The $BPD_{50/90}$ for prevention of clinical FMD (any lesions) was 3.1×10^{10} / 5.5×10^{10} PU. All vaccinates were rRT-PCR positive for FMDV RNA in the oronasal cavity. The majority (16/18; 89%) of AdtA24 vaccinated steers developed NSP antibodies at 14 dpcc (Table 1). The two NSP negative, vaccinated steers in the T1 high dose group were also completely protected against pedal and oronasal lesions (data not shown).

Efficacy – Study 2
On 7 dpv (day of contact challenge with 10 T1 IDL challenged 'seeder' steers with lesions on all hooves), 100% of T2 1° vaccinated and exposed steers had FMDV VNT titers (GMT = 1.5 ± 0.2 log_{10}). Additionally, 75% (3/4) of T4 AdtA24 2° vaccinates (Room 1) had FMDV VNT titers (GMT = 0.9 ± 0.2 log_{10}) at 5 dpv, the first day of contact challenge with T2 1° vaccinated and exposed steers (Table 2).

All ten T1 IDL challenged seeder steers developed clinical disease by four days post challenge (Table 3). All six T3 1° naïve contact-exposed steers developed clinical FMD by 7 dpcc with lesions on all hooves, and

Table 1 Efficacy Study 1. Summary of outcomes based on clinical and laboratory results

Treatment Group	N	Percent Protected from Lesions (21 dpcc)		Geometric mean FMDV A24/Cruzeiro/BRA/55 VNT titer (log_{10}) ± SD on 7 dpv/0 dpcc (range)	Percent Positive for FMDV A24/Cruzeiro/BRA/55 VNT on 7 dpv/0 dpcc	Percent Protected from FMDV RNA in oral and nasal cavities (0–5 dpcc)	Percent Positive for FMDV NSP Antibodies
		Pedal only	Pedal and Oronasal				
T1: 1° vaccinated AdtA24 5×10^{10} PU (high dose) Contact Challenge	6	83%	50%	$2.2 \pm 0.2^{a,b}$ (1.8–2.4)	100%	0%	0% - 0 dpcc 67% - 14 dpcc
T2: 1° vaccinated AdtA24 1.25×10^{10} PU (medium dose) Contact Challenge	6	100%	33%	1.5 ± 0.5^{a} (0.9–2.1)	100%	0%	0% - 0 dpcc 100% - 14 dpcc
T3: 1° vaccinated AdtA24 3.125×10^{9} PU (low dose) Contact Challenge	6	67%	0%	1.1 ± 0.5^{b} (0.6–1.8)	67%	0%	0% - 0 dpcc 100% - 14 dpcc
T4: 1° naïve Contact Challenge (control)	4	0%	0%	0.6 ± 0.0*	0%	0%	ND
T5 (IDL challenged seeder steers) 1 day prior to contact with T1-T4	8	0%	0%	0.6 ± 0.0*	0%	0%	ND

Dpcc days post contact challenge, *DPV* days post vaccination, *VNT* virus neutralization test, *1°* primary, *PU* particle units, *IDL* intradermolingual challenge, *ND* Not Determined
*A positive VNT is ≥0.9 log_{10}. [a,] $p = 0.01$ for T1 > T2. [b,] $p = < 0.001$ for T1 > T3. $p = 0.1$ for T2 and T3

Table 2 Efficacy Study 2: Summary of FMDV Geometric mean virus neutralization titers (GMT) in cattle

Treatment Group	FMDV A24/Cruzeiro/BRA/55 GMT (± std. dev.; log_{10}) Days Post-Vaccination/Post Contact Challenge (% seropositive)			
	7/0	14/7	21/14	24/17
12 T2: 1° Vaccinated and Exposed to 10 IDL challenged seeder cattle for 2–3 days	1.5 ± 0.2** (100%)	1.7 ± 0.2 (100%)	2.0 ± 0.4** (100%)	1.9 ± 0.2** (100%)
6 T3: 1° naïve and Exposed to 10 IDL challenged seeder cattle for 2–3 days	0.6 ± 0.0 (0%)	1.4 ± 0.5 (83%)	2.6 ± 0.2 (100%)	2.8 ± 0.4 (100%)
	FMDV A24/Cruzeiro/BRA/55 GMT (± std. dev.; log_{10}) Days Post-Vaccination/Post Contact Challenge (% seropositive)			
	5/−2	12/5	19/12	22/15
4 T4: 2° Vaccinated; Intermingled with 6 T2: 1° Vaccinated and Exposed cattle in Room 1 for 35 days	0.9 ± 0.2* (75%)	1.5 ± 0.4** (100%)	1.3 ± 0.2** (100%)	1.7 ± 0.4** (100%)
4 T5: 2° naïve; Intermingled with 6 T2: 1° Vaccinated and Exposed cattle in Room 2 for 35 days	0.6 ± 0.0 (0%)	0.6 ± 0.0 (0%)	0.6 ± 0.0 (0%)	0.6 ± 0.0 (0%)
4 T6: 2° naïve; Intermingled with 6 T3: 1° naïve and Exposed cattle in Room 3 for 35 days	0.6 ± 0.0 (0%)	0.6 ± 0.0 (0%)	2.0 ± 0.2** (100%)	2.9 ± 0.3** (100%)

All are two-tailed T-test comparisons within the specified time period
Vaccinated cattle received 5×10^{10} particle units of AdtA24
1° primary, *2°* secondary, *IDL* intradermolingual challenge
*different at $p = 0.05$; **different at $p \leq 0.01$

all had oronasal lesions. In addition, each T3 1° naïve contact-exposed steer had at least one FMDV-positive plasma and oronasal fluid sample during the first five dpcc. Similarly, all four T6 2° naïve steers co-mingled with T3 1° naïve and contact-exposed steers developed clinical FMD by 7 dpcc and had at least one FMDV-positive plasma and oronasal fluid sample by 9 dpcc.

In contrast, all 12 of the AdtA24 T2 1° vaccinated and contact-exposed steers were completely protected against clinical FMD and viremia (Table 3). However, each T2 1° vaccinated and exposed steer had at least one

Table 3 Efficacy Study 2. Summary of protection based on clinical and laboratory results

Treatment Group	N	Percent Protection from Outcomes					Percent Positive for Antibodies to FMDV NSPs
		Clinical FMD (1–15 dpcc)	FMDV or FMDV RNA in plasma (0–7, 9 dpcc)	FMDV RNA in oronasal fluid (0, 2, 4 dpcc)	FMDV RNA in probang (27, 34, 41 dpcc)	FMDV in probang (27, 34, 41 dpcc)	
T1: IDL challenged seeder steers	10	0%	ND	ND	ND	ND	ND
T2: 1° AdtA24 5×10^{10} PU vaccinated; Intermingled with 10 IDL challenged 'seeder steers' for 2–3 days	12	100% No oronasal lesions	100%	0%	18%	27%	9%[a] - 0 dpcc 91% -30 dpcc
T3: 1° naïve; Intermingled with 10 IDL challenged 'seeder steers' for 2–3 days	6	0%	0%	0%	17%	17%	0% - 0 dpcc 100%-30 dpcc
T4: 2° AdtA24 5×10^{10} PU vaccinated; Intermingled with 6 T2: 1° vaccinated and exposed steers (Room 1)	4	100% No oronasal lesions	100%	100%	100%	100%	0% - 0 and 30 dpcc
T5: 2° naïve; Intermingled with 6 T2: 1° vaccinated and exposed steers (Room 2)	4	100% No oronasal lesions	100%	75%	50%	100%	0% - 0 and 30 dpcc
T6: 2° naïve; Intermingled with 6 T3: 1° naïve and exposed steers (Room 3)	4	0%	0%	0%	25%	25%	0% - 0 dpcc 100%-30 dpcc

Dpcc days post contact challenge, *NSP* nonstructural protein, *1°* primary, *2°* secondary, *IDL* intradermolingual challenge, *PU* particle units
[a]one false positive (consistent with reported diagnostic specificity rates for this assay [36, 37])

PCR-positive FMDV oronasal fluid sample at either 2 or 4 days post-contact exposure to the 10 T1 IDL challenged 'seeder' steers. In addition, 73% of T2 1° vaccinated and exposed steers had at least one FMDV-positive probang sample following contact exposure to the 10 T1 IDL challenged 'seeder' steers.

All T4 2° vaccinated and exposed steers were completely protected against clinical FMD, viremia, oronasal infection and remained probang-negative following contact exposure to T2 1° vaccinated and contact-exposed steers (Table 3). Notably, following co-mingling with T2 1° vaccinated and contact-exposed steers, none of the four T5 2° naïve steers became infected, as evidenced by the absence of clinical FMD, viremia, and FMDV positive probang samples.

All 27 Room 2 air samples collected during the secondary contact exposure study phase with all four T5 2° naïve and six T2 1° vaccinated and contact-exposed steers were FMDV negative by PCR (Fig. 2). In Room 1 containing all four T4 2° vaccinated and exposed steers and six T2 1° vaccinated and contact-exposed steers, 86% of 28 air samples collected during this same time period were PCR negative, and the remaining 14% were borderline positive (Ct = 38.5- < 40). In contrast, 48% of 28 Room 3 air samples were PCR positive; none of the steers were vaccinated: four T6 2° naïve steers and six T3 1° naïve contact-exposed steers.

Eleven of twelve (91%) of T2 1° vaccinated and contact-exposed steers, although fully protected against clinical FMD, developed FMDV NSP antibodies at 30 dpcc (Table 3). In contrast, during this same period, no T4 2° vaccinated and contact-exposed, protected steers or T5 2° naïve, protected steers were NSP antibody positive following co-mingling with T2 1° vaccinated and contact-exposed steers. All four T6 2° naïve, non-protected steers in Room 3 developed FMDV NSP antibodies following 43 days co-mingling with T3 1° naïve contact-exposed steers.

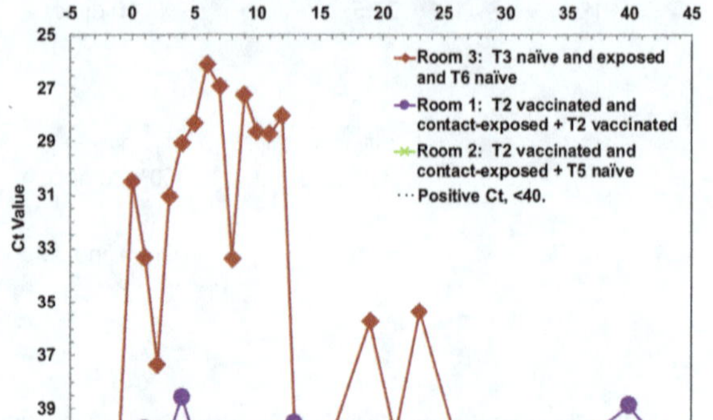

Fig. 2 Efficacy Study 2: Detection of FMDV nucleic acid in air filters collected from animal rooms. FMDV nucleic acid in air samples that were collected on air filters from each of the three animal rooms, were detected by rRT-PCR, and a C_t value < 40 was scored positive. Air filters were collected daily for the first 18 days and then on alternate days to 43 days. The experimental design is diagramed in Fig. 1b

Discussion

The ability of a non-adjuvanted AdtA24 recombinant subunit vaccine to confer protection against clinical FMD in immunized cattle at 7 dpv following subsequent direct contact exposure to previously FMDV-infected, naïve 'seeder' steers was assessed in two independent studies. Collectively across all vaccine doses tested, the AdtA24 vaccine conferred 62% protection (21 fully protected/34 vaccinated, FMDV exposed) against clinical FMD. The higher protection against clinical FMD observed in the second efficacy study (100%) compared to the first efficacy study (50%) with the highest vaccine dose (5×10^{10} PU) may be due to AdtA24 vaccine lot differences and the presence of non-neutralizing antibody antigenic vaccine components (i.e., pentamers) produced in AdtA24 virus vaccine production and purification in the second lot. These two studies also show AdtA24 vaccine DIVA capability prior to contact exposure. However, additional studies designed to validate the AdtA24 DIVA attribute under repeated vaccination and sampling at longer time points post-vaccination are necessary.

In Efficacy Study 1, on 7dpv/0 dpcc, 89% (16/18) of T1-T3 immunized steers had vaccine dose-dependent FMDV VNT titers, with the statistically highest GMT in the highest dose group (T1) (Table 1). The estimated $BPD_{50/90}$ of $3.1 \times 10^{10}/5.5 \times 10^{10}$ PU against any vesicular lesions in this study was comparable to results obtained in steers vaccinated with AdtA24 and directly infected intradermolingually 7 days later with FMDV A24 ($BPD_{50/90}$ to prevent clinical FMD was $1.0 \times 10^{10}/5.6 \times 10^{10}$ PU) [15]. Since an AdtA24 vaccine formulated in ENABL® adjuvant significantly lowered the vaccine protective dose in the IDL direct challenge model [18], future studies should be conducted to determine if an AdtA24/ ENABL® formulation can also lower the $BPD_{50/90}$ values reported in this study.

In Efficacy Study 2 (Fig. 1b), a more complex study design was used to evaluate the ability of direct contact challenge exposed AdtA24 primary vaccinates to transmit FMDV to produce clinical or subclinical FMD to other AdtA24 secondary vaccinates as well as to naïve, non-vaccinated cohorts. We acknowledge the limitations in this laboratory research experimental design for Efficacy Study 2, specifically the tightly controlled, very high air exchange rate, and intentional animal movement/ room re-distribution compared to the natural feedlot, pasture or dairy parlor setting. The onset of clinical FMD observed in the non-vaccinated steers in contact with FMDV-infected steers was consistent with the 1–6 day onset reported in a previous study [24]. Under the research conditions and experimental design used herein, the contact transmission model clearly demonstrated that naïve, non-vaccinated steers with active clinical FMD readily transmitted FMDV to other naïve, non-vaccinated steers, resulting in clinical FMD. AdtA24 vaccinated steers failed to develop clinical FMD. Notably, despite evidence of FMDV in AdtA24 1° vaccinated steers' oronasal fluid and probang samples, these steers did not transmit clinical or subclinical FMD to AdtA24 2° vaccinated steers or to 2° naïve, non-vaccinated steers, all of which remained FMDV seronegative by VNT and NSP antibody assays. Air samples collected for 43 days following co-mingling of AdtA24 1° vaccinated, contact-exposed steers with 2° naïve non-vaccinated steers were consistently negative, or in the case of the room with AdtA24 2° vaccinated steers, were sporadically borderline positive. The rRT-PCR values obtained from air samples in rooms with infected cattle were consistent with the values reported in another cattle study during 0–12 dpcc [25]. The consistently lower Ct values in room 3 compared to room 1 suggest that the AdtA24 vaccine may help reduce the FMD virus environment load during a natural outbreak. Results also support the conclusion that detection of rRT-PCR-positive oronasal or probang samples at approximately 4–6 weeks post-contact exposure in these disease-free 'carrier' AdtA24-vaccinated, donor steers is unlikely to play a role in FMDV transmission or FMD outbreak control efforts. The epidemiological importance of persistently infected cattle ("carrier state") remains a controversial topic for discussion and further research [26, 27]. However, our results are consistent with conclusions drawn by other FMD researchers [28, 29].

Based on our results, we expect that AdtA24-vaccinated cattle would be protected from contact transmission of FMDV from other FMDV-infected hosts, such as sheep, pigs, goats, and buffalo. A variety of studies have demonstrated the effectiveness of other types of FMDV vaccines in preventing transmission of FMDV among animals [5, 10–12, 14, 30–35].

Conclusion

In summary, using a simulated natural FMDV infection route, we demonstrated that the replication-deficient AdtA24 FMD DIVA vaccine was effective at preventing clinical FMD and viremia following direct contact transmission exposure. Under field conditions following a FMD outbreak in a previous FMD-free country, we expect that AdtA24 and other AdtFMD serotype/subtype DIVA vaccines will be effective in reducing FMDV transmission from vaccinated to naïve steers, leading to a reduction in both disease outbreak magnitude and duration.

Abbreviations

AdtA24: Replication-deficient human adenovirus vectored FMDV A24/Cruzeiro/BRA/55 vaccine; $BPD_{50/90}$: Estimated 50%/90% bovine protective dose; Ct: Cycle threshold; DIVA: Differentiate infected from vaccinated animals; dpcc: Days post contact challenge; dpv: Days post-vaccination; FFB: Final formulation buffer; FMD: Foot-and-mouth disease; FMDV: Foot-and-mouth disease virus; GMT: Geometric mean virus neutralization test titer; IDL: Intradermolingual; NSP: Nonstructural protein; PIADC: Plum Island Animal Disease Center; PU: Particle units; rRT-PCR: Real-Time Reverse Transcriptase-Polymerase Chain Reaction; USDA: United States Department of Agriculture; VNT: Virus neutralization test

Acknowledgements

We thank M. Grubman, A. Zsak, M. Moraes, H. Duque, K. Addorisio, W. Hurtle, T. Hester, and K. Floyd for their technical assistance, and K. Apicelli for preparing Fig. 1a and b. We thank the PIADC Animal Research Branch for their professional support and assistance.

Funding

GenVec, Inc., Leidos, Inc., and The McConnell Group, Inc. were funded through separate agreements with the U.S. Department of Homeland Security (DHS) Science and Technology Directorate (S&T) under Award Numbers HSHQPD-07-X-00003, GS-23F-8006H, and HSHQDC-8-C-00011. This research was supported in part by an appointment of M. Pisano to the PIADC Research Participation Program administered by the Oak Ridge Institute for Science and Education (ORISE) through an interagency agreement, HSHQPM-14-X-00001, between the U.S. Department of Energy (DOE) and the U.S. DHS S&T. ORISE is managed by ORAU under DOE contract number DE-AC05-06OR23100. DHS S&T, as the funding source, had no involvement in the study design; collection, analysis and interpretation of data; writing of the report; and in the decision to submit the article for publication. All opinions expressed are the authors' and do not necessarily reflect the policies and views of DHS, ARS, GenVec, Inc., Leidos, Inc., The McConnell Group, Inc., DOE, or ORAU/ORISE.

Authors' contributions

JGN, DAB, and MR conceived the studies. DE, DEB, BTB prepared and analyzed the vaccine constructs. CS, JB, LZ conducted the animal studies, and JB, MP, LZ, and EH performed the laboratory analyses. BJK and DAB wrote the manuscript, and BJK and JB performed the statistical analyses. All authors read and approved the manuscript.

Consent for publication

Not applicable.

Competing interests

DE, DEB, and BTB were employed by GenVec Inc. when the studies were performed. DEB and JGN are inventors on a U.S. patent describing AdtA24.

Author details

[1]U.S. Department of Homeland Security Science and Technology Directorate, Plum Island Animal Disease Center, P.O. Box 848, Greenport, NY 11944, USA. [2]The McConnell Group, Inc., Plum Island Animal Disease Center, P.O. Box 848, Greenport, NY 11944, USA. [3]Leidos, Plum Island Animal Disease Center, P.O. Box 848, Greenport, NY 11944, USA. [4]Plum Island Animal Disease Center Research Participation Program, Oak Ridge Institute for Science and Education, Oak Ridge, TN, USA. [5]U.S. Department of Agriculture, Agricultural Research Service, Foreign Animal Disease Research Unit, Plum Island Animal Disease Center, P.O. Box 848, Greenport, NY 11944, USA. [6]GenVec, Inc., 910 Clopper Road, Suite 220N, Gaithersburg, MD 20878, USA. [7]BioQuest Associates, LLC, Plum Island Animal Disease Center, P.O. Box 848, Greenport, NY 11944, USA.

References

1. Grubman MJ, Rodriguez LL, De Los Santos TB. Foot-and-mouth disease. In: Ehrenfeld E, Domingo E, Roos RP, editors. The Picornaviruses. American Society for Microbiology; 2010. p. 397–410.
2. Alexandersen S, Zhang Z, Donaldson AI, Garland AJ. The pathogenesis and diagnosis of foot-and-mouth disease. J Comp Pathol. 2003;129(1):1–36.

References

1. Grubman MJ, Rodriguez LL, De Los Santos TB. Foot-and-mouth disease. In: Ehrenfeld E, Domingo E, Roos RP, editors. The Picornaviruses. American Society for Microbiology; 2010. p. 397–410.
2. Alexandersen S, Zhang Z, Donaldson AI, Garland AJ. The pathogenesis and diagnosis of foot-and-mouth disease. J Comp Pathol. 2003;129(1):1–36.
3. Paton DJ, Gubbins S, King DP. Understanding the transmission of foot-and-mouth disease virus at different scales. Curr Opin Virol. 2017;28:85–91.
4. Cox SJ, Barnett PV. Experimental evaluation of foot-and-mouth disease vaccines for emergency use in ruminants and pigs: a review. Vet Res. 2009; 40(3):13.
5. Donaldson AI, Kitching RP. Transmission of foot-and-mouth disease by vaccinated cattle following natural challenge. Res Vet Sci. 1989;46(1):9–14.
6. Doel TR, Williams L, Barnett PV. Emergency vaccination against foot-and-mouth disease: rate of development of immunity and its implications for the carrier state. Vaccine. 1994;12(7):592–600.
7. Salt JS, Barnett PV, Dani P, Williams L. Emergency vaccination of pigs against foot-and-mouth disease: protection against disease and reduction in contact transmission. Vaccine. 1998;16(7):746–54.
8. Barnett PV, Cox SJ, Aggarwal N, Gerber H, McCullough KC. Further studies on the early protective responses of pigs following immunisation with high potency foot and mouth disease vaccine. Vaccine. 2002;20(25–26):3197–208.
9. Parida S, Fleming L, Oh Y, Mahapatra M, Hamblin P, Gloster J, Doel C, Gubbins S, Paton DJ. Reduction of foot-and-mouth disease (FMD) virus load in nasal excretions, saliva and exhaled air of vaccinated pigs following direct contact challenge. Vaccine. 2007;25(45):7806–17.
10. Cox SJ, Voyce C, Parida S, Reid SM, Hamblin PA, Paton DJ, Barnett PV. Protection against direct-contact challenge following emergency FMD vaccination of cattle and the effect on virus excretion from the oropharynx. Vaccine. 2005;23(9):1106–13.
11. Cox SJ, Voyce C, Parida S, Reid SM, Hamblin PA, Hutchings G, Paton DJ, Barnett PV. Effect of emergency FMD vaccine antigen payload on protection, sub-clinical infection and persistence following direct contact challenge of cattle. Vaccine. 2006;24(16):3184–90.
12. Cox SJ, Parida S, Voyce C, Reid SM, Hamblin PA, Hutchings G, Paton DJ, Barnett PV. Further evaluation of higher potency vaccines for early protection of cattle against FMDV direct contact challenge. Vaccine. 2007; 25(44):7687–95.
13. Mayr GA, Chinsangaram J, Grubman MJ. Development of replication-defective adenovirus serotype 5 containing the capsid and 3C protease coding regions of foot-and-mouth disease virus as a vaccine candidate. Virology. 1999;263(2):496–506.
14. Mayr GA, O'Donnell V, Chinsangaram J, Mason PW, Grubman MJ. Immune responses and protection against foot-and-mouth disease virus (FMDV) challenge in swine vaccinated with adenovirus-FMDV constructs. Vaccine. 2001;19(15–16):2152–62.
15. Schutta C, Barrera J, Pisano M, Zsak L, Grubman MJ, Mayr GA, Moraes MP, Kamicker BJ, Brake DA, Ettyreddy D, Butman BT, Neilan JG. Multiple efficacy studies of an adenovirus-vectored foot-and-mouth disease virus serotype A24 subunit vaccine in cattle using homologous challenge. Vaccine. 2016; 34(27):3214–20.
16. Barrera J, Brake DA, Kamicker BJ, Purcell C, Kaptur R Jr, Schieber T, Lechtenberg K, Miller TD, Ettyreddy D, Brough DE, Butman BT, Colby M, Neilan JG. Safety profile of a replication-deficient human adenovirus-vectored foot-and-mouth disease virus serotype A24 subunit vaccine in cattle. Transbound Emerg Dis. 2017; https://doi.org/10.1111/tbed.12724.
17. Brake DA, McIlhaney M, Miller T, Christianson K, Keene A, Lohnas G, Purcell C, Neilan J, Schutta C, Barrera J, Burrage T, Brough DE, Butman BT. Human adenovirus-vectored foot-and-mouth disease vaccines: establishment of a vaccine product profile through in vitro testing. Dev Biol (Basel). 2012;134:123–33.
18. Barrera J, Schutta C, Pisano M, Grubman MJ, Brake DA, Miller T, Kamicker BJ, Olutunmbi F, Ettyreddy D, Brough DE, Butman BT, Neilan JG. Use of ENABL® adjuvant to increase the potency of an adenovirus-vectored foot-and-mouth disease virus serotype a subunit vaccine. Vaccine. 2018;36(8):1078–84.
19. LaRocco M, Krug PW, Kramer E, Ahmed Z, Pacheco JM, Duque H, Baxt B, Rodriguez LL. Correction for LaRocco et al., A Continuous Bovine Kidney Cell Line Constitutively Expressing Bovine alphaVbeta6 Integrin Has Increased Susceptibility to Foot-and-Mouth Disease Virus. J Clin Microbiol. 2015;53(2):755.
20. LaRocco M, Krug PW, Kramer E, Ahmed Z, Pacheco JM, Duque H, Baxt B, Rodriguez LL. A continuous bovine kidney cell line constitutively expressing bovine alphavbeta6 integrin has increased susceptibility to foot-and-mouth disease virus. J Clin Microbiol. 2013;51(6):1714–20.
21. Callahan JD, Brown F, Osorio FA, Sur JH, Kramer E, Long GW, Lubroth J, Ellis SJ, Shoulars KS, Gaffney KL, Rock DL, Nelson WM. Use of a portable real-time reverse transcriptase-polymerase chain reaction assay for rapid detection of foot-and-mouth disease virus. J Am Vet Med Assoc. 2002;220(11):1636–42.
22. Mohamed F, Swafford S, Petrowski H, Bracht A, Schmit B, Fabian A, Pacheco JM, Hartwig E, Berninger M, Carrillo C, Mayr G, Moran K, Kavanaugh D, Leibrecht H, White W, Metwally S. Foot-and-mouth disease in feral swine: susceptibility and transmission. Transbound Emerg Dis. 2011;58(4):358–71.
23. Doel TR. Potency assessment of inactivated viral vaccines. In: Vaccine manual. The production and quality control of veterinary vaccines for use in developing countries. Food and Agriculture Organization of the United Nations: Rome, Italy; 1997.
24. Graves JH, McVicar JW, Sutmoller P, Trautman R. Contact transmission of foot-and-mouth disease from infected to susceptible cattle. J Infect Dis. 1971;123(4):386–91.
25. Christensen LS, Brehm KE, Skov J, Harlow KW, Christensen J, Haas B. Detection of foot-and-mouth disease virus in the breath of infected cattle using a hand-held device to collect aerosols. J Virol Methods. 2011;177(1):44–8.
26. Bronsvoort BM, Handel IG, Nfon CK, Sorensen KJ, Malirat V, Bergmann I, Tanya VN, Morgan KL. Redefining the "carrier" state for foot-and-mouth disease from the dynamics of virus persistence in endemically affected cattle populations. Sci Rep. 2016;6:29059.
27. Stenfeldt C, Eschbaumer M, Rekant SI, Pacheco JM, Smoliga GR, Hartwig EJ, Rodriguez LL, Arzt J. The foot-and-mouth disease carrier state divergence in cattle. J Virol. 2016;90(14):6344–64.
28. Tenzin, Dekker A, Vernooij H, Bouma A, Stegeman A. Rate of foot-and-mouth disease virus transmission by carriers quantified from experimental data. Risk Anal. 2008;28(2):303–9.
29. Charleston B, Bankowski BM, Gubbins S, Chase-Topping ME, Schley D, Howey R, Barnett PV, Gibson D, Juleff ND, Woolhouse ME. Relationship between clinical signs and transmission of an infectious disease and the implications for control. Science. 2011;332(6030):726–9.
30. Golde WT, Pacheco JM, Duque H, Doel T, Penfold B, Ferman GS, Gregg DR, Rodriguez LL. Vaccination against foot-and-mouth disease virus confers complete clinical protection in 7 days and partial protection in 4 days: use in emergency outbreak response. Vaccine. 2005;23(50):5775–82.
31. Eble PL, Bouma A, Weerdmeester K, Stegeman JA, Dekker A. Serological and mucosal immune responses after vaccination and infection with FMDV in pigs. Vaccine. 2007;25(6):1043–54.
32. Orsel K, de Jong MC, Bouma A, Stegeman JA, Dekker A. The effect of vaccination on foot and mouth disease virus transmission among dairy cows. Vaccine. 2007;25(2):327–35.
33. Orsel K, Dekker A, Bouma A, Stegeman JA, de Jong MC. Vaccination against foot and mouth disease reduces virus transmission in groups of calves. Vaccine. 2005;23(41):4887–94.
34. Madhanmohan M, Yuvaraj S, Nagendrakumar SB, Srinivasan VA, Gubbins S, Paton DJ, Parida S. Transmission of foot-and-mouth disease virus from experimentally infected Indian buffalo (Bubalus bubalis) to in-contact naive and vaccinated Indian buffalo and cattle. Vaccine. 2014;32(39):5125–30.
35. Graves JH, McKercher PD, Farris HE Jr, Cowan KM. Early response of cattle and swine to inactivated foot-and-mouth disease vaccine. Res Vet Sci. 1968; 9(1):35–40.
36. Brocchi E, Bergmann IE, Dekker A, Paton DJ, Sammin DJ, Greiner M, Grazioli S, De Simone F, Yadin H, Haas B, Bulut N, Malirat V, Neitzert E, Goris N, Parida S, Sørensen K, De Clercq K. Comparative evaluation of six ELISAs for the detection of antibodies to the non-structural proteins of foot-and-mouth disease virus. Vaccine. 2006;24(47–48):6966–79.
37. Paton DJ, de Clercq K, Greiner M, Dekker A, Brocchi E, Bergmann I, Sammin DJ, Gubbins S, Parida S. Application of non-structural protein antibody tests in substantiating freedom from foot-and-mouth disease virus infection after emergency vaccination of cattle. Vaccine. 2006;24(42–43):6503–12.

On-farm storage of livestock vaccines may be a risk to vaccine efficacy: a study of the performance of on-farm refrigerators to maintain the correct storage temperature

Paul D. Williams[1*] and Gustavo Paixão[2,3]

Abstract

Background: Livestock vaccines (LV) are often stored on-farm, in a refrigerator (fridge), prior to use and little is documented about the storage conditions during this period. As the quality of a vaccine can be impaired by storage at an incorrect temperature, the present study aimed to evaluate the on-farm performance of farm fridges to maintain the correct storage temperature. From January to August 2014, temperature data loggers were placed on selected farm fridges used to store LV ($n = 20$) in South-West England.

Results: Temperature recording data was available from 17 of the 20 farms. Fifty-nine percent of farm fridges had at least one temperature recording above 8 °C, 53% had at least one recording below 2 °C and 41% at or below 0 °C. Internal fridge temperatures attained 24 °C and dropped to − 12 °C as an absolute maximum and minimum respectively. Fridges tested spent an average of 16% of the total time recorded above 8 °C. Time of the year significantly influenced the percentage of time above 8 °C. External and internal temperatures were found to be positively correlated ($p < 0.001$). Statistical significant differences in internal and external temperatures were found between March and August.

Conclusions: The majority of fridges in this study would have failed to keep any stored LV within the recommended storage temperature range. If LV are going to be stored on-farm prior to use, then urgent improvements in this part of the cold-chain are required in order to insure vaccine efficacy is not compromised.

Keywords: Vaccine storage, Cold chain, Veterinary vaccines, Livestock, Temperature monitoring

Background

Livestock vaccines (LV) are crucial tools for animal and public health. They are a cost-effective method to prevent animal disease, enhance the efficiency of food production, and reduce or prevent transmission of zoonotic and foodborne infections to people [1]. Proper usage and storage of LV are essential to achieve maximal vaccine safety and efficacy [2]. Vaccines should always be stored as per manufacturer instructions and general recommendations [3]. For the majority of vaccines, especially those used in cattle, sheep and pigs, the recommended storage temperature (RST) is between 2 °C and 8 °C [4]. Vaccines stored at different temperatures could result in potency loss and impaired efficacy [5–7]. Furthermore, emphasis is being increased nowadays on vaccine management to protect vaccines from freezing [8, 9] as cold chain practices tend to prioritize protecting vaccine from heat damage. Very often the risk of vaccine exposure to temperatures below freezing point is considered greater than heat exposure [10–12].

Vaccines thermal sensitivity can be explained by the complex nature of the three-dimensional structure of the antigen [13]. There are clear data regarding effects of temperature oscillation in human vaccines and therefore multiple recommendations to ensure optimal potency [14]; but there is little information regarding the tolerance levels for most commonly used LV, except for some specific vaccines, like the foot and mouth disease [7]. Vaccines can be classified into two general groups:

* Correspondence: paul.williams9@merck.com
[1]MSD Animal Health, Walton Manor, Walton, Milton Keynes MK7 7AJ, UK
Full list of author information is available at the end of the article

inactivated and live vaccines. Live vaccines are made of weakened, attenuated versions of infectious viruses, bacteria, fungus or parasites that can replicate in vivo. Live vaccines do not normally require adjuvants to boost the immune response but are more sensitive to potency loss during storage and distribution, especially at elevated temperatures [13]. Inactivated vaccines on the other hand often require adjuvants to boost the immune response. They are typically more stable to moderate heat exposure than live vaccines, yet more sensitive to freezing [15], especially when containing adjuvant with aluminum salts, which may aggregate on freezing, lowering the adjuvant effect [16, 17].

The end of the cold chain, where the vaccine is stored prior to use, is pointed as a critical stage due to the widespread use of domestic refrigerators, especially in developing countries [18]. To address this issue, World Health Organization (WHO) establishes guidelines for manufacturers of refrigerators intended to store vaccines to use in humans in order to ensure performance standards [19]. Stand-alone units, freeze or refrigerate only, and frost-free or automatic defrost cycle are important features on units intended to store vaccines. Ideally, units should be dedicated to storage of vaccines and temperature monitoring should be performed with calibrated devices and digital data loggers [20]. In regards to animal health, there are no guidelines available in terms of refrigerators requirements.

In the United Kingdom, LV are often stored on-farm, in domestic refrigerators, prior to use and administered by farm workers [21, 22]. The objective of the present study is to evaluate the LV storage associated risk when stored on-farm before use.

Methods

Data recording

Between 15th January and 25th August 2014, 3 temperature data loggers (EL-USB-2-LCD, Lascar Electronics, UK) were each placed on 20 non-randomly selected farms from 3 large animal veterinary practices in South West England (Somerset, Devon and Dorset). Two data loggers were placed inside of the fridge used to store LV used on the farm. One data logger was placed on the uppermost shelf of the fridge, the other on the lowest. Both data loggers were placed towards the back of the fridge. The remaining data logger was placed outside of the fridge, but in the same room as where the fridge was located. The data loggers were setup to record the temperature every 30 min after placement. At each farm the approximate number of animals on the farm and an estimated age of the fridge was recorded, and if the fridge was used for any other storage purposes beside that of LV.

Data analysis

Descriptive statistical analysis was performed in Microsoft Excel 2010 Microsoft Corporation, Redmond, WA, USA, 2010. One-way variance and regression analysis was done in JMP, Version 7.0. SAS Institute Inc., Cary, NC, 2007. Pearson's correlation factor Tukey's test was used to compare means when significantly different ($p < 0.05$).

Further analysis of the individual data logger temperature recordings from inside the fridges was undertaken using a script written using Microsoft Visual Basic for Applications, Microsoft Corporation, Redmond, WA, USA, 2010. This script processed all individual temperature recordings for each internal data logger and categorised them into "Events". An Event occurred when two or more consecutive temperature recordings were below or above a defined temperature parameter: above 8 °C, below 2 °C and equal or below 0 °C; meaning there could be up to 3 different Event types for each data logger; "Above 8 °C", "Below 2 ° C" and "At or below 0 °C". The number of consecutive 30-min recordings outside the temperature parameter determined the Event duration. Each Event occurrence would provide an opportunity for any vaccine stored in the fridge at that time to equilibrate with the temperature in the fridge.

Results and discussion

Of the 20 farms, complete temperature recordings were available from 17 farms. On Farm 1 the data loggers from inside the fridge were missing at the end of the study, Farm 8 stopped storing vaccines on-farm and Farm 15 could not be contacted after initially agreeing to take part in the study. Dairy farms composed the majority of farms present in the study (8/17) (Table 1). Of those, 75% of fridges were located in the office adjacent to the milking parlour. All fridges present in the study were classified as common domestic fridges, with no power backup or temperature logger. Dairy farms also had a higher proportion of older fridges (5/8) compared to other farm types (3/9). Seventy-one percent (12/17) of the fridges tested were not dedicated to vaccine storage. This was most noticeable in the beef and sheep farms, where the fridge was also used for domestic purposes. When possible, farmers should have a dedicated vaccine storage refrigerator. This could minimize the frequency of openings, reducing temperature fluctuations, and ensure appropriate biosecurity [20].

The minimum and maximum external temperatures recorded during the study period were 1.5 °C in January and 33.0 °C in July respectively. There was a marked variation in the mean external temperatures recorded between each farm, on a monthly basis; as would be expected, there was an increase in the median external temperature as the study progressed from January to August (Fig. 1). All fridges were located in the same

Table 1 Farm and fridge details for which temperature recordings were available ($n = 17$)

Farm No	Farm details		Fridge details			
	Type	No Animals	Age (Years)	Location	Vaccine only	Other use
2	Dairy	140 cows	< 10	Farm office	Yes	–
3	Dairy	250 cows	> 10	Farm washroom	No	Colostrum, milk test kits
4	Dairy	280 cows	< 10	Parlour office	Yes	–
5	Dairy	350 cows	< 1	Parlour office	Yes	–
6	Dairy	420 cows	> 10	Parlour office	Yes	–
7	Dairy	270 cows	> 10	Parlour office	No	Medicines
9	Dairy	500 cows	> 10	Parlour office	No	Medicines
10	Dairy	250 cows	> 10	Parlour office	No	Drinking water
11	Pig	2000 sows	> 10	Workshop	No	Medicines
12	Pig	950 sows	< 10	Staff room	Yes	–
13	Sheep	500 ewes	< 10	House kitchen	No	House food
14	Beef and Sheep	360 cows &1700 ewes	> 10	House porch	No	Beer
16	Beef and Sheep	50 cows & 500 ewes	< 10	House outside larder	No	Household food
17	Sheep	370 ewes	< 5	House kitchen	No	Household food
18	Sheep	100 ewes	< 5	House kitchen	No	Household food
19	Sheep	60 ewes	> 10	House kitchen	No	Household food
20	Beef and Sheep	60 cows & 320 ewes	< 10	House kitchen	No	Household food

geographical region so the marked variation in monthly temperatures was mostly likely due to their individual location on farm. A fridge is designed to operate within a specific temperature range and if placed in an environment where the external temperature is outside this range it may not operate as intended. A properly functioning refrigerator can only lower the temperature of its internal environment, not raise it. As the external temperature during the study did not drop to 0 °C or below, it was not possible to observe what impact such a low external temperature might have had on the internal temperature of a fridge.

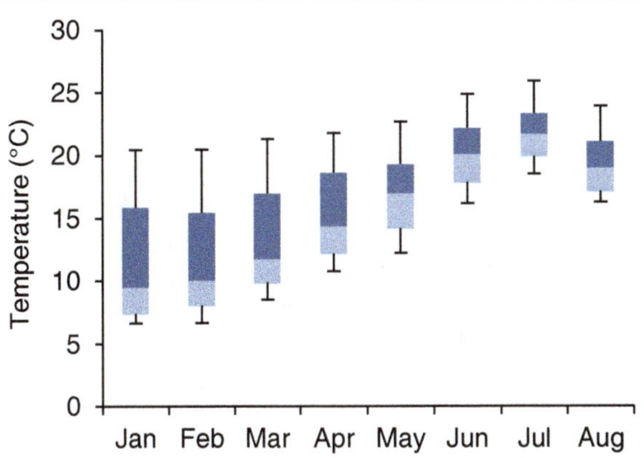

Fig. 1 Box plot showing farm variation in mean monthly external temperature. Boxes represent interquartile range and whiskers span all data points within 1.5 times interquartile range of the nearer quartile

Figure 2 shows the maximum and minimum internal fridge temperatures recorded. Throughout every month of the study, an average of 59% (10/17) of the farms had at least one temperature recording above 8 °C, 53% (9/17) had at least one recording below 2 °C and 41% (7/17) at or below 0 °C. The maximum internal fridge temperature appeared to be affected by the external temperature, with an increase in the number of fridges recording at least one internal temperature greater than 8 °C between May and August. Within those recordings, temperatures had reached 24 °C, as a maximum recorded

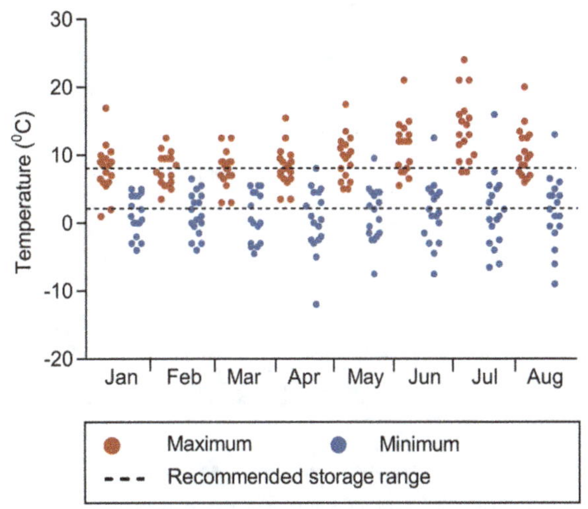

Fig. 2 Maximum and minimum internal fridge individual temperatures recorded on a monthly basis

temperature in July on Farm 9, and dropped to – 12 °C, as minimum recorded temperature in April, on Farm 16. Even though some of these individual recordings do not correspond to sustained events, it is clear that temperature can deviate considerably from the RST.

Figure 3 displays a graphical presentation of the temperature recordings from a selection of farms. Farm 7 had one of the better performing fridges during the study period. Although there are individual temperature recordings outside the 2 and 8 °C storage range, the trend in temperature recordings is between these two values, as demonstrated by the daily rolling average. The Farm 2 fridge also performed well up to the point of a dramatic temporary increase in internal temperature recordings from 04:45 on 11th July to 00:45 on 16th July. Retrospective questioning of farm staff did not identify the cause of this, but either the fridge door being left open or an interruption to the fridge power supply seem most likely. The Farm 10 fridge internal temperature increased in line with increasing external temperature. As already noted, this increase in fridge temperature with increasing external temperature was recorded in several other fridges. The Farm 4 fridge recordings were consistently well below 0 °C for much of the study period. The Farm 9 fridge internal temperature tracked the external temperature throughout the study period. The farm staff were notified that the fridge did not appear to be working, despite being plugged in, at the start of the study period but it was not replaced during the study. In different degrees, external temperature seems to have affected the internal temperature of the fridges tested.

Fridges subject to study recorded sustained temperatures above and below the RST (Table 2). Fridges tested on our study spent an average of 16% of the total time recorded above 8 °C. Time of the year significantly influenced the percentage of time above 8 °C ($p = 0.0135$, $n = 136$); summer months contributed more for this phenomenon: during July and August, the farm fridges had spent an average of 31% of their time above the RST, contrasting with 5% during January and February. Moreover, the same units

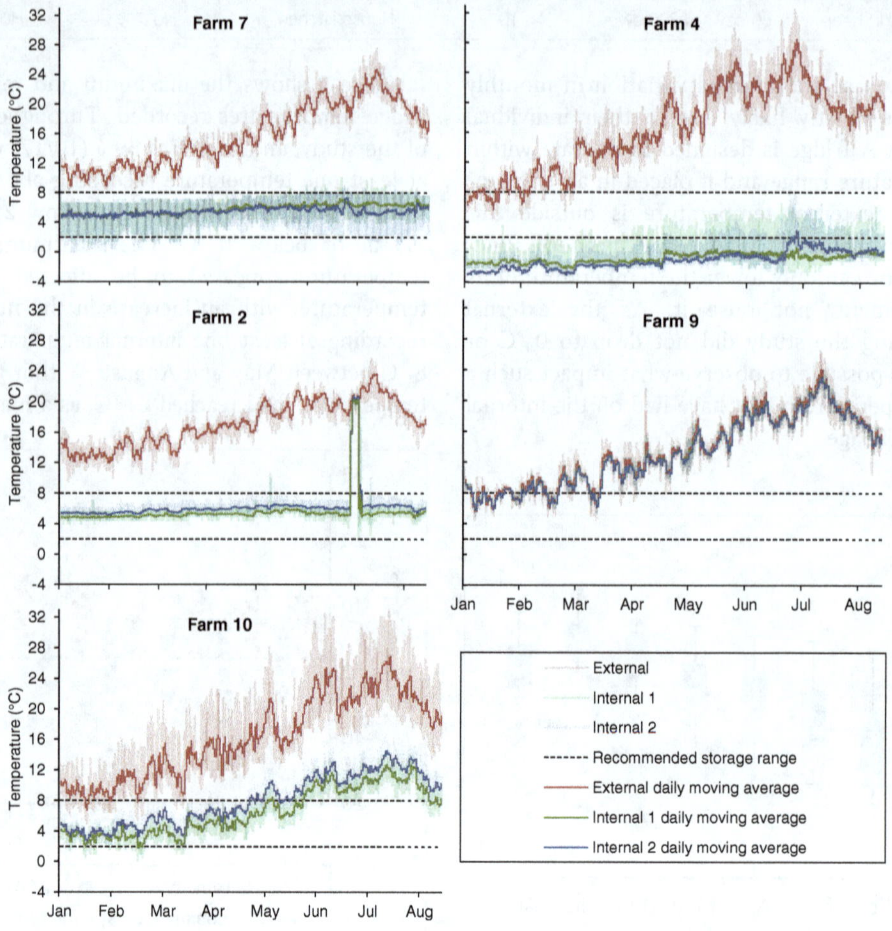

Fig. 3 Temperature recordings from five selected farms. Shaded areas represent individual recordings whereas the solid-line represents a daily moving average. External is the data logger placed outside of the fridge, Internal 1 the data logger placed on the uppermost shelf in the fridge and Internal 2 the lowermost. Squared dot line represents the recommended storage temperature range of 2 to 8 °C

Table 2 Summation of all Events, expressed as percentage (%) of the total minutes recorded in a given month. Data is only shown for farms for which there was at least one Event occurrence

Farm No	Jan	Feb	Mar	Apr	May	Jun	Jul	Aug
a) Events above 8 °C								
2							17%	
6		1%			2%	13%	53%	69%
9	26%	46%	59%	99%	100%	100%	100%	100%
10					45%	97%	100%	97%
11	29%	16%	5%		2%			
12		1%				2%	27%	39%
13				9%	20%	34%	31%	68%
16			14%				10%	48%
18	4%	4%	14%	16%	43%	69%	55%	37%
19	33%	19%	6%	24%	85%	100%	100%	99%
b) Events at or below 0 °C								
3	54%	38%	16%	7%	18%	14%	1%	
4	98%	97%	95%	94%	87%	81%	80%	87%
11					1%	1%	1%	1%
13							5%	1%
14	100%	87%	60%	15%	6%			
16				4%	25%	54%	41%	14%
20			1%	1%			1%	

tested spent an average of 16% of the time below 2 °C and 9% at or below 0 °C. These results suggest that external temperatures are positively correlated with the percentage of time recorded above 8 °C ($r = 0.2523$, $p = 0.003$, $n = 136$) and negatively correlated with the percentage of time below 2 °C ($r = -0.2271$, $p = 0{,}008$, $n = 136$). Table 3 shows significant differences ($p < 0.05$) in external and internal temperatures between months, except for January and February ($p = 0.2027$), where external and internal temperature means were similar. Although significant differences in monthly external temperatures are expected, following environmental temperature fluctuations in temperate climates, internal fridge temperatures shouldn´t have been significantly different. This finding can be explained by the inability of the fridges to maintain their internal temperature within the RST. Furthermore, monthly internal temperature means tend to follow external temperatures means. Contrarily, internal temperature SD appear to be negatively correlated with external temperatures SD ($r = -0.8752$, $p = 0.0044$, $n = 8$). This may be due to the higher variance of a fridge's capability to maintain internal temperature within the RST on hotter months. The higher external temperature SD observed on cooler months could be explained by the higher temperature differences recorded amongst the rooms where the fridges were located.

Table 3 Descriptive statistics of external and internal temperatures within the different months. Means with different superscript letters in a column are significantly different ($p < 0.05$)

		External temperature			Internal temperature		
Month	*n*	Mean	SD	SEM	Mean	SD	SEM
Jan	13,447	11.8^{a}	5.1	0.044	4.1^{a}	2.8	0.024
Feb	24,192	11.9^{a}	5.0	0.032	4.0^{a}	2.8	0.018
Mar	26,784	13.4^{b}	4.8	0.030	4.2^{b}	2.9	0.018
Apr	25,920	15.2^{c}	4.0	0.025	4.6^{c}	3.0	0.018
May	26,784	17.0^{d}	3.8	0.023	5.0^{d}	3.2	0.012
Jun	25,920	20.3^{e}	3.4	0.021	5.7^{e}	4.0	0.025
Jul	26,784	21.8^{f}	3.2	0.019	6.2^{f}	4.7	0.028
Aug	26,265	19.1^{g}	3.1	0.019	5.9^{g}	3.9	0.024
p value		< 0.05			< 0.05		

The fact that farms were not randomly selected predisposes the study to selection bias. Also, as the study was undertaken for only part of the year, it was not possible to determine how the remaining months would have impacted the results. The number of farms that participated was limited, making the study subject to minor statistical confidence. However, the group of farms included in the study was broad spectrum in the sense they include different farmed species and stock sizes, reflecting the reality of South West England. Finally, this study only shows temperature variances when stored in a farm fridge and vaccines can be exposed to sub-optimal temperatures during transportation and administration. The period of 30 min between recordings was chosen as the most frequent interval available to capture temperature recordings throughout the study period, based on data logger storage capacity. Personal communication with the Technical Department, Lascar Electronics, indicated it typically takes 20 min for the contents of a normally packaged vaccine vial to equilibrate with its external environmental temperature. Based on this, a minimum possible duration of 30 min, was established to categorize Events. Each Event occurrence would provide an opportunity for any vaccine stored in the fridge at that time to equilibrate with the temperature in the fridge.

Despite the limitations, the findings from this research confirm anecdotal reports that on-farm vaccine storage is often being neglected by UK farmers. Improvements related with on-farm refrigerators used to store vaccines are strongly advised. Many of these improvements can be easily done without great financial investment, but educating and motivating farmers for the need to change is required. Minimizing the vaccine storage time on-farm should be promoted by veterinarians and suitably qualified persons.[1] In situations where vaccine is being stored on farm then the routine temperature monitoring of fridges is recommended. This could be done with simple maximum-minimum thermometers or digital loggers similar to those used in this study, but both must be checked on at least a daily basis. Digital loggers are available with buffered probes, which can send automatic alerts remotely via SMS or email to forewarn of potential temperature deviation, therefore, allowing action to be taken before a vaccine is exposed to a potentially damaging temperature. Although these are more expensive, their use could be justified where larger quantities of vaccine are being stored. Vaccine vial monitors, visual freeze indicators or a "shake test" may also be used to determine if a vaccine has been exposed to potentially damaging storage temperatures. Vaccine vial monitors trace if the vaccine has suffered cumulative heat impact by showing clear visual change; the reactions vary in accordance with the category of vaccine to which they are assigned [14]. Visual freeze indicators provide a visual indication of exposure to freezing [23]. Additionally, the "shake test" enables visual detection of whether an aluminium-based freeze-sensitive vaccine has been affected by freezing [24].

In this study, it was also demonstrated that external temperatures influence a fridge's internal temperature and consequently the ability of the fridge to maintain the temperature within the RST. Therefore, placing the farm's fridge in a controlled temperature room could improve a fridge's capability of stabilizing its internal temperature. The results from this research go in line with other recent studies where weaknesses of domestic fridges used to store human vaccines, a common finding in developing countries, were also been found [9, 25]. More comprehensive studies, with a larger number of fridges are needed in order to fully understand the scale of the problem.

Conclusions

All of the fridges in this study failed to maintain their internal temperature within the RST, at some point during study period. The internal temperature recorded and the total time recorded outside the RST were influenced by external temperature. More importantly, the majority of fridges present in this study were inadequate to provide proper vaccine storage, having had at least one sustained event outside the RST. In sum, LV are at risk of losing potency and efficacy when stored on-farm prior to use. Despite the many variables that play a crucial role in farm animal vaccination, there is a real need to improve on-farm vaccine storage conditions or implement alternative measures in order to minimize the risk of a vaccine losing potency and to ensure its retains efficacy.

Endnotes

[1]Suitably qualified person (SQP) is a phrase used to describe a person, without a degree in veterinary or pharmacy, who is permitted to prescribe and supply veterinary medicines classified as prescription-only (POM-VPS and NFA-VPS), in the UK.

Abbreviations

LV: Livestock vaccines; RST: Recommended storage temperature

Acknowledgements

The authors wish to thank Dr. Kristen Reyher for bringing both authors together, Professor Rita Payan-Carreira for her helpful suggestions, and to all the farmers who participated in this work.

Funding

MSD Animal Health funded the purchase of the data loggers used in this study. No other funding exists.

Authors' contributions

PW collected, processed and analysed the temperature logger's data. GP studied the background research and performed the statistical analysis. Both authors had contributed equally to the research. Both authors read and approved the final manuscript.

Competing interests

The author's declare that they have no competing interests.

Author details

[1]MSD Animal Health, Walton Manor, Walton, Milton Keynes MK7 7AJ, UK. [2]School of Veterinary Science, University of Bristol, Langford House, Langford, Bristol BS40 5DU, UK. [3]Present address: Animal and Veterinary Research Centre (CECAV), Universidade de Trás-os-Montes e Alto Douro, 5001-801 Vila Real, Portugal.

References

1. Roth JA. Veterinary vaccines and their importance to animal health and public health. Procedia Vaccinol. 2011;5:127–36.
2. Roth JA. Mechanistic bases for adverse vaccine reactions and vaccine failures. Adv Vet Med. 1999;41:681–700.
3. VMD. Veterinary guidance note no 3. Veterinary directorate. 2014. https://www.gov.uk/government/publications/retailers-of-veterinary-medicines-vmgn-3. Accessed 15 Oct 2016.
4. VMD. Product information database. Defra. 2015. http://www.vmd.defra.gov.uk/productinformationdatabase/search.aspx. Accessed 15 Oct 2016.
5. Sheikh MA, Tasneem K, Zafar MS, Butt IA, Shakoor AR. Effect of storage on the prevalent alum-precipitated Haemorrhagic Septicaemia vaccine in Pakistan and preparation of a more efficient oil adjuvant vaccine using dense culture of Pasteurella multocida Roberts type 1 on an improved culture medium. J Vet Med. 1995;42:28–34.
6. Okwor E, Eze D, Uzuegbu M. The effect of storage conditions on the potency of Newcastle disease vaccine La Sota. Int J of Poult Sci. 2009;8(10): 999–1002.
7. El-Sayed E, El-Din WMG, Rizk SA, El-Aty MA. Effect of different storage temperatures on the efficacy of the bivalent foot and mouth disease oil vaccine. J Adv Vet Res. 2012;2(3):198–205.
8. Matthias DM, Robertson J, Garrison MM, Newland S, Nelson C. Freezing temperatures in the vaccine cold chain: a systematic literature review. Vaccine. 2007;25(20):3980–6.
9. Lloyd J, Lydon P, Ouhichi R, Zaffran M. Reducing the loss of vaccines from accidental freezing in the cold chain: the experience of continuous temperature monitoring in Tunisia. Vaccine. 2015;33(7):902–7.
10. Techathawat S, Varinsathien P, Rasdjarmrearnsook A, Tharmaphornpilas P. Exposure to heat and freezing in the vaccine cold chain in Thailand. Vaccine. 2007;25(7):1328–33.

11. Kartoglu U, Nelaj E, Maire D. Improving temperature monitoring in the vaccine cold chain at the periphery: an intervention study using a 30-day electronic refrigerator temperature logger (fridge-tag). Vaccine. 2010;28(24):4065–72.
12. Kumru OS, Joshi SB, Smith DE, Middaugh CR, Prusik T, Volkin DB. Vaccine instability in the cold chain: mechanisms, analysis and formulation strategies. Biologicals. 2014;42(5):237–59.
13. Kartoglu U, Milstien J. Tools and approaches to ensure quality of vaccines throughout the cold chain. Expert Rev Vaccines. 2014;13(7):843–54.
14. QSS. Temperature sensitivity of vaccines. In: WHO, editor. Immunization, vaccines and biologicals. Geneva, Switzerland: WHO Press; 2006. [WHO/IVB/06.10].
15. Pickering LK, Wallace G, Rodewald L. Too hot, too cold: issues with vaccine storage. Pediatrics. 2006;118(4):1738–9.
16. Kurzatkowski W, Kartoglu U, Staniszewska M, Gorska P, Krause A, Wysocki MJ. Structural damages in adsorbed vaccines affected by freezing. Biologicals. 2013;41(2):71–6.
17. Clapp T, Siebert P, Chen D, Braun LJ. Vaccines with aluminum-containing adjuvants: optimizing vaccine efficacy and thermal stability. J Pharm Sci. 2011;100(2):388–401.
18. Martin-de-Nicolas A, McColloster P. Vaccine refrigerator regulator with Data Logger & Back-up Power Supply. Procedia Vaccinol. 2014;8:89–93.
19. PQS. In: WHO, editor. Refrigerator or combined refrigerator water-pack freezer: compression cycle; 2010. [WHO/PQS/E003/RF01.2].
20. CDC. Vaccine storage and handling. In: Hamborsky J, Kroger A, Wolfe CS, editors. Epidemiology and prevention of vaccine-preventable diseases. 13th ed. Washington D.C.: Public Health Foundation; 2015.
21. Meadows D. A study to investigate the use and application of BVDV vaccine in UK cattle. Cattle Practice. 2010;18(3):203–15.
22. Cresswell E, Brennan ML, Barkema HW, Wapenaar W. A questionnaire-based survey on the uptake and use of cattle vaccines in the UK. Vet Rec Open. 2014;1(1):e000042.
23. Angoff R, Wood J, Chernock MC, Tipping D. Visual indicators on vaccine boxes as early warning tools to identify potential freeze damage. Infect Dis Clin Pract. 2015;23(4):184–9.
24. Kartoglu U, Ozguler NK, Wolfson LJ, Kurzatkowski W. Validation of the shake test for detecting freeze damage to adsorbed vaccines. B World Health Organ. 2010;88(8):624–31.
25. Yakum MN, Ateudjieu J, Walter EA, Watcho P. Vaccine storage and cold chain monitoring in the North West region of Cameroon: a cross sectional study. BMC Res Notes. 2015;8:145.

Evaluation of the humoral immune response induced by vaccination for canine distemper and parvovirus

Beatriz Vila Nova[1], Eva Cunha[2], Nuno Sepúlveda[3,4], Manuela Oliveira[1,2], Berta São Braz[1,2], Luis Tavares[1,2], Virgílio Almeida[1,2] and Solange Gil[1,2*]

Abstract

Background: Canine Distemper Virus (CDV) and Canine Parvovirus (CPV) lead to infections with high mortality rates in dogs. These viruses affect unvaccinated dogs or dogs with incomplete vaccination protocols. Vaccination plays an important role in reducing death rates, preventing clinical cases and controlling the spread of virus However, the efficacy of vaccination might be affected by different factors including vaccine scheduling and the neutralization of the vaccine targets by maternal antibodies. In face of these factors, the main goals of this study are (i) to investigate the antibody responses of puppies undergoing different primary vaccination protocols against CPV and CDV and (ii) to estimate the time until seroreversion in adult dogs unvaccinated for at least 3 years.

Results: Antibody protection against CDV and CPV was evaluated in a total of 20 dogs: 5 puppies that initiated immunization at 6 weeks after birth (group A), 8 animals that started vaccination between 8 and 12 weeks of age (group B), and 7 adult dogs that have not been vaccinated for at least 3 years (group C). Blood samples were collected from each animal, with 3 to 4 weeks apart. Antibody responses were measured using indirect ELISA. In the second immunization point, no significant differences were found between the seroconversion of groups A and B for each viral infection ($p = 0.81$ and 0.20 for CDV and CPV, respectively). In the third immunization, there was evidence for a shorter time to achieve a protective titer against CPV in group B when compared to group A ($p = 0.015$). Similar evidence was not found for CDV (p-value $= 0.41$). In Group C, the average time until seroveversion was estimated at 2.86 years and 7.63 years for CDV and CPV, respectively.

Conclusion: Vaccine response to CDV and CPV is specific in each individual. Effective immune protection in primary vaccination depends mainly on the initial titer of maternal antibodies acquired by the neonate. Other factors such as environmental exposure, immunization schedules and immune system activity influence the duration of immunity in adult dogs. The variability found reinforces the need to determine individual humoral immunity levels in order to assess vaccine efficacy.

Keywords: CDV, CPV, Vaccination, Humoral immunity, Maternal antibodies, Seroprevalence, Seroreversion

* Correspondence: solange@fmv.ulisboa.pt
[1]Faculty of Veterinary Medicine, University of Lisbon, Av. Universidade Técnica, 1300-477 Lisbon, Portugal
[2]CIISA- Centre for Interdisciplinary Research in Animal Health, Faculty of Veterinary Medicine, University of Lisbon, Av. Universidade Técnica, 1300-477 Lisbon, Portugal
Full list of author information is available at the end of the article

Background

Canine parvovirus (CPV) and Canine Distemper Virus (CDV) cause life-threatening infections with a major impact on the canine population [1, 2]. These viruses are distributed worldwide affecting both domestic and wildlife mammals [2]. In dogs, CPV is an important enteric pathogen because of the associated high morbidity and mortality rates [3]. It can affect dogs of any age, but severe infections are most likely to occur between 6 weeks and 6 months after birth [3]. Since CPV is a DNA virus without an envelope, it is highly resistant to adverse environmental conditions and persistent on fomites and cage floors for more than a year [4]. CPV inactivation can be achieved by agents include sodium hypochlorite and potassium peroxymonosulfate [4, 5].

Infections by CDV show a range of symptoms in dogs including fever, respiratory, enteric and neurological signs [6, 7]. In these infections, young dogs with age between 3 and 6 months are more like to show clinical symptoms than older ones [6]. In contrast to CPV, CDV can be easily inactivated using UV radiation, heat, desiccation, oxidizing agents, detergents and lipid solvents [6].

Vaccination has proven successful to prevent future CPV and CDV infections [8–10]. Current recommendations suggest that puppies should have the first (or primary) vaccination scheduled between the first 6 and 8 weeks of age, followed by several boosts administered in intervals of 3 or 4 weeks until 16 weeks of age. At this point, maternal antibodies are expected to have declined so their chance of interfering with the vaccine antigen is low [11–13]. The number of vaccine boosts required during this phase might vary with age at which the vaccination protocol began [10]. For example, if the first vaccination has been administered 16 weeks after birth, a single dose may be sufficient to achieve protection [10]. In adult dogs, vaccination should be carried out every 3 years [10].

Vaccination stimulates both humoral response via antibody production and cellular responses via B and T lymphocytes [14]. The duration of immunity is mainly dependent on the degree of immunological memory developed [12, 14, 15]. However, it is unclear whether a vaccinated dog is fully protected throughout its life or whether revaccination is always necessary [16]. To clarify these issues, it is important to quantify the rate by which vaccinated animals become sero-naive again, the so-called seroreversion rate (SRR) [14]. Under the assumption that serum antibody titer is correlated with protective immunity, antibody quantification may be seen as a way to assess the immune protection in vaccinated and unvaccinated animal [17, 18].

The pharmaceutical industry has been developing tests for antibody quantification associated with CPV and CDV exposure in canines [19]. These tests should be performed within 3 to 4 weeks after vaccine administration to assess the necessity of further vaccination steps [10]. This evaluation is essential to reduce the number of necessary immunization shots and to detect possible vaccine failures, thus, decreasing the chance of having a large pool of susceptible animals in the population [20].

From an animal health perspective, the improvement of current vaccine protocols is important to reduce the high incidence of CPV and CDV in the canine population. In this scenario, this work has the objective of investigating the seroconversion to CPV and CDV in two groups of puppies undergoing two different primary vaccination protocols. It also aims to evaluate the serological status associated with CPV and CDV in a group of adult dogs unvaccinated for at least 3 years and to estimate the respective seroreversion rate.

Results

All dogs included in this study were dewormed and evaluated by a veterinarian from the Veterinary Teaching Hospital (VTH, Faculty of Veterinary Medicine, University of Lisbon) before each vaccination. Only dogs deemed healthy were allowed to start the vaccination protocol. Dogs deemed unhealthy at the vaccination appointment, dogs that failed the immunization schedule, dogs that started vaccination after 12 weeks of age and dogs whose age was unknown, were excluded from the study.

The above exclusion criteria discarded 64 out of 84 available dogs of different races, sex and ages. The study was then carried out in 20 dogs with following distribution across three vaccination groups: A ($n = 5$), B ($n = 8$) and C ($n = 7$) (Tables 1 and 2).

Group A consisted of five dogs from the same litter that started vaccination at 6 weeks and were followed for humoral protection evaluation until 12 weeks of age (Table 1). Group B encompassed eight older puppies from different origins, which began vaccination at 8 to 12 weeks. This group enabled the analysis of antibody protection beyond the 16 weeks of age. In these groups, there was no data on immune status of the respective parents. It was also unknown the amount of colostrum ingested by each puppy. Group C referred to seven adult animals unvaccinated for at least 3 years (Table 2). The age of these animals varied from 3.7 to 18 years old with an average of 9.7 years. Six out of seven dogs were vaccinated before this study. The average time since vaccination was 7.2 years with a range from 3 to 12 years.

In order to assess humoral response/seroconversion, blood samples were collected before and after vaccination in groups A and B. There was then a total of 39 blood samples. Antibody quantification was performed using indirect ELISA [10]. In Group C, a single blood sample per dog was collected for serological screening.

Table 1 Ages of dogs in group A and B at the time of sample collection and vaccination. Three blood samples were collected from each animal at the time of vaccination

GROUP	DOG (ID)	Age (weeks) 1st sample	Age (weeks) 2nd sample	Age (weeks) 3rd sample
A	A1	6,3	9,3	10,7
	A2	6,3	9,3	10,7
	A3	6,3	9,3	10,7
	A4	6,3	9,3	10,7
	A5	6,3	9,3	10,7
B	B1	8,9	11,9	15,6
	B2	8,7	13,1	20,7
	B3	11,7	15,9	19,9
	B4	8,9	13,3	16,7
	B5	11,1	15,4	21,4
	B6	11,1	15,4	21,4
	B7	9,6	13,9	18,9
	B8	8	12	16

In group A, all dogs were unprotected against CDV before vaccination using TiterCHEK titres less than 1:16 (TITERCHEK® CDV-CPV, Zoetis). Three weeks after the first immunization (9.3 weeks), 80% of the dogs already showed a protective CDV SN titer and this percentage increased to 100% after the second vaccination (10.7 weeks) (Fig. 1).

With respect to CPV, there was a single animal (20%) who was protected before vaccination. This animal showed a TiterCHEK titre equivalent to a 1:80 (TITERCHEK® CDV-CPV, Zoetis). After the first vaccination at 9.3 weeks, none of the animals were protected and, after the second vaccination (10.7 weeks), only one dog (20%; one out of five) developed protection (Fig. 1). The remaining 80% of the puppies were still unprotected after the administration of two vaccine doses.

In group B, two animals (B4 and B7) received the first vaccine 3 weeks before the collection of first blood sample. On average the first sample was obtained at 9.8 weeks after birth, the second at 14.2 and the third at 17.8. In this group, CDV evaluation before vaccination revealed a protective antibody level in two out of eight dogs. However, one dog (B4) had been previously vaccinated. After the first vaccination, all dogs showed CDV protection with higher values than the protection baseline, which was maintained after the second vaccination (Fig. 2).

Table 2 Ages of dogs and time elapsed since last vaccination in group C at the time of sample collection

Dog (ID)	Age (years)	Time elapsed since last vaccination (in years)
C1	3,7	3
C2	7	5
C3	6	6
C4	18	8
C5	9	9
C6	16	12
C7	8	Never vaccinated

Concerning CPV, one dog showed protective HI titers before vaccination (B7). However, after the first vaccination, 50% (4/8) of the animals revealed HI titers higher than 1:80. After the second vaccination, all animals had protective titers against this virus (Fig. 2).

In the second immunization point, no significant differences were found between the seroconversion of groups A and B for each viral infection ($p = 0.81$ and 0.20 for CDV and CPV, respectively). However, in the third immunization point, there was evidence for higher seroconversion against CPV in group B ($p = 0.015$). This result suggested a shorter time to achieve a protective titer against CPV in this group when compared to group A ($p = 0.015$). Similar evidence was not found for CDV (p-value = 0.41). Both groups appeared then to require the same amount of time to acquire immunity against this virus.

In Group C, there was only one animal (14.3%) that was protected against both viruses (Fig. 3). Three dogs of this group (C2, C5 and C6) had protective titers against CPV only. The unvaccinated dog n° 7 was unprotected against both virus as well as dogs C3 and C4. Overall, 57 and 14% of dogs were protected against CPV and CDV, respectively. Using data of the vaccinated animals from this group, SRR was estimated at 0.350 for CDV. This estimate predicted an average time of 2.86 years to seroreversion. The respective seroconversion rate (SCR) was estimated at zero, a value consistent with the lack of information to estimate natural exposure to that virus in vaccinated animals. With respect to

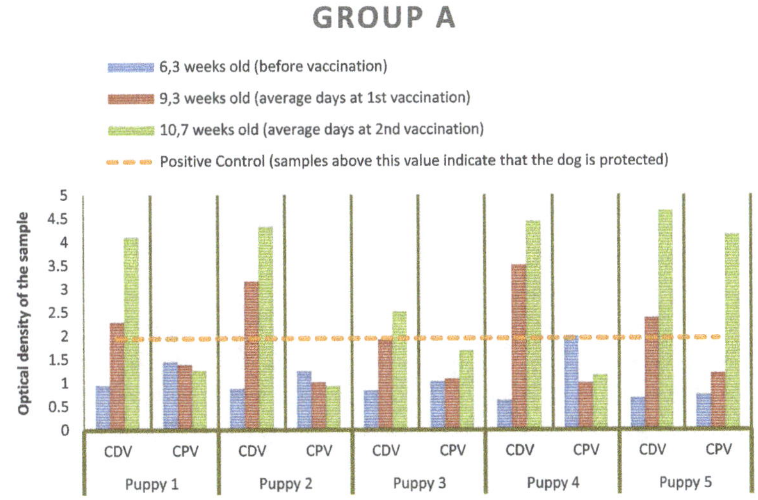

Fig. 1 Results for CDV and CPV after measurement of the optical densities of the group A samples in the spectrophotometer. The dashed line corresponds to the optical density of the positive control so that all samples above the dashed line are positive

CPV, the estimate of SRR was 0.131, which implied an average of 7.63 years to seroreversion. In this case, the seroconversion rate is estimated at 0.21, a value associated with an average of 4.76 years between infections.

Discussion

Vaccination is usually seen as part of a comprehensive health program for both humans and animals in the fight against infectious diseases and in the prevention of future outbreaks [14]. To achieve measurable impacts in the population, immunization schedules should be optimized according to the specific context of each animal, including its species, age, habitat, lifestyle, effectiveness of available vaccines and the underlying disease prevalence [10, 13].

In group A, only one dog had a protective titer for CPV prior to vaccination. This result was consistent with a persistence of maternal antibodies in this animal. After the second vaccination, only puppy n° 5 was protected for CPV. Regarding this dog, the vaccine protocol for CDV and CPV could have ended at 10 weeks of age. In contrast, almost all dogs were antibody-protected against CDV after the first vaccination. The variability of the maternal antibodies level may be explained by the amount of colostrum ingested by the puppies and by the mother's antibodies titer [11, 13, 17]. In this case, the titer was the same for all puppies and therefore the amount of colostrum ingested by each puppy might be the only variable to consider. Therefore, the only protected puppy against CPV in the first assessment probably ingested more colostrum. It is

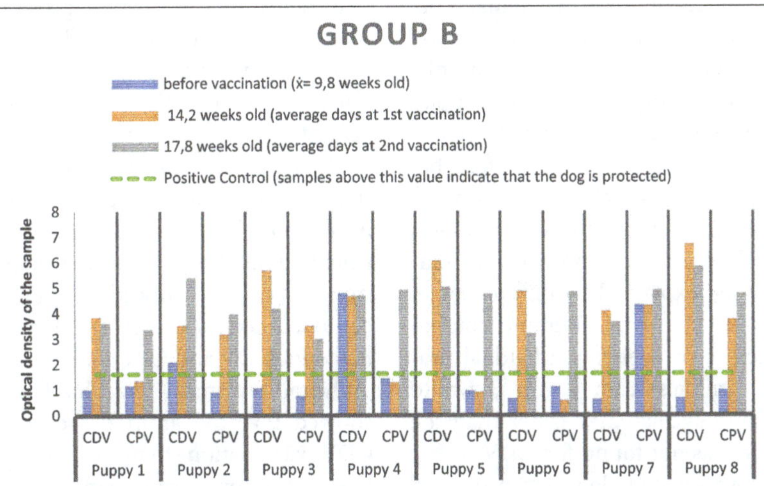

Fig. 2 Results for CDV and CPV after measurement of the optical densities of the group B samples in the spectrophotometer. The dashed line corresponds to the optical density of the positive control so that all samples above the dashed line are positive

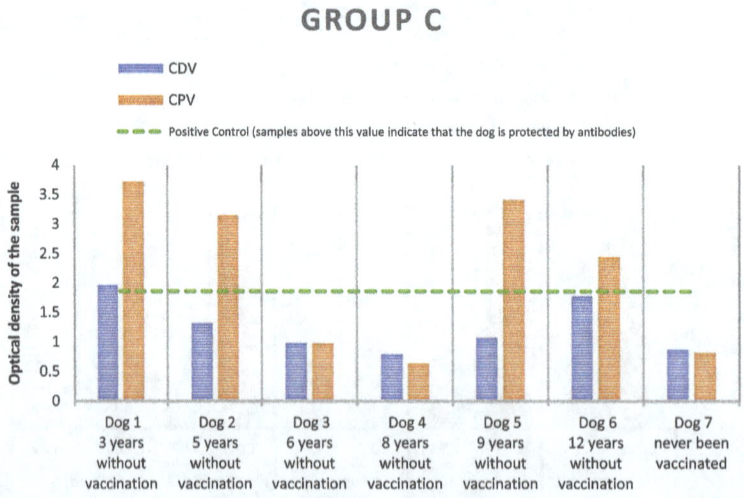

Fig. 3 Results for CDV and CPV after measurement of the optical densities of the group C samples in the spectrophotometer. The dashed line corresponds to the optical density of the positive control so that all samples above the dashed line are positive

likely that the maternal antibodies titer was low for CDV, not allowing for an effective transfer of antibodies through colostrum. Despite the fact that only one puppy was protected against CPV, none of the puppies responded to the first CPV immunization. These puppies probably had maternal antibodies against CPV higher than 1:20, which hindered vaccination success [11].

Group B consisted of slightly older dogs, which started the vaccination protocol after 8 weeks of age. All dogs in this group developed an immune response to CDV after the first vaccine administration. Four weeks after the second administration, which matched with more than 16 weeks of age, all puppies were protected against both CDV and CPV, thus, ending primary vaccination protocol successfully. This suggests a low level of maternal antibodies at the start of the vaccination protocol, which were insufficient to neutralize the vaccine antigen at this age. With respect to CDV, there were no changes between the results obtained after the first and the second immunizations, revealing that only one vaccine administration could have been enough to protect these puppies against CDV infection. Regarding CPV, a single puppy showed a protective titer (higher than 1:80) before beginning the vaccination protocol, revealing a previous effective immune response, contrary to the other puppy, which also had been submitted to a previous vaccination. This variation may be explained by differences in maternal antibody titers, vaccine type, immune competence, environmental factors or even by individual biological differences [21]. Animals from group B would appear to achieve immunity against CPV faster than the group A. Similar evidence was not found for CDV.

In group C, only one vaccinated dog was protected against both viruses (Table 2 and Fig. 3). Three other vaccinated dogs had a protective humoral immunity against CPV. Yet, they did not present antibody protection against CDV. As previously described, CPV is ubiquitous and very resistant to adverse conditions and disinfectants. In contrast, CDV is extremely susceptible to environmental conditions [4–6]. This results in an increased natural exposure to CPV, leading to more frequent antibody boosts and a quicker development of immune protection when compared to the less-frequent CDV. In fact, the occasional exposure to CDV might not be sufficient to generate strong immune responses that, ultimately, lead to a protective antibody titer [22, 23]. This interpretation is in line with a zero estimation for SCR, a common proxy of exposure frequency. However, this group was very heterogeneous in terms of age, environmental exposure, immunization schedules and immune system activity [21]. Therefore, the respective results should be interpreted with caution. However, there is evidence of a long-term protective immunity induced by core viral vaccines in adult dogs that had not been revaccinated for more than 9 years [12, 14, 15]. In fact, our results suggest that the duration of antibody immunity against CPV is longer than the one against CDV in these adult dogs. Unfortunately, there was no information on the type of vaccines used and immunization schedules in order to understand this result better. Additional heterogeneity in antibody-induced immunity can also be derived from vaccines produced by different manufacturers, as demonstrated by a serological survey on 780 dogs vaccinated for CDV and CPV [23].

Overall, primary vaccination results for puppies showed that the antibody response occurred earlier to CDV vaccination than to CPV. These results suggest that during primary vaccination the response is individual and mostly dependent on the initial titer of maternal antibodies acquired by the neonate [11, 13]. Also, the use of multivalent vaccines may induce different immune responses against the immunogenic agents [24]. In some dogs, a single administration may be sufficient to provide protection, namely against CDV. Therefore, the use of monovalent vaccines may be advisable in individual cases rather than the administration of multivalent ones [24].

The variability found reinforces the importance of determining the antibody immunity of each animal [19]. ELISA tests provide an advantageous tool to confirm protection levels during consultation at a relatively low cost [19]. These tests should be primarily used to validate vaccine efficacy induced by primary vaccination, but also to assist the veterinarian in establishing dog-specific vaccination protocols [18, 20]. These tests may help to identify dogs susceptible to these infectious diseases as well as to reduce the frequency of necessary vaccination doses. As suggested by Twark & Dodds (2000), these tests should be implemented as a routine similarly to what occurs in the poultry and the pig industry [25]. This would lead to a better control of core viral diseases, such as those caused by CDV and CPV infections.

Conclusion

Timely vaccination protocols are essential to prevent infectious diseases, such as those caused by CPV and CDV. Besides optimization of vaccination schedules, other factors including dogs' age, protective antibody titer or even vaccine type should not be neglected in assessing the effectiveness of a given vaccine. In this scenario, the present study reinforces the evidence that antibody response to vaccination is specific to each animal. This variation supports the necessity of assessing individual humoral immunity before vaccination. This evaluation can be easily performed using ELISA assays during consultation at the veterinary clinic.

Methods

All puppies from 6 to 12 weeks of age submitted to primary vaccination and adult dogs unvaccinated for at least 3 years, presented at VTH, were selected to this study. All dogs included in this study were dewormed and evaluated by a veterinarian prior to each vaccination and considered healthy and able to initiate the vaccine protocol. Animals were distributed by three groups: A – puppies which started the vaccine protocol at 6 weeks; B - puppies which started the vaccine protocol at 8 to 12 weeks; C - adult animals, unvaccinated for at least 3 years. Primary vaccination in group A was performed using the multivalent Nobivac® Puppy DP vaccine (MSD Animal Health Lda., Paço de Arcos, Portugal); for group B was used the multivalent Nobivac ® DHPPi vaccine (MSD Animal Health Lda., Paço de Arcos, Portugal).

Blood samples were collected (0.5 or 1 ml) from the lateral saphenous vein, prior to the administration of the first vaccine, and in the subsequent vaccine boosters.

Three blood samples were collected from each animal of groups A and B at the time of the vaccination consultations, 3 to 4 weeks apart. The first blood sample was collected before vaccination, allowing the evaluation of maternal antibodies in vaccine effectiveness. The remaining samples enabled the determination of the puppy's immune response to vaccination. In adult dogs, which were unvaccinated for more than 3 years, only one blood sample was collected to investigate their humoral immunity status for CPV and CDV. Each sample was then centrifuged (6000 rpm for 10 min). Plasma was collected and stored in the freezer at – 20 °C until further use.

Unhealthy dogs, dogs that missed scheduled immunization appointments, or started vaccination after 12 weeks of age, or whose age was unknown were excluded from this study.

All procedures involving the manipulation of these dogs were performed after owner's written consent and approval by the Committee for Ethics and Animal Welfare (CEBEA) of the Faculty of Veterinary Medicine – University of Lisbon, Portugal. All dogs that participated in this study were client-owned animals which joined the study during their current vaccination schedule protocol at VTH. All sampled animals stayed with their owners after each sample collection.

Antibody evaluation

The antibody response was evaluated using a rapid test based on the indirect ELISA technique for antibody detection (TiterCHEK® CDV/CPV, Synbiotics Corporation, San Diego, USA). Results from samples were compared with the positive control provided, as well as with the negative control. For CDV, a positive result indicates a SN titer equal to or greater than 1:16, and a negative result a SN titer of less than 1:16 [20]. For CPV, a positive test result indicates a HI titer of 1:80 or higher, and a negative HI titer of less than 1:80 [20]. According to the test's manufacturer, a comparative colorimetric evaluation by direct observation is sufficient to detect the positivity of a sample; however, this observation was further supported with a quantitative measurement of the absorbance on a spectrophotometer (FLUOstar optima BMT Labtech) to increase evaluation objectivity. A standard sample was used and evaluated at different wavelengths to determine which one should be applied. Readings were performed at 405 nm.

Statistical analysis

The seroprevalences of groups A and B were compared with each other at the equivalent immunisation schedule using a Pearson's chi-square test for two-way frequency table. To compare the induced immunizations against CDV and CPV, the respective data was transformed into a frequency vector (f1,f2,f3) where f1 is the frequency of animals in which transition from seronegative to seropositive (e.g., seroconversion) for CDV and CPV occurred in the same time interval, f2 is the frequency of animals in which seroconversion for CDV occurred earlier than for CPV, f3 is the frequency of animals in which seroconversion for CPV occurred earlier for CDV. It was then tested whether both viruses would induce the same time for seroconversion. This hypothesis was statistically translated into $f2 = f3$, or equivalently, $f2/(f2 + f3) = 0.5$. A Binomial test using the number of trials equal to f2 + f3 was used to formally test the hypothesis $p = 0.5$.

The statistical analysis of the group associated with adult dogs aimed to estimate the average time until a vaccinated animal becomes seronegative for each virus. With that purpose, a simple reversible catalytic model was fit to the corresponding data. In general, this model describes the stochastic transitions between seropositivity and seronegativity as function of age [26]. The respective transition rates are the so-called SCR and SRR assumed to be constant over time. The former rate is the frequency by which a seronegative animal becomes seropositive upon natural exposure to the infection, while the latter rate is the frequency by which a seropositive animal returns to a seronegative state in absence of recurrent exposure. In this study, it was assumed that (i) animals were all seropositive after vaccination, (ii) the time vaccination was the instant zero of the model, (iii) time since vaccination was the age variable of the model and (iv) serological outcomes of the individual were derived from independent Bernoulli trials. This model was then estimated using the maximum likelihood method, as described elsewhere [26]. Finally, for each virus, the average time to seroreversion was estimated as the inverse of the SRR estimate.

The whole statistical analysis was performed in the R software version 3.3.2. All statistical tests were carried out at 5% significance level. The sero-aid package was specifically used to fit the reversible catalytic model to the data. This package is available from NS upon request.

Abbreviations

CDV: Canine Distemper Virus; CEBEA: Committee for Ethics and Animal Welfare (Faculty of Veterinary MedicineUniversity of Lisbon); CPV: Canine Parvovirus; HI: Hemagglutination Inhibition; SCR: Seroconversion rate; SN: Serum Neutralizing; SRR: Seroreversion rate; VTH: Veterinary Teaching Hospital

Acknowledgements

The authors want to thank to FCT, the CIISA - Centre for Interdisciplinary Research in Animal Health, Faculty of Veterinary Medicine, University of Lisbon, Portugal and Zoetis®Portugal for supporting this work.

Funding

This study was financed by the Fundação para a Ciência e a Tecnologia (FCT), Portugal (Project UID/CVT/00276/2013; Fellowship SFRH/BD/131384/2017), CIISA - Centre for Interdisciplinary Research in Animal Health, Faculty of Veterinary Medicine, University of Lisbon, Portugal and Zoetis®Portugal. The funding bodies had no role in the design of the study or collection, analysis, and interpretation of data or in writing the manuscript.

Authors' contributions

BVN performed the experiments and analyzed the data. EC helped to perform the experiments, analyze the data and to write the manuscript. NS – performed the statistical analysis and helped drafting and revising the manuscript. MO helped to perform the experiments and to analyze the data. BSB helped to perform the experiments and to analyze the data. LT contributed to the analysis and interpretation of data. VA helped to analyze the data and helped to draft and revise the manuscript. SG conceived the study and participated in its coordination, helped to draft the manuscript and supervised throughout. All authors read and approved the final manuscript.

Authors' information

BVN – DVM. EC - DVM, Researcher at FMV. NS – BSc, MSc, PhD, Assistant Professor at LSHTM, MO – MSc, DVM, PhD, Assistant Professor at FMV. BSB - DVM, PhD, Assistant Professor at FMV. LT - DVM, PhD, Full Professor at FMV. VA - DVM, PhD, Associate Professor at FMV. SG - DVM, PhD, Assistant Professor at FMV.

Consent for publication

Not applicable.

Competing interests

The authors declare that they have no competing interests.

Author details

[1]Faculty of Veterinary Medicine, University of Lisbon, Av. Universidade Técnica, 1300-477 Lisbon, Portugal. [2]CIISA- Centre for Interdisciplinary Research in Animal Health, Faculty of Veterinary Medicine, University of Lisbon, Av. Universidade Técnica, 1300-477 Lisbon, Portugal. [3]London School of Hygiene and Tropical Medicine, London, UK. [4]Centro de Estatística e Aplicações da Universidade de Lisboa, Lisbon, Portugal.

References

1. Greene CE, Decaro N. Canine viral enteritis. In: Greene CE, editor. Infectious diseases of the dog and cat. 4th ed. Philadelphia: Saunders Elsevier Co; 2012. p. 67–75.
2. Greene CE, Levy JK. Immunoprophylaxis. In: Greene CE, editor. Infectious diseases of the dog and cat. 4th ed. Philadelphia: Saunders Elsevier Co; 2012. p. 1163–204.
3. Miranda C, Thompson GJ. Canine parvovirus: the worldwide occurrence of antigenic variants. Gen Virol. 2016;97(9):2043–57. https://doi.org/10.1099/jgv.0.000540.
4. Goddard A, Leisewitz A. Canine Parvovirus. Vet Clin Small Anim. 2010;40:1041–53. https://doi.org/10.1016/j.cvsm.2010.07.007.
5. Crawford PC, Sellon RK. Canine viral diseases. In: Ettinger SJ, Feldman EC, editors. Veterinary internal medicine. 7th ed. Canada: Saunders Elsevier Co; 2010. p. 958–62.
6. Martella V, Elia G, Buonavoglia C. Canine Distemper Virus. Vet Clin Small Anim. 2008;38:787–97. https://doi.org/10.1016/j.cvsm.2008.02.007.
7. Loots A, Mitchell E, Dalton D, Kotzé A, Venter E. Advances in canine distemper virus pathogenesis research: a wildlife perspective. J Gen Virol. 2017;98(3):311–21. https://doi.org/10.1099/jgv.0.000666.
8. Thiry E, Horzinek MC. Vaccination guidelines: a bridge between official requirements and the daily use of vaccines. Rev Sci Tech. 2007;26(2):511–7.
9. Greene CE, Vandevelde M. Canine distemper. In: Greene CE, editor. Infectious diseases of the dog and cat. 4th ed. Philadelphia: Saunders Elsevier Co; 2012. p. 25–42.

10. Day MJ, Horzinek MC, Schultz RD, Squires RA. WSAVA Guidelines for the vaccination of dogs and cats – compiled by the vaccination guidelines Group of the World Small Animal Veterinary Association. J Small Anim Pract. 2016;57:1–45.
11. Pollock RV, Carmichael LE. Maternally derived immunity to canine parvovirus infection: transfer, decline, and interference with vaccination. J Am Vet Med Assoc. 1982;180(1):37–42.
12. Schultz RD, Thiel B, Mukhtar E, Sharp P, Larson LJ. Age and long-term protective immunity in dogs and cats. J Comp Pathol. 2010;142:102–8. https://doi.org/10.1016/j.jcpa.2009.10.009.
13. Mila H, Grellet A, Desario C, Feugier A, Decaro N, Buonavoglia C, Chastant- Maillard S. Protection against canine parvovirus type 2 infection in puppies by colostrum-derived antibodies. J Nutr Sci. 2014; 3(e54):1–4. https://doi.org/10.1017/jns.2014.57.
14. Day MJ. Vaccination. In: Day MJ, editor. Clinical immunology of the dog and cat. 2nd ed. Bristol: Manson Publishing; 2012. p. 413–30.
15. Jensen W, Totten J, Lappin M, Schultz R. Use of serologic tests to predict resistance to canine distemper virus-induced disease in vaccinated dogs. J Vet Diagn Investig. 2015;27(5):576–80. https://doi.org/10.1177/1040638715602291.
16. Abdelmagid O, Larson L, Payne L, Tubbs A, Wasmoen T, Schultz R. Evaluation of the efficacy and duration of immunity of a canine combination vaccine against virulent parvovirus, infectious canine hepatitis virus, and distemper virus experimental challenges. Vet Ther. 2004;5(3):173–86.
17. Böhm M, Thompson H, Weir A, Hasted AM, Maxwell NS, Herrtage ME. Serum antibody Titres to canine parvovirus, adenovirus and distemper virus in dogs in the UK which had not been vaccinated for at least three years. Vet Rec. 2004;154(15):457–63. https://doi.org/10.1136/vr.154.15.457.
18. Litster A, Pressler B, Volpe A, Dubovi E. Accuracy of a point-of-care ELISA test kit for predicting the presence of protective canine parvovirus and canine distemper virus antibody concentrations in dogs. Vet J. 2012;193(2): 363–6. https://doi.org/10.1016/j.tvjl.2012.01.027.
19. Litster A, Nichols J, Volpe A. Prevalence of positive antibody test results for canine parvovirus (CPV) and canine distemper virus (CDV) and response to modified live vaccination against CPV and CDV in dogs entering animal shelters. Vet Microbiol. 2012;157(1–2):86–90. https://doi.org/10.1016/j.vetmic.2011.12.030.
20. Coyne MJ, Burr JH, Yule TD, Harding MJ, Tresnan DB, McGavin D. Duration of immunity in dogs after vaccination or naturally acquired infection. Vet Rec. 2001;149:509–15. https://doi.org/10.1136/vr.149.17.509.
21. Tizard I, Ni Y. Use of serologic testing to assess immune status of companion animals. J Am Vet Med Assoc. 1998;213(1):54–60.
22. Olson P, Finnsdóttir H, Klingeborn B, Hedhammar A. Short Communications: Duration of antibodies elicited by canine distemper virus. Vet Rec. 1997;141:654–5.
23. Almendra C, Pinto O, Carmichael L, Tavares L. Determinação dos níveis de imunidade humoral induzidos pela vacinação contra a Esgana e a Parvovirose caninas. RPCV. 2005;100:75–84.
24. Wilson S, Illambas J, Siedek E, Thomas A, King V, Stirling C, Plevová E, Salt J, Sture G. The administration of a single dose of a multivalent (DHPPiL4R) vaccine prevents clinical signs and mortality following virulent challenge with canine distemper virus, canine adenovirus or canine parvovirus. Trials Vaccinol. 2017;3(1):107–13. https://doi.org/10.1016/j.trivac.2014.05.002.
25. Twark L, Dodds WJ. Clinical use of serum parvovirus and distemper virus antibody titers for determining revaccination strategies in healthy dogs. J Am Vet Med Assoc. 2000;217(7):1021–4.
26. Sepúlveda N, Stresman G, White MT, Drakeley CJ. Current mathematical models for analyzing anti-malarial antibody data with an eye to malaria elimination and eradication. J Immunol Res. 2015;2015:1–21.

Safety and immunogenicity of an attenuated Chinese pseudorabies variant by dual deletion of TK&gE genes

Jichun Wang[1,2], Zengcai Song[3], Aimin Ge[4], Rongli Guo[2,5], Yongfeng Qiao[1,2], Mengwei Xu[1,2], Zhisheng Wang[1,2], Yamei Liu[1,2], Yating Zheng[1,2], Hongjie Fan[3] and Jibo Hou[1,2*]

Abstract

Background: Since the outbreak of a new emerging virulent pseudorabies virus mutant in Chinese pig herds, intensive research has been focused on the construction of novel gene deletion vaccine based on the variant virulent viruses. An ideal vaccine candidate is expected to have a balanced safety and immunogenicity.

Results: From the infectious clone of PRV AH02LA strain, a TK deletion mutant was generated through two-step Red mutagenesis. After homologous recombination with a transfer vector, a TK&gE dual deficient mutant PRV ($PRV^{\Delta TK\&gE\text{-}AH02}$) was generated, and its structure verified by PCR, RFLP and sequencing. Growth kinetics test showed that $PRV^{\Delta TK\&gE\text{-}AH02}$ reached a titer of $10^{7.5}$ $TCID_{50}$ /mL on ST cells.
The $PRV^{\Delta TK\&gE\text{-}AH02}$ at a dose of $10^{6.0}$ $TCID_{50}$ /animal was not virulent in mice or 1-day-old piglets with maternal PRV antibodies. No clinical signs or virus shedding were detected in 28~ 35-day-old piglets without maternal PRV antibodies after nasal or intramuscular administration with a dose of $10^{6.0}$ $TCID_{50}$, although it caused one death of four 1-day-old piglets without maternal PRV antibodies. In the efficiency test of $PRV^{\Delta TK\&gE\text{-}AH02}$, all four 28~ 35-day-old piglets without PRV antibody in the challenge control showed typical clinical symptoms and virus shedding, and two died at 4~ 5 days post challenge. All piglets in $10^{5.0}$, $10^{4.0}$ and $10^{3.0}$ $TCID_{50}$/dose $PRV^{\Delta TK\&gE\text{-}AH02}$ groups provided complete protection against challenge at only 7 days post intramuscular vaccination. More importantly, $PRV^{\Delta TK\&gE\text{-}AH02}$ stopped virus shedding in these piglets. In contrast, all four piglets in PRV Bartha K61 vaccine group developed high body temperature (≥40.5 °C) and viral shedding, despite they had mild or even no clinical symptoms.

Conclusions: The constructed TK&gE dual deletion mutant $PRV^{\Delta TK\&gE\text{-}AH02}$ can reach high titers on ST cells. The live vaccine of $PRV^{\Delta TK\&gE\text{-}AH02}$ is highly safe, and can not only provide clinical protection but also stops virus shedding. This study suggests that $PRV^{\Delta TK\&gE\text{-}AH02}$ might work as a promising vaccine candidate to combat the PRV variant emerging in Chinese herds since 2011.

Keywords: Pseudorabies virus emerging variant, TK&gE dual deletion, Attenuation, Live vaccine, Safety, Immunogenicity

* Correspondence: houjiboccvv@163.com
[1]National Research Center of Engineering and Technology for Veterinary Biologicals/Institute of Veterinary Immunology & Engineering, Jiangsu Academy of Agricultural Sciences, Nanjing 210014, Jiangsu, China
[2]Jiangsu Co-innovation Center for Prevention and Control of Important Animal Infectious Diseases and Zoonoses, Yangzhou, China
Full list of author information is available at the end of the article

Background

Since 2011, a new emerging pseudorabies virus(PRV) variant has swept many Chinese pig herds, leading to infection or disease of variable severity [1–4]. Several studies have shown that PRV Bartha K61 vaccine can only provide clinical protection against the new PRV mutants, but fail to stop virus shedding in piglets post challenge [5]. It is therefore urgent to develop a more efficacious vaccine in order to eradicate the virulent PRV variant. Since successful eradication of pseudorabies in many nations have been achieved via the application of gene deletion DIVA(differentiating infected from vaccinated animals) vaccines [6–9], gene deletion mutants of the emerging PRV may be promising vaccine candidates for infection control and eradication [10].

Expectedly, PRV glycoprotein E (gE) gene is one target of deletion for differentiation purpose [11, 12]. For further attenuation, thymidine kinase(TK), glycoprotein I(gI) and/or glycoprotein G(gG) genes were also chosen as targets for deletion to generate gE&gI, TK&gE, TK&gE&gI or TK&gG deletion mutants [6, 13]. Several mutants of gE, gE&gI or gE&gI&TK deletion from the new variant have been generated and evaluated for safety and immunogenicity [11, 12, 14–19]. However, the safety and/or immunogenicity of these mutants is far from being satisfactory. TK is associated with virulence and reactivation from latent infection of PRV, and therefore the deletion of TK leads to attenuation of virulent PRV [20, 21]. As known, gE can form complexes with gI to obtain neuro-tropism and reactivation. It is proposed that gI will lose this function without gE, while immune stimulation by gI will be reserved. A TK&gE dual deletion mutant of the wild-type PRV TNL strain, which was isolated from a commercial pig farm in southern Taiwan in 1976, has been generated and proposed potential vaccine candidate with safety, efficacy and DIVA capability [22]. To our knowledge, no TK&gE deletion mutant from the new emerging Chinese variant has been reported so far.

Therefore, in this study, a TK&gE dual deletion mutant was constructed using a bacterial artificial chromosome clone of the emerging PRV AH02LA strain. Safety and immunogenicity of this mutant was evaluated in regard to its potency as a vaccine candidate for the control or eradication of the new emerging pseudorabies virus in Chinese pig herds.

Methods

Cells and viruses

Swine testicular (ST) cells (CVCC:CL27, from China Veterinary Culture Collection Center), and primary or secondary chicken embryo cells (CECs) made from 10 days SPF chicken embryo (from Beijing Merial Vital Laboratory Animal Technology Co., Ltd.) were cultured in Dulbecco's Modified Eagle Medium(DMEM, Gibco) supplemented with 2~ 10% newborn calf serum(NCS, Gibco), 100 U/mL penicillin and 100 μg/mL streptomycin at 37 °C, 5% CO_2 atmosphere. The PRV AH02LA strain was isolated and identified in our lab(CGMCC No. 10891) [23]. The gE deletion mutant(LA-A^B) from AH02LA strain was constructed in our lab as reported previously [23]. The PRV Bartha K61 strain was kindly provided by Professor Ping Jiang at the Nanjing Agricultural University, China. Virus cultures and stocks were prepared using CECs or ST cells and were frozen in aliquots at -70 °C after three round of freeze-thawing(- 70 °C and 37 °C). Virus titers were determined by $TCID_{50}$ on ST cells following the Reed-Muench method. Viral Deoxyribonucleic acid(DNA) was extracted from infected cells by the sodium dodecyl sulfate(SDS)-proteinase K method. Transfection of plasmid, virus or bacterial artificial chromosome(BAC) DNA were performed using Lipofectamine® 3000 (Invitrogen) following manual of supplier.

Bacterial manipulation

The BAC of PRV AH02LA strain(BAC^{PRV-G}), constructed previously in our lab [23], was used for generation of TK&gE deletion mutant. Plasmid and BAC DNAs were prepared with commercial kits (QIAGEN). Restriction fragment length polymorphism(RFLP) analyses of PRV BAC or BAC mutants was conducted using the restriction endonucleases *Kpn* I (Takara) as described earlier [24]. Electroporation was performed to transform plasmid or BAC DNA as previously described [24].

PCR and sequencing

To conduct *En Passant* recombination, a pair of primers (PRV ΔTK En pa F/R) for amplification of kanamycin resistance gene was designed with 60 bp homologous sequences (Fig. 1a)(Table 1) [25]. Primers of PRV ΔTK check F/R were used for check of correct insertion of kanamycin resistance gene and correct deletion of TK gene (Table 1). Primers(PRV BAC H1 F and PRV BAC H2 R) were designed from a reference sequence (GenBank:NC_006151.1) to amplify a DNA fragment including upstream and downstream homologous arms, the intact gI gene and part of gE gene(1299 bp to 1735 bp of gE ORF) (Fig. 1d) (Table 1) using isolated PRV LA-A^B strain DNA as template. The correct deletion of gE was verified with a pair of primers(PRV ΔgE check F/R)(Table 1). The primers used for sequencing gI gene were prepared as described previously(GeneScript, Nanjing China). [26]

Construction of PRV BAC deletion mutants

The PRV BAC TK deletion mutant was constructed from BAC^{PRV-G} following *En Passant* protocol as described previously (Fig. 1a, b and c) [27]. Briefly, after

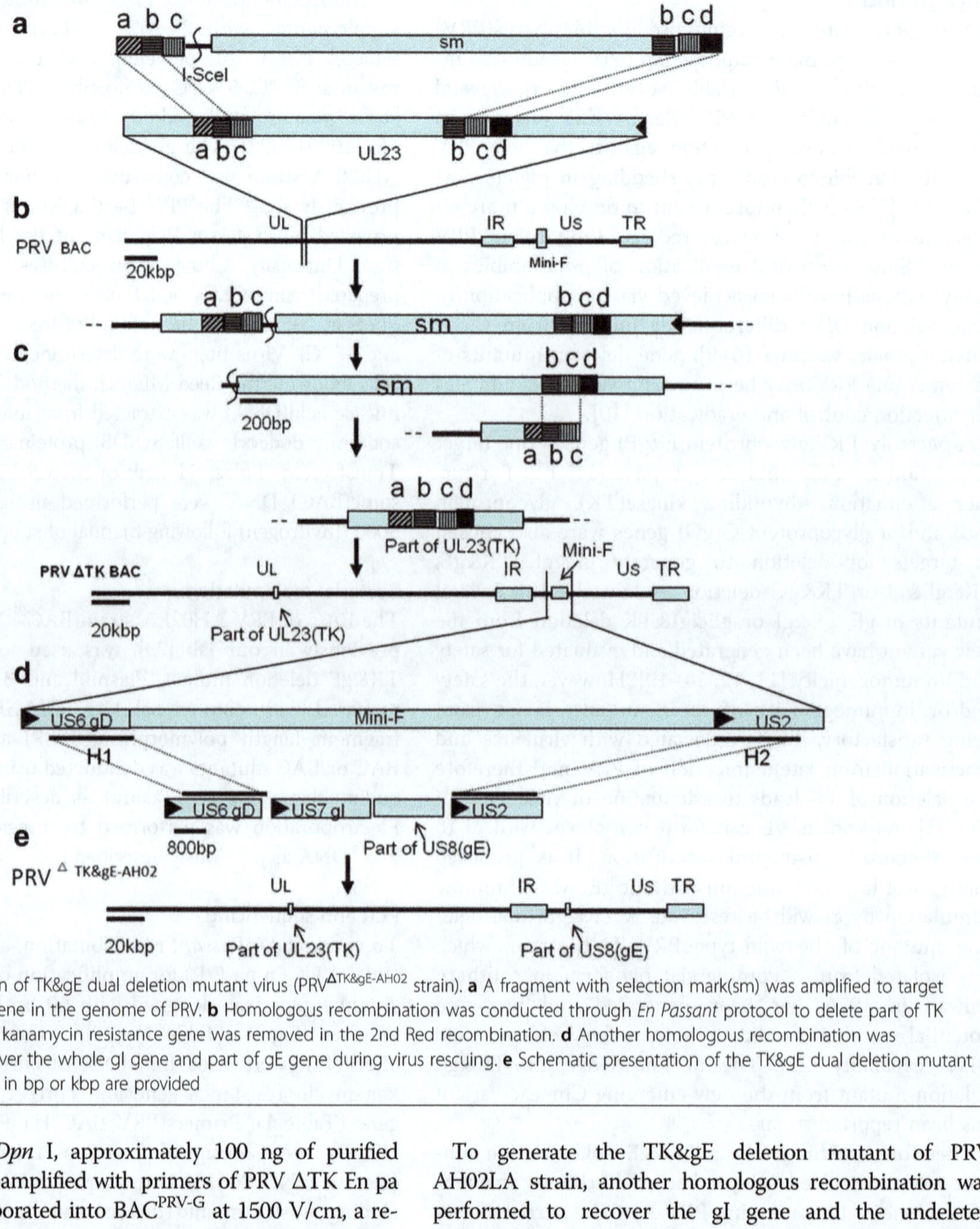

Fig. 1 Construction of TK&gE dual deletion mutant virus (PRV$^{\Delta TK\&gE\text{-}AH02}$ strain). **a** A fragment with selection mark(sm) was amplified to target part of UL23(TK) gene in the genome of PRV. **b** Homologous recombination was conducted through *En Passant* protocol to delete part of TK gene. **c** The sm of kanamycin resistance gene was removed in the 2nd Red recombination. **d** Another homologous recombination was performed to recover the whole gI gene and part of gE gene during virus rescuing. **e** Schematic presentation of the TK&gE dual deletion mutant was shown. Scales in bp or kbp are provided

digestion with *Dpn* I, approximately 100 ng of purified DNA fragments amplified with primers of PRV ΔTK En pa F/R was electroporated into BAC$^{PRV\text{-}G}$ at 1500 V/cm, a resistance and a capacitance of 25F(Precision Pulse, ECM630 BTX). Colonies with resistance to both chloramphenicol(34 μg/mL) and kanamycin(50 μg/mL) were checked through PCR with a pair of primers(PRV ΔTK check F/R) and through RFLP after digestion with *Kpn* I. One correct colony consistent with prediction from reference sequence of PRV ZJ01 strain (GenBank:KM061380.1) was used for the 2nd Red recombination to remove the kanamycin resistance gene (Fig. 1c). Colonies sensitive to kanamycin but resistant to chloramphenicol were double checked for the correct deletion of TK gene through PCR and RFLP as described above.

To generate the TK&gE deletion mutant of PRV AH02LA strain, another homologous recombination was performed to recover the gI gene and the undeleted sequences of gE (Fig. 1d). Briefly, PCR was carried out using primers PRV BAC H1 F and PRV BAC H2 F R (Table 1) and the PRV LA-A^{B} DNA as template. Primary CECs were co-transfected with approximately 1 μg of PRV BAC DNA and 100ngof DNA fragment from the PCR reaction using Lipofectamine® 3000 (Invitrogen™). Non-fluorescent virus plaques were purified after several round of picking and plating to obtain a homogeneous virus populations. Selected viruses were confirmed for correct deletion of TK gene and gE gene by PCR and sequencing using primers(PRV ΔTK check F/R and PRV ΔgE check F/R) (Table 1), and the recovery of gI gene were checked as described previously [23].

Table 1 Primers for PCR or sequencing

Primer	Sequence(5'- 3')	Positions
PRV ΔTK En pa F	CGGTATTTACGATGCGCAGACCCGGAAGC AGAACGGCAGCGCTCACGGCCCTGCGCA ACGGGATGACGACGATAAGTAGGGATAAC	59,655
PRV ΔTK En pa R	GTTGACCAGCATGGCGTAGACGTTGCGC AGGGCCGTGAGCGCTGCCGTTCTGCTTC CGGGGGGTAATGCCAGTGTTACAACCA	60,081
PRV ΔTK check F	CGGATCTACCTCGACGGCGCCTA	59,524
PRV ΔTK check R	TTGTACGCGCCGAAGAGGGTGT	/
PRV BAC H1 F	GTACCCGTACACCGAGTCGT	121,170
PRV BAC H2 R	TTGTGGACCCGCGCGAACAT	126,648
PRV ΔgE check F	AGCCCCGGGAAGATAGCCAT	123,141
PRV ΔgE check R	ATCGCGGAACCAGACGTCGAAG	125,157
PRV gD part F	GGTGCGCGCACCTGCTGTACTTTA	121,385
PRV gD part R	AGATGTAGACGCACACGCCCACCAG	122,191

Positions indicate the position of the first base of 5' terminal on the reference genome sequence NC_006151.1. "/" indicate the primer is not on the genome of PRV but the Kanamycin resistance mark gene

Multistep growth kinetics

Multistep growth kinetics of parental AH02LA, gE deletion mutant (LA-A^{B} strain), and TK&gE dual deletion mutant (PRV$^{\Delta TK\&gE\text{-}AH02}$) viruses were conducted following the methods as described previously with slight modifications [24]. Briefly, supernatant and cell-associated virus titers were determined before infection and at 6, 12, 24, 36, 48 and 72 h post infection (P.I.) on monolayers (1×10^{6} cells) of ST cells with a multiplicity of infection (MOI)of 0.01. Viruses from supernatant or released from cells by three freeze-thaw cycles were titrated on fresh ST cells. Three independent experiments were conducted and one-way ANOVA (SPSS software package 17.0, IBM SPSS, Chicargo, IL, USA) was employed for statistical analysis.

Preparation of vaccine

PRV$^{\Delta TK\&gE\text{-}AH02}$, PRV LA-A^{B} and Bartha K61 viruses were propagated on ST cells using a 5 l bioreactor, each virus stock was titrated by $TCID_{50}$ following the Reed-Muench method on ST cells. All vaccines were confirmed to be free of bacteria and fungi following standard method as described in "People's Republic of China Veterinary Pharmacopoeia, 2015 edition", and were stored at -70 °C until use.

Test of vaccine safety of PRV$^{\Delta TK\&gE\text{-}AH02}$

Twenty one-day-old PRV gB antibody negative piglets (from Zhengzhuquan Pig Breeding Farm in Pukou district, Nanjing, China), free of porcine reproductive and respiratory syndrome virus (PRRSV), porcine parvovirus (PPV), porcine circovirus 2(PCV2) and classical swine fever virus (CSFV), were divided into 5 groups. In group A(N) and B(N) piglets were inoculated intranasally(I.N.) with PRV$^{\Delta TK\&gE\text{-}AH02}$ and PRV LA-A^{B} respectively with a dose of $10^{7.0}TCID_{50}$, while in group C(N) and D(N) intramuscularly (I.M.) respectively. Group E(N) was inoculated 2 mL PBS as placebo control (Table 2). Clinical signs were monitored daily for 14 days. Serum samples were collected for PRV gB and gE antibodies test at 14 days P.I..

Twenty one-day-old PRV gB antibody positive/gE antibody negative piglets(from Zhengzhuquan Pig Breeding Farm in Pukou district, Nanjing, China), also free of

Table 2 Groups division and results of antibodies, clinical signs in safety test

Groups			A(N)	B(N)	C(N)	D(N)	E(N)
Inoculation route			I.N.		I.M.		
PRV strain tested			PRV$^{\Delta TK\&gE\text{-}AH02}$	LA-A^{B}	PRV$^{\Delta TK\&gE\text{-}AH02}$	LA-A^{B}	
ELISA antibodies against PRV gB or gE	B.I.	gB+	0^{a}/4^{b}	0/4	0/4	0/4	0/4
	14d P.I.	gB+	3/3	/	4/4	1/1	0/4
		gE+	0/3	/	0/4	0/1	0/4
Morbidity			2/4	4/4	1/4	4/4	0/4
Mortality			1/4	4/4	0/4	3/4	0/4
Groups			A(P)	B(P)	C(P)	D(P)	E(P)
Inoculation route			I.N.		I.M.		
PRV strain tested			PRV$^{\Delta TK\&gE\text{-}AH02}$	LA-A^{B}	PRV$^{\Delta TK\&gE\text{-}AH02}$	LA-A^{B}	
ELISA antibodies against PRV gB or gE	B.I.	gB+	4/4	4/4	4/4	4/4	4/4
	14d P.I.	gB+	4/4	4/4	4/4	4/4	4/4
		gE+	0/4	0/4	0/4	0/4	0/4
Morbidity			0/4	0/4	0/4	0/4	0/4
Mortality			0/4	0/4	0/4	0/4	0/4

I.N. means intranasally, *I.M.* means intramuscularly, *gB+* means antibodies against PRV gB positive, *gE+* means antibodies against PRV gE positive, *B.I.* means before inoculation, *P.I.* means post inoculation. "a" indicates the number of piglets positive;"b" indicates the number of piglets in the group

PRRSV, PPV, PCV2 and CSFV, were divided into 5 groups of A(P), B(P), C(P), D(P) and E(P). All piglets were treated and monitored exactly as those PRV gB antibody negative piglets (Table 2).

Safety of PRV mutants in mice (Balb/c mice, from Nanjing biomedical research institute of Nanjing University,Nanjing, China) was also tested. $PRV^{\Delta TK\&gE\text{-}AH02}$, PRV LA-$A^{B}$ and parental PRV AH02LA were separately used to inoculate mice subcutaneously with doses of $10^{6.0}$, $10^{5.0}$, $10^{4.0}$ and $10^{3.0}$ $TCID_{50}$ respectively (Table 2). LD_{50} of each strain for mice were determined following Reed-Muench method. The euthanasia of survived mices mere performed usingy compressed CO2 gas.

Test of vaccine efficacy of $PRV^{\Delta TK\&gE\text{-}AH02}$

Twenty four 28~ 35-day-old piglets(from Zhengzhuquan Pig Breeding Farm in Pukou district, Nanjing, China) were randomly divided into 6 groups (A-F). All piglets were antibody negative for PRV gB and gE, and free of PRRSV, PPV, PCV2 and CSFV. Piglets in group A, B and C were vaccinated with $PRV^{\Delta TK\&gE\text{-}AH02}$ strain with $1 \times 10^{3.0}$, $1 \times 10^{4.0}$ and $1 \times 10^{5.0}$ $TCID_{50}$ /dose respectively, group D piglets with live Bartha K61 of $1 \times 10^{5.0}$ $TCID_{50}$ /dose, and groups E and F piglets were dosed with PBS only(Table 3). All inoculations were given intramuscularly(I.M.) at 2 mL/pig. At 1 week post vaccination(P.V.), groups A, B, C, D and E were challenged intranasally (I.N.) with $2LD_{50}$ PRV AH02LA per piglet. Group F piglets were not challenged, serving as a negative control. Clinical signs, body temperature and virus shedding were monitored and recorded daily from vaccination to 14 days P.C.. Serum samples from all piglets were collected for PRV gB and gE antibodies test before vaccination, and at 7 days post vaccination (P.V.), and 14 days post challenge (P.C.). All survived piglets were euthanized by injection of pentobarbital. The presence of lung lesions for survived or died piglets was noted at the end of the test.

Test for serological antibodies

ELISA tests were performed using PRV gE or gB antibody detection kit (IDEXX, Maine, USA) following the manufacturer's instructions. In safety experiment, all 1-day-old piglets were tested for serum antibodies against PRV gB and gE, and then divided into PRV negative group or positive group accordingly. At 14 days post vaccination, serum samples of all piglets were collected for test of PRV gB and gE antibodies again. In efficacy experiment, serum samples of all piglets were collected before vaccination, at 7 days post vaccination (before challenge) and at 14 days P.C. for test of PRV gB and gE antibodies.

Detection of virus shedding

Nasal swab samples were collected daily from all piglets in efficacy experiment from inoculation of vaccines to

Table 3 Group division and results of antibodies, clinical signs and lung lesions in efficacy test

Groups			A	B	C	D	E	F
Virus tested			$PRV^{\Delta TK\&gE\text{-}AH02}$			Bartha K61	/	/
Dosage ($TCID_{50}$)			10^3	10^4	10^5	10^5	/	/
Inoculation route			Intramuscularly					
ELISA antibodies against PRV gB or gE	B.V.	gB+	0[a]/4[b]	0/4	0/4	0/4	0/4	0/4
		gE+	0/4	0/4	0/4	0/4	0/4	0/4
	7d P.V.	gB+	4/4	4/4	4/4	4/4	0/4	0/4
		gE+	0/4	0/4	0/4	0/4	0/4	0/4
	14 d P.C.	gB+	4/4	4/4	4/4	4/4	0/4	0/4
		gE+	4/4	4/4	4/4	4/4	1/1	0/4
Clinical signs P.V.			0/4	0/4	0/4	0/4	0/4	0/4
Fever frequency (≥40.5 °C) P.V.			0/4	0/4	0/4	0/4	0/4	0/4
Virus shedding P.V.			0/4	0/4	0/4	0/4	/	/
Fever frequency (≥40.5 °C) P.C.			0/4	0/4	0/4	4/4	4/4	0/4
Clinical signs P.C.	Morbidity		0/4	0/4	0/4	0/4	4/4	0/4
	Duration (days)		/	/	/	/	4~ 9	/
	Mortality		0/4	0/4	0/4	0/4	3/4	0/4
Virus shedding P.C.	Frequency		0/4	0/4	0/4	4/4	4/4	0/4
	Duration (days)		/	/	/	3~ 5	2~ 9	/
Lung lesions			0/4	0/4	0/4	2/4	4/4	0/4

B.V. means before vaccination, *P.V.* means post vaccination, *P.C.* means post challenge, *gB+* means antibodies against PRV gB positive, *gE+* means antibodies against PRV gE positive, "a" indicates the number of piglets positive; "b" indicates the number of piglets in the group

14 days P.C.. Treatment and titration of nasal swab samples were performed following the method as described earlier. Viral DNA isolated from titration cells with typical cytopathogenic effects (CPE) was used as template to amplify a specific fragment of 813 bp in gD gene with a pair of primers(PRV gD part F/R) (Table 1).

Experiments involving virulent PRV were conducted under Biosafety Level 2+ containment. All animal tests were approved by the Experimental Animal Committee of the Jiangsu Academy of Agriculture Sciences and were conducted in accordance with the "Guidelines for Experimental Animals" of the Ministry of Science and Technology (Beijing, China). All animals were fed with complete formula feed and free access to drinking water.

Results

Generation of mutant PRV BAC with TK deletion

Based on BAC $^{PRV\text{-}G}$, we targeted a 347 bp fragment in TK gene. With a first Red recombination, 120 ng of gel-purified DNA of PCR product was electroporated into BAC$^{PRV\text{-}G}$. The PCR product was amplified with a pair of primers(PRV ΔTK check F/R) that specified the homologous sequences to allow recombination. As a result the sequences from position 184 to 530 of TK gene was replaced with a kanamycin resistance cassette. Several colonies with resistance to chloramphenicol and kanamycin were obtained and verified through PCR with a pair of primers(PRV ΔTK check F/R)(data not shown) and through RFLP after digestion with *Kpn* I(Fig. 2), which showed a band of 5975 bp missed and an additional band of 6639 bp present after the first recombination. One of the verified clones, named BAC$^{PRV\Delta TK/gE/gI\&K+}$, was selected to perform the 2nd Red recombination for removal of the kanamycin resistance cassette. Colonies with resistance to chloramphenicol, but sensitive to kanamycin were selected and one of them, named BAC $^{PRV\Delta TK/gE/gI}$, was successfully confirmed through PCR with a pair of primers(PRV ΔTK check F/R)(data not shown) and through RFLP after digestion with *Kpn* I(Fig. 2), which showed a

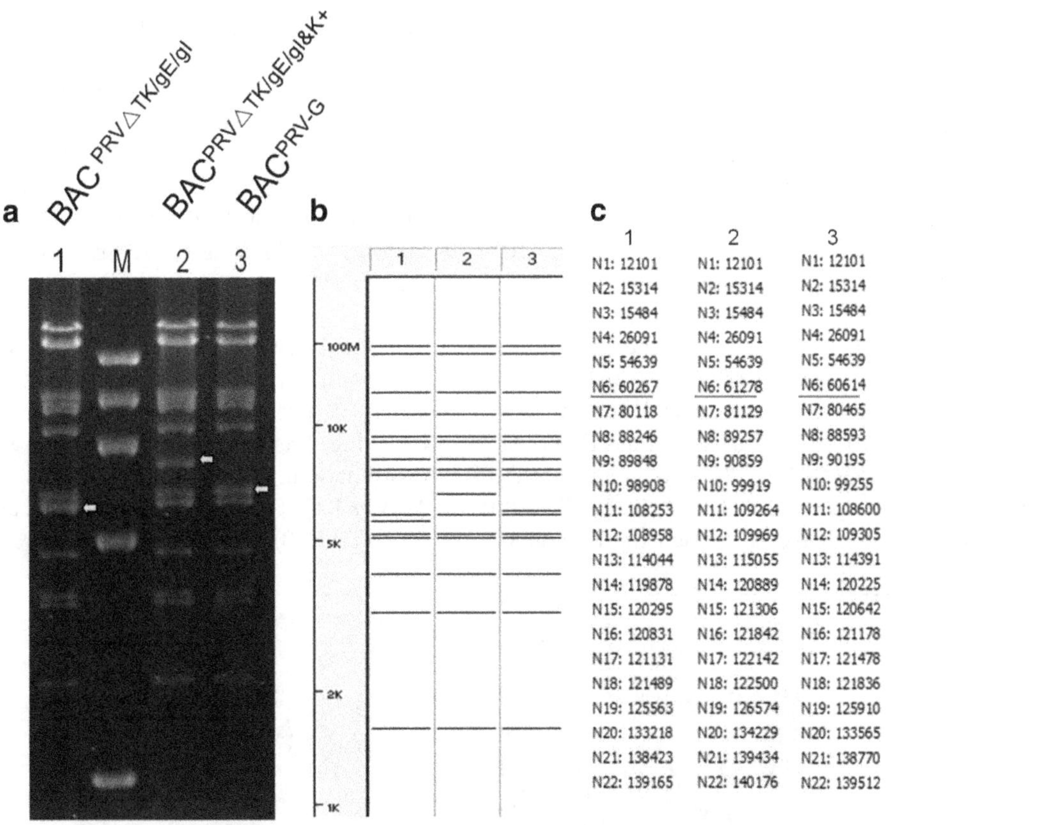

Fig. 2 Restriction fragment length polymorphism (RFLP) of BAC$^{PRV\text{-}G}$ and its TK deletion mutants. **a** RFLP pattern of BAC $^{PRV\Delta TK/gE/gI}$, BAC$^{PRV\Delta TK/gE/gI\&K+}$ and BAC$^{PRV\text{-}G}$. Lane 1, 2 and 3 are BAC $^{PRV\Delta TK/gE/gI}$, BAC$^{PRV\Delta TK/gE/gI\&K+}$ and BAC$^{PRV\text{-}G}$ respectively after digestion with *Kpn* I. The arrow (lane 2) shows an additional band of 6639 bp and a 5975 bp band missed when compared to lane 3. The arrow(lane 1) showed an additional band of 5628 bp and a missing band of 6639 bp when compared to lane 2. M is 1Kb DNA marker. **b** Predicted RFLP pattern with PRV ZJ01 strain (GenBank:KM061380.1) as a reference. Lane 1, 2 and 3 are prediction of BAC $^{PRV\Delta TK/gE/gI}$, BAC$^{PRV\Delta TK/gE/gI\&K+}$ and BAC$^{PRV\text{-}G}$ respectively digested with *Kpn* I. **c** *Kpn* I sites were cited in lane 1, 2 and 3 for BAC $^{PRV\Delta TK/gE/gI}$, BAC$^{PRV\Delta TK/gE/gI\&K+}$ and BAC$^{PRV\text{-}G}$ respectively. Sites underlined with red lines indicate the changed position of *Kpn* I restriction site leading to the bands changing accordingly

missing band of 6639 bp and instead an additional 5628 bp band present. Finally, the sequencing of the resulting PCR products after removal of kanamycin resistance cassette confirmed the successful deletion of a fragment from position 184 to 530 of TK gene in the genome of $BAC^{PRV\text{-}G}$.

Reconstitution of a TK&gE dual deletion PRV from cloned DNA

After co-transfection of BAC $^{PRV\Delta TK/gE/gI}$ DNA with a DNA fragment that was amplified with primers PRV BAC H1 F and PRV BAC H2 F R (Table 1) using PRV LA-A^B DNA as template, non-fluorescing plaques were observed under UV illumination at 488 nm (Fig. 3). The recombinant virus was purified after several round of picking and plating, and designated $PRV^{\Delta TK\&gE\text{-}AH02}$. The deletion of TK and gE and the recovery of gI were verified by PCR using primers of PRV ΔTK check F/R and PRV ΔgE check F/R respectively (Table 1). Sequencing with appropriate primers revealed the correct deletion of the 347 bp fragment in TK gene and the deletion of the 1286 bp fragment(position 13 to 1298) in gE gene and successful recovery of gI gene.

Growth kinetics of the $PRV^{\Delta TK\&gE\text{-}AH02}$ virus

Multistep growth kinetics for the PRV AH02LA, LA-A^B, and $PRV^{\Delta TK\&gE\text{-}AH02}$ viruses were determined on ST cells and the differences of titers at 48 h P.I. were statistically analyzed. For supernatant virus, peak titers for AH02LA, LA-A^B, and $PRV^{\Delta TK\&gE\text{-}AH02}$ were $10^{8.81}$, $10^{8.71}$, and $10^{8.19}$ $TCID_{50}$ /mL respectively. At 48 hpi the titers of $PRV^{\Delta TK\&gE\text{-}AH02}$ were not significantly different from LA-A^B ($p = 0.212$), while significantly different from AH02LA($P = 0.042$). For cell- associated virus, peak titers of AH02LA, LA-A^B, and $PRV^{\Delta TK\&gE\text{-}AH02}$ were $10^{8.71}$, $10^{8.49}$, and $10^{7.81}$ $TCID_{50}$ /mL respectively. At 48 hpi the titers of $PRV^{\Delta TK\&gE\text{-}AH02}$ were significantly different from LA-A^B ($p = 0.016$), and AH02LA($P = 0.001$). The results indicate that even though the mutant virus $PRV^{\Delta TK\&gE\text{-}AH02}$ can not propagate on ST cells as efficiently as LA-A^B or AH02LA strain after deletion of TK gene, it reaches titers of more than $10^{8.00}TCID_{50}$/mL (Fig. 4).

Safety of the $PRV^{\Delta TK\&gE\text{-}AH02}$ vaccine

For 1-day-old PRV antibody negative piglets, 2 of 4 piglets in group A(N) showed typical clinical signs of PR from 3 days after inoculation intranasally with $PRV^{\Delta TK\&gE\text{-}AH02}$, and one of the two ill piglets died at 7 days P.I. All the 4 piglets in group B(N) showed typical clinical signs of PR from 2 to 3 days after intranasal vaccination with PRV LA-A^B and all died at 3 to 5 days P.I.. In groups C(N) and D(N), 1 out of 4 and 4 out of 4 showed PR signs from 3 to 4 days post vaccination intramuscularly with PRV $PRV^{\Delta TK\&gE\text{-}AH02}$ or LA-A^B. No animal died in group C(N),while 3 out of 4 died in group D(N) at 4 to 7 days P.I.. No PRV gE antibodies was detected in all survived piglets. All animals in placebo control group(E(N)) were healthy during the whole test(Table 2)(Fig. 5).

For 1-day-old PRV antibody positive piglets, neither $PRV^{\Delta TK\&gE\text{-}AH02}$ (group A(P) and C(P)) nor LA-A^B (group B(P) and D(P)) showed any virulence post inoculation either intranasally or intramuscularly(Fig. 5). No PRV gE antibody was detected in all animals at 14d P.I. (Table 2).

The virulence to mice was reduced after deletion of gE gene and attenuated further after TK&gE dual deletion. LD_{50} to mice of AH02LA was $10^{3.66}TCID_{50}$, and went up to $10^{5.29}TCID_{50}$ for LA-A^B strain, while $PRV^{\Delta TK\&gE\text{-}AH02}$ did show virulence to mice at a dose of $10^{6.00}TCID_{50}$.

Immunogenicity of the $PRV^{\Delta TK\&gE\text{-}AH02}$ vaccine

In group E (challenge control), all piglets showed clinical signs of pseudorabies infection including sneezing, coughing, nasal discharge, respiratory distress, lack of coordination, circling and paralysis from 2 days to 11 days P.C.. One piglet died at 8 days and two at 10 days P.C. (Table 3) (Fig. 5). Body temperatures of all these

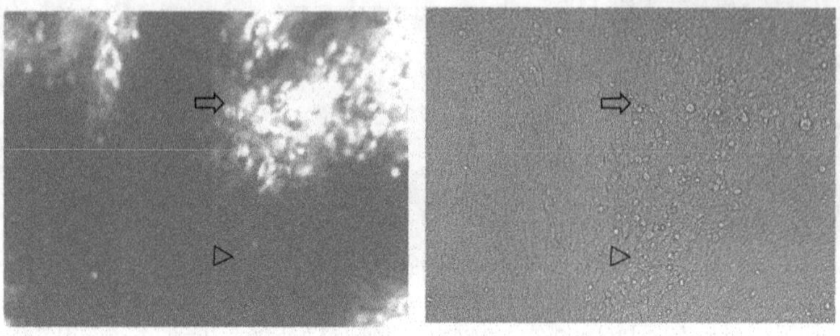

Fig. 3 Plaques of TK&gE dual deletion mutant virus. Plaques are shown under UV excitation(left) or phase control(right). Arrow shows the plaque of rescued virus from BAC $^{PRV\Delta TK/gE/gI}$. Arrowhead shows the plaque of TK&gE dual deletion mutant virus ($PRV^{\Delta TK\&gE\text{-}AH02}$) after replacement of mini-F sequences through another homologous recombination. Individual panels present views of 600 × 600 μm

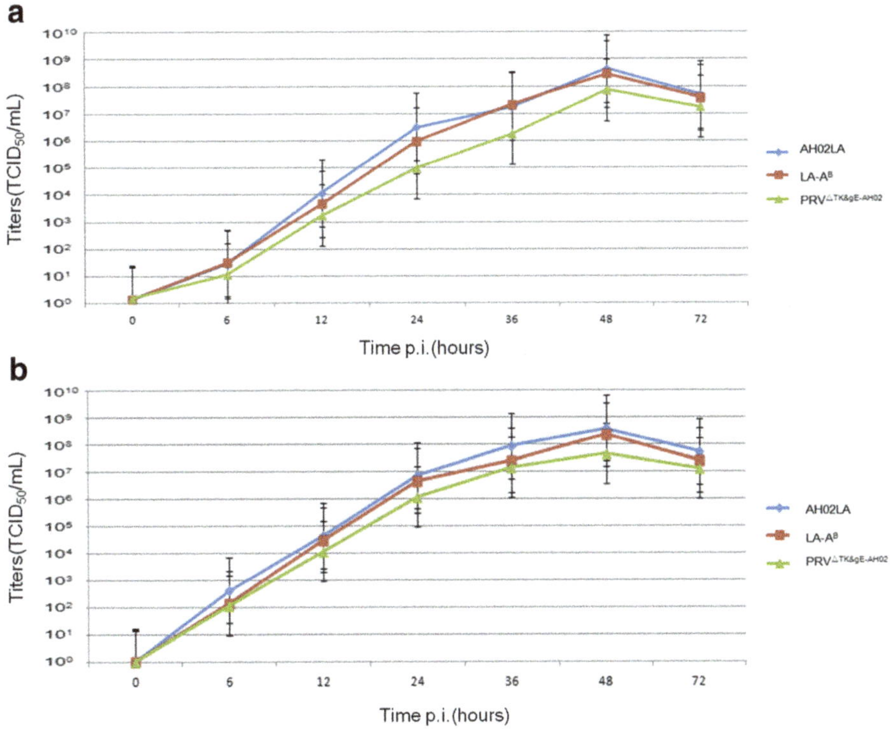

Fig. 4 Multi-step growth kinetics of AH02LA, LA-A^B and PRV$^{\Delta TK\&gE\text{-}AH02}$ on ST cells Titers of infected-cell supernatants (**a**) and cell-associated virus(**b**) of AH02LA, LA-A^B and PRV$^{\Delta TK\&gE\text{-}AH02}$ were tested at 0, 6, 12, 23, 36, 48 and 72 h post infection with an MOI of 0.01. Shown are means of titers in three independent experiments. Standard deviation are shown with the error bar

piglets reached over 40.5 °C and lasted for 4~ 10 days (data not shown). All piglets shed virus from 2 or 3 days P.C. and lasting for 5~ 7 days till death or 6~ 10 days for the surviving piglets. PCR using primers((PRV gD part F/R)(Table 1)) with the DNA of isolated virus as template amplified a specific fragment of 813 bp as suspected (data not shown). All piglets showed severe lung lesions from hemorrhaging and congestion (Table 3). All animals in group F(placebo control) were healthy during the whole test(Table 3).

At 7 days post vaccination(P.V.), gB antibodies in all piglets vaccinated with the PRV$^{\Delta TK\&gE\text{-}AH02}$ strain or Bartha K61 strain were detected positive. All piglets in vaccination groups A, B, C and D or survived piglets in group E were positive for gE antibodies at 14 days P.C. (Table 3). All animals in group F(placebo control) were gE and gB negative during the whole test(Table 3).

All piglets in the vaccinated groups (A, B, C and D) were protected against lethal challenge(Fig. 5). No fever, virus shedding or other clinical symptoms were observed in group A, B and C vaccinated with PRV$^{\Delta TK\&gE\text{-}AH02}$ strain. While all four piglets in group D vaccinated with Bartha K61 strain showed fevers of ≥40.5 °C and virus shedding was detected for 3~ 5 days, even though no other clinical signs were observed in this group(Table 3). Special fragments of 813 bp were amplified through PCR with DNA of isolated virus as template and with primers(PRV gD part F/R). No lung lesions were observed in piglets of groups A, B or C at 14 days P.C., while 2 out of 4 piglets in group D and all group E piglets presented lesions from hemorrhage and/or congestion after death or euthanization at 14 days P.C.(Table 3).

Discussion

Owing to the implementation of DIVA based vaccine [9], PRV eradication has been achieved with remarkable success [6]. Some developed countries including USA and several European nations have declared PRV free in domestic swine populations. In China, PRV was well controlled through intensive vaccination of traditional vaccines including Bartha K61 until late 2011, when a novel PRV variant with enhanced virulence emerged in several pig herds [2, 3]. AH02LA strain was isolated from the brain of a dead 1-day-old piglet in a pig farm during a PR outbreak in Anhui province of China in 2012 [23]. Sequence analysis reveals that AH02LA strain belongs to the same clade as the other new PRV variants isolated after 2011 in China [23, 28], and has significant mutations in gB, gD and gC genes when compared to the most popular vaccine strain Bartha K61 strain. Specially, gB (GenBank: KR605319) of AH02LA contains a 4 amino acid(aa)

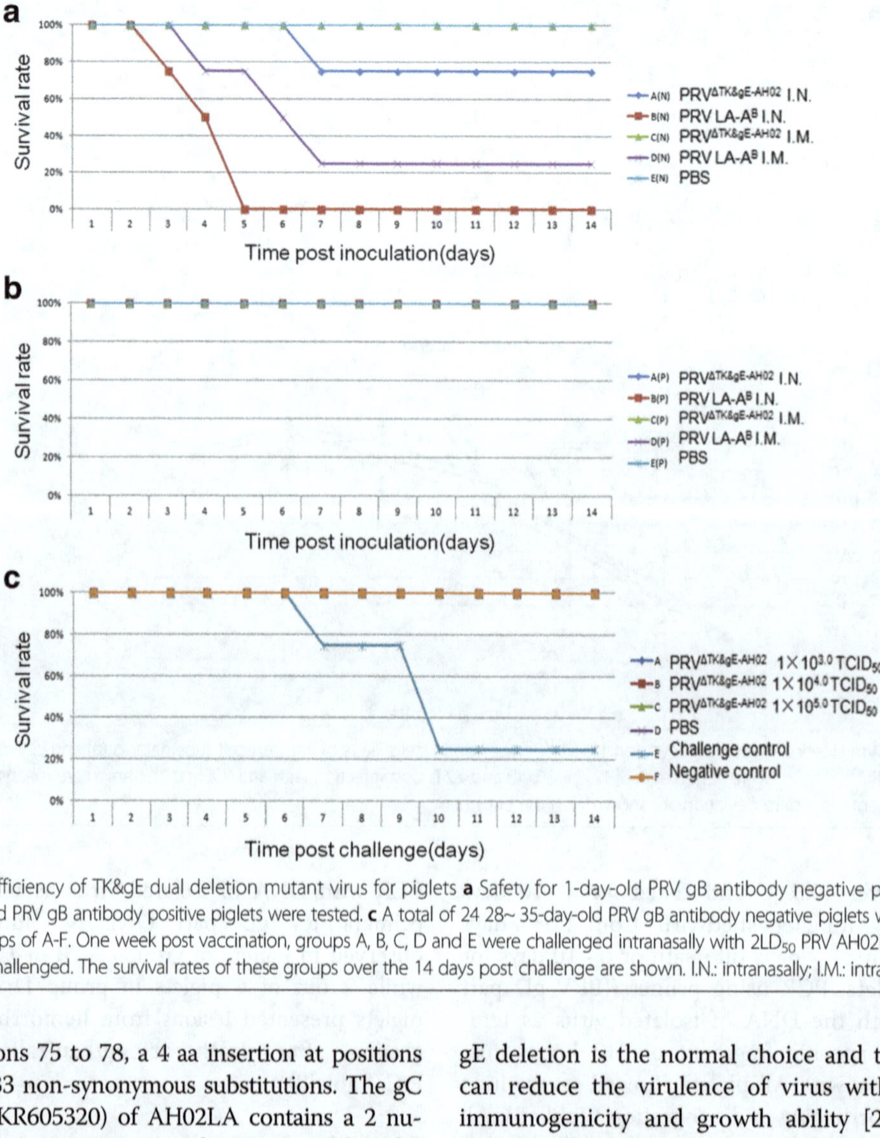

Fig. 5 Safety and efficiency of TK&gE dual deletion mutant virus for piglets **a** Safety for 1-day-old PRV gB antibody negative piglets were tested. **b** Safety for 1-day-old PRV gB antibody positive piglets were tested. **c** A total of 24 28~ 35-day-old PRV gB antibody negative piglets were randomly divided into six groups of A-F. One week post vaccination, groups A, B, C, D and E were challenged intranasally with $2LD_{50}$ PRV AH02LA per piglet. Group F piglets were not challenged. The survival rates of these groups over the 14 days post challenge are shown. I.N.: intranasally; I.M.: intramuscularly

deletion at positions 75 to 78, a 4 aa insertion at positions 121 to 124, and 33 non-synonymous substitutions. The gC gene (GenBank: KR605320) of AH02LA contains a 2 nucleotide insertion at position 176 and 177, a 7 nucleotides insertions at position 184 to 190 and a 12 nucleotide insertion at position 196 to 207, leading to a 7 aa insertion, several aa changes, and 35 non-synonymous substitutions. The gD (GenBank:KR605321) of AH02LA contains a 2 aa insertion at positions 275 and 276 and 9 non-synonymous substitutions. gD, gB and gC are the major neutralizing stimulation antigens of PRV, the reduced protection efficiency of Bartha K61 vaccines against AH02LA strain might be closely associated with the mutations in these three genes. Theoretically, gene deletion mutants from homologous virulent virus could provide better protection.

To avoid the potential threat of the latent infection of PRV to porcine herds, the eradication strategy has been a direct selection of many countries or pig farms. DIVA vaccines have played an important role for control of disease and efficient reduction of virus shedding post infection with virulent strain. For differentiation purpose, gE deletion is the normal choice and the absence of gE can reduce the virulence of virus without affecting its immunogenicity and growth ability [29, 30]. However, absence of gE along can not be used as a live vaccine without further attenuation by an additional deletion of TK gene. In this study, a live vaccine candidate of TK&gE dual deletion strain($PRV^{\Delta TK\&gE\text{-}AH02}$ strain) from the emerging PRV AH02LA strain was constructed successfully. Safety and efficacy tests demonstrated significant attenuation of the $PRV^{\Delta TK\&gE\text{-}AH02}$ strain virus and complete protection at 7 only days post vaccination. The $PRV^{\Delta TK\&gE\text{-}AH02}$ strain had stopped virus shedding against challenge by virulent AH02LA strain, suggesting that it is superior to the Bartha K61 strain for the eradication of virulent virus. It is worth noting that the $PRV^{\Delta TK\&gE\text{-}AH02}$ strain exhibited impaired replication in ST cells due to the deletion of TK and reached significantly reduced titers when compared to AH02LA or LA-A^B strain. Nevertheless, the peak titer of $PRV^{\Delta TK\&gE\text{-}AH02}$ strain still reached $10^{8.0}$ $TCID_{50}$ /mL which is sufficient for the production of a live vaccine.

In practice, 1-day-old piglets are inoculated intranasally(I.N.) with live vaccine in porcine farms that suffered from PRV emerging variants infection or under the threat of the infection. The safety test of $PRV^{\Delta TK\&gE\text{-}AH02}$ strain for 1-day-old piglets demonstrated that both $PRV^{\Delta TK\&gE\text{-}AH02}$ strain and $LA\text{-}A^{B}$ strain are safe for PRV antibody positive piglets. However, although $PRV^{\Delta TK\&gE\text{-}AH02}$ strain showed less virulence than $LA\text{-}A^{B}$ in piglets without PRV antibody, it caused lethal infection after inoculation I.N. or I.M. These results indicate that further attenuation might be necessary to improve the safety of $PRV^{\Delta TK\&gE\text{-}AH02}$. However, since farm pig herds are PRV antibody positive due to intensive vaccination of PRV vaccine and newborn piglets are surely PRV antibody positive after intake of sow's colostrum, indicating that the $PRV^{\Delta TK\&gE\text{-}AH02}$ strain should be safe for 1-day-old inoculation in farm pig herds.

Bacterial artificial chromosome(BAC) of PRV is a useful tool for the study of the virus [31–33]. After the construction of the first PRV BAC of Becker strain, a few of other PRV genomes have been maintained in BACs as infectious clones [14, 34, 35]. The infectious clone of the PRV AH02LA strain($BAC^{PRV\text{-}G}$) was previously constructed in our lab and was used in this study to generate the TK deletion BAC mutant by *En Passant* protocol. Additionally, this BAC can be used for the mechanistic analysis of the high virulence of this variant and the construction of other viral vectored vaccines.

Conclusion

A TK&gE dual deletion mutant($PRV^{\Delta TK\&gE\text{-}AH02}$ strain) was generated successfully based on the BAC of the virulent PRV AH02LA strain. The $PRV^{\Delta TK\&gE\text{-}AH02}$ strain was highly attenuated for 1-day-old piglets or mice. Live vaccine made of $PRV^{\Delta TK\&gE\text{-}AH02}$ strain is safe for 4~5 week-old PRV antibody negative piglets and can provide complete protection against lethal challenge with the emerging PRV virulent strain AH02LA at only 7 days post vaccination. Most importantly, $PRV^{\Delta TK\&gE\text{-}AH02}$ can stop virus shedding post lethal challenge and thus might be a promising vaccine candidate for the eradication of emerging virulent mutants of PRV in China.

Abbreviations

aa: Amino acid; BAC: Bacterial artificial chromosome; CEC: Chicken embryo cell; CPE: Cytopathogenic effects; CSFV: Classical swine fever virus; DIVA: Differentiating infected from vaccinated animals; DNA: Deoxyribonucleic acid; ELISA: Enzyme-linked immunosorbent assay; gB: Glycoprotein B; gC: Glycoprotein C; gD: Glycoprotein D; gE: Glycoprotein E; gG: Glycoprotein G; gI: Glycoprotein I; I.M.: Intramuscularly; I.N.: Intranasally; LD_{50}: 50% lethal dose; MOI: Multiplicity of infection; P.C.: Post challenge; P.I.: Post infection; P.V.: Post vaccination; PCR: Polymerase chain reaction; PCV2: Porcine circovirus 2; PPV: Porcine parvovirus; PRRSV: Porcine reproductive and respiratory syndrome virus; PRV: Pseudorabies virus; RFLP: Restriction fragment length polymorphism; $TCID_{50}$: 50% tissue culture infectious dose; TK: Thymidine kinase; UV: Ultraviolet

Acknowledgements

We thanks professor Nikolaus Osterrieder at the Free University of Berlin for kindly providing *E.coli* GS1783.

Funding

This study was supported by the Special Fund for Agro-Scientific Research in the Public Interest (201303046), Program for Independence and Innovation in Agricultural Sciences of Jiangsu Province (CX(12)3061 and CX(14)2084), and the Natural Science Foundation of Jiangsu Province (BK20131334).

Authors' contributions

JW HF and JH designed the generation TK&gE dual deletion mutant. JW, YQ, ZW and AG contributed to the design and performance of animal tests. JW, ZS and RG constructed the TK deleted PRV BAC and the TK&gE deleted virus. ZS, AG, YQ, MX, ZW, YL and YZ investigated the related properties of the vaccine and performed the animal experiments and related tests. All authors read and approved the final manuscript.

Consent for publication

Not applicable.

Competing interests

The authors declare that they have no conflicts of interest.

Author details

[1]National Research Center of Engineering and Technology for Veterinary Biologicals/Institute of Veterinary Immunology & Engineering, Jiangsu Academy of Agricultural Sciences, Nanjing 210014, Jiangsu, China. [2]Jiangsu Co-innovation Center for Prevention and Control of Important Animal Infectious Diseases and Zoonoses, Yangzhou, China. [3]College of Veterinary Medicine, Nanjing Agricultural University, Nanjing 210095, China. [4]Shandong Vocational Animal Science and Veterinary College, Weifang 261061, China. [5]Institute of Veterinary Medicine, Jiangsu Academy of Agricultural Sciences, Nanjing 210014, Jiangsu, China.

References

1. An T, Peng J, Tian Z, Zhao H, Li N, Liu Y, et al. Pseudorabies virus variant in bartha-k61-vaccinated pigs, China, 2012. Emerg Infect Dis. 2013;19(11):1749–55.
2. Wu R, Bai C, Sun J, Chang S, Zhang X. Emergence of virulent pseudorabies virus infection in northern China. J Vet Sci. 2013;14(3):363–5.
3. Yu X, Zhou Z, Hu D, Zhang Q, Han T, Li X, et al. Pathogenic pseudorabies virus, China, 2012. Emerg Infect Dis. 2014;20(1):102–4.
4. Hu D, Zhang Z, Lv L, Xiao Y, Qu Y, Ma H, et al. Outbreak of variant pseudorabies virus in Bartha-K61-vaccinated piglets in Central Shandong Province, China. J Vet Diagn Investig. 2015;27:600–5.
5. Zhou J, Li S, Wang X, Zou M, Gao S. Bartha-k61 vaccine protects growing pigs against challenge with an emerging variant pseudorabies virus. Vaccine. 2017;35:1161–6.
6. Freuling CM, Muller TF, Mettenleiter TC. Vaccines against pseudorabies virus(PrV). Vet Microbiol. 2017;206:3–9.
7. Müller T, Hahn E, Tottewitz F, Kramer M, Klupp B, Mettenleiter T, et al. Pseudorabies virus in wild swine: a global perspective. Arch Virol. 2011; 156(10):1691–705.
8. Lyman M, Demmin G, Banfield B. The attenuated pseudorabies virus strain Bartha fails to package the tegument proteins Us3 and VP22. J Virol. 2003; 77(2):1403–14.
9. Lomniczi B, Watanabe S, Ben-Porat T, Kaplan A. Genome location and identification of functions defective in the Bartha vaccine strain of pseudorabies virus. J Virol. 1987;61(3):796–801.
10. Sun Y, Luo Y, Wang CH, Yuan J, Li N, Song K, et al. Control of swine pseudorabies in China: opportunities and limitations. Vet Microbiol. 2016;183:119–24.
11. Wang C, Yuan J, Qin H, Luo Y, Cong X, Li Y, et al. A novel gE-deleted pseudorabies virus (PRV) provides rapid and complete protection from lethal challenge with the PRV variant emerging in Bartha-K61-vaccinated swine population in China. Vaccine. 2014;32(27):3379–85.
12. Wang T, Xiao Y, Yang Q, Wang Y, Sun Z, Zhang C, et al. Construction of a gE-deleted pseudorabies virus and its efficacy to the new-emerging variant PRV challenge in the form of killed vaccine. Biomed Res Int. 2015;2015:684945.
13. Ferrari M, Brack A, Romanelli M, Mettenleiter T, Corradi A, Dal Mas N, et al. A study of the ability of a TK-negative and gI/gE-negative pseudorabies virus (PRV) mutant inoculated by different routes to protect pigs against PRV infection. J Vet Med B Infect Dis Vet Public Health. 2000;47(10):753–62.

14. Gu Z, Dong J, Wang J, Hou C, Sun H, Yang W, et al. A novel inactivated gE/gI deleted pseudorabies virus (PRV) vaccine completely protects pigs from an emerged variant PRV challenge. Virus Res. 2015;195:57–63.
15. Hu RM, Zhou Q, Song WB, Sun EC, Zhang MM, He QG, et al. Novel pseudorabies virus variant with defects in TK, gE and gI protects growing pigs against lethal challenge. Vaccine. 2015;33:5733–40.
16. Zhang C, Guo L, Jia X, Wang T, Wang J, Sun Z, et al. Construction of a triple gene-deleted Chinese pseudorabies virus variant and its efficacy study as a vaccine candidate on suckling piglets. Vaccine. 2015;33:2432–7.
17. Cong X, Lei JL, Xia SL, Wang YM, Li Y, Li S, et al. Pathogenicity and immunogenicity of a gE/gI/TK gene-deleted pseudorabies virus variant in susceptible animals. Vet Microbiol. 2016;182:170–7.
18. Tong W, Li G, Liang C, Liu F, Tian Q, Cao Y, et al. A live, attenuated pseudorabies virus strain JS-2012 deleted for gE/gI protects against both classical and emerging strains. Antivir Res. 2016;130:110–7.
19. X C, JL L, SL X, YM W, Y L, S L, et al. Pathogenicity and immunogenicity of a gE/gI/TK gene-deleted pseudorabies virus variant in susceptible animals. Vet Microbiol. 2016;182:170–7.
20. Enquist LW, Husak PJ, Banfield BW, Smith GA. Infection and spread of alphaherpesviruses in the nervous system. Adv Virus Res. 1998;51:237–347.
21. Ferrari M, Gualandi GL, Corradi A, Monaci C, Romanelli MG, Tosi G, et al. Experimental infection of pigs with a thymidine kinase negative strain of pseudorabies virus. Comp Immunol Microbiol Infect Dis. 1998;21:291–303.
22. Wu CY, Liao CM, Chi JN, Chien MS, Huang C. Growth properties and vaccine efficacy of recombinant pseudorabies virus defective in glycoprotein E and thymidine kinase genes. J Biotechnol. 2016;229:58–64.
23. Wang J, Guo R, Qiao Y, Xu M, Wang Z, Liu Y, et al. An inactivated gE-deleted pseudorabies vaccine provides complete clinical protection and reduces virus shedding against challenge by a Chinese pseudorabies variant. BMC Vet Res. 2016;12:277.
24. Wang J, Osterrieder N. Generation of an infectious clone of duck enteritis virus and generation of a vectored DEV expressing hemagglutinin of H5N1 avian influenza virus. Virus Res. 2011;159(1):23–31.
25. Tischer B, Smith G, Osterrieder N. En passant mutagenesis: a two step markerless red recombination system. Methods Mol Biol. 2010;634:421–30.
26. Gu Z, Dong J, Wang J, Hou C, Sun H, Yang W, et al. A novel inactivated gE/gI deleted pseudorabies virus (PRV) vaccine completely protects pigs from an emerged variant PRV challenge. Virus Res. 2014;14:00371–2.
27. Osterrieder N. Construction and characterization of an equine herpesvirus 1 glycoprotein C negative mutant. Virus Res. 1999;59:165–77.
28. Ye C, Zhang Q, Tian Z, Zheng H, Zhao K, Liu F, et al. Genomic characterization of emergent pseudorabies virus in China reveals marked sequence divergence: evidence for the existence of two major genotypes. Virology. 2015;483:32–43.
29. Bouma A. Determination of the effectiveness of pseudorabies marker vaccines in experiments and field trials. Biologicals. 2005;33:241–5.
30. Casal J, Planasdemunt L, Varo JA, Martin M. The use of different vaccination schedules for sows to protect piglets against Aujeszky's disease. J Vet Med B Infect Dis Vet Public Health. 2004;51:8–11.
31. Shizuya H, Birren B, Kim U, Mancino V, Slepak T, Tachiiri Y, et al. Cloning and stable maintenance of 300-kilobase-pair fragments of human DNA in Escherichia coli using an F-factor-based vector. Proc Natl Acad Sci U S A. 1992;89:8794–7.
32. Warden C, Tang Q, Zhu H. Herpesvirus BACs: past, present, and future. J Biomed Biotechnol. 2011;2011:124595.
33. Tischer B, Kaufer B. Viral bacterial artificial chromosomes: generation, mutagenesis, and removal of mini-f sequences. J Biomed Biotechnol. 2012; 2012:472537. Epub 2012 Feb 23
34. Yin W, Yin L, Ye W, Sun X, Yao H, Zhang M, et al. Construction of an infectious clone of pseudorabies virus strain ZJ genome maintained as a bacterial artificial chromosome [Article in Chinese]. Bing Du Xue Bao. 2010; 26(4):330–5.
35. Smith GA, Enquist LW. Construction and transposon mutagenesis in Escherichia coli of a full-length infectious clone of pseudorabies virus, an alphaherpesvirus. J Virol. 1999;73:6405–14.

25

Evaluation and optimization of a conventional SPCE for FMD post-vaccination monitoring

Yeong-Lim Kang[1], Ji-Yun Jeong[1], Hwi-Yeon Choi[1], Yanhong Zhang[2], Yumei Liu[2], Ho-Jong Lee[1], Jong-Chul Choi[1], So-Hyun Lee[1], Beom-Joo Lee[1], Sang-Won Lee[1], Joong-Bok Lee[1], Ki-hyun Cho[3*] and Seung-Yong Park[1*]

Abstract

Background: Foot-and-mouth disease (FMD) can be controlled by either stamping out or vaccination, a choice which depends on both the economic importance of the livestock sector as well as the disease status. In FMD-free countries with vaccination, such as Korea, vaccination programs should guarantee prevention against transmission of FMD. Monitoring of vaccination programs is also essential for ensuring sufficient coverage that will limit the transmission of FMDV. There are several methods to screen FMD virus (FMDV) structural protein (SP) antibodies including SPCE (Solid-phase competitive ELISA), LPBE (Liquid-phase blocking ELISA), and VNT (Virus neutralization test). Among these, SPCE is widely used for serological monitoring since VNT—the gold standard method—has certain practical limitations, such as high costs in terms of time and labor. However, whether SPCE can ensure the vaccination status of individual animals and whole farms is unclear. In this study, SPCE, LPBE and VNT were compared with respect to correlation with each other and sensitivity at commercial pig farms.

Results: The positive results obtained by PrioCHECK SPCE differed from those obtained by LPBE and VNT. The sensitivity of SPCE relative to those of the other tests was fairly low. The raw data of SPCE were most highly correlated with those of VNT with XJ strain, while their positivity and negativity were most highly correlated with LPBE. The results of ROC analysis proposed new cut-off for PrioCHECK SPCE higher than the previous 50% inhibition.

Conclusions: The high false positive rate of PrioCHECK SPCE suggested that high seropositivity by SPCE may not guarantee a true vaccination coverage. Adjusting the cut-off percentage (%) inhibition value for SPCE is needed to address this problem, and it is highly recommended that routine FMDV serological monitoring programs using PrioCHECK SPCE should be combined with alternative methods such as LPBE or VNT.

Keywords: Foot-and-mouth disease, Serological monitoring, Vaccination coverage, Solid-phase competitive ELISA, Liquid-phase blocking ELISA, Virus neutralization test

* Correspondence: vet10@naver.com; paseyo@konkuk.ac.kr
[3]Veterinary Epidemiology Division, Animal and Plant Quarantine Agency, 177, Hyeoksin 8-ro, Gimcheon, Gyeongsangbuk-do 39660, Republic of Korea
[1]Laboratory of Veterinary Immunology, College of Veterinary Medicine, Konkuk University, 120 Neungdong-ro, Gwangjin-gu, Seoul 05029, Republic of Korea
Full list of author information is available at the end of the article

Background

Foot-and-mouth disease (FMD) is a viral disease caused by the FMD virus (FMDV), which belongs to the genus *Aphthovirus* in the Picornaviridae family [1]. The contagious nature of the virus and its various serotypes make it a major threat to animal husbandry worldwide [2]. Rapid and precise diagnosis is a prerequisite for preventing the spread of this disease. One diagnostic approach is to detect FMDV-specific antibodies; serological monitoring tests usually detect antibodies against either non-structural proteins (NSPs) [3–7] or structural protein (SPs). Solid-phase competition enzyme-linked immunosorbent assay (ELISA) (SPCE) [8–10], liquid-phase blocking ELISA (LPBE) [11, 12], and the virus neutralization test (VNT) [13] are typically used for SP antibody screening. They are performed in support of four main purposes: 1) to certify individual animals prior to import or export; 2) to confirm suspected cases of FMD; 3) to substantiate absence of infection; and 4) to demonstrate the efficacy of vaccination [14].

In FMD-free countries with vaccination, such as Korea, SPCE is adopted as a screening method for evaluating herd immune status after FMD vaccination because the gold standard method, VNT, is time and labor consuming. In Korea, there is a cut-off value of vaccination coverage by SPCE according to the relevant regulations, and farms with less than this value are subject to a fine. Despite these efforts, FMD has still been detected in premises with sufficient vaccination coverage above the cut-off value. Moreover, it is unclear whether SPCE is an appropriate method to certify individual animals and whether it demonstrates efficacy for the evaluation of vaccination status.

In the present study, we investigated whether PrioCHECK SPCE is appropriate for determining the FMD vaccination status of farms by comparing the vaccination coverage and correlation to those obtained by other SP antibody test methods and by assessing the relative sensitivity and specificity of the assay.

Results

SP antibody response after vaccination

To compare the performance of the three SP antibody tests, we evaluated vaccination coverage and antibody response based on logarithmic titers determined by each assay. Results of LPBE were confirmed by performing the assay using reagents from the World Reference Laboratory for Foot-and-Mouth Disease (data not shown).

The development of SP antibody was compared among the three methods used in the study (Fig. 1a–c). In the case of SPCE, the antibody level was highest 12 weeks after the vaccination in group I (Fig. 1a), whereas the level peaked after 8 weeks in group II (Fig. 1b). In group III, the antibody response was highest 8 weeks after the second vaccination (Fig. 1c).

Interestingly, the percentage of positive reactions before vaccination was above 50% when tested by SPCE, but it was below 20% when tested by LPBE and VNT in all groups (Fig. 1d–f). No NSP antibody was detected in any of the samples (data not shown). However, there were no significant differences between LPBE or VNT with XJ strain (VNT/XJ) and SPCE titers except for group II at 8 weeks of age. SPCE differed significantly from VNT/GX at 20 and 24 weeks of age in group I, at 8, 16, 20 and 24 weeks of age in group II, and at 24 weeks of age in group III. At market age, the mean vaccination coverage of SPCE were 88.56, 87.98 and 100% for each group.

Scatter plots and calculated regression lines for each assay

To further investigate the correlation between PrioCHECK SPCE and other assays and obtain regression lines, scatter plots were generated that showed logarithmic titers of SPCE on the x-axis and those of LPBE or VNT on the y-axis. The results for four positive and three negative reference serum samples obtained by SPCE were highly correlated with those obtained by LPBE ($R^2 = 0.973$, $P < 0.0001$) (Fig. 2a). However, not all the field samples that tested positive by SPCE were positive by LPBE ($R^2 = 0.517$) (Fig. 2b). Nevertheless, we observed a trend that all but seven samples, positive by LPBE, had a $\log_{10}$ titer > 0.85 by SPCE. On the contrary, LPBE titers of samples positive by SPCE ranged from 1.51 to 3.61.

In the scatter plots for SPCE and VNT, R^2 was higher when SPCE was matched with VNT/XJ ($R^2 = 0.579$) than when it was matched with VNT/GX ($R^2 = 0.438$) (Fig. 2c, d). Most serum samples positive by VNT had a $\log_{10}$ titer > 0.85 by SPCE, except six and two samples of the XJ and GX strain, respectively. On the other hand, VNT titers of sera positive by SPCE ranged from 0.3 to 3.46.

Correlation and relative sensitivity of SPCE compared to other tests

We calculated the Pearson correlation coefficient between PrioCHECK SPCE and other SP tests by comparing the data at the individual level. Overall, the highest correlation coefficient was between VNT/XJ and VNT/GX ($r = 0.803$, $P < 0.001$) (Table 1). SPCE showed the highest correlation with VNT/XJ ($r = 0.761$), followed by LPBE ($r = 0.719$) and VNT/GX ($r = 0.662$).

The relative sensitivity and specificity of SPCE were compared with LPBE, VNT/XJ and VNT/GX (Table 2). A total of 25, 19, and 9 samples confirmed positive by LPBE, VNT/XJ, and VNT/GX, respectively, were negative by SPCE. Conversely, 147, 164, and 342 samples positive by

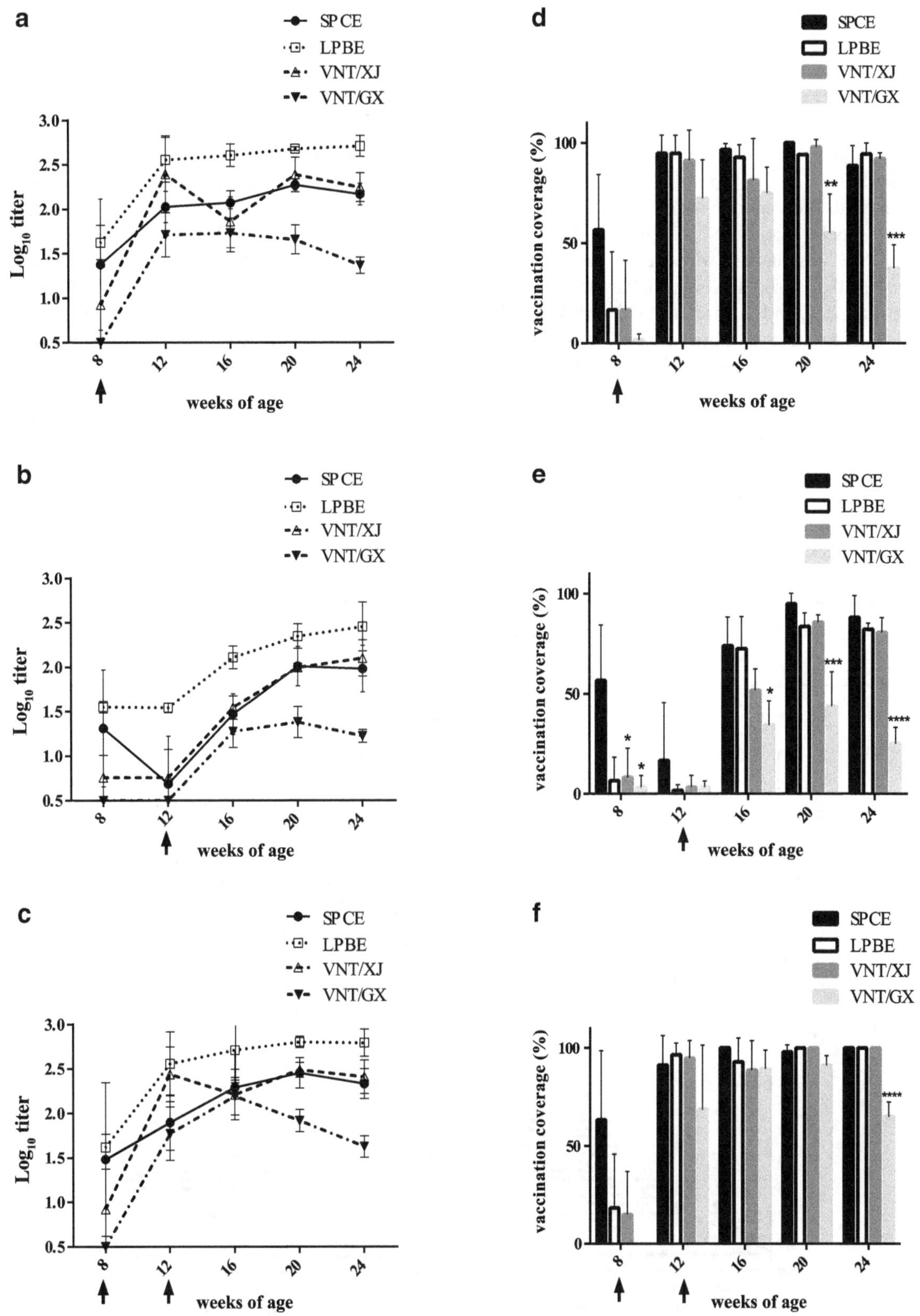

Fig. 1 (See legend on next page.)

(See figure on previous page.)
Fig. 1 a–f Progression of antibody response (**a**–**c**) and vaccination coverage (**d**–**f**) determined by SPCE, LPBE, and VNT. Data for group I (**a**, **d**), group II (**b**, **e**), and group III (**c**, **f**) are shown. The arrow indicates the timing of vaccination. Results of SPCE are expressed as PI, while those of LPBE and VNT are expressed as a logarithmic titer. Criteria for positivity by SPCE, LPBE, and VNT are 50%, 1/64 (1.81 $\log_{10}$), and 1/45 (1.65 $\log_{10}$), respectively. The results of average titer are presented as mean ± SD ($n = 60$). *$P < 0.05$, **$P < 0.01$, ***$P < 0.001$

SPCE were negative by LPBE, VNT/XJ, and VNT/GX, respectively.

SPCE showed the highest concordance with LPBE, followed by VNT/XJ and VNT/GX (Table 2). Cohen's kappa of SPCE was highest with LPBE. False negative rates were less than 10%. However, the false positive rate was more than 20%, and in case of SPCE with VNT/GX, it was 50.4%. It means that more than half of pigs identified as positive by SPCE screening did not have sufficient antibodies for protection.

Standardization of cut-off value for SPCE

To decrease false positive rate of PrioCHECK SPCE, we determined the optimal cut-off for PI of SPCE in 1/10 dilution and generated receiver operated characteristic (ROC) curves using the results obtained by other SP tests as standards (Fig. 3). Because the results of PrioCHECK SPCE were expressed as PI in general, PI results, not $\log_{10}$ titer, were used in this time. The area under the curve (AUC), sensitivity, and specificity were also calculated, and the optimal cut-off value was determined to obtain the maximum sensitivity and specificity.

The AUC was largest when the standard was VNT/XJ, followed by LPBE and VNT/GX ($P < 0.0001$) (Fig. 3). The optimal cut-off for SPCE was 63.55% when compared with LPBE, with a sensitivity of 0.801 and specificity of 0.800. For VNT/XJ, the cut-off value was 67.23% and the sensitivity and specificity were 0.834 and 0.829, respectively. For VNT/GX, the cut-off value was 76.83% and the sensitivity and specificity were 0.753 and 0.753, respectively.

Discussion

In this study, we compared PrioCHECK SPCE with LPBE and VNT in terms of their potential to demonstrate efficacy for the evaluation of vaccination status at the herd level and certification of animals at the individual level. All these methods detected SP antibodies

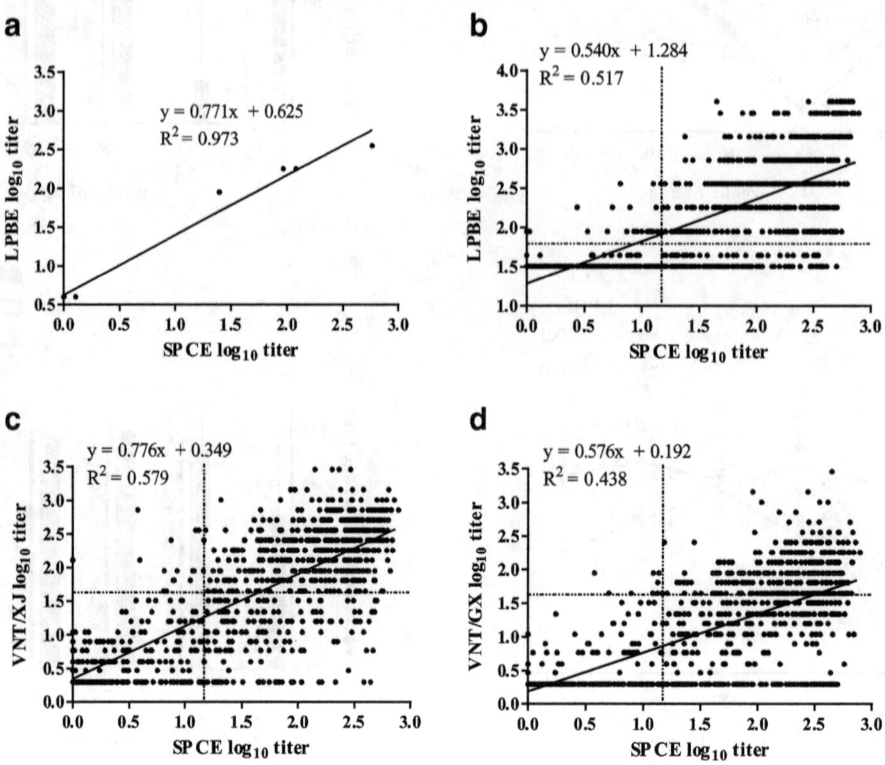

Fig. 2 a–d Scatter plots and calculated regression lines between SPCE and LPBE (**a**, **b**) and between SPCE and VNT (**c**, **d**). Scatter plots show PI ratio of SPCE on the x-axis and logarithmic titer of LPBE or VNT on the y-axis. Dotted line represents the cut-off value for each test (1.17, SPCE; 1.81, LPBE; and 1.65, VNT)

Table 1 The Pearson correlation among SP antibody test methods

	SPCE	LPBE	VNT/XJ	VNT/GX
SPCE	1	0.719	0.761	0.662
LPBE		1	0.783	0.777
VNT/XJ			1	0.803
VNT/GX				1

*All correlation values are significant at a confidence level of 0.001 (2-tailed)

generated 5–8 days after FMDV infection or vaccination in pigs [15]. However, there was disparity among the results, possibly due to the antigen used in each assay, that is, the vaccine strains O/Mya-98/XJ/2010 and O/Cathay/GX/09–7 for VNT and O/SEA/Mya-98 for LPBE.

We expected a high correlation between LPBE and VNT since the former was considered a replacement assay for the latter [16]. A high correlation coefficient proved this to some degree.

The antibody responses measured by SPCE are consistent with those reported in previous studies [17, 18]. More specifically, the vaccination coverage of group I was higher than that of group II at market age. Additionally, both groups had the highest vaccination coverage at 20 weeks of age. These results, along with previous findings by our group and others [17, 19], suggest that vaccination at 8 weeks of age achieves the highest vaccination coverage as detected by SPCE.

The antibody titer and vaccination coverage determined by SPCE were relatively similar to those determined by LPBE and VNT at 4–12 weeks after vaccination and differed from the values measured before and 16 weeks after vaccination. The significant difference in the results obtained during the late period of vaccination poses a potential threat since SPCE was performed immediately before the animals were taken to the market and vaccination is usually performed only once from 8 to 12 weeks of age in many countries. Moreover, vaccination coverage by SPCE was above 50% even before the vaccination. It suggests that SPCE is less specific than other SP test methods since there was no infection during the study, supported by the absence of NSP antibody.

One of the characteristics of PrioCHECK SPCE was the high false positive rate and relatively low correlation coefficient compared to the other test methods. As a general rule of thumb, specific tests are needed to rule in diagnoses, and highly sensitive tests are needed to rule them out. [20] Thus, the results of SPCE do not fully reflect the protective capacity of sera, unlike LPBE and VNT, which measure the neutralizing capacity. In addition, a high false positive rate can be a serious problem in FMD-endemic countries, given the highly contagious nature of FMDV.

Our study showed that almost 60% of the serum samples were positive for PrioCHECK SPCE before vaccination. Therefore, 50% inhibition is inadequate as a cut-off value; the results of the ROC analysis suggested 63.55% inhibition as a minimum value. We also found that 1:10 is the optimal dilution for PrioCHECK SPCE because there was no overlap between positive and negative sera (data not included). It was demonstrated previously that 30% inhibition at 1:5 dilution was the optimal cut-off for differentiating positive from negative serum [9], and that 60% inhibition was a proper cut-off for SPCE [10]. Further studies are needed to establish a definitive standard.

Conclusions

This study evaluated and optimized PrioCHECK type O SPCE for post-vaccination monitoring. The positive results obtained by SPCE were higher than those obtained by LPBE and VNT, especially at 8 weeks of age. SPCE showed a relatively high false positive rate compared with LPBE and VNT, suggesting that positivity by PrioCHECK SPCE is not sufficient to certify animals and to confirm the implementation of vaccination. Adjusting the cut-off PI value for SPCE may be a possible solution to this problem. The raw data of PrioCHECK SPCE had the highest correlation with VNT/XJ, while the positivity and negativity were highly correlated with LPBE. Nevertheless, correlations between SPCE and other tests were lower than those among other tests. It is highly recommended that routine FMDV post-vaccination monitoring and corresponding regulatory programs using PrioCHECK SPCE

Table 2 Comparison of sensitivity and specificity of SPCE with LPBE, VNT/XJ and VNT/GX

Method		LPBE		VNT/XJ		VNT/GX	
	Result	Positive	Negative	Positive	Negative	Positive	Negative
SPCE	Positive	531	147	514	164	336	342
	Negative	25	251	19	257	9	267
Cohen's kappa		0.612		0.596		0.340	
Overall concordance (%)		82.0		80.8		63.2	
False positive (%)		21.7		24.2		50.4	
False negative (%)		9.1		6.9		3.3	

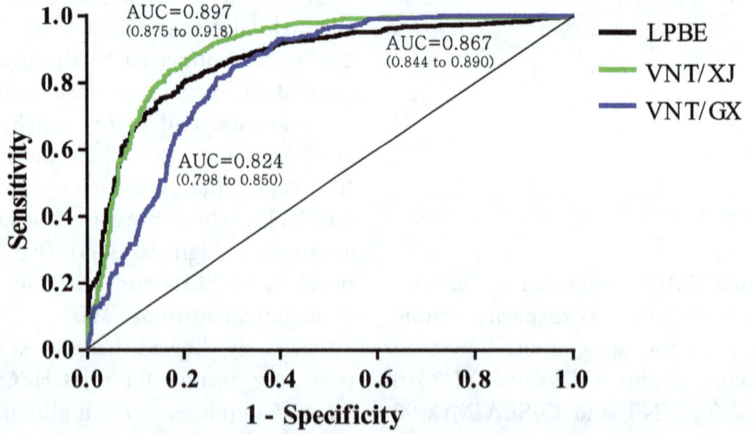

Fig. 3 ROC curve analysis of results of individual SP antibody tests. The AUC is shown for each graph, with the 95% confidence interval in parentheses

should be combined with alternative methods such as LPBE or VNT.

Methods

Animals

The pigs used in this study were kept on three farrow-to-finish commercial farms in Pocheon, Gyeonggi province. Routine vaccination programs for porcine circovirus type 2 virus, classical swine fever virus, FMDV, and *Mycoplasma hyopneumoniae* were carried out. Infectious diseases such as porcine epidemic diarrhea and FMD were not detected. On each farm, 60 piglets were raised and selected at the age of 7 weeks; these pigs were divided into three groups based on the results of PrioCHECK SPCE antibody level against FMD type O. Each group consisted of 20 pigs for each farm and the average antibody levels were similar among the groups. After this study, all pigs of market age were sent to the abattoir and slaughtered humanely. They were stunned with electricity and bled without consciousness according to the Article 10 of Animal Protection Law of Republic of Korea.

Vaccination and sample collection

Animals were vaccinated with inactivated FMD type O bivalent vaccine consisting of O/Mya-98/XJ/2010 and O/Cathay/GX/09–7 strains in oil adjuvant (Jinyu Baoling Bio-pharmaceutical Co., Hohhot, China). These strains were selected based on their genetic homology to field strains isolated in Korea and neighboring countries. The vaccine was formulated to contain at least six times the 50% protective dose.

A single dose (2 ml) of the vaccine was injected intramuscularly into group I (8 weeks old) and group II (12 weeks old). Group III was vaccinated twice at 8 and 12 weeks old. These schedules were designed to analyze antibody response after vaccination in the presence of maternally derived antibodies. Blood samples were collected at 8, 12, 16, 20, and 24 weeks of age in all three groups to evaluate SP antibody titers. The sample size fluctuated during the experimental period because some of the pigs died. Serum samples were stored at – 20 °C or – 70 °C until the analysis.

SPCE

FMDV type O SP antibody levels were determined using the PrioCHECK FMDV Type O Antibody ELISA kit (Prionics AG, Schlieren-Zurich, Switzerland) according to the manufacturer's instructions. PrioCHECK SPCE was chosen because it is most frequently adopted as a primary screening method in Korea. Briefly, a microtiter plate coated with FMD type O antigen was incubated with a 1/10 dilution of serum for 1 h at room temperature. After washing, a predetermined dilution of conjugate was added, and the plate was incubated for 1 h at room temperature. The plate was washed and the chromogenic substrate 3,3′,5,5′-tetramethylbenzidine (TMB) was added. The results were expressed as percentage inhibition (PI) relative to the maximum optical density at 450 nm. FMDV type O SP antibodies were considered to be absent and present in the serum if the PI was < 50 and ≥ 50%, respectively. Additionally, serum samples were 1:2 serially diluted and the 50% endpoint titers were calculated.

LPBE

LPBE was performed using a commercial kit (Lanzhou Veterinary Research Institute, Lanzhou, China) according to the manufacturer's manual. The assay is based on specific blocking of a defined amount of FMDV antigen by antibodies in the test serum in liquid phase. Briefly, a mixture of viral antigen (O/SEA/Mya-98) and diluted test serum was incubated overnight at 4 °C in liquid phase. The mixture was transferred to a trapping antibody-coated immune plate and incubated for 1 h at 37 °C. After washing, the plate was incubated with FMDV type O guinea pig antibody for 30 min at 37 °C. The plate was washed, rabbit anti-guinea pig IgG conjugated with horseradish peroxidase was added, and incubated for 30 min at 37 °C. After washing, the chromogenic substrate, TMB, was added. The results were expressed as the 50% endpoint titer, that is, the dilution at which the reaction of the test serum yields an optical density equivalent to half of the reaction (antigen) control wells. If the titer was equal to or above 1/64 (1.81 $\log_{10}$), samples were considered to be positive.

VNT

Serum samples were tested for virus-neutralizing antibodies against FMDV vaccine strains (O/Mya-98/XJ/2010 and O/GX/09–7) according to the standard protocol of the Animal and Plant Quarantine Agency (Gimcheon, Korea). Two-fold dilutions of the sample were distributed across the plate, starting from a 1/2 dilution. Previously titrated virus was added within $\log_{10}$ 1.5–2.5 $TCID_{50}$ per well. After 1 h incubation at 37 °C, LFBK cell suspension was added at 2.5×10^4 cells per well. Plates were incubated at 37 °C for 3 days. Titers were expressed as the final dilution that inhibited virus growth in 100% of the wells. A titer of ≥1/45 (1.65 $\log_{10}$) and < 1/16 of the final serum dilution in the serum/virus mixture was considered positive and negative, respectively.

Statistical analysis

Data are presented as mean ± standard deviation. The Pearson correlation coefficient was calculated using Prism v.6.0 software (Graph Pad Inc., La Jolla, CA, USA). Scatter plots were generated using the same program. Group means were compared by the one-way analysis of variance with multiple comparisons. Cohen's kappa of the assay was calculated by comparing the number of true positives and true negatives. Receiver Operating Characteristic (ROC) curves that illustrate the diagnostic ability of assay were drawn. The optimal cut-off value and the sensitivity and specificity were determined using the ROC curves.

Abbreviations

AUC: Area under curve; ELISA: Enzyme-linked immunosorbent assay; FMD: Foot-and-mouth disease; FMDV: FMD virus; LPBE: Liquid-phase blocking ELISA; NSP: Non-structural protein; PI: Percentage inhibition; ROC: Receiver operated characteristic; SP: Structural protein; SPCE: Solid phase competition ELISA; TCID: Tissue culture infective dose; VNT: Virus neutralization test

Acknowledgements

The authors would like to thank Chang-Seon Song and In-Soo Choi for assistance with revision of the manuscript, and Sang-Oh Lee for technical assistance.

Funding

This work was supported by Korea Institute of Planning and Evaluation for Technology in Food, Agriculture, Forestry (IPET) through Technology Commercialization Support Program, funded by Ministry of Agriculture, Food and Rural Affairs (MAFRA) (112157-3). We would also like to acknowledge the financial support from the R&D Convergence Program of National Research Council of Science & Technology (NST) of Republic of Korea (Grant No. CAP-16-02-KIST).

Authors' contributions

YLK performed the trial, the laboratory analyses, the statistical analyses and wrote the manuscript. JYJ, HYC, HJL, JCC, SHL and BJL performed the trial and the laboratory analyses. YZ and YL were responsible for performing VNT and LPBE. SWL, JBL, KHC and SYP designed the study protocol, reviewed the manuscript and assisted with the interpretation of the data. All authors contributed to the final discussion and revisions of the manuscript. All authors read and approved the final manuscript.

Consent for publication

Not applicable.

Competing interests

The authors declare that they have no competing interests.

Author details

[1]Laboratory of Veterinary Immunology, College of Veterinary Medicine, Konkuk University, 120 Neungdong-ro, Gwangjin-gu, Seoul 05029, Republic of Korea. [2]Jinyu Baoling Bio-pharmaceutical Co., Ltd., Hohhot 010030, Inner Mongolia, China. [3]Veterinary Epidemiology Division, Animal and Plant Quarantine Agency, 177, Hyeoksin 8-ro, Gimcheon, Gyeongsangbuk-do 39660, Republic of Korea.

References

1. Belsham GJ. Distinctive features of foot-and-mouth disease virus, a member of the picornavirus family; aspects of virus protein synthesis, protein processing and structure. Prog Biophys Mol Biol. 1993;60(3):241–60.
2. Krystynak RH, Charlebois PA. The potential economic impact of an outbreak of foot-and-mouth disease in Canada. Can Vet J. 1987;28(8):523–7.
3. Berger HG, Straub OC, Ahl R, Tesar M, Marquardt O. Identification of foot-and-mouth disease virus replication in vaccinated cattle by antibodies to non-structural virus proteins. Vaccine. 1990;8(3):213–6.
4. Bergmann IE, de Mello PA, Neitzert E, Beck E, Gomes I. Diagnosis of persistent aphthovirus infection and its differentiation from vaccination response in cattle by use of enzyme-linked immunoelectrotransfer blot analysis with bioengineered nonstructural viral antigens. Am J Vet Res. 1993; 54(6):825–31.
5. Neitzert E, Beck E, de Mello PA, Gomes I, Bergmann IE. Expression of the aphthovirus RNA polymerase gene in Escherichia coli and its use together with other bioengineered nonstructural antigens in detection of late persistent infections. Virology. 1991;184(2):799–804.
6. Sorensen KJ, Madsen KG, Madsen ES, Salt JS, Nqindi J, Mackay DK. Differentiation of infection from vaccination in foot-and-mouth disease by the detection of antibodies to the non-structural proteins 3D, 3AB and 3ABC in ELISA using antigens expressed in baculovirus. Arch Virol. 1998; 143(8):1461–76.
7. Lubroth J, Brown F. Identification of native foot-and-mouth disease virus non-structural protein 2C as a serological indicator to differentiate infected from vaccinated livestock. Res Vet Sci. 1995;59(1):70–8.
8. Chenard G, Miedema K, Moonen P, Schrijver RS, Dekker A. A solid-phase blocking ELISA for detection of type O foot-and-mouth disease virus antibodies suitable for mass serology. J Virol Methods. 2003;107(1):89–98.
9. Mackay DK, Bulut AN, Rendle T, Davidson F, Ferris NP. A solid-phase competition ELISA for measuring antibody to foot-and-mouth disease virus. J Virol Methods. 2001;97(1–2):33–48.
10. Paiba GA, Anderson J, Paton DJ, Soldan AW, Alexandersen S, Corteyn M, Wilsden G, Hamblin P, MacKay DK, Donaldson AI. Validation of a foot-and-mouth disease antibody screening solid-phase competition ELISA (SPCE). J Virol Methods. 2004;115(2):145–58.

11. Hamblin C, Barnett IT, Hedger RS. A new enzyme-linked immunosorbent assay (ELISA) for the detection of antibodies against foot-and-mouth disease virus. I. Development and method of ELISA. J Immunol Methods. 1986;93(1):115–21.
12. Hamblin C, Kitching RP, Donaldson AI, Crowther JR, Barnett IT. Enzyme-linked immunosorbent assay (ELISA) for the detection of antibodies against foot-and-mouth disease virus. III. Evaluation of antibodies after infection and vaccination. Epidemiol Infect. 1987;99(3):733–44.
13. Golding SM, Hedger RS, Talbot P. Radial immuno-diffusion and serum-neutralisation techniques for the assay of antibodies to swine vesicular disease. Res Vet Sci. 1976;20(2):142–7.
14. Health WOfA. OIE terrestrial manual 2012. In: Foot and mouth disease (infection with foot and mouth disease virus); 2012.
15. Alexandersen S, Zhang Z, Donaldson AI, Garland AJ. The pathogenesis and diagnosis of foot-and-mouth disease. J Comp Pathol. 2003;129(1):1–36.
16. Ferris NP, Kitching RP, Oxtoby JM, Philpot RM, Rendle R. Use of inactivated foot-and-mouth disease virus antigen in liquid-phase blocking ELISA. J Virol Methods. 1990;29(1):33–41.
17. Kim AY, Tark D, Kim H, Kim JS, Lee JM, Kwon M, Bae S, Kim B, Ko YJ. Determination of optimal age for single vaccination of growing pigs with foot-and-mouth disease bivalent vaccine in South Korea. J Vet Med Sci. 2017;79(11):1822–5.
18. Lee HS, Lee NH, Seo MG, Ko YJ, Kim B, Lee JB, Kim JS, Park S, Shin YK. Serological responses after vaccination of growing pigs with foot-and-mouth disease trivalent (type O, a and Asia1) vaccine. Vet Microbiol. 2013; 164(3–4):239–45.
19. Dekker A, Chenard G, Stockhofe N, Eble PL. Proper timing of foot-and-mouth disease vaccination of piglets with maternally derived antibodies will maximize expected protection levels. Front Vet Sci. 2016;3:52.
20. Stevenson M. An Introduction to Veterinary Epidemiology. Palmerston North: Massey University; 2008.

26

Supplementation of dietary germanium biotite enhances induction of the immune responses by foot-and-mouth disease vaccine in cattle

Myunghwan Jung[1], Min-Kyoung Shin[1], Seung-Bin Cha[1], Seung Won Shin[1], Anna Yoo[1], Won-Jung Lee[1], Hong-Tae Park[1], Jong-Hyeon Park[2], Byounghan Kim[2], Yeon-Kwon Jung[3] and Han Sang Yoo[1,4*]

Abstract

Background: After the recent outbreak of foot-and-mouth disease (FMD) in Korea, a vaccination policy has been applied to control the disease. In addition, several non-specific immune stimulators have been used without any scientific evidence that they would enhance the immune response after FMD vaccination and/or protect against FMD. Based on the current situation, the aim of this study was to evaluate the effect of the non-specific immune stimulator germanium biotite on FMD vaccination and immune responses in cattle. To achieve our goal, immune responses to FMD vaccination, such as levels of IgG and IgA, antibody duration, and virus-neutralizing titers were investigated after germanium biotite feeding. The PBMC typing and proliferative response after stimulation with mitogens, the cytokines expression level of PBMC, and the lysozyme activity in the serum were measured to evaluate the immune enhancing effects of germanium biotite following its administration.

Results: Following the first vaccination, high level of IgG (at 4 weeks) and IgA (at 2 and 31 weeks) titers in serum and saliva were observed in the germanium biotite-feeding group ($p < 0.05$). The germanium biotite group also showed high and longstanding inhibition percentage value in ELISA assay at 31 weeks ($p < 0.05$). Generally, higher virus-neutralizing antibody titers were observed in the feeding group at 20 and 31 weeks after vaccination. Following the feeding germanium biotite, the germanium biotite group showed increased subpopulation of $CD4^+$ lymphocytes and MHC I^+II^+ cells in PBMCs at 23 week, responding to stimulation of ConA. The levels of IFN-γ (at 3 and 8 weeks), IL-1α (at 3, 11, and 23 weeks), IL-1β (at 3, 8, and 11 weeks), and IL-4 (at 8 and 11 weeks) gene expression were also significantly increased in the feeding group ($p < 0.01$ and $p < 0.05$). Feeding with germanium biotite increased the lymphocytes' proliferative response to the stimulation of ConA and LPS at 23 weeks and lysozyme activity at 9 weeks after feeding.

Conclusions: These results suggest that germanium biotite feeding could increase the protection against FMD virus infection via the induction of higher humoral and cellular immune responses in cattle.

Keywords: FMD, Germanium biotite, Immune responses, Cattle

* Correspondence: yoohs@snu.ac.kr
[1]Department of Infectious Diseases, College of Veterinary Medicine, Seoul National University, Seoul 151-742, South Korea
[4]Institute of Green Bio Science and Technology, Seoul National University, Pyeongchang 232-916, South Korea
Full list of author information is available at the end of the article

Background

Foot-and-mouth disease (FMD) is a highly contagious and economically important disease that affects cloven-hoofed animals, and it is characterized by appetite loss, an increase in body temperature, and vesicles in the mouth, tongue, hooves, and nipples [1,2]. The disease is caused by the FMD virus (FMDV), which is a small, icosahedral, non-enveloped RNA virus classified within the *Aphthovirus* genus as a member of *Picornaviridae*. The clinical severity of the disease varies with the strain of FMDV, infection dose, species, and individual susceptibility of the host [3]. The disease can be transmitted via direct or indirect contact between FMDV-infected animals and susceptible animals [2].

Due to its high mutation rate, this virus exists as seven distinct serotypes (O, A, C, Asia 1, South African territories [SAT]1, SAT2, and SAT3) as well as numerous and constantly evolving subtypes, which shows a spectrum of antigenic diversity [2,3]. Therefore, one major problem in controlling FMD is antigenic variation, as infection or vaccination with one FMDV serotype does not protect against other serotypes, and it may even fail to protect fully against other subtypes within the same serotype [4-6]. This problem has been raised by the experimental and field data of previous researchers on vaccination, including both single and multivalent vaccines [3,7,8].

Despite the powerful effects of vaccines, which have mitigated enormous FMD outbreaks, the current vaccines have many problems to overcome such as the long time required to induce antibodies and short duration of immunity when applying them to emergency and routine vaccination programs [6-9]. Therefore, strategies to improve the immune response to vaccination have included using higher vaccine doses or increasing the number of doses, using different routes of administration, accelerating the dosing schedule, and using adjuvants such as antigen delivery systems and various immunostimulators [10].

The immune response against FMDV is related to circulating humoral antibody titers; this is considered the most important factor in conferring protection against FMD [4]. The importance of cell-mediated immunity also has been recognized in the induction of humoral immunity and the clearance of FMDV. T-cell responses mediated by $CD4^+$ cells are required for protective immunity against FMDV as they participate in the production of antiviral antibodies [11]. Subsets of the $CD4^+$ major histocompatibility complex (MHC) class II-restricted T-cells respond to activation by antigen-presenting cells and antigens by producing a T helper type 1 (Th1, IFN-γ) and T helper type 2 (Th2; IL-4, IL-5, and IL-13) responses [12]. Several studies have also demonstrated the presence of FMD-specific MHC II-restricted responses in cattle and pigs [11-13]. The antiviral responses of $CD8^+$ T-cells were also detected following FMDV infection in previous studies [14,15]. These antiviral responses were through direct cytotoxicity or release of cytokines such as IFN-γ following vaccination, and that the antiviral responses were almost 100 times higher following re-stimulation [15]. MHC class I-restricted $CD8^+$ T-cells also showed specific immune response to FMDV as memory cells; however, the correlation between FMDV-specific $CD8^+$ T-cell recognition and protection remains to be defined [14,15]. In addition, the innate immune systems, as well as adaptive immune, play an important role in immune responses to FMDV infection [16,17]. The innate immune system, characterized by non-specific responses, is associated with early protection against FMD and is involved in the formation of adaptive immune response to FMDV infection [16,17].

Germanium biotite, as a well-known feed supplement, is a common phyllosilicate mineral that contains potassium, magnesium, iron, aluminum, and silicate. It has been reported that the effects of non-specific immune stimulating of biotite are associated with the immune cells being stimulated by silicates [18-20]. Fibrogenic silicates (SiO_2) activated proinflammatory macrophages, and aluminosilicates (Al_2SiO_5) improved immune-cell differentiation [21]. Aluminosilicates act as a nonspecific immunostimulator that is similar to a superantigen [22]. Superantigens are a class of extremely potent T-cell mitogens, and have a high affinity to regions of MHC II molecules [23]. Indeed, proinflammatory macrophages, which belong to MHC class II antigen–presenting cells, are activated by fibrogenic silicate particulates [21]. Thus, previous studies have suggested that germanium biotite has a potential as a new supplement for immunostimulators, prophylactic agents, and remedial agents [20].

Since the devastating FMD outbreak in Korea at the end of 2010, cattle, pigs, and some small ruminants have been vaccinated with a trivalent FMD vaccine (O1 Manisa, A Malaysia 97, and Asia1 Shamir) at least 6 protective dose 50% (PD_{50}). [24]. To improve the vaccine efficacy, several non-specific immune stimulators have been used in Korea without any scientific understanding of their effects. Therefore, as a first step to understanding the immunological mechanism and improve the vaccine's efficacy, we examined the effects of a non-specific immune stimulator, germanium biotite, in relation to the FMD vaccine in cattle.

Results

Antibody responses to FDMV

In the analysis of the duration of antibody levels and the secretion of IgA after FMD vaccination, the inhibition percentage (PI) values started to increase with the first vaccination, and the values were significantly increased by a booster vaccination at 4 weeks, with the highest PI values at 10 weeks, and this continued steadily up to 28 weeks, regardless of whether the germanium biotite was administered. However, the values decreased at 31 weeks in the control group when the re-booster vaccination was required, while the values continued at 31 weeks in the germanium biotite group (Figure 1A).

FMDV-specific IgA in the saliva of the germanium biotite group was generally higher than in the control group, although there were no significant differences between the groups at some points during this experiment (Figure 1B). However, IgA could not be detected in the feces of the two groups with the kit used (data not shown).

In the analysis of the early response of IgG, both groups showed a steady increase in the IgG antibody level up to 3 weeks after vaccination; after this point, the level decreased (Figure 1C). The IgG level in the germanium biotite group was higher than in the control group, although the difference was not significant. However, there was a significantly higher IgG antibody level at 4 weeks after vaccination when the booster vaccination was required ($p < 0.05$, Figure 1C).

Virus neutralization antibody against the heterologous FMDV strain

As shown in Table 1, the sera of the control group had a titer of less than 16 at both points. On the other hand, while the germanium biotite group had a VN titer of 16 or less at 20 weeks after vaccination, the VN titer in the group was found to have increased at 31 weeks after vaccination.

Analysis of peripheral blood mononuclear cell subpopulation

Changes in the subpopulations of five different lymphocytes were analyzed based on the administration of the germanium biotite. At 23 weeks, $CD4^+$ lymphocytes and $MHCI^+II^+$ cells in the germanium biotite group were significantly higher than in the control group ($p < 0.01$), while $CD79a^+$, $CD3^+$, and $CD8^+$ lymphocytes exhibited no differences between the two groups (Table 2).

Analysis of cytokine gene expression

The gene expression of IFN-γ, IL-1α, IL-1β, and IL-4 was significantly higher in the germanium biotite group during this experiment (Figure 2). The significant high levels of IFN-γ were determined in the germanium biotite group at 3 and 8 weeks, compared to the control ($p < 0.01$). In case of IL-1α and IL-1β, significant differences were observed at 3, 11, and 23 weeks and at 3, 8, and 11 weeks, respectively ($p < 0.05$ and $p < 0.01$). The germanium biotite group also showed significant high levels of IL-4 at 8 and 11 weeks, compared to the control ($p < 0.01$). However, there were no noticeable differences in the expression levels of IL-6 and IL-10 between the two groups although a significant difference in IL-6 expression was observed at 3 week. The germanium biotite feeding induced a significant increase in IFN-γ gene expression at a relatively early stage and in IL-4 at a late stage, while increases in IL-1α and IL-1β gene expression were observed throughout the experimental period.

Lymphocyte proliferation

Higher lymphocyte proliferation in the germanium biotite group was observed by LPS and ConA stimulation at 23 weeks compared to the control (Figure 3A, $p < 0.05$).

Lysozyme activity

Of the three points at which the lysozyme activity was measured in the serum, significantly higher lysozyme activity was observed in the germanium biotite group at 9 weeks after starting the feeding (Figure 3B, $p < 0.05$). The increase was observed at a relatively early stage after germanium biotite feeding.

Discussion

The current FMD vaccines that are used in cattle need to be administered every 6 months, in accordance with the duration of the antibody, to protect against the disease [5,6,25,26]. The diversity of FMD serotypes has also raised issues related to the efficacy of the current FMD vaccines. Furthermore, there is considerable argument about whether the trivalent vaccines show protective abilities against the Andong strain through the cross-reactivity of antibodies induced by trivalent vaccination [24]. Based on the current knowledge of FMD vaccines, the need for additional materials and/or methods has been raised with a view to overcoming the problem. Therefore, non-specific immune stimulators have received attention as a possible solution to this issue. In the disastrous FMD outbreak in Korea in 2010 [24], many non-specific immune stimulators were used without any scientific evidence that they would enhance protection against FMDV infection. Although non-specific immune stimulators have been used, their efficiency is still controversial. Therefore, we evaluated the effect of a non-specific immune stimulator, germanium biotite, for FMD vaccination in cattle.

Previous studies reported that a re-booster vaccination was needed 6 months after the booster vaccination based on the decrease of antibody titer against FMDV [5,6,25,26]. Coinciding with these previous studies, this study observed a decreased PI value in the control group at 31 weeks. However, the germanium biotite group showed a continued high level of PI value for 31 weeks. In order to elevate the antibody level, a booster vaccination was needed 4 weeks after the first vaccination. At that time, the germanium biotite group showed a high level of IgG antibody compared to the control. This

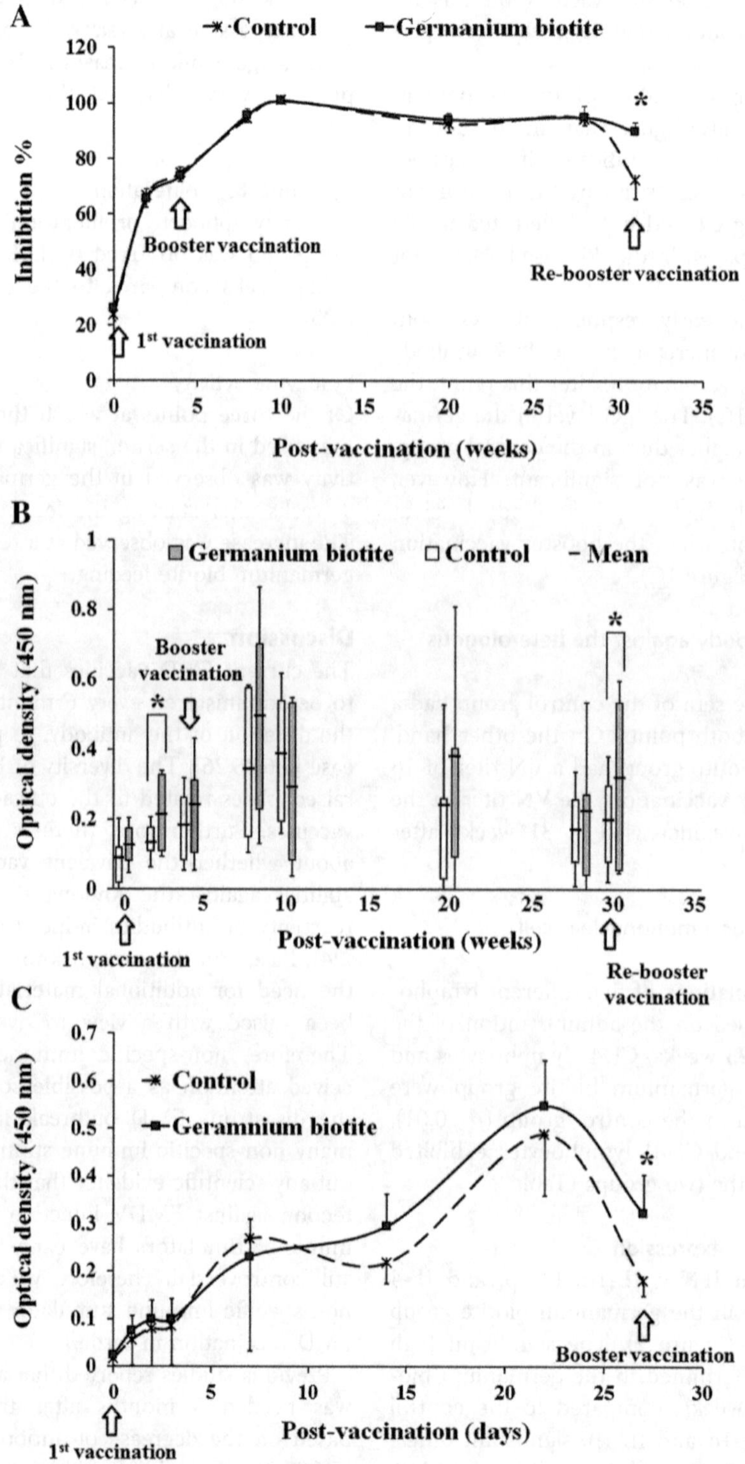

Figure 1 Humoral immune responses after vaccination with Decivac FMD DOE trivalent vaccine in cattle. A. Inhibition percentage (PI) of the antibody against FMDV serotype O in both the germanium biotite-feeding group and the non-feeding group after vaccination. The high PI value indicates a high level of antibody titer, and the sera that showed more than 50% of the PI value were considered to be seropositive in the ELISA assays. **B.** The FMDV serotype O-specific IgA response in the saliva of cattle of the germanium biotite and the control groups after vaccination with Decivac FMD DOE trivalent vaccine. **C.** Induction of FMDV serotype O-specific IgG in the cattle of the germanium biotite and control groups after vaccination with Decivac FMD DOE trivalent vaccine.

Table 1 Virus neutralization antibody titers in sera after vaccination

Group	Samples	20 weeks	31 weeks
Control	1	<16	<16
	2	<16	<16
	3	<16	<16
	4	<16	<16
	5	<16	<16
	6	<16	<16
	7	<16	<16
Germanium biotite	1	<16	16
	2	16	<16
	3	16	32
	4	16	26
	5	16	<16
	6	16	<16
	7	<16	26
	8	<16	32

The selected sera were taken from the same cattle in each collection date. All cattle were 6-month-old when the first vaccination was conducted. The sera selected from the germanium biotite group show a higher virus neutralization antibody titer than the control group.

experimental result closely matches with previous studies' findings on the improvement of antibody production by germanium biotite [18,19]. Furthermore, germanium biotite feeding showed a high level of IgA in the saliva, which could provide a beneficial effect when it comes to protecting against FMDV infection in cattle [27]. In addition, the IgG response suggested that the point at which to administer the booster injection in the FMD vaccine program for cattle is the same as indicated in previous studies [6,26]. However, the increase in antibody duration suggests that the current FMD vaccine program should be reconsidered in animals fed germanium biotite. In this study, sampling of sera after 31 weeks from only first and boosting vaccinated cattle was limited, due to national FMD control policy by which re-booster vaccination carried out every 6 months in cattle. The decline point of PI 6 month after booster vaccination could not be identified. Therefore, the investigation of PI value changes for a longer period should be conducted in the future study to determine the re-booster vaccination timing.

Along with these antibody responses, a VN test was performed using the Andong strain, which is an isolate from the recent outbreak in Korea in 2010. Following the vaccination, 20 weeks was the mid-point of the period showing a high PI value and 31 weeks was the time point that showed a difference in PI values between the two experiment groups. To ensure the reliability of VN test and reduce the variation, cattle in Farm B were selected and sera of half the number of scale of each group in Farm B were taken from the same cattle in each collection date. As shown in Table 1, all experimental groups showed a low VN titer. These low VN titers might be due to using the heterologous FMDV. The immunological relationship between the O1 Manisa vaccine and the Andong strains was relatively low or moderate (r-value of approximately 0.3) [28]. A previous study considered an r-value in the range of 0.3–1.0 as indicative of reasonable levels of cross-reactivity [29]. Therefore, the low VN titers observed in this study could be explained by the low level of the r-value between the two strains. However, in comparison with the control group, the increase of VN antibodies in the germanium biotite group suggests that protectivity against FMDV infection might be increased through the supplementation of germanium biotite [3,6,9].

Although the importance of antibodies in protection against FMDV infection is well known [3,6,9], a specific antibody does not guarantee sterile immunity or clinical protection against FMDV infection [9,25]. Moreover, protection against FMDV infection has been observed in the absence of a detectable specific humoral response [30]. Therefore, it is reasonable to consider a possible protective role for innate immune responses in FMD infection and for control of the disease [12,13,26,31]. In this study, high lysozyme activity—indicating macrophage activity—was observed in the germanium biotite group compared to the control group. This result corresponds with the findings of previous studies, which that the macrophage activation effects of silicate (SiO_2) and aluminosilicate (Al_2SiO_5), which are major components of germanium

Table 2 Subsets of peripheral blood mononuclear cells after mitogen stimulation

	Before administration		23 weeks after administration		Stimulators
	Control	Germanium biotite	Control	Germanium biotite	
$CD79a^+$	8.40% (±0.17)	7.90% (±0.14)	6.70% (±0.53)	4.70% (±1.01)	LPS
$CD3^+$	59.50% (±0.49)	57.80% (±0.53)	93.50% (±0.04)	93.10% (±0.28)	ConA
$CD4^+$	14.10% (±0.72)	13.00% (±0.22)	15.40% (±0.58)	23.80% (±0.52)**	ConA
$CD8^+$	12.50% (±0.74)	10.40% (±1.30)	14.30% (±1.40)	10.20% (±1.21)	ConA
MHC I^+, II^+	43.00% (±0.45)	37.50% (±0.12)	8.80% (±0.17)	10.20% (±0.15)**	ConA

The data were expressed as mean ± standard deviation (SD) (**$p < 0.01$ compared to the control group at each time point).

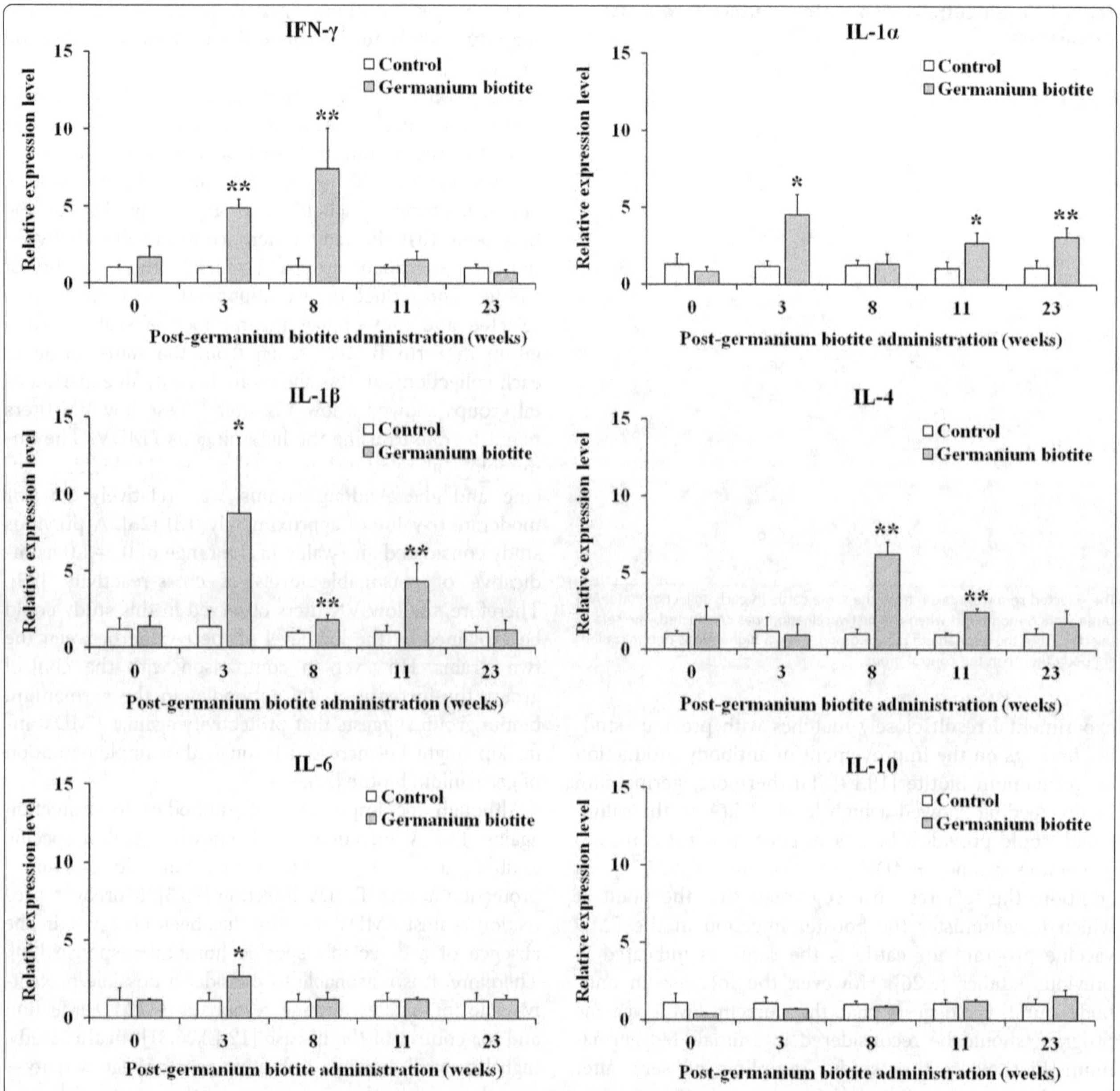

Figure 2 Analysis of gene expression of cytokines IFN-γ, IL-1α, IL-1β, IL-4, IL-6, and IL-10. Total RNA were purified from peripheral blood mononuclear cells separated from cattle vaccinated and fed with the germanium biotite supplement or without the supplement.

biotite [18,19,21]. Along with macrophage activation, a high proliferative response of T and B lymphocytes to the mitogen stimulation was observed in the germanium biotite group compared to the control group, thereby indicating that the marker level of lymphocyte activity in the germanium biotite group was higher than in the control group. Through the analysis of PBMC subset stimulation with ConA and LPS, it can be presumed that the proliferative responses of the T lymphocytes were predominately associated with $CD4^+$ and $MHCI^+$ II^+ cells, as the $CD4^+$ and $MHCI^+$ II^+ cells were significantly increased at 23 weeks after stimulation with ConA. The important role of $CD4^+$ T-cells in the induction of the antibody response in ruminants following infection or vaccination with a virus or a viral peptide has been demonstrated [11,12]. Furthermore, MHC II–restricted T-cells (CD4) play an important role in the immune responses to the FMDV antigen and the activation of macrophages [31]. These results show the increase of activation markers for innate immune responses associated with cell-mediated immunity in the germanium biotite group. In addition, previous studies reported that the cross-reactivities against a heterologous virus were mainly induced by T-cell responses to FMDV vaccination [13]. Therefore, it could be postulated

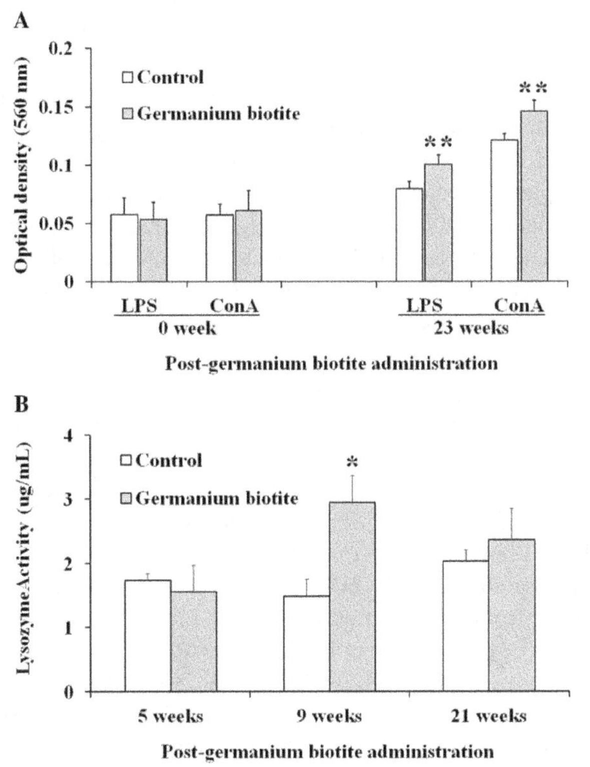

Figure 3 Proliferation of peripheral blood mononuclear cells (PBMCs) and lysozyme activity of sera. A. PBMCs were separated from the vaccinated cattle that were fed with the germanium biotite supplement or without the supplement at 0 and 23 weeks. The proliferation of the PBMCs was estimated after stimulation with LPS or ConA. **B**. The lysozyme activities of the sera from the vaccinated cattle that were fed with the germanium biotite supplement or without the supplement were measured based on the dissolution ability against *Micrococcus lysodeikticus*.

that the increase of VN titer against Andong strain in the germanium biotite group compared to the control might result from enhanced T-cell responses due to germanium biotite feeding.

The increase of the expression of the IFN-γ, IL-1α, IL-1β, and IL-4 genes in the germanium biotite group was in agreement with the results that demonstrated the activation of immune cells associated with cell-mediated immune responses. The increase of the IFN-γ expression level and the $CD4^+$ T-cell subpopulation in our results is closely correlated with a previous report that indicated that $CD4^+$ T-cells were the major proliferating phenotype and IFN-γ producing cells [12]. The induction of IFN-γ expression has been observed in antigen-specific T-cell activation [32], MHC II–restricted T-cells (CD4) [5], and activation of macrophages [31]. This immune cell activation induced by IFN-γ expression could also be observed in our results through the increases in the $CD4^+$ and $MHCI^+$ II^+ cell subpopulations, lysozyme activity, and lymphocyte proliferation level. In addition, the antiviral activity of IFN-γ against FMDV contributed to the control of FMDV replication and the spread of the virus within the host via activation of NK cells and macrophages [33]. IL-1α and IL-1β are mainly produced in activated macrophages and promote Th2 immune cells, which represent the major source of IL-4 [34]. IL-4 also promotes Th2 cell growth and enhances MHC II expression in B-cells [34]. These results suggest that germanium biotite induces Th1 and Th2 responses through the activation of macrophages and CD4+ class II MHC–restricted T-cells [1,34]. Considering these results, it can be presumed that supplementation of germanium biotite may activate cell-mediated immunity, thereby enhancing the induction of the immune responses by FMD vaccination and the protectivity against FMDV infection. However, the effects of germanium biotite on T-cell activation through FMDV specific T-cell responses could not be investigated. Therefore, an inquiry on the effects of germanium biotite on immune responses to FMDV vaccination through a comparative study of T-cell responses using FMDV antigen were needed to evaluate the specific effects in a further research.

In addition, a large difference in the appearance of the MHC II subpopulation was observed in the experiment cattle between two time points, before and after the administration of the germanium biotite. Previous studies showed that the MHC II subpopulation in the PBMCs of Holstein at 5–7 and 15–16 months could be estimated at about 32.2% and 10.7%, respectively [35,36]. Based on these reports, it can be presumed that the significant difference in this study could be caused by the age change in the experiment calves.

Conclusions

The results of this study suggest an enhancement of the immune responses to FMD vaccination through the supplementation of dietary germanium biotite such as IgG, IgA, and VN antibodies. It can be presumed that these enhancements are induced by the immunostimulating effects of the germanium biotite, including the activation of macrophages and CD4+ class II MHC–restricted cells, as well as the induction of cytokines, which can activate Th1 and Th2 immune cells. In conclusion, the findings of this study indicate that dietary germanium biotite could be used to improve the efficacy of the FMD vaccine.

Methods

Experimental animals and vaccination

This experiment was carried out with 89 cattle from 6–8 months in age (Korean Native Cattle) at three different farms, which were located in different provinces in Korea. Forty-five cattle were raised with feed supplemented with 0.5% germanium biotite (SoltoB, Seobong

BioBestech Co, Seoul, Korea; germanium biotite group) from 1 week before vaccination to the end of the experiment, while the rest were raised without supplementation (control group). Control and germanium biotite groups were arranged at each farm (Table 3). All the cattle were intramuscularly vaccinated with 2 ml of Decivac FMD DOE trivalent vaccine (InterVet, Germany). A booster vaccination was given 4 weeks after the first vaccination, according to the national vaccination policy of Korea. Samples of blood, saliva, and feces were collected before vaccination and up to 6 months after the second vaccination. Feces and saliva were collected by swabbing with a cotton swab. Bleeding was carried out from the jugular vein. Sera were collected and stored at −20°C until use after inactivation at 56°C for 30 min. The cotton swabs were immersed in 1 ml of PBS for 1 h at 4°C, and the supernatants were collected after centrifugation at 1,500 × g for 15 min at 4°C; the supernatants were stored at −20°C and used as samples for the ELISA analysis of FMDV-specific IgA.

The germanium biotite consisted of silicon dioxide (61.90%), aluminum dioxide (23.19%), iron oxide (3.97%), sodium oxide (3.36%), calcium oxide (<2%), magnesium oxide (<2%), titanium oxide (<2%), and 36 ppm germanium. All procedures in the animal experiment in this study were approved by the Institution Animal Care and Use Committee (IACUC) of Seoul National University (SNU-111210-1).

Measurement of antibody against FMDV

The antibody titers against FMDV were measured using the PrioCHECK FMDV type O ELISA kit (Prionics, Switzerland) following the manufacturer's protocols. The serotype O antibody titer using this ELISA kit is the criterion for assessing seropositivity in the national policy of Korea. The antibody titer against FMDV was indicated by the PI value. The high PI value presents a high level of antibody titer, and the sera that showed more than 50% of the PI value were considered to be seropositive in the ELISA assays. FMDV-specific IgG in the serum were measured using the PrioCHECK FMDV type O ELISA kit (Prionics) with 1:40 diluted serum and horseradish peroxidase (HRP)-conjugated sheep anti-bovine IgG (Bethyl, USA). In addition, FMDV-specific IgA in the saliva and feces was measured using the PrioCHECK FMDV type O ELISA kit (Prionics) with 1 x samples extracted by PBS from cotton swabs and HRP-conjugated rabbit anti-bovine IgA (Bethyl). All procedures for detecting FMDV-specific IgG and IgA followed the manufacturer's protocols with a 1:3,000 dilution of each immunoglobulin-specific conjugate.

Analysis of VN antibody titer

The VN titer was measured in eight randomly selected sera from the germanium biotite and seven sera from the control groups of Farm B at 20 and 31 weeks after vaccination (Tables 1 and 3). Fifty microliters of twofold serially diluted bovine sera were reacted with 50 μl of the FMDV Andong strain (100TCID$_{50}$), a serotype O FMDV Korean isolate from the 2010 outbreak, at 37°C for 1 h. After incubation, 50 μl of complete Dulbecco's Modified Eagle Medium (Gibco, USA) with 5% fetal bovine serum containing 1 × 10^4 LFBK cells/ml was added to the reaction mixture. After incubation of the reaction mixtures at 37°C for 48 h, the VN titer was determined as the final dilution of serum showing no cytopathic effect.

Analysis of PBMC subsets

Among the 89 cattle, analysis of the peripheral lymphocyte profiles was conducted with ten Korean native cattle (IACUC permission no. SNU-111210-1). Five of them were fed with a commercial feed supplemented with 0.5% germanium biotite (germanium biotite group), while the rest were fed without the supplement (control group). PBMCs were cultured from the heparinized whole blood of the experiment cattle using the Histopaque®-1077 Hybri-Max™ (Sigma, USA) system, as described by the manufacturer. The PMBCs were then stimulated with DPBS (Gibco), ConA (5 g/ml, Sigma) for CD3, CD4, CD8, and MHC I and II and LPS (5 g/ml, Sigma) for CD79a staining for 96 h

Table 3 Experiment design for grouping, sampling, and analysis

Farms	Number of cattle		Samples	Analysis of
	Control	Germanium biotite		
A	26	22	Serum, saliva, feces	Inhibition percentage, ELISA for antibody levels (IgG and IgA), lysozyme activity
B	13	18	Serum, saliva, feces	Inhibition percentage, ELISA for antibody levels (IgG and IgA), lysozyme activity, virus neutralization test
C	5	5	Serum, saliva, feces, PBMC	Inhibition percentage, ELISA for antibody levels (IgG and IgA), lysozyme activity, PBMC (phenotype, cytokines, proliferation)

Among 89 cattle at 6–8 months of age, 45 cattle were raised with feeds supplemented with 0.5% germanium biotite from 1 week before vaccination to the end of experiment (germanium biotite group) and the rest of them were raised without supplementation (control group).

Table 4 Antibodies used to detect the cell surface markers

Target	Antibody	Company
CD79a	PE-conjugated mouse anti-bovine CD79a	Abcam, UK
CD3	FITC-conjugated hamster anti-bovine CD3	Abcam
CD4	PE-conjugated mouse anti-bovine CD4	US Biological, USA
CD8	PE-conjugated mouse anti-bovine CD8	LifeSpan BioSciences, USA
MHC I	FITC-conjugated mouse anti-bovine MHC I	Novus Biological, USA
MHC II	Mouse anti-bovine MHC II[a]	Abcam
Fc receptor blocking	Polyclonal mouse IgG fraction	Abcam
	Monoclonal Armenian hamster IgG fraction	Abcam

[a]Mouse anti-bovine MHC II antibody was conjugated with PE using an EasyLink B-Phycoerythrin conjugation kit (Abcam).

to characterize the phenotype of PBMC responding to stimulation with mitogens. The procedures for cell fixation and antibody reaction to detect the cell markers were performed as previously reported [37] using the DPBS with 0.2% Tween® 20 (Sigma) as the permeabilisation solution. To prevent a non-specific reaction of the Fc receptor with the detection antibodies, the fixed cells were reacted with normal Ig from the antibody-producing host for 10 min and reacted with fluorescein isothiocyanate (FITC) or phycoerythrin (PE)-conjugated cell surface marker detection antibodies. After the reaction, the number of cells reacting with the FITC or PE conjugate was analyzed using Flow cytometric analysis (BD, USA). The monoclonal antibodies used for the staining of the cells surface markers are listed in Table 4.

Analysis of cytokine gene expression in PBMC

Total RNAs were extracted from PBMCs with the RNeasy mini kit (Qiagen, USA), and cDNAs were synthesized with the reverse transcription kit (Qiagen). The relative expression levels of IFN-γ, IL-1α, IL-1β, IL-4, IL-6, and IL-10 were quantitated using the Rotor-Gene SYBR Green PCR kit (Qiagen) and Rotor-Gene Q (Qiagen), as previously reported [38]. The expression levels were normalized by β-actin expression using the $2^{-\Delta\Delta C}{}_{T}$ method [39].

Analysis of PBMC proliferation

A lymphocyte proliferation assay was conducted with the PBMCs collected from the experiment cattle. Ninety microliters of PBMCs (5×10^6 cells/ml) in a 96-well plate were incubated with ConA (5 μg/ml) and LPS (5 μg/ml) at 37°C for 96 h in a 5% CO_2 atmosphere. Absorbance at 560 nm was measured 2 h after the addition of 10 μl of 10× Prestoblue (Invitrogen, USA). Proliferation of the PBMCs was compared based on this absorbance.

Analysis of lysozyme activities

Lysozyme activities in the serum were measured based on the dissolution ability against *Micrococcus lysodeikticus* (Sigma) [40]. The activity was calculated based on the standard curve generated from the serially diluted lysozyme solution.

Statistical analysis

The data were expressed as mean ± standard deviation (SD). A student's *t*-test and repeated measures of ANOVA were performed for statistical analysis of the data. All statistical analyses of data were carried out using SPSS version 19.0 software (SPSS, USA). A probability value of $p < 0.05$ was considered significant.

Abbreviations

ConA: Concanavalin A; FITC: Fluorescein isothiocyanate; FMD: Foot-and-mouth disease; FMDV: Foot-and-mouth disease virus; HRP: Horseradish peroxidase; IACUC: Institution Animal Care and Use Committee; LPS: Lipopolysaccharide; MHC: Major histocompatibility complex; PBMC: Peripheral blood mononuclear cell; PE: Phycoerythrin; PI: Inhibition percentage; SAT: South African territories; Th1: T helper type 1; Th2: T helper type 2; VN: Virus neutralization.

Competing interests

Effects of the germanium biotite in FMD vaccination are applying to patent in Korea.

Authors' contributions

MJ was involved in sampling, sample processing, data analysis and drafting of manuscript. MKS was involved in sampling and participated in the studies of ELISA for antibodies. SBC and SWS carried out sampling and participated in study of cytokine. AY carried out sampling. WJL and HTP participated in the analysis of PBMC and in study of cytokines analysis. JHP and BK carried out virus neutralization test with a Korea isolate of FMDV. YKJ carried out development of germanium biotite. HSY was involved in experimental design and supervision of the experiments and manuscript revision. All authors read and approved the final manuscript.

Acknowledgements

This study was supported by Ministry of Agriculture, Food and Rural Affairs (IPET 111104–1), BK21 for Veterinary Science and Research Institute for Veterinary Science, Seoul National University, Korea.

Author details

[1]Department of Infectious Diseases, College of Veterinary Medicine, Seoul National University, Seoul 151-742, South Korea. [2]Foot and Mouth Disease Division, Animal and Plant Quarantine Agency, Anyang, Gyeonggido 430-757, South Korea. [3]Seobong BioBestech Co., Ltd, Hyechon Bldg. #401, 831 Yeoksam-dong, Kangnam-gu, Seoul 135-792, South Korea. [4]Institute of Green Bio Science and Technology, Seoul National University, Pyeongchang 232-916, South Korea.

References

1. Sobrino F, Sáiz M, Jiménez-Clavero MA, Núñez JI, Rosas MF, Baranowski E, Ley V: **Foot-and-mouth disease virus: a long known virus, but a current threat.** *Vet Res* 2001, **32:**1–30.
2. OIE: *OIE Terrestrial Manual 2012.* Paris: OIE; 2011.
3. Cox SJ, Barnett PV: **Experimental evaluation of foot-and-mouth disease vaccines for emergency use in ruminants and pigs: a review.** *Vet Res* 2009, **40:**13–42.
4. Nagendrakumar SB, Srinivasan VA, Madhanmohan M, Yuvaraj S, Parida S, Di Nardo A, Horsington J, Paton DJ: **Evaluation of cross-protection between O_1 Manisa and O_1 Campos in cattle vaccinated with foot-and-mouth disease virus vaccine incorporating different payloads of inactivated O_1 Manisa antigen.** *Vaccine* 2011, **29:**1906–1912.
5. Parida S: **Vaccination against foot-and-mouth disease virus: strategies and effectiveness.** *Expert Rev Vaccines* 2009, **8:**347–365.
6. Park JH: **Requirements for improved vaccines against foot-and-mouth disease epidemics.** *Clin Exp Vaccine* 2013, **2:**8–18.
7. Elnekave E, Li Y, Zamir L, Even-Tov B, Hamblin P, Gelman B, Hammond J, Klement E: **The field effectiveness of routine and emergency vaccination with an inactivated vaccine against foot and mouth disease.** *Vaccine* 2013, **31:**879–885.
8. Höhlich BJ, Wiesmüller KH, Haas B, Gerner W, Correa R, Hehnen HR, Schlapp T, Pfaff E, Saalmüller A: **Induction of an antigen-specific immune response and partial protection of cattle against challenge infection with foot-and-mouth disease virus (FMDV) after lipopeptide vaccination with FMDV-specific B-cell epitopes.** *J Gen Virol* 2003, **84:**3315–3324.
9. McCullough KC, Bruckner L, Schaffner R, Fraefel W, Müller HK, Kihm U: **Relationship between the anti-FMD virus antibody reaction as measured by different assays, and protection *in vivo* against challenge infection.** *Vet Microbiol* 1992, **30:**99–112.
10. Li R, Sakwiwatkul K, Yutao L, Hu S: **Enhancement of the immune responses to vaccination against foot-and-mouth disease in mice by oral administration of an extract made from *Rhizoma Atractylodis Macrocephalae* (RAM).** *Vaccine* 2009, **27:**2094–2098.
11. Gerner W, Carr BV, Wiesmüller KH, Pfaff E, Saalmüller A, Charleston B: **Identification of a novel foot-and-mouth disease virus specific T-cell epitope with immunodominant characteristics in cattle with MHC serotype A31.** *Vet Res* 2007, **38:**565–572.
12. Oh Y, Fleming L, Statham B, Hamblin P, Barnett P, Paton DJ, Park JH, Joo YS, Parida S: **Interferon-γ induced by *in vitro* re-stimulation of CD4+ T-cells correlates with *in vivo* FMD vaccine induced protection of cattle against disease and persistent infection.** *PLoS One* 2012, **7:**e44365.
13. Doel T: **Natural and vaccine induced immunity to FMD.** *Curr Top Microbiol Immunol* 2005, **288:**103–131.
14. Oh Y, Reid S, Cox S, Statham R, Mahapatra M, Anderson J, Barnett P, Charleston B, Paton D, Parida S: **Interferon-γ production *in vitro* from whole blood of foot-and-mouth disease virus (FMDV) vaccinated and infected cattle after incubation with inactivated FMDV.** *Vaccine* 2006, **24:**964–969.
15. Guzman E, Taylor G, Charleston B, Skinner MA, Ellis SA: **An MHC-restricted CD8+ T-cell response is induced in cattle by foot-and-mouth disease virus (FMDV) infection and also following vaccination with inactivated FMDV.** *J Gen Virol* 2008, **89:**667–675.
16. Grubman MJ, Moraes MP, Segundo DS, Pena L, De Los Santos T: **Evading the host immune response: how foot-and-mouth disease virus has become an effective pathogen.** *FEMS Immunol Med Microbiol* 2008, **53:**8–17.
17. Summerfield A, Guzylack-Piriou L, Harwood L, McCullough KC: **Innate immune responses against foot-and-mouth disease virus: current understanding and future directions.** *Vet Immunol Immunopathol* 2009, **128:**205–210.
18. Jung BG, Toan NT, Cho SJ, Ko J, Jung YK, Lee BJ: **Dietary aluminosilicate supplement enhances immune activity in mice and reinforces clearance of porcine circovirus type 2 in experimentally infected pigs.** *Vet Microbiol* 2010, **143:**117–125.
19. Jung BG, Lee JA, Lee BJ: **Antiviral effect of dietary germanium biotite supplementation in pigs experimentally infected with porcine reproductive and respiratory syndrome virus.** *J Vet Sci* 2013, **14:**135–141.
20. Jung M, Jung BG, Cha SB, Shin MK, Lee WJ, Shin SW, Lee JA, Jung YK, Lee BJ, Yoo HS: **The effects of germanium biotite supplement as a prophylactic agent against respiratory infection in calves.** *Pak Vet J* 2012, **32:**319–324.
21. Holian A, Uthman MO, Goltsova T, Brown SD, Hamilton RF Jr: **Asbestos and silica-induced changes in human alveolar macrophage phenotype.** *Environ Health Perspect* 1997, **105:**1139–1142.
22. Aikoh T, Tomokuni A, Matsukii T, Hyodoh F, Ueki H, Otsuki T, Ueki A: **Activation-induced cell death in human peripheral blood lymphocytes after stimulation with silicate *in vitro*.** *Int J Oncol* 1998, **12:**1355–1359.
23. Mollick JA, Cook RG, Rich RR: **Class II MHC molecules are specific receptors for staphylococcus enterotoxin A.** *Science* 1989, **244:**817–820.
24. Park JH, Lee KN, Ko YJ, Kim SM, Lee HS, Shin YK, Sohn HJ, Park JY, Yeh JY, Lee YH: **Control of foot-and-mouth disease during 2010–2011 epidemic, South Korea.** *Emerg Infect Dis* 2013, **19:**655–659.
25. Zheng H, Guo J, Jin Y, Yang F, He J, Lv L, Zhang K, Wu Q, Liu X, Cai X: **Engineering foot-and-mouth disease viruses with improved growth properties for vaccine development.** *PLoS One* 2013, **8:**e55228.
26. Cox SJ, Aggarwal N, Statham RJ, Barnett PV: **Longevity of antibody and cytokine responses following vaccination with high potency emergency FMD vaccines.** *Vaccine* 2003, **21:**1336–1347.
27. Doel T: **Optimisation of the immune response to foot-and-mouth disease vaccines.** *Vaccine* 1999, **17:**1767–1771.
28. Park JN, Lee SY, Chu JQ, Lee YJ, Kim RH, Lee KN, Kim SM, Tark DS, Kim B, Park JH: **Protection to homologous and heterologous challenge in pigs immunized with vaccine against foot-and-mouth disease type O caused an epidemic in East Asia during 2010/2011.** *Vaccine* 2014, **32:**1882–1889.
29. Barnett P, Samuel A, Statham R: **The suitability of the 'emergency' foot-and-mouth disease antigens held by the International Vaccine Bank within a global context.** *Vaccine* 2001, **19:**2107–2117.
30. Sanz-Parra A, Jimenez-Clavero MA, Garcıa-Briones MM, Blanco E, Sobrino F, Ley V: **Recombinant viruses expressing the foot-and-mouth disease virus capsid precursor polypeptide (P1) induce cellular but not humoral antiviral immunity and partial protection in pigs.** *Virology* 1999, **259:**129–134.
31. Boehm U, Klamp T, Groot M, Howard J: **Cellular responses to interferon-γ.** *Annu Rev Immunol* 1997, **15:**749–795.
32. Carr BV, Lefevre EA, Windsor MA, Inghese C, Gubbins S, Prentice H, Juleff ND, Charleston B: **CD4+ T-cell responses to foot-and-mouth disease virus in vaccinated cattle.** *J Gen Virol* 2013, **94:**97–107.
33. Zhang Z, Hutching G, Kitching P, Alexandersen S: **The effects of gamma interferon on replication of foot-and-mouth disease virus in persistently infected bovine cells.** *Arch Virol* 2002, **147:**2157–2167.
34. Elgert KD: *Immunolgy.* 2nd edition. Hoboken: John Wiley & Sons Inc.; 2009.
35. Griebel PJ, Qualtiere L, Davis WC, Lawman MJP, Babiuk LA: **Bovine peripheral blood leukocyte subpopulation dynamics following a primary bovine herpesvirus-1 infection.** *Viral Immunol* 1987, **1:**267–286.
36. Burton JL, Kehrli ME: **Effects of dexamethasone on bovine circulating T lymphocyte populations.** *J Leukoc Biol* 1996, **59:**90–99.
37. Gerner W, Käser T, Pintarič M, Groiß S, Saalmüller A: **Detection of intracellular antigens in porcine PBMC by flow cytometry: A comparison of fixation and permeabilisation reagents.** *Vet Immunol Immunopathol* 2008, **121:**251–259.
38. Konnai S, Usui T, Ohashi K, Onuma M: **The rapid quantitative analysis of bovine cytokine genes by real-time RT-PCR.** *Vet Microbiol* 2003, **94:**283–294.
39. Livak KJ, Schmittgen TD: **Analysis of relative gene expression data using real-time quantitative PCR and the $2^{-\Delta\Delta CT}$ method.** *Methods* 2001, **25:**402–408.
40. Kreukniet MB, Nieuwland MGB, Van der Zijpp AJ: **Phagocytic activity of two lines of chickens divergently selected for antibody production.** *Vet Immunol Immunopathol* 1994, **44:**377–387.

Efficacy of multivalent, modified-live virus (MLV) vaccines administered to early weaned beef calves subsequently challenged with virulent *Bovine viral diarrhea virus* type 2

Manuel F Chamorro[1], Paul H Walz[2*], Thomas Passler[1], Edzard van Santen[4], Julie Gard[1], Soren P Rodning[3], Kay P Riddell[2], Patricia K Galik[2] and Yijing Zhang[2]

Abstract

Background: Vaccination of young calves against *Bovine viral diarrhea virus* (BVDV) is desirable in dairy and beef operations to reduce clinical disease and prevent spread of the virus among cattle. Although protection from clinical disease by multivalent, modified-live virus (MLV) vaccines has been demonstrated, the ability of MLV vaccines to prevent viremia and viral shedding in young calves possessing passive immunity is not known. The purpose of this study was to compare the ability of three different MLV vaccines to prevent clinical disease, viremia, and virus shedding in early weaned beef calves possessing maternal immunity that were vaccinated once at 45 days prior to challenge with virulent BVDV 2.

Results: At 45 days following vaccination, calves that received vaccines B and C had significantly higher BVDV 1 and BVDV 2 serum antibody titers compared with control calves. Serum antibody titers for BVDV 1 and BVDV 2 were not significantly different between control calves and calves that received vaccine D. Following BVDV 2 challenge, a higher proportion of control calves and calves that received vaccine D presented viremia and shed virus compared with calves that received vaccines B and C. Rectal temperatures and clinical scores were not significantly different between groups at any time period. Calves that received vaccines B and C had significantly higher mean body weights at BVDV 2 challenge and at the end of the study compared with control calves.

Conclusions: Moderate to low maternally-derived BVDV antibody levels protected all calves against severe clinical disease after challenge with virulent BVDV 2. Vaccines B and C induced a greater antibody response to BVDV 1 and BVDV 2, and resulted in reduced viremia and virus shedding in vaccinated calves after challenge indicating a greater efficacy in preventing virus transmission and reducing negative effects of viremia.

Keywords: Early weaning, BVDV, MLV, Vaccine, Antibody titres, Virus, Isolation, Shedding

Background

Bovine viral diarrhea virus (BVDV) is an important cause of respiratory, enteric, and reproductive disease in cattle and has been associated with major economic losses in cattle operations worldwide [1]. Vaccination of young calves against BVDV reduces the number of acute infections in the herd and limits spread of virus among cattle populations [1,2]; however, effective vaccination of young calves against BVDV can be challenging due to the presence of maternally-derived BVDV antibodies at the time of vaccination [3]. Although maternally-derived BVDV antibodies can provide protection against acute BVDV infection and clinical disease, humoral immune responses to vaccination might be adversely affected [4]. Concentration of maternally-derived BVDV antibodies and age of calf at the time of vaccination are important factors in the induction of adequate immune responses following BVDV immunization [5-7]. Calves with moderate

* Correspondence: walzpau@auburn.edu
[2]Department of Pathobiology, College of Veterinary Medicine, Auburn University, Auburn, AL, USA
Full list of author information is available at the end of the article

to high maternally-derived BVDV antibody levels at vaccination do not usually respond with an increase in BVDV antibodies but are protected against clinical disease, have a slower decay rate of maternal immunity, and develop anamnestic antibody responses following BVDV challenge [8-10]. Calves with low maternally-derived BVDV antibody levels respond to vaccination by increasing BVDV antibody titers. The priming of naive B and T cells, the induction of specific cell mediated immune memory responses, and the induction of anamnestic antibody responses have been identified as the main source of protection of young calves vaccinated in the presence of maternally-derived antibodies and subsequently challenged with virulent BVDV [11-15].

Early weaned beef calves possess variable levels of maternally-derived BVDV antibodies at 2–4 months of age and therefore could benefit from vaccination prior to stress of weaning and shipment. A single dose of a multivalent, MLV BVDV vaccine was demonstrated to be effective in protecting young calves possessing different levels of maternal immunity against acute BVDV infection [16]. In addition to prevention of clinical disease, vaccination should limit the spread of BVDV by reducing virus shedding and horizontal transmission, a desirable outcome of vaccination in herds or units where populations of highly stressed cattle are commingled. However, experimental studies comparing different multivalent MLV vaccines containing BVDV in their ability to prevent viremia and viral shedding in young calves possessing maternally-derived immunity that subsequently undergo challenge with virulent BVDV are limited. The objective of this study was to evaluate the ability of three different commercially available, multivalent MLV vaccines containing BVDV to prevent clinical disease and reduce shedding of virus when administered to early weaned beef calves subsequently challenged with virulent BVDV 2 at 45 days after vaccination.

Results

Four groups of early weaned beef calves were vaccinated (B, C, and D) or received phosphate saline (A) at weaning at a median calf age of 72.2 days. The calves were born from cows that had been previously vaccinated at least once during the last 2 years with a MLV vaccine. The vaccine used in the cows during the previous 2 years was the same vaccine used in experimental calves from group D. Forty five days after weaning calves were challenged with BVDV 2 1373. Evaluation of clinical responses to challenge and sample collection was performed from day 0 (challenge day) until day 28.

Serum virus neutralization titers

Thirty days prior to vaccination (day –75) and at a median calf age of 44 days, the mean levels of maternally-derived BVDV 1 NADL and BVDV 2 125c serum antibodies were similar between groups (Table 1). At vaccination (day –45), a significant effect of time (day) was detected ($P = 0.0001$) as decay of maternally-derived antibodies for BVDV 1 NADL and BVDV 2 125c occurred in all groups; however, mean levels of BVDV 1 and BVDV 2 antibodies were not significantly different ($P > 0.05$) between groups. Forty-five days after vaccination, which corresponded to the time of BVDV 2 challenge (day 0), a significant effect of group and time (day) was detected ($P = 0.0001$ and $P = 0.0001$, respectively). Groups B and C calves had mean levels of serum BVDV 1 NADL antibodies significantly greater than controls ($P = 0.0033$ and $P = 0.0002$, respectively). Additionally, on day 0, mean levels of BVDV 1 NADL antibodies were similar between group D and the control group ($P = 0.2641$). With respect to BVDV 2 125c, group C calves had mean levels of antibodies significantly greater than the control group ($P = 0.0368$). Twenty eight days following challenge, a significant effect of time (day) was detected ($p = 0.0001$) with respect to the levels of BVDV 2 125c. The mean BVDV 2 125c serum antibody levels increased similarly in all groups ($P > 0.05$); in contrast, time (day) and group effects were significant ($P = 0.0001$ and $P = 0.0001$, respectively) for BVDV 1 NADL mean antibody levels as these were higher in group B and C calves compared to the control group ($P < 0.00001$). When antibodies to the challenge strain BVDV 2 1373 were examined at day 0, a significant effect of group and time (day) was detected ($P = 0.0001$ and $P = 0.0001$). Calves from groups B and C had greater levels of antibodies compared with control calves ($P = 0.05$ and $P = 0.025$, respectively). At day 28 after challenge, a significant ($P = 0.0001$) effect of time (day) was detected as all groups had increased and similar levels of antibodies to the challenge BVDV strain ($P > 0.05$).

Among vaccinated groups, seroconversion, as defined as a 4-fold or greater rise in antibody titers to BVDV 1 NADL after vaccination (at day 0) was observed in 16.6% of the calves from group B, 50% of the calves from group C, and 9% of the calves from group D. Similarly, seroconversion to BVDV 2 125c after vaccination was observed in 16.6% of the calves from group B, 8.3% of the calves from group C, and 9% of the calves from group D. None of the calves in group A (control) seroconverted to BVDV 1 NADL or BVDV 2 125c. The proportion of calves that seroconverted to BVDV 2 125c after vaccination was not significantly different between groups ($P > 0.05$); however, a higher proportion of calves from group C (50%) seroconverted to BVDV 1 NADL with a fourfold increase in antibody titers.

Virus isolation

Virus positive samples in serum and WBC samples were detected more frequently and for a longer time in the

Table 1 Geometric mean (95% CI) of virus neutralizing serum antibody titers to BVDV 1, BVDV 2, and BVDV 2 1373 from vaccinated (B, C, and D) and unvaccinated (A) calves at each time period

		Day of Study			
Virus	Group	−75	−45	0	28
BVDV 1 NADL	A	157.58 (31.12 – 831.74)	60.12 (14.52 – 250.73)	15.03 (5.93 – 38.05)	35.75 (17.38 – 74.02)
	B	135.29^{NS} (28.64 – 639.14)	67.64^{NS} (17.50 – 259.57)	**107.63*** (62.68 – 183.54)	**861.07*** (377.41 - 1951)
	C	222.86^{NS} (67.64 – 765.36)	101.12^{NS} (30.27 – 337.79)	**202.25*** (110.66 – 369.64)	**680.28*** (225.97 - 2048)
	D	194.01^{NS} (45.56 – 903.88)	95.67^{NS} (22.47 – 407.31)	36.25^{NS} (12.04 – 108.38)	57.70^{NS} (12.99 – 213.78)
BVDV 2 125c	A	107.63 (23.10 - 498)	47.83 (13.08 – 173.64)	14.22 (4.08 – 49.18)	608.87 (292.03 – 1260.69)
	B	101.12^{NS} (23.26 – 439.58)	60.12^{NS} (15.67 – 232.32)	42.52^{NS} (22.47 – 80.44)	809^{NS} (455.08 – 1438.15)
	C	128^{NS} (38.85 – 418.76)	85.03^{NS} (26.53 – 272.47)	**60.12*** (26.35 – 138.14)	1820.34^{NS} (955.42 – 3468.26)
	D	128^{NS} (40.78 – 398.93)	90.50^{NS} (31.34 – 259.57)	29.85^{NS} (15.24 – 58.89)	286.02^{NS} (149.08 – 1541.37)
BVDV 2 1373	A	_	_	16.91 (5.02 – 56.44)	861.07 (424.61 – 1734.13)
	B	_	_	**76.10*** (47.50 – 121.09)	643.59^{NS} (352.13 – 1176.26)
	C	_	_	**93.05*** (49.18 – 176.06)	1530.72^{NS} (617.37 – 3795.30)
	D	_	_	56.10^{NS} (28.44 – 11.43)	544.95^{NS} (245.57 – 1200.98)

NS, *Means within BVDV strain and Day of Study are not significantly different (NS) from the control group A or are significantly different (*) based on Dunnett's test at $P = 0.05$.

control group compared with groups, B, C, and D (Figure 1). The total proportion of calves that tested positive to BVDV 2 in serum and WBC samples after challenge (days 0 to 28) was higher in the control group (90%) and group D (54.5%) compared with groups B (16%) and C (25%) (Table 2). A significant effect of group and time (day) was detected on days 6, 8, 10, and 14 after challenge with BVDV 2 1373 (P = 0.0001 and P = 0.0001, respectively). On day 6 post-challenge, the control group had a higher proportion of calves with positive BVDV samples (58.3%) compared with groups B (8.3%) and C (8.3%) (P < 0.05) but not with group D (36.3%). Additionally, at days 8, 10, and 14 post-challenge, a higher proportion of calves in the control group had BVDV positive samples compared with calves in groups B, C, and D. The proportion of viremic calves (calves with positive serum or WBC samples) that shed virus after challenge (calves whose nasal swab samples tested positive to BVDV by virus isolation) was higher in the control group (72.7%) compared with groups B (0) and C (0) and D (33.3%) (P < 0.05).

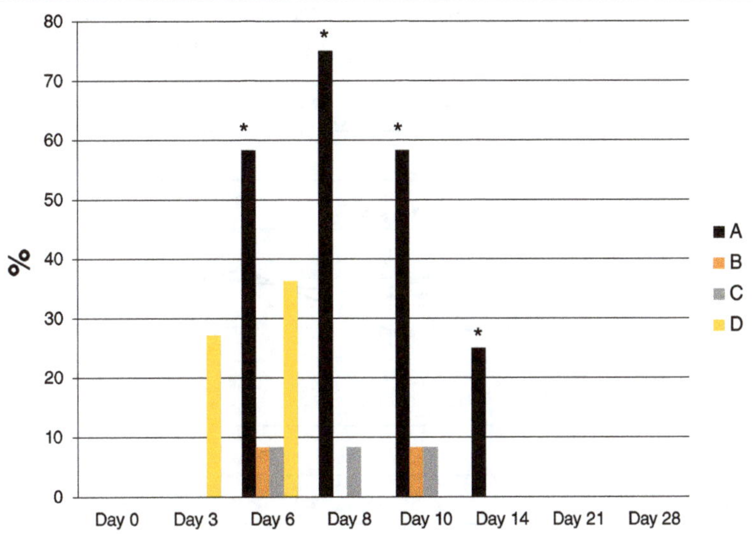

Figure 1 Total proportion of calves with a positive virus isolation result in WBC and serum samples at each time point after challenge with BVDV 2 1373. The proportion of vaccinated (B, C and D) and control (A) calves with positive virus isolation WBC or serum samples at each time point (day) after challenge with BVDV 2 1373 was higher and more frequent in the control group (A) compared with groups B and C and D. The star *sign refers to statistical significance (P < 0.05).

Table 2 Total number and proportion of calves (%) that became viremic and shed virus in nasal secretions after challenge (days 0 to 28) with BVDV 2 1373 in each group

Group	Number of viremic¥ calves (%)	Number of viremic calves that shed virus (%)
A	11 (90)*	8 (72.7)*
B	2 (16.6)	0
C	3 (25)	0
D	6 (54.5)*	2 (33.3)

¥, viremic calves = calves with a BVDV positive sample in WBC or serum.
A higher proportion of control (A) and group D calves became viremic and shed virus after challenge compared with calves from groups B and C. The star *sign refers to statistical significance (P < 0.05).

Clinical scores and body weight

There were no detectable adverse vaccine reactions in any of the calves. One calf in group D was euthanized on the day prior to challenge with BVDV 2 1373 due to rectal prolapse. Vaccinated and control calves demonstrated clinical protection against challenge with virulent BVDV 2 1373 as only one calf in the control group developed mild diarrhea and anorexia on day 14 post-challenge. The proportion of calves with clinical scores of ≥ 2 for respiratory, diarrhea, and depression parameters was similar between groups (P > 0.05). A mild increase in body temperature, nasal secretion, and loose feces was observed in all calves after challenge independent of group designation. A significant effect of time (day) on rectal temperatures was observed (P < 0.00001). On day 8, the mean rectal temperatures of all groups were increased compared with other days post-challenge.

The average body weight at weaning (day -45) was not significantly different between groups (A = 206.56 +/- 3.53, B = 207.25 +/- 8.33, C = 214.08 +/- 9.25, D = 188.41 +/- 10.08); however, a significant effect of group and time (day) was detected at day 0 and at the end of the study (P = 0.0001 and P = 0.0001, respectively). Calves from group B and C had significantly higher mean body weights at both time points compared with control calves (B = 257.5 +/- 13.14, C = 257.5 +/- 11.87 vs. A = 242.5 +/- 11.08 and B = 345 +/- 15.72, C = 333.75 +/- 12.17 vs. A = 267.91 +/- 12.63, respectively). At the same times (day 0 and end of the trial), the mean body weights of calves from group D were not significantly different compared with control calves (240 +/- 15.25 vs. 242.5 +/- 11.08 and 300.90 +/- 14.7 vs. 267.91 +/- 12.63, respectively) (P = 0.568 and P = 0.262, respectively).

Hematology

A significant effect of time (day) but not group was detected in the mean WBC counts, as mean WBC decreased in all groups from day 0 (challenge) until day 6 post-challenge (P = 0.0001); however, significant differences were not observed between groups (P > 0.05). On day 8 post-challenge, a significant effect of group and time (day) was detected. The mean WBC count from Group D calves was significantly higher compared with control calves (P = 0.007). At the same time, the mean WBC from calves in groups B and C were not significantly different compared to control calves (Figure 2). Effects of group and time (day) were not detected in platelet counts at any time point after challenge with BVDV 1373 (Figure 3).

Discussion

High levels of BVDV-specific antibodies from colostrum or vaccination effectively protect calves against severe clinical disease induced by challenge with virulent BVDV [3,9]; however, prevention of viremia and virus shedding are variable in cattle vaccinated with MLV vaccines and subsequently challenged with virulent BVDV [17-19]. In

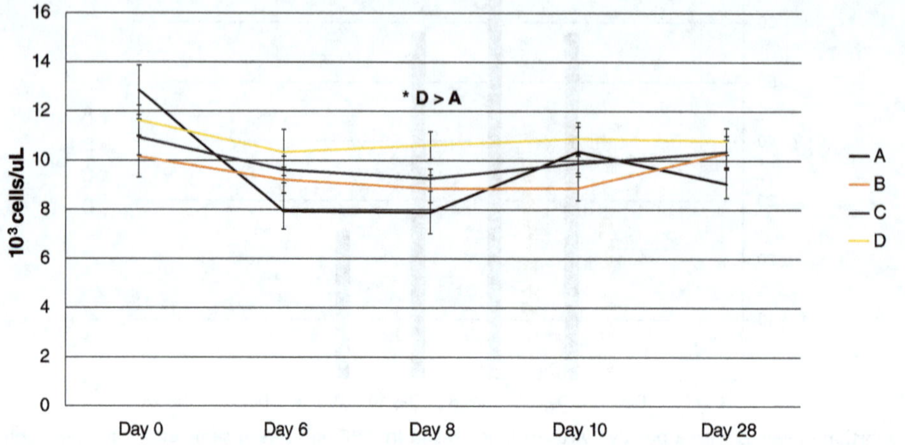

Figure 2 Mean white blood cell count (+/–SEM) after challenge with BVDV 2 1373. Mean WBC between vaccinated (B, C, and D) and control (A) calves after challenge. In all calves mean WBC decreased until day 6 after challenge. At day 8 after challenge calves from group D had higher mean WBC compared with the control group (P = 0.007).

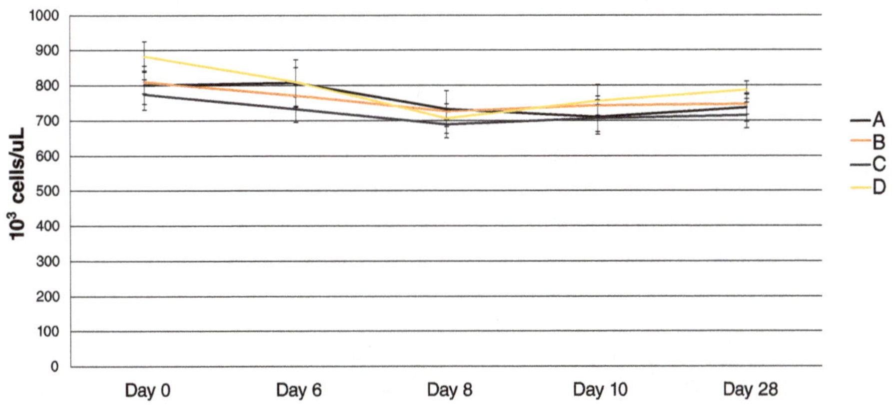

Figure 3 Mean platelet count (+/−SEM) after challenge with BVDV 2 1373. Mean platelet count after challenge with BVDV 2 1373 was not significantly different between vaccinated (B, C, and D) and control (A) calves.

the current study, calves from all groups had similar clinical scores and rectal temperatures, and mortality was not observed after challenge with virulent BVDV 2 1373. This could be associated with protection offered by maternally-derived BVDV antibodies in vaccinated and unvaccinated calves as has been previously reported [11], or could have resulted from lower virulence of the challenge virus than in previous reports [20]. Pestiviruses constantly undergo genetic change due to the poor proof-reading capability of the RNA-dependent RNA polymerase, resulting in variability of phenotypic characteristics such as host-cell tropism and virulence [21]. Repeated passage in cell culture was previously reported to result in attenuation of a BVDV isolate, and may have occurred with the BVDV 1373 used in this study [22].

Interestingly, only calves from group D had an increased white blood cell count compared with control calves at day 8 post-challenge. Prevention of leukopenia is one of several parameters used to evaluate response to vaccination after challenge with BVDV [9,11], and in this case the lack of a decrease in WBC counts observed in group D could have been related to the effects of vaccination or to the presence of high levels of specific maternal antibodies. Despite their ability to reduce clinical disease, maternally-derived BVDV antibodies were not as effective in preventing viremia and viral shedding in calves from the control group as 11/12 (90%) of the calves became viremic and of those 8/11 (72.2%) shed virus after challenge. For this study, we chose VI as our testing method in order to document clinically relevant shedding of live virus [23]. Prior to challenge, the geometric mean of serum BVDV 2 1373 antibody titers of control calves was significantly lower compared with titers from groups B and C (16.91 vs. 76.10 and 93.05, respectively). Low serum antibody titers prior to challenge with BVDV have been associated with an increased risk of viremia and clinical disease as demonstrated in previous studies [3,4]. Other reports have indicated that calves with serum maternally-derived BVDV antibody titers < 64 before challenge with virulent BVDV have a higher risk of developing clinical disease and systemic spread of the virus compared to calves with greater antibody titers [3,8].

Antibody response to vaccination with MLV BVDV vaccines of young calves in the presence of maternally-derived BVDV antibodies has produced variable results. Previous studies have demonstrated that 40 to 90-day-old calves with maternally-derived antibody titers ≤ 32 against BVDV 1 and BVDV 2 prior to vaccination seroconvert after vaccination [5-7,10]; additionally, these calves can develop an anamnestic response when a second dose of vaccine is administered [5,10]. In contrast, similar studies have demonstrated that 3 to 56-day-old calves with BVDV 1 and BVDV 2 maternally-derived antibody titers ≥ 32 prior to vaccination usually do not seroconvert to vaccination and clinical protection against challenge with BVDV is variable [4,9,13]. In our study, a small proportion of calves vaccinated at weaning, at a median age of 72.2 days, seroconverted to BVDV 2 after vaccination. In contrast, 50% of calves from group C seroconverted to BVDV 1 suggesting a greater ability of the vaccine C to overcome maternal interference to BVDV 1. The higher levels of antibodies to BVDV 1 NADL and BVDV 2 1373 before challenge, the lower proportion of viremia, and the absence of viral shedding after challenge observed in calves from groups B and C suggests that vaccination with B and C may have primed B cell responses to increase specific antibody production or may have delayed the normal decay of maternal BVDV antibodies [6-8,10]. Additionally, the higher levels of antibodies at challenge could have reduced viremia and prevented viral shedding in calves from the same groups. The reduction of viremia and viral shedding is a highly desirable outcome of vaccination since this could prevent BVDV transmission in operations such as feedlots and stocker units where high numbers of cattle from multiple origins are commingled.

The higher proportion of calves with viremia and virus shedding observed in group D could have been a consequence of the presence of more specific maternal antibodies induced by previous vaccination of the dams with vaccine D. The presence of more specific BVDV antibodies induced by vaccine D on colostra from the dams could have exerted a more efficient blockage of humoral cell responses of calves vaccinated with D. Similar results were detected in a recent study in which lower antibody levels to BVDV 1a, BVDV 1b, and BVDV 2 and a higher proportion of viremia after BVDV 2 challenge were observed in calves 42 days after vaccination with D [19]. Protection against viremia and virus shedding after experimental challenge with BVDV of calves vaccinated with MLV BVDV vaccines has been commonly associated with activation of T cell mediated immune responses independent of the induction of an adequate antibody response [11,13,14]. A previous study reported the depletion of CD4+ lymphocytes in calves acutely infected with BVDV could prolong the duration of viral shedding [24]. Additionally, in another study, 80% of calves vaccinated at 3 days of age with a MLV BVDV vaccine and challenged 7-9 months later with virulent BVDV 2 became viremic after challenge; however, calves were protected against severe clinical disease in the absence of antibody responses at initial vaccination [17]. This indicates that induction of specific T cell memory responses after early vaccination may not always prevent viremia and virus shedding in young calves after challenge with BVDV. In the current study we did not evaluate BVDV-specific T cell responses to vaccination and challenge; however, it is possible that a stronger activation of T cell memory responses in calves vaccinated with D that became viremic could have reduced the duration of viremia to only 2 days; additionally, T cell memory responses in groups B and C could have been associated with the reduced proportion of calves with viremia and nasal shedding.

Previous reports have demonstrated that acute BVDV infection in young calves can result in decreased weight gains and decreased performance [9,11]. In the current study, control calves had lower mean body weights at day 0 and at the end of the study compared with calves from groups B and C. Mean body weights of control and group D calves were similar during the study. It is possible that vaccines B and C had a positive effect on weight gain after vaccination as previously reported [25]. Additionally, the higher frequency of viremia in control and group D calves could have had a negative effect on performance and weight gain. Another study demonstrated that young calves vaccinated with a MLV BVDV vaccine and subsequently challenged with virulent BVDV have higher mean body weights and average daily gains compared with non-vaccinated calves [9]. The higher mean body weights observed in calves from groups B and C at the end of the study suggest that higher levels of BVDV antibodies before challenge and prevention of viremia could have a positive effect on performance, although this observation would need further research using larger numbers of experimental subjects. Prevention of weight loss could be a highly desirable outcome of vaccination programs for early weaned beef calves.

Conclusions

Vaccination of young calves possessing maternally-derived immunity with multivalent MLV vaccines was demonstrated to be beneficial in reducing viremia and virus shedding following BVDV challenge at 45 days after vaccination. Moderate to low levels of maternally-derived BVDV antibodies protected early weaned beef calves against severe clinical disease induced by challenge with virulent BVDV 2. Decay of maternally-derived BVDV antibodies was observed in all groups and just a small proportion of calves seroconverted to BVDV 2 after vaccination; however, the ability of MLV BVDV vaccines to prime B cell responses, induce antibody production, or delay the decay of maternal immunity could result in reduced numbers of viremic calves and prevent virus shedding as was observed in calves from groups B and C in the present study. Reduction of viremia and BVDV shedding could result in decreased BVDV transmission and disease by increasing calf-herd immunity and reducing environmental load of free virus as has been suggested by a previous study [26]. Additionally, MLV BVDV vaccines that reduce viremia after BVDV challenge could have a positive effect on calf performance and would be of most benefit when establishing health programs for early weaned beef calves.

Methods

Animals

Forty-eight crossbred steer calves born and raised at the Upper Coastal Plain Agricultural Research Center, Winfield, AL were utilized in this study. Calves were born in September-October 2012 to cows that had received at least one dose of a modified-live BVDV vaccine D[a] prior to breeding during the 2 years previous to the start of the study. At birth, calves were identified by an ear tattoo and ear tag. All calves remained with their dams and consumption of colostrum occurred under natural conditions in the pasture. A blood sample for detection of neutralizing antibodies against BVDV 1 and BVDV 2 was collected from all calves at day −75 of the study at a median calf age of 44 days to determine the initial maternally-derived BVDV antibody levels.

Experimental design

All calves were early weaned on study day −45, which corresponded to calf ages between 62–92 days (2–3 months) with a median age of 72.2 days. To prepare for early weaning, creep feeding was offered for 3 weeks prior to weaning in order to train calves to the weaning diet. The weaning diet was an energy dense (65-75% of total digestible nutrients), relatively high protein (14-17%), and highly palatable ration to meet all nutritional requirements of young growing calves. Calves were stratified by initial maternally-derived BVDV 2 serum antibody titers and assigned by the use of a random number generator [b] to 1 of 4 different vaccination groups. The stratification by initial levels of BVDV 2 antibodies ensured that each group received similar numbers of calves with different levels of maternally-derived BVDV 2 antibody levels. All calves underwent abrupt weaning on day −45 of the study and were vaccinated according to their assigned treatment group A (n = 12), B (n = 12), C (n = 12), or D (n = 12). Following vaccination, calves were separated in isolated pastures to prevent transmission of vaccine strains between groups. During this time, daily observation of the calves was performed to evaluate for adverse vaccine reactions. Forty-four days after weaning, calves were transported 192 miles to the North Auburn BVDV Unit located in Auburn, AL. Upon arrival to the North Auburn BVDV Unit, calves were rested and given access to fresh water, hay, and supplement. On the next day (day 0), all calves were challenged with virulent BVDV 2 1373 and placed in the same pasture for the remainder of the study. Clinical evaluation and sampling of calves was performed until day 28 after challenge. All calf protocols were reviewed and approved by the Institutional Animal Care and Use Committee of Auburn University (PRN # 2012–2157).

Vaccines

All vaccines used were commercially available, USDA-licensed stock material and were administered to calves at weaning (day −45). Group A was the control group and received 2 mL of 0.9% phosphate buffered saline subcutaneously once. Group B received 2 mL of vaccine B[c] subcutaneously once, group C received 2 mL of vaccine C[d] subcutaneously once, and group D received 2 mL of vaccine D[a] subcutaneously once. All vaccines were modified-live and multivalent containing modified-live types 1 and 2 of BVDV, parainfluenza virus 3, bovine herpesvirus 1, and bovine respiratory syncytial virus. All calves in this study were under 6 months of age and vaccination with vaccines B, C, and D was considered off-label.

BVDV challenge

Forty-five days after vaccination (day 0), all calves were experimentally inoculated with the noncytopathic (NCP) BVDV 2 strain 1373. The NCP BVDV 2 strain 1373 has been previously used in experimental BVDV inoculation of calves and shown to induce severe clinical disease, leukopenia, and thrombocytopenia [27]. The BVDV 2 strain 1373 was propagated in Madin-Darby bovine kidney (MDBK) cells in minimum essential medium [j] (MEM), supplemented with 10% equine serum, L-glutamine, penicillin G (100 units/ml), and streptomycin (100 μg/ml). Virus was harvested from cells by a single freeze-thaw method, aliquoted, and stored (−80°C) until needed. Aliquots were enumerated using the method of Reed and Muench [28], prior to inoculation of calves. All calves were inoculated by intranasal aerosol administration of 1×10^6 $TCID_{50}$ of the BVDV 2 strain 1373.

Sample and data collection

Daily clinical observations were performed by the same person, who was blinded to study group allocation, on days 0, 3, 6, 8, 10, 14, 21, and 28. Additionally, individual rectal temperatures, serum, whole blood, and deep nasal swab samples were collected on those same days. Whole blood samples were subjected to hematologic analysis on day 0 prior to challenge and on days 6, 8, 10, and 28 after challenge for individual white blood cell and platelet counts.

During sampling days, each calf was scored prior to handling for signs of abnormal respiration, diarrhea, and depression using a scale of 0 to 3, with the absence of a clinical sign scored as 0 and the most severe clinical sign scored as 3 [17]. Briefly, an abnormal respiratory score was given if an animal presented with a cough, labored breathing, nasal, or ocular discharge. Nasal and ocular discharges were judged as being serous, mucous, or mucopurulent. Diarrhea scores were judged as being normal feces, pasty feces, runny feces, or severe diarrhea with or without blood. Depression scores ranged from no depression, mild depression, moderate depression, or severe depression. In addition to visual examination, individual body weights were obtained on day −45 (vaccination/weaning day), day 0 (challenge day), and days 14, and 28 after challenge using a portable livestock electric scale [f] that was validated prior to and after each weighing.

Virus Isolation (VI)

Whole blood, serum, and deep nasal swab samples collected on days 0, 3, 6, 8, 10, 14, 21, and 28 after challenge were used for BVDV VI using the immunoperoxidase monolayer assay with techniques previously described [29]. Briefly, the isolated samples were suspended in 24-well plates and subsequently seeded in 50 μL culture medium. The cell suspension was subjected to co-cultivation on 25 cm^3 flasks containing monolayers of MDBK cells and was incubated for 24 hours at 38.5°C and 5% CO_2. Following cultivation, 50 μl of the cell culture supernatant was inoculated in triplicate into wells on 96-well microtiter plates containing monolayers of MDBK cells in culture medium. After 96 hours of incubation at 38.5°C and 5% CO_2, all samples were frozen at −80°C and subsequently thawed to detect BVDV using the immunoperoxidase monolayer assay as previously described [29].

Virus Neutralization (VN)

The standard virus neutralization microtiter assay was used to detect antibodies against BVDV in serum of calves collected on days −75, −45, 0 (prior to challenge), and 28 [28]. The BVDV 1 cytopathic strain NADL and BVDV 2 cytopathic strain 125c were used. For samples collected on days 0 and 28, the challenge BVDV 2 1373 non-cytopathic strain was also used. Briefly, following heat inactivation at 56°C for 30 minutes, serial 2-fold dilutions (1:2 to 1:4096) were made in 50 μL of culture medium. For each dilution, 3 wells of a 96-well plate were inoculated with an equal volume (50 μL) of culture medium containing 100–500 $TCID_{50}$ of the test strain. After inoculation, the plate was incubated at 38.5°C in a humidified atmosphere of 5% CO_2 and room air for 1 hour. Then, 2.5×10^3 MDBK cells in 50 μL of culture medium were added to each well. Plates were incubated for 72 hours and evaluated visually for cytopathic effect for the BVDV 1 and 2 cytopathic strains [29,30] or by staining the plates using the immunoperoxidase assay for the BVDV 2 1373 non-cytopathic strain. The geometric mean of antibody titers was calculated from the endpoint Log_2 titers of the animals in each group. Seronegativity to BVDV 1 and BVDV 2 was defined as a serum antibody titer less than 2 which equates to a Log_2 antibody titer of 0.

Statistical analysis

All statistical analyses were performed using the GLIMMIX procedure in the SAS 9.3 software package [g]. To detect changes in Log_2 transformed antibody levels, virus isolation, rectal temperatures, white blood cell counts, platelet counts, and body weights, a repeated measures generalized linear mixed model [Response = Group + Time (day) + Group * Day] was performed using an appropriate distribution function. The repeated nature of this experiment, viz. multiple observations on the same experimental unit = animal over time, implies non-independence of residuals. Hence, the residual variance was modelled to arrive at a reasonable residual covariance structure using Akaike's Information criterion corrected for small sample sizes (AICc) to determine the best structure. A first-order autoregressive structure with heterogeneous variances (ARH 1) was most commonly fitted. This structure allows for a separate residual variance at each time point and a correlation among time points that diminishes with the lag. Because clinical scores for respiratory distress and diarrhea were binary in nature (only scores 1 and 2 were given) the binary distribution function was used in the abovementioned procedure; this analysis approach is commonly referred to as logistic regression. No analysis was performed for clinical depression score as all scores equalled zero. Dunnett's test for multiple comparisons was used to detect differences between vaccinated groups and the control group; a probability of $P \leq 0.05$ was considered statistically significant for all tests. The FREQ procedure in the abovementioned software package [h] was used to analyze the proportion of calves with viremia and virus shedding with a χ^2 test.

Endnotes

[a]Bovi-Shield Gold 5, Zoetis Animal Health, Florham Park, NJ
[b]Microsoft Excel 2010, Redmond, WA
[c]BRD-Shield, Novartis Animal Health, Larchwood, IA
[d]Express 5, Boehringer Ingelheim Vetmedica, Ridgefield, Conn.
[e]Powder River Cattle & Livestock Equipment, Provo, UT
[f]True-test Inc. Mineral Wells, TX
[g]SAS Institute Inc., Cary, NC
[h]PROC FREQ SAS 9.2, SAS Institute Inc., Cary, NC

Abbreviations

BVDV: Bovine viral diarrhea virus; MLV: Modified- live virus; CP: Cytopathic; NCP: Non-cytopathic; VI: Virus isolation; VN: Virus neutralization.

Competing interests

The authors declare that they have no competing interests.

Authors' contributions

MFC, PHW, and TP developed the experimental design of this study and co-wrote the manuscript. EvS performed the statistical analysis of the data and revised the manuscript. KPR, JG, and SPR collaborated with animal experiments, sampling, and data collection. PG and YZ performed laboratory testing. All authors read and approved the final manuscript.

Acknowledgements

The authors would like to thank Mr. George Fincher and Mr. Steven Ledbetter for animal care assistance.

Funding

Funds for this research project were obtained from the Alabama Agricultural Experimental Station, Auburn, AL.

Author details

[1]Department of Clinical Sciences, College of Veterinary Medicine, Auburn University, Auburn, AL, USA. [2]Department of Pathobiology, College of Veterinary Medicine, Auburn University, Auburn, AL, USA. [3]Department of Animal Sciences, College of Agriculture, Auburn University, Auburn, AL, USA. [4]Department of Crop, Soils, and Environmental Sciences, College of Agriculture and Alabama Agricultural Experiment Station, Auburn University, Auburn, AL, USA.

References

1. Houe H. Epidemiology of bovine viral diarrhea virus. Vet Clin North Am Food Anim Pract. 1995;11:521–47.
2. Ridpath JF. Immunology of BVDV vaccines. Biologicals. 2013;41:14–9.
3. Cortese VS, West KH, Hassard LE, Carman S, Ellis JA. Clinical and immunologic responses of vaccinated and unvaccinated calves to infection with a virulent type-II isolate of bovine viral diarrhea virus. J Am Vet Med Assoc. 1998;213:1312–9.

4. Ellis J, West K, Cortese V, Konoby C, Weigel D. Effect of maternal antibodies on induction and persistence of vaccine-induced immune responses against bovine viral diarrhea virus type II in young calves. J Am Vet Med Assoc. 2001;219:351–6.
5. Menanteau-Horta AM, Ames TR, Johnson DW, Meiske JC. Effect of maternal antibody upon vaccination with infectious bovine rhinotracheitis and bovine virus diarrhea vaccines. Can J Comp Med. 1985;49:10–4.
6. Munoz-Zanzi CA, Thurmond MC, Johnson WO, Hietala SK. Predicted ages of dairy calves when colostrum-derived bovine viral diarrhea virus antibodies would no longer offer protection against disease or interfere with vaccination. J Am Vet Med Assoc. 2002;221:678–85.
7. Fulton RW, Briggs RE, Payton ME, Confer AW, Saliki JT, Ridpath JF, et al. Maternally derived humoral immunity to bovine viral diarrhea virus (BVDV) 1a, BVDV1b, BVDV2, bovine herpesvirus-1, parainfluenza-3 virus bovine respiratory syncytial virus, Mannheimia haemolytica and Pasteurella multocida in beef calves, antibody decline by half-life studies and effect on response to vaccination. Vaccine. 2004;22:643–9.
8. Howard CJ, Clarke MC, Brownlie J. Protection against respiratory infection with bovine virus diarrhoea virus by passively acquired antibody. Vet Microbiol. 1989;19:195–203.
9. Platt R, Widel PW, Kesl LD, Roth JA. Comparison of humoral and cellular immune responses to a pentavalent modified live virus vaccine in three age groups of calves with maternal antibodies, before and after BVDV type 2 challenge. Vaccine. 2009;27:4508–19.
10. Woolums AR, Berghaus RD, Berghaus LJ, Ellis RW, Pence ME, Saliki JT, et al. Effect of calf age and administration route of initial multivalent modified-live virus vaccine on humoral and cell-mediated immune responses following subsequent administration of a booster vaccination at weaning in beef calves. Am J Vet Res. 2013;74:343–54.
11. Ridpath JF, Neill JD, Endsley J, Roth JA. Effect of passive immunity on the development of a protective immune response against bovine viral diarrhea virus in calves. Am J Vet Res. 2003;64:65–9.
12. Endsley JJ, Roth JA, Ridpath J, Neill J. Maternal antibody blocks humoral but not T cell responses to BVDV. Biologicals. 2003;31:123–5.
13. Zimmerman AD, Boots RE, Valli JL, Chase CC. Evaluation of protection against virulent bovine viral diarrhea virus type 2 in calves that had maternal antibodies and were vaccinated with a modified-live vaccine. J Am Vet Med Assoc. 2006;228:1757–61.
14. Endsley JJ, Quade MJ, Terhaar B, Roth JA. Bovine viral diarrhea virus type 1- and type 2-specific bovine T lymphocyte-subset responses following modified-live virus vaccination. Vet Ther. 2002;3:364–72.
15. Endsley JJ, Ridpath JF, Neill JD, Sandbulte MR, Roth JA. Induction of T lymphocytes specific for bovine viral diarrhea virus in calves with maternal antibody. Viral Immunol. 2004;17:13–23.
16. Step DL, Krehbiel CR, Burciaga-Robles LO, Holland BP, Fulton RW, Confer AW, et al. Comparison of single vaccination versus revaccination with a modified-live virus vaccine containing bovine herpesvirus-1, bovine viral diarrhea virus (types 1a and 2a), parainfluenza type 3 virus, and bovine respiratory syncytial virus in the prevention of bovine respiratory disease in cattle. J Am Vet Med Assoc. 2009;235:580–7.
17. Stevens ET, Brown MS, Burdett WW, Bolton MW, Nordstrom ST, Chase CC. Efficacy of a non-adjuvanted, modified-live virus vaccine in calves with maternal antibodies against a virulent bovine viral diarrhea virus type 2a challenge seven months following vaccination. Bovine Pract. 2011;45:23–31.
18. Palomares RA, Givens MD, Wright JC, Walz PH, Brock KV. Evaluation of the onset of protection induced by a modified-live virus vaccine in calves challenge inoculated with type 1b bovine viral diarrhea virus. Am J Vet Res. 2012;73:567–74.
19. Ridpath JF, Dominowski P, Mannan R, Yancey Jr R, Jackson JA, Taylor L. Evaluation of three experimental bovine viral diarrhea virus killed vaccines adjuvanted with combinations of Quil A cholesterol and dimethyldioctadecylammonium (DDA) bromide. Vet Res Commun. 2010;34:691–702.
20. Stoffregen BL, Bolin SR, Ridpath JF, Pohlenz J. Morphologic lesions in type 2 BVDV infections experimentally induced by strain BVDV2-1373 recovered from a field case. Vet Microbiol. 2000;77:157–62.
21. Moya A, Elena SF, Bracho A, Miralles R, Barrio E. The evolution of RNA viruses: A population genetics view. Proc Natl Acad Sci U S A. 2000;97:6967–73.
22. Deregt DL, Jacobs RM, Carman PS, Tessaro SV. Attenuation of a virulent type 2 bovine viral diarrhea virus. Vet Microbiol. 2004;100:151–61.
23. Dubey P, Mishra N, Rajukumar K, Behera SP, Kalaiyarasu S, Nema RK, et al. Development of a RT-PCR ELISA for simultaneous detection of BVDV-1, BVDV-2 and BDV in ruminants and its evaluation on clinical samples. J Virol Methods. 2014;213C:50–6.
24. Howard CJ, Clarke MC, Sopp P, Brownlie J. Immunity to bovine virus diarrhoea virus in calves: the role of different T-cell subpopulations analysed by specific depletion in vivo with monoclonal antibodies. Vet Immunol Immunopathol. 1992;32:303–14.
25. Tait Jr RG, Downey ED, Mayes MS, Park CA, Ridpath JF, Garrick DJ, et al. Evaluation of response to bovine viral diarrhea virus type 2 vaccination and timing of weaning on yearling ultrasound body composition, performance, and carcass quality traits in Angus calves. J Anim Sci. 2013;91:5466–76.
26. Thurmond MC, Munos-Zansi CA, Hietala SK. Effect of calfhood vaccination on tranmission of bovine viral diarrhea virus under typical drylot dairy conditions. J Am Vet Med Assoc. 2001;219:968–75.
27. Brock KV, Widel P, Walz P, Walz HL. Onset of protection from experimental infection with type 2 bovine viral diarrhea virus following vaccination with a modified-live vaccine. Vet Ther. 2007;8:88–96.
28. Reed LJ, Muench H. A simple method of estimating fifty per cent endpoints. Am J Hyg. 1938;27:493–7. **71**:5–6822.
29. Walz PH, Givens MD, Cochran A, Navarre CB. Effect of dexamethasone administration on bulls with a localized testicular infection with bovine viral diarrhea virus. Can J Vet Res. 2008;72:56–62.
30. Larska M, Polak MP, Liu L, Alenius S, Uttenthal A. Comparison of the performance of five different immunoassays to detect specific antibodies against emerging atypical bovine pestivirus. J Virol Methods. 2013;187:103–9.

PERMISSIONS

All chapters in this book were first published in VR, by BioMed Central; hereby published with permission under the Creative Commons Attribution License or equivalent. Every chapter published in this book has been scrutinized by our experts. Their significance has been extensively debated. The topics covered herein carry significant findings which will fuel the growth of the discipline. They may even be implemented as practical applications or may be referred to as a beginning point for another development.

The contributors of this book come from diverse backgrounds, making this book a truly international effort. This book will bring forth new frontiers with its revolutionizing research information and detailed analysis of the nascent developments around the world.

We would like to thank all the contributing authors for lending their expertise to make the book truly unique. They have played a crucial role in the development of this book. Without their invaluable contributions this book wouldn't have been possible. They have made vital efforts to compile up to date information on the varied aspects of this subject to make this book a valuable addition to the collection of many professionals and students.

This book was conceptualized with the vision of imparting up-to-date information and advanced data in this field. To ensure the same, a matchless editorial board was set up. Every individual on the board went through rigorous rounds of assessment to prove their worth. After which they invested a large part of their time researching and compiling the most relevant data for our readers.

The editorial board has been involved in producing this book since its inception. They have spent rigorous hours researching and exploring the diverse topics which have resulted in the successful publishing of this book. They have passed on their knowledge of decades through this book. To expedite this challenging task, the publisher supported the team at every step. A small team of assistant editors was also appointed to further simplify the editing procedure and attain best results for the readers.

Apart from the editorial board, the designing team has also invested a significant amount of their time in understanding the subject and creating the most relevant covers. They scrutinized every image to scout for the most suitable representation of the subject and create an appropriate cover for the book.

The publishing team has been an ardent support to the editorial, designing and production team. Their endless efforts to recruit the best for this project, has resulted in the accomplishment of this book. They are a veteran in the field of academics and their pool of knowledge is as vast as their experience in printing. Their expertise and guidance has proved useful at every step. Their uncompromising quality standards have made this book an exceptional effort. Their encouragement from time to time has been an inspiration for everyone.

The publisher and the editorial board hope that this book will prove to be a valuable piece of knowledge for researchers, students, practitioners and scholars across the globe.

LIST OF CONTRIBUTORS

Paolo Martelli, Roberta Saleri, Giulia Ferrarini, Elena De Angelis, Valeria Cavalli, Michele Benetti, Luca Ferrari, Elena Canelli and Paolo Borghetti
Department of Veterinary Science, University of Parma, Via del Taglio, 10 - 43126 Parma, Italy

Paolo Bonilauri
Istituto Zooprofi lattico Sperimentale della Lombardia edell' Emilia Romagna (IZSLER), Via Pitagora, 2-42100 Reggio, Emilia, Italy

Elena Arioli and Antonio Caleffi
Veterinary Practitioner, 46100 Mantua, Italy

Heiko Nathues
Swine Clinic, Department of Clinical Veterinary Medicine, Vetsuisse Faculty, University of Bern, Bremgartenstrasse 109a, CH-3012 Bern, Switzerland

Annelies Michiels, Ioannis Arsenakis and Dominiek Maes
Department of Reproduction, Obstetrics and Herd Health, Faculty of Veterinary Medicine, Ghent University, Merelbeke, Belgium

Filip Boyen and Freddy Haesebrouck
Department of Pathology, Bacteriology and Avian Diseases, Faculty of Veterinary Medicine, Ghent University, Merelbeke, Belgium

Roman Krejci
CEVA Santé Animale, Cedex, Libourne, France

Hana Kudlackova, Radek Tesarik, Martin Faldyna and Jan Matiasovic
Department of Immunology, Veterinary Research Institute, Hudcova296/70, 62100 Brno, Czech Republic

Jan Gebauer
Department of Immunology, Veterinary Research Institute, Hudcova296/70, 62100 Brno, Czech Republic
Department of Experimental Biology, Faculty of Science, Masaryk University, Kotlarska267/2, 611 37 Brno, Czech Republic

Alena Osvaldova
Department of Immunology, Veterinary Research Institute, Hudcova296/70, 62100 Brno, Czech Republic
Faculty of Veterinary Medicine, University of Veterinary and Pharmaceutical Sciences, Palackeho 1/3, 612 42 Brno, Czech Republic

Marcel Kosina
Bioveta a. s., Komenskeho212/12, 683 23 Ivanovice na Hane, Czech Republic

Kamil Kovarcik
Department of Virology, Veterinary Research Institute, Hudcova296/70, 62100 Brno, Czech Republic

R. M. S. Pimburage
Ministry of Health, No.555/5, Elvitigala Mawatha, Colombo 05, Sri Lanka

M. Gunatilake
Department of Physiology, Faculty of Medicine, University of Colombo, No.25, Kynsey Road, Colombo 08, Sri Lanka

O. Wimalaratne and K. A. D. N. Perera
Department of Rabies Research and Vaccine Quality Control, Medical Research Institute, Colombo 08, Sri Lanka

A. Balasuriya
Faculty of Medicine, General Sir John Kotelawala Defense University, Kandawala Road, Rathmalana, Sri Lanka
Enric Vidal and Bernat Pérez de Val
IRTA, Centre de Recerca en Sanitat Animal (CReSA, IRTA-UAB), Campus de la Universitat Autònoma de Barcelona, Bellaterra, 08193 Barcelona, Catalonia, Spain

Mariano Domingo
IRTA, Centre de Recerca en Sanitat Animal (CReSA, IRTA-UAB), Campus de la Universitat Autònoma de Barcelona, Bellaterra, 08193 Barcelona, Catalonia, Spain
Departament de Sanitat i Anatomia Animals, Universitat Autònoma de Barcelona, Bellaterra, 08193 Barcelona, Catalonia, Spain

Claudia Arrieta-Villegas
Departament de Sanitat i Anatomia Animals, Universitat Autònoma de Barcelona, Bellaterra, 08193 Barcelona, Catalonia, Spain

Miriam Grasa
Associació de Ramaders de Cabrum de Catalunya, 25400 Les Borges Blanques, Lleida, Catalonia, Spain

Irene Mercader
Departament d'Agricultura, Ramaderia, Pesca i Alimentació de la Generalitat de Catalunya, 08007 Barcelona, Catalonia, Spain

Rodrigo Puentes, Laureana De Brun, Agustina Algorta and Valeria Da Silva
Immunology Area - Department of Microbiological Sciences, Faculty of Veterinary, University of the Republic (UdelaR), Montevideo, Uruguay

Silvia Llambí
Genetics Area, Faculty of Veterinary, University of the Republic (UdelaR), Montevideo, Uruguay

Florencia Mansilla
Centre of Veterinary Sciences and Agronomic Investigations, INTA, Virology Institute, Buenos Aires, Argentina

Alejandra V. Capozzo
Centre of Veterinary Sciences and Agronomic Investigations, INTA, Virology Institute, Buenos Aires, Argentina
CONICET – National Council of Scientific and Technological Research, Buenos Aires, Argentina

Gustavo Sacco
Independent Veterinary Practice, Florida, Uruguay

M. Arregui and L. E. Samartino
Centre of Veterinary Sciences and Agronomic Investigations, INTA, Virology Institute, Buenos Aires, Argentina

M. N. Aznar
Centre of Veterinary Sciences and Agronomic Investigations, INTA, Virology Institute, Buenos Aires, Argentina
Research Unit of Epidemiology and Risk Analysis applied to veterinary sciences (UREAR-ULg), Center for Fundamental and Applied Research for Animal and Health (FARAH), Faculty of Veterinary Medicine, University of Liege, PC 4000 Liege, Belgium

C. Saegerman
Research Unit of Epidemiology and Risk Analysis applied to veterinary sciences (UREAR-ULg), Center for Fundamental and Applied Research for Animal and Health (FARAH), Faculty of Veterinary Medicine, University of Liege, PC 4000 Liege, Belgium

M. F. Humblet
Department for Occupational Safety and Health, Biosafety and Biosecurity Unit, University of Liege, PC 4000 Liege, Belgium

Xiaoyu Niu, Bingqian Zhang, Xianglong Yu, Xin Zhang, Yanguo Dou, Yi Tang and Youxiang Diao
College of Animal Science and Technology, Shandong Agricultural University, Daizong Road 61, Tai'an, Shandong 271018, China

T. Almeras, P. Schreiber, S. Fournel, V. Martin, C. S. Nicolas, C. Fontaine, C. Lesbros and S. Gueguen
Virbac, 13ème rue, LID, 06511 Carros, France

Chuanmin Liu, Libin Wen, Qi Xiao and Kongwang He
Institute of Veterinary Medicine, Jiangsu Academy of Agricultural Sciences, 50 Zhong-ling Street, Xuanwu District, Nanjing 210014, China
Key laboratory of Veterinary Biological Engineering and Technology, Ministry of Agriculture, 50 Zhong-ling Street, Xuanwu District, Nanjing 210014, China
National Center for Engineering Research of Veterinary Bio-products, 50 Zhong-ling Street, Xuanwu District, Nanjing 210014, China
Jiangsu Co-innovation Center for Prevention and Control of Important Animal Infectious Diseases and Zoonoses, 12 Wen-Hui East Road, Hanjiang District, Yangzhou 225009, China

Tomislav Bedeković, Ivana Šimić, Nina Krešić, Ivana Lojkić and Željko Mihaljević
Croatian Veterinary Institute, Savska cesta 143, 10000 Zagreb, Croatia

Peter Hostnik
University of Ljubljana, Veterinary Faculty, Gerbičeva 60, 1115 Ljubljana, Slovenia

Ivana Lohman Janković and Ivica Sučec
Veterinary Directorate, Planinska 2a, 10000 Zagreb, Croatia

Kibrom Mebrahtu
Jinka Agricultural Research Center, Department of Animal Health, Southern Ethiopian Nations, Nationalities and People's Regional State, Jinka, Ethiopia

S. Teshale
Addis Ababa University College of Veterinary Medicine and griculture, Bishoftu Ethiopia, Department of Clinical Studies, Ethiopia

Wendimeneh Esatu and Tadios Habte
Ethiopian Institute of Agriculture, Debre Zeit Agricultural Research Center, Bishoftu, Ethiopia

Esayas Gelaye
National Veterinary Institute, Bishoftu, Ethiopia

Panagiotis D. Tassis, Ioannis Tsakmakidis, Dimitrios Koulialis and Eleni D. Tzika
Farm Animals Clinic, School of Veterinary Medicine, Aristotle University of Thessaloniki, St. Voutyra 11, 54627 Thessaloniki, Greece

Vassileios G. Papatsiros
Clinic of Medicine, Faculty of Veterinary Science, University of Thessaly, Trikalon 224, Karditsa, Greece

Tom Nell
Animal Health, Clinical Study Team Biologicals, Boxmeer 5830 AA, the Netherlands

Georgia Brellou
Laboratory of Pathology, School of Veterinary Medicine, Aristotle University of Thessaloniki, University Campus, 54124 Thessaloniki, Greece

Zineb Boumart, Samira Daouam, Lamya Rafi, Khalid Omari Tadlaoui and Mehdi El Harrak
Research and Development Virology, Multi-Chemical Industry, Lot. 157, Z I, Sud-Ouest (ERAC) B.P.: 278, Mohammedia 28810, Morocco

Imane Belkourati and Eeva Tuppurainen
Capripoxvirus Reference Laboratory, The Pirbright Institute, Ash Road, Pirbright, Woking, Surrey GU24 0NF, United Kingdom

Yumeng Shen, Weiwei Hu and Qian Yang
Veterinary College, Nanjing Agricultural University, Weigang 1, Nanjing, Jiangsu 210095, People's Republic of China

Yanna Wei and Zhixin Feng
Institute of Veterinary Medicine, Jiangsu Academy of Agricultural Sciences, Key Laboratory of Veterinary Biological Engineering and Technology, Ministry of Agriculture, National Center for Engineering Research of Veterinary Bio-products, Nanjing 210014, People's Republic of China

F. Ghzal, Y. Naouli, K. O. Tadlaoui and M. EL Harrak
Research and Development Virology, Multi-Chemical Industry, Lot. 157, Z I, Sud-Ouest (ERAC) B.P: 278, Mohammedia 28810, Morocco

S. Daouam
Research and Development Virology, Multi-Chemical Industry, Lot. 157, Z I, Sud-Ouest (ERAC) B.P: 278, Mohammedia 28810, Morocco
Laboratory of Virology, Hygiene & Microbiology, Faculty of Sciences & Technics, University Hassan II Mohammedia-Casablanca, 20650 Mohammedia, Morocco

M. M. Ennaji
Laboratory of Virology, Hygiene & Microbiology, Faculty of Sciences & Technics, University Hassan II Mohammedia-Casablanca, 20650 Mohammedia, Morocco

C. Oura
School of Veterinary Medicine, University of the West Indies, St. Augustine, Trinidad and Tobago

Steffen Ortmann, Ad Vos, Antje Kretzschmar, Nomusa Walther and Christiane Kaiser
IDT Biologika GmbH, Am Pharmapark, 06861 Dessau Rosslau, Germany

Thomas Müller and Conrad Freuling
Institute of Molecular Virology and Cell Biology, Friedrich-Loeffler-Institute, Südufer 10, 17493 Greifswald, Insel Riems, Germany

Ivana Lojkic
Department of Virology, Croatian Veterinary Institute, Svaská cesta 143, 10000 Zagreb, Croatia

Christian Visscher, Jasmin Mischok, Saara Sander and Josef Kamphues
Institute for Animal Nutrition, University of Veterinary Medicine Hannover, Foundation, Bischofsholer Damm 15, D-30173 Hannover, Germany

Marion Schmicke
Clinic for Cattle, University of Veterinary Medicine Hannover, Foundation, Bischofsholer Damm 15, D-30173 Hannover, Germany

Eva-Ursula Peitzmeier and Isabel von dem Busche
Tierarztpraxis Dr. Peitzmeier, Meente 24, D-32479 Hille, Germany

Karl Rohn
Institute for Biometry, Epidemiology and Information Processing, University of Veterinary Medicine Hannover, Foundation, Bünteweg 2, D-30559 Hannover, Germany

Salvador Oliver-Ferrando, Sergio López-Soria and Marina Sibila
IRTA, Centre de Recerca en Sanitat Animal (CReSA, IRTA-UAB), Campus de la Universitat Autònoma de Barcelona, 08193 Bellaterra, Spain

Joaquim Segalés
UAB, Centre de Recerca en Sanitat Animal (CReSA, IRTA-UAB), Campus de la Universitat Autònoma de Barcelona, 08193 Bellaterra, Spain
Departament de Sanitat I Anatomia Animals, Facultat de Veterinària, UAB, 08193 Bellaterra, Spain

Antonio Callén
Veterinarian, Zaragoza, Spain

Olivier Merdy
Agronomist, Lyon, France

François Joisel
Private veterinary consultant, Lyon, France

Anqiang Lai, Guozhong Dong and Daijun Song
College of Animal Science and Technology, Southwest University, Beibei, Chongqing 400716, People's Republic of China

Tan Yang and Xiaolong Zhang
Sichuan Giant Star Company's Experimental Station, Leshan, Sichuan 614800, People's Republic of China

John G. Neilan, Christopher Schutta, Laszlo Zsak and Max V. Rasmussen
U.S. Department of Homeland Security Science and Technology Directorate, Plum Island Animal Disease Center, Greenport, NY 11944, USA

José Barrera
The McConnell Group, Inc., Plum Island Animal Disease Center, Greenport, NY 11944, USA
Leidos, Plum Island Animal Disease Center, Greenport, NY 11944, USA

Barbara J. Kamicker and Melia Pisano
Leidos, Plum Island Animal Disease Center, Greenport, NY 11944, USA
Plum Island Animal Disease Center Research Participation Program, Oak Ridge Institute for Science and Education, Oak Ridge, TN, USA

Ethan Hartwig
U.S. Department of Agriculture, Agricultural Research Service, Foreign Animal Disease Research Unit, Plum Island Animal Disease Center, Greenport, NY 11944, USA

Bryan T. Butman, Damodar Ettyreddy and Douglas E. Brough
GenVec, Inc., 910 Clopper Road, Suite 220N, Gaithersburg, MD 20878, USA

David A. Brake
BioQuest Associates, LLC, Plum Island Animal Disease Center, Greenport, NY 11944, USA

Paul D. Williams
MSD Animal Health, Walton Manor, Walton, Milton Keynes MK7 7AJ, UK

Gustavo Paixão
School of Veterinary Science, University of Bristol, Langford House, Langford, Bristol BS40 5DU, UK
Animal and Veterinary Research Centre (CECAV), Universidade de Trás-os-Montes e Alto Douro, 5001-801 Vila Real, Portugal

Beatriz Vila Nova
Faculty of Veterinary Medicine, University of Lisbon, Av. Universidade Técnica, 1300-477 Lisbon, Portugal

Manuela Oliveira, Berta São Braz, Luis Tavares, Virgílio Almeida and Solange Gil
Faculty of Veterinary Medicine, University of Lisbon, Av. Universidade Técnica, 1300-477 Lisbon, Portugal
CIISA- Centre for Interdisciplinary Research in Animal Health, Faculty of Veterinary Medicine, University of Lisbon, Av. Universidade Técnica, 1300-477 Lisbon, Portugal

Eva Cunha
CIISA- Centre for Interdisciplinary Research in Animal Health, Faculty of Veterinary Medicine, University of Lisbon, Av. Universidade Técnica, 1300-477 Lisbon, Portugal

Nuno Sepúlveda
London School of Hygiene and Tropical Medicine, London, UK
Centro de Estatística e Aplicações da Universidade de Lisboa, Lisbon, Portugal

Jichun Wang, Yongfeng Qiao, Mengwei Xu, Zhisheng Wang, Yamei Liu, Yating Zheng and Jibo Hou
National Research Center of Engineering and Technology for Veterinary Biologicals/Institute of Veterinary Immunology & Engineering, Jiangsu Academy of Agricultural Sciences, Nanjing 210014, Jiangsu, China
Jiangsu Co-innovation Center for Prevention and Control of Important Animal Infectious Diseases and Zoonoses, Yangzhou, China

Rongli Guo
Jiangsu Co-innovation Center for Prevention and Control of Important Animal Infectious Diseases and Zoonoses, Yangzhou, China
Institute of Veterinary Medicine, Jiangsu Academy of Agricultural Sciences, Nanjing 210014, Jiangsu, China

Hongjie Fan and Zengcai Song
College of Veterinary Medicine, Nanjing Agricultural University, Nanjing 210095, China

Aimin Ge
Shandong Vocational Animal Science and Veterinary College, Weifang 261061, China

Yeong-Lim Kang, Ji-Yun Jeong, Hwi-Yeon Choi, Ho-Jong Lee, Jong-Chul Choi, So-Hyun Lee, Beom-Joo Lee, Sang-Won Lee, Joong-Bok Lee and Seung-Yong Park
Laboratory of Veterinary Immunology, College of Veterinary Medicine, Konkuk University, 120 Neungdong-ro, Gwangjin-gu, Seoul 05029, Republic of Korea

Yanhong Zhang and Yumei Liu
Jinyu Baoling Bio-pharmaceutical Co., Ltd., Hohhot 010030, Inner Mongolia, China

Ki-hyun Cho
Veterinary Epidemiology Division, Animal and Plant Quarantine Agency, 177, Hyeoksin 8-ro, Gimcheon, Gyeongsangbuk-do 39660, Republic of Korea

Index

A

Actinobacillus Pleuropneumoniae, 2, 14, 22, 112-114, 117

Animal Tuberculosis, 44

Apparent Total Tract Digestibility, 143, 148

Aujeszky's Disease, 2, 12, 111, 123, 154, 208

Aujeszky's Disease Virus, 2, 111, 154

Avian Reovirus, 68, 71, 75

B

Bacillus Calmette-guérin, 44, 48

Biopro Elisa, 95-100

Border Disease Virus, 119, 123

Bovine Brucellosis, 57-58, 63, 67

Bovine Leukemia Virus, 50, 55-56

Brucella Abortus, 57-58, 67

Bunyaviridae, 131, 135

C

Canine Distemper Virus, 190-191, 196-197

Canine Parvovirus, 190, 196-197

Capripoxvirus, 118

Cl13t Vaccine, 131-134

Coccidiosis, 163-164, 169-172

Contact Transmission Model, 174, 181

D

Dendritic Cells, 124, 128-130

Direct Contact Transmission Challenge Model, 174

Diva Vaccine, 23, 31-32, 181

Duck Reovirus, 68, 75

E

Elisa, 2, 4-8, 12-13, 15-17, 21, 23-24, 26-27, 29, 31-32, 42, 46-47, 50-56, 69-73, 75, 115, 132, 134, 157, 159-160, 166, 178, 190-191, 195, 197, 201-202, 207, 209-210, 214-216

Enzootic Bovine Leucosis, 50

Enzootic Pneumonia, 13, 20-22, 109-110, 114, 116, 124, 128-129

Enzyme-linked Immunosorbent Assay, 87, 160, 166, 207, 210, 215-216

Erysipelothrix Rhusiopathiae, 3, 12, 111, 144

F

Feline Calicivirus, 76-78, 82, 84-85

Foot And Mouth Disease, 50-51, 56, 67, 182-183, 188

G

Goose Reovirus, 68-69, 75

H

Herpestes Auropunctatus, 136, 141-142

Immunoaffinity Chromatography, 24-25, 27, 31-32

Indian Mongoose, 136-138, 140-142

L

Lawsonia Intracellularis, 143-144, 147, 151-152

Liquid-phase Blocking Elisa, 209-210, 216

Livestock Vaccines, 183

M

Mass Spectrometry, 23, 25-26, 30-32

Methionine, 25, 28, 163, 165-166, 168-169, 171-173

Mucosa-associated Lymphoid Tissue, 129

Mycobacterium Bovis Bcg Vaccine, 44, 48

Mycobacterium Caprae, 44-45, 49

Mycoplasma Hyopneumoniae, 3, 13-17, 19, 21-22, 109-110, 116-117, 124, 129-130, 214

N

Newcastle Disease, 69, 102-103, 106, 108, 165, 188

Nitric Oxide, 86, 93-94, 146

O

Oral Vaccination, 48, 95, 98, 108, 136-137, 140-142

P

Peripheral Blood Mononuclear Cell, 51, 53

Phlebovirus, 131, 135 Piglets, 1-4, 8, 10-14, 16, 18-24, 29-30, 32, 86, 109-117, 125, 130, 143-151, 153-162, 198-199, 201-202, 204-208, 214, 216

Porcilis Pcv M Hyo, 109, 116

Porcine Circovirus Type 2, 1-2, 12, 86, 93-94, 109, 116-117, 125, 152, 161-162, 214

Porcine Circovirus-associated Disease, 12, 93

Porcine Epidemic Diarrhea, 130, 214

Porcine Parvovirus, 3, 12, 86, 91, 93-94, 111, 144, 154, 201, 207

Porcine Reproductive And Respiratory Syndrome Virus, 21-22, 93-94, 151-152, 160

Pseudorabies Virus, 198-199, 207-208

R

Rabies, 34-43, 85, 94-98, 100-101, 136-142

Rapid Fluorescent Focus Inhibition Test, 34-35, 42, 96

Replication-deficient Human Adenovirus, 174, 181-182

Retrovirus, 50

Rift Valley Fever, 131, 134-135

Rift Valley Fever Vaccine, 131, 135

S

S-nitroso-acetylpenicillamine (SNAP), 86

S-nitrosoglutathione, 86, 93

Salmonella Enterica Serovar Typhimurium, 23, 32

Salmonella Typhimurium, 23-25, 30, 32-33, 151

Sheeppox, 118, 122-123

Sheeppox Virus, 118, 122

Single Intradermal Comparative Cervical Tuberculin, 45

Spbn Gasgas, 136-138, 140

Swine Industry, 124, 128, 152, 154

Swine Influenza Virus, 3, 112, 154

V

Veterinary Vaccines, 182-183, 188

Virus Neutralization, 36-39, 43, 97, 101, 119, 122, 176, 178-179, 181, 209-210, 215

Virus Neutralization Test, 43, 97, 101, 176, 178, 181, 209-210, 215

Vitality Index, 153, 155-156, 158, 160

Z

Zoonotic Disease, 34, 40

Zoonotic Viral Disease, 131